Outpatient Regenerative Medicine

Mario Goisis
Editor

Outpatient Regenerative Medicine

Fat Injection and PRP as Minor Office-based Procedures

Springer

Editor
Mario Goisis
Maxillo-Facial and Aesthetic Surgeon
Go Easy Clinic
Milan
Italy

ISBN 978-3-319-44892-3   ISBN 978-3-319-44894-7 (eBook)
https://doi.org/10.1007/978-3-319-44894-7

Library of Congress Control Number: 2019933362

This Springer imprint is published by the registered company Springer Nature Switzerland AG
The registered company address is: Gewerbestrasse 11, 6330 Cham, Switzerland

To my young assistants, Pietro and Matteo

Foreword

The gradual aging of the population and improved living conditions in many geographical areas have made regenerative medicine more and more relevant over the last few decades. Besides their traditional areas of application (e.g., reconstruction after trauma or injury), regenerative approaches have become increasingly more pertinent in antiaging or simply aesthetic medicine. The branches that avail themselves of regenerative approaches are numerous and include plastic surgery, odontostomatology, otolaryngology, orthopedics, dermatology, gynecology, and many others besides. The exponential increase of professionals, meetings, and training centers, together with strong links with the industrial world, has meant that the scientific level too of regenerative approaches has progressively reached high levels of excellence. The most advanced regenerative techniques emerging from research centers and supported by a wealth of first-class technologies are now being widely used in medicine. Regenerative techniques are based on three main pillars: stem-cells, growth factors, and scaffolds. The development of these, which may also be used in combination, is by no means simple and requires optimization by means of recourse to technologies that must be, at once, effective and safe while also being simple to carry out. Only the simplicity of the procedures involved can actually ensure their widespread use outside of operating theaters. Finally, we must remember that it is mandatory that all operators have a thorough and correct knowledge of the macroscopic and microscopic anatomy of the areas of the body which they intend treating. This aspect, above all, appears to be one of the prerequisites essential for correct treatment and achieving lasting results. All these considerations lead us to stress the need for the development of appropriate training courses capable of meeting the growing demands of a technologically highly advanced and rapidly evolving sector that is also making a huge contribution to the knowledge of the regenerative mechanisms of tissue.

Andrea Sbarbati
Department of Neuroscience, Biomedicine and Movement
Human Anatomy and Histology Section
University of Verona
Verona, Italy

Foreword

Surgery has always made use of fat grafts for reconstructive and aesthetic purposes. Starting from the early 1980s, the introduction of standardized techniques, like Coleman's, led to the achievement of excellent results reported in numerous scientific publications. So, today, many years after its first introduction, adipose tissue may be considered, without a shadow of doubt, the safest filler and the scientifically most validated medium of tissue regeneration. Today, the real challenge is to simplify and make harvesting and injection techniques more and more efficient. The future of lipofilling, by means of microfat and nanofat techniques, will most probably involve the integration and progressive replacement of injection techniques by hyaluronic acid and fillers.

Francesco Nicoletti
Multidisciplinary Department of Medical-Surgical
and Dental Specialties, Plastic Surgery Unit
Università degli Studi della Campania "Luigi Vanvitelli"
Naples, Italy

Contents

Part I

General Aspects

Introduction

1

Mario Goisis and Sara Izzo

The famous Pala di Brera (also known as the Montefeltro Altarpiece or Brera Altarpiece) was painted, using tempera on wood, in 1472–1474 by the Italian Renaissance master Piero della Francesca (Fig. 1.1). It is housed in one of Milan's the Pinacoteca di Brera, and was commissioned by Federico III da Montefeltro, Duke of Urbino, to celebrate his conquest of several castles.

Federico was a great "condottiero" (warlord or captain at arms) of the Renaissance, and is shown kneeling on the right-hand side of the painting. Piero portrayed the Duke in profile, a position recollective of coins and medals. His profile is one of the most famous in history, because of the empty space above the nose.

The reason was that during a tournament Federico was injured with a lance, losing his right eye. According to the legend, he uttered, "Never mind, I'll see better with one eye than with a hundred!" So, he decided to have the upper part of his nose cut away, in order to see better with his left eye. This might well be the first case of rhinoplasty we know about.

At the centre of the painting, hanging on a chain from the ceiling of the apse, is an egg, emblem of the promise of immortality and regeneration.

We like to think about regenerative medicine as the chain portrayed in the Pala di Brera.

In fact, during transfer of fat, injection of stem-cells and production of PRP, many different steps are required. For example, in the case of fat grafting we have to harvest the fat, process it, and, finally inject it into the recipient sites. These steps may be considered the four different links of a chain. Because a chain is only as strong as its weakest link, the creation of a procedure, optimal from start to finish, is mandatory.

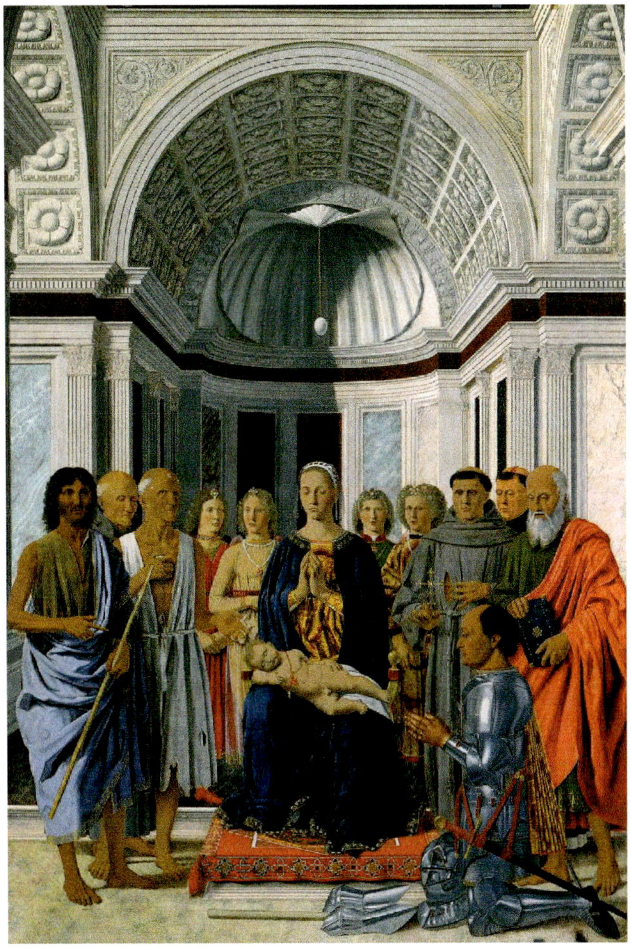

Fig. 1.1 The Montefeltro Altarpiece or Brera Altarpiece. (Courtesy of the Pinacoteca di Brera Museum, Milan, Italy http://pinacotecabrera.org/)

In fact, if one link of the chain is weak, then all the procedures will be compromised. In the case of Piero's chain, the egg may fall. In the case of the transfer of fat, the fat cells will not survive and will not regenerate themselves in the recipient area.

M. Goisis (✉)
Department of Plastic Surgery, University of Campania "Luigi Vanvitelli", Naples, Naples, Italy

Maxillo-Facial and Aesthetic Surgeon, Go Easy Clinic, Milan, Italy

S. Izzo
Department of Plastic Surgery, University of Campania "Luigi Vanvitelli", Naples, Naples, Italy

M. Goisis (ed.), *Outpatient Regenerative Medicine*, https://doi.org/10.1007/978-3-319-44894-7_1

Fat Harvesting

2

Andrea Sbarbati, Giamaica Conti, Sara Izzo, and Giovanni Francesco Nicoletti

2.1 Introduction

The fat grafting procedure may be divided into three separate phases: fat harvesting, fat processing, and fat injection into recipient sites [1]. When speaking of fat harvesting, we refer to the surgical procedure which permits us to obtain adipose tissue through the use of suction cannulas or, rarely, through en bloc surgical excision of fat. Processing techniques involve centrifugation, filtration, Telfa rolling, and cleansing of the fat to remove anaesthesia, oil, blood, and other components in the harvested adipose tissue. Injection techniques differ much, depending on the selection of different syringes and cannulas or needles for injecting the fat in the recipient area. Within each phase of fat grafting, there are many variations in techniques and numerous discussions in favour of one rather than another. It is mandatory to construct an optimal procedure from start to finish.

2.2 The Influence of the Size of Fat Particle

Fat particles may be defined as intact globules of adipocytes, interconnected by means of mesenchymal tissue. It should be noted that the structure of the individual fat particle does not occur naturally within the native tissue but is produced, rather, during the harvesting process. En bloc surgical excision of adipose tissue produces the largest fat particles.

In the case of liposuction by cannulas, the range of fat particles is directly related to the diameter of the cannula and the size of the cannula ports, with larger sizes separating larger particles. The theory that the size of adipose particles may have a direct influence on the survival of fat is described in many scientific studies.

In 1893, in Germany, Gustav Neuber described the transfer of lipoma specimens from the forearm to fill facial contour deficiencies produced by tuberculosis. He dissected fragments of fat from the abdomen in "bean or almond sizes." These fragments were reported to survive [2]. In 1937, Gurney reviewed fat transplants averaging 1.7 mm^3 over a period of 12 months and reported that "grafts were viable for at least 1 year" [3]. During the mid-1950s, Peer, in the journal *Plastic and Reconstructive Surgery* reported that "walnut sized fat grafts" seemed to have lost 45% of their original volume after 1 year, which may have been due to trauma during grafting, trimming, or to lack of blood supply [4].

Modern liposuction with a cannula was first described by Fischer and Fischer in Italy in 1974: this technique extended the success of fat grafting techniques significantly [5, 6]. Kato et al. recently published a pioneering study, emphasizing the significance of the size of fat particles in grafting. The authors demonstrated that within a particle, the adipocytes which survive are placed closer to the external part of the fat lobule. Based upon histological findings, fat particles may be divided into three different sections:

- Surviving section: the layer closest to the surface of the lobule. In this section all adipocytes survive.
- Regenerating section: the middle layer, where the adipocytes die but are replaced by proliferating stem-cells.
- Necrotic section: the central core of the fat particle, which presents with necrosis, oil cysts, and fibrosis.

The limits of the surviving and regenerating zones occurred normally at 100–300 μm and 600–1200 μm from the surface, respectively (Fig. 2.1).

A. Sbarbati (✉) · G. Conti
Department of Neuroscience, Biomedicine and Movement, Human Anatomy and Histology Section, University of Verona, Verona, Italy
e-mail: andrea.sbarbati@univr.it; giamaica.conti@univr.it

S. Izzo · G. F. Nicoletti
Department of Plastic Surgery, University of Campania "Luigi Vanvitelli", Naples, Italy
e-mail: giovannif.nicoletti@unicampania.it

M. Goisis (ed.), *Outpatient Regenerative Medicine*, https://doi.org/10.1007/978-3-319-44894-7_2

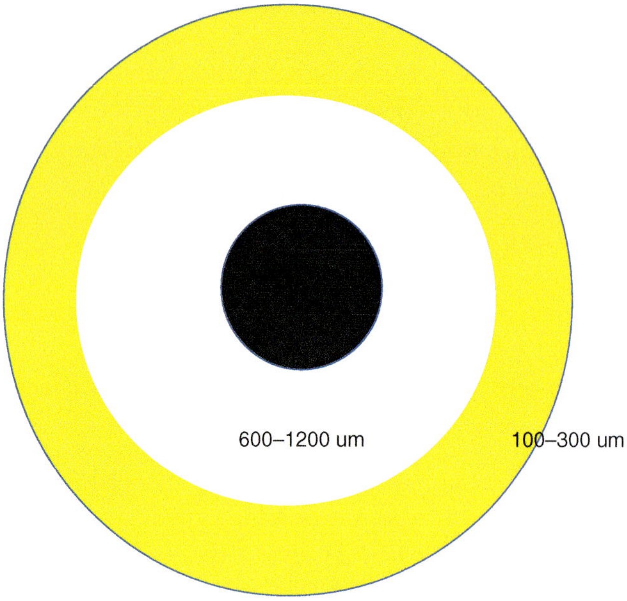

Fig. 2.1 Yellow: the surviving section 100–300 μm which is the layer closest to the surface where all the adipocytes survive. White: regenerating section 600–1200 μm which is the middle layer where the adipocytes die but are replaced by proliferating stem-cells. Black: the necrotic section, the central core of the fat particle dominated by necrosis, oil cysts, and fibrosis. (Published by kind permission of ©Mario Goisis 2018. All Rights Reserved)

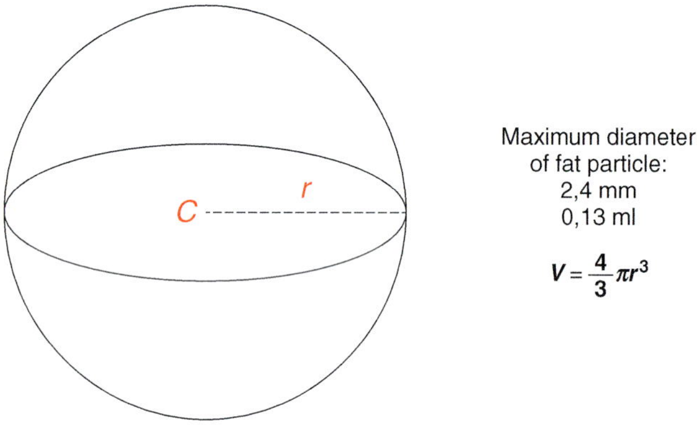

Fig. 2.2 Maximum diameter of a fat particle according to the limitations of diffusion described by Kato et al. (Published by kind permission of ©Mario Goisis 2018. All Rights Reserved)

Prior to the restoration of the blood supply, fat particles largely survive by diffusion of nutrients. As the diameter of adipose lobules becomes larger, the central zone of necrosis will ideally expand according to the limitations of diffusion (Fig. 2.2). Therefore, one may surmise that the size of fat particles may influence, ultimately, how much of the grafted fat survives [7].

2.3 Diameters of Cannulas and Port Sizes and Their Influence on Fat and Stem-Cell Viability

Shiffman and Mirrafati compared cannulas ranging from 2.5 to 3.7 mm in diameter, to establish if these an influenced cellular viability. They did not observe any significant difference [8]. When comparing a 2-mm- versus a 4-mm-diameter cannula, Leong et al. evaluated the state of the fat harvested. The study does not assert significant differences in metabolism [9]. According to Klein's definition, a micro-cannula has an inside diameter of 2.0 mm or less.

Trivisonno et al. studied whether the small size of a micro-cannula might reduce the collection of well-organized fat, which is mostly composed of mature adipocytes, and improve the harvesting of more superficial layers of adipose tissue, which are related to a higher percentage of ADSC. They compared (1) a rounded-tip cannula having a length of 170 mm, a diameter of 3 mm, and a single elliptic suction port on the side near its distal end (port diameter, 3 × 9 mm) and (2) a rounded-tip infiltration cannula having a length of 170 mm, a diameter of 2 mm, and 5 round ports positioned spirally along the sides of the distal cannula shaft (each port diameter, 1 mm).

Using the 3 mm cannula, they isolated nearly 1.4×10^5 cells/mL, a quantity similar to that described by several authors [10].

Fat harvested using a micro-cannula was associated with a higher number of stromal and vascular cells, and obtained a higher rate of survival. The main problem reported by Trivisonno et al. was related to the longer treatment times required for treatment using the micro-cannula compared to those needed when employing a standard cannula. In fact, aspiration of fat with a micro-cannula yielded smaller volumes of aspirated tissue with each stroke and, therefore, proved more time-consuming (approximately two times slower compared to manual suction with the larger cannula) [11].

Alharbi et al. [12] compared fat harvesting with the Coleman cannula (3 mm diameter, one-hole blunt tip) and fat harvesting using a 2 mm, multi-perforated hole blunt tip cannula. They used the different cannulas on contralateral areas of the same patients. The study established that growth-factor concentrations, cell-migration from pieces of fatty tissue, and adherence-rates of ASCs increased using the smaller cannula.

The authors concluded that these better results were due to the smaller sizes and different surface/volume ratios of pieces of the fatty tissue harvested with the smaller cannula.

2.4 A Newly-Patented Micro-Cannula

Goisis (Imcas 2015) described a newly-patented micro-cannula. This cannula has a small diameter (2 mm) with a blunt tip and six ports placed along the sides of the distal cannula shaft (each port is of a diameter of 1 mm). These ports are arranged in spirally with the angle of patency aligned along the axis of the cannula (Figs. 2.3 and 2.4). The ports have a rectangular shape, with a raised edge arranged parallel to the axis of the cannula and a depressed edge placed in front of the raised edge.

The main advantages of a cannula designed in such a way are related to faster times of treatment compared with those of other micro-cannulas: the aspiration of fat is performed with a rotational movement (see Figs. 2.5, 2.6, and

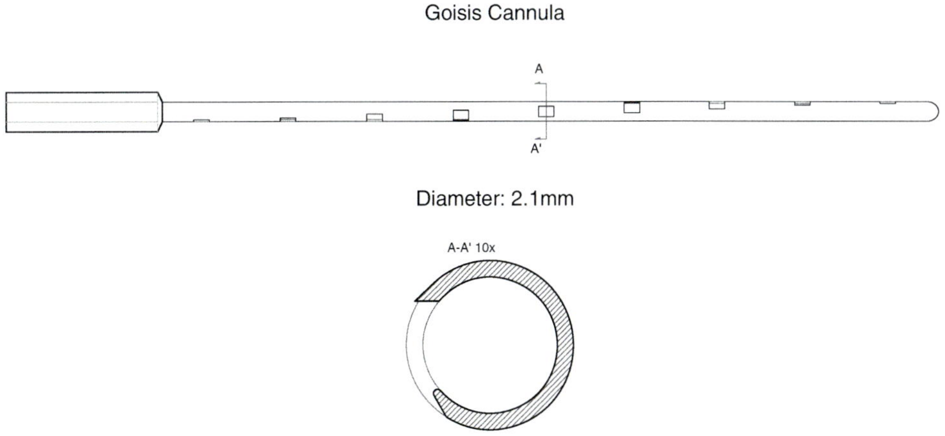

Fig. 2.3 The design of the cannula (published by kind permission of ©Mario Goisis 2018. All Rights Reserved)

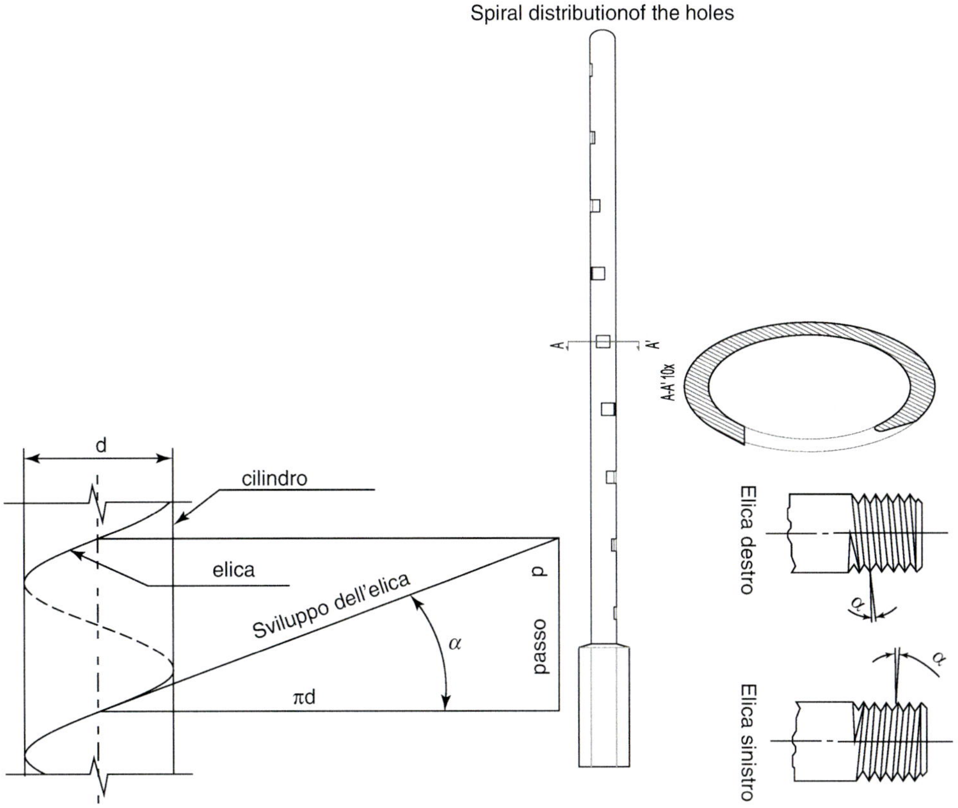

Fig. 2.4 The suction ports are arranged spirally

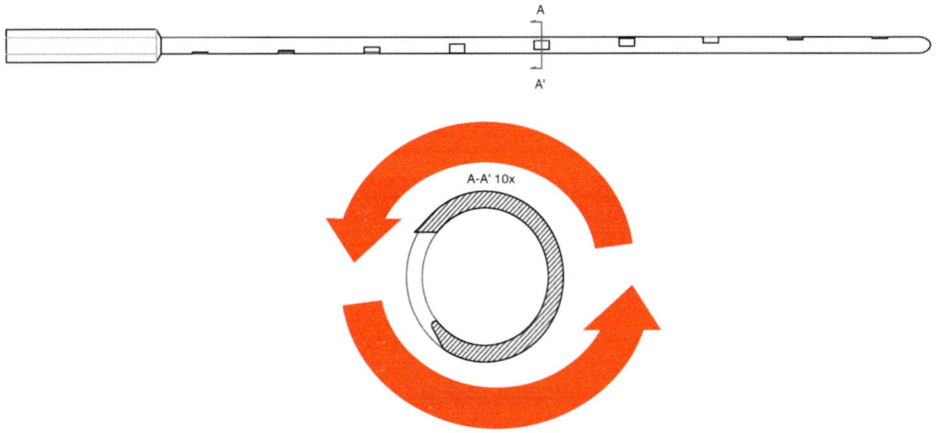

Fig. 2.5 The particularity of the rotational movement to be performed to harvest the fat. The rotational movement, which increases fat harvesting, is efficient, thanks to the depressed edge of the port holes, which facilitates the entrance of the fat into the cannula. Furthermore, the raised-barbed edge at the front of the depressed edge increases dissection of fat tissue and better aspiration of adipocytes. (Published by kind permission of ©Mario Goisis 2018. All Rights Reserved)

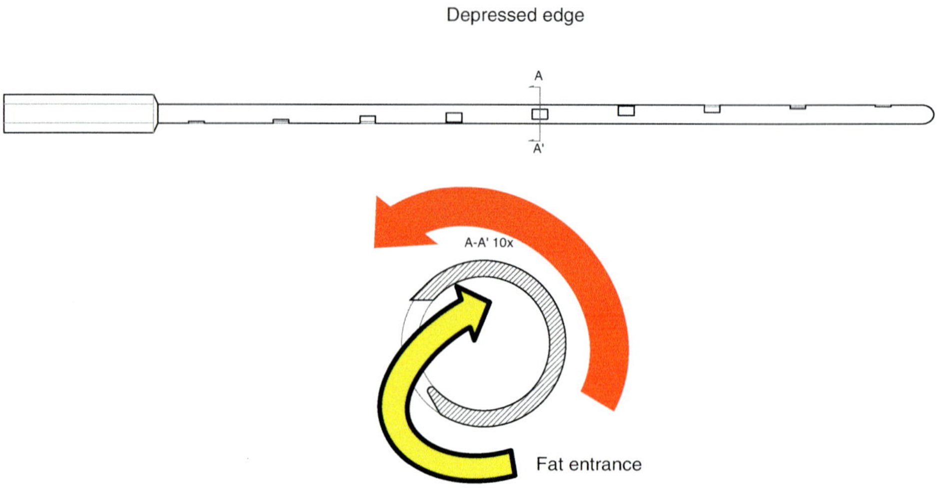

Fig. 2.6 The depressed edge of the holes increases the entrance of the fat into the cannula. (Published by kind permission of ©Mario Goisis 2018. All Rights Reserved)

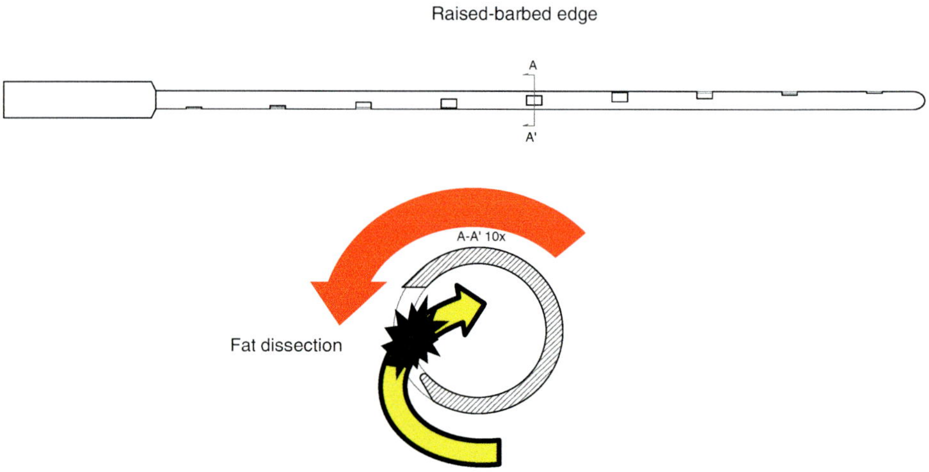

Fig. 2.7 The raised-barbed edge at the front of the depressed edge increases dissection of fat tissue, with better aspiration of adipocytes. (Published by kind permission of ©Mario Goisis 2018. All Rights Reserved)

2.7). The depressed edge promotes the entrance of fat into the hole. The raised edge facilitates the dissection of the fat particles. This way, the shape of the multiple ports yields a large volume of aspirated tissue with each rotational stroke. The use of the Goisis cannula is, therefore, several times more efficient compared to the Coleman harvesting cannula (approximately twice as fast as the Coleman 3-mm cannula).

Histological examinations performed on 547 samples demonstrated that the fat cells harvested with the Goisis cannula were associated with a higher number of stromal and vascular components, when compared with fat harvested using the traditional Coleman (Figs. 2.8, 2.9, 2.10, and 2.11). The quality of the aspirate is finer, thus lending itself to lipofilling procedures using a small cannula for infiltration to the donor site. The micro-cannula reduces incidences of patient trauma, discomfort, and skin irregularities and minimises the risk of vascular injury due to multiple reduced-size ports. Because the insertion requires less force and is more precise, the micro-cannula affords superior manual control, improved superficial removal of fat (reducing the risk of accidental injuries to deeper tissues), and fewer scars due to the micro-incisions required.In a Study presented by Goisis et al. Imcas 2019 (Goisis et al., comparing protocols, IMCAS 2019) the

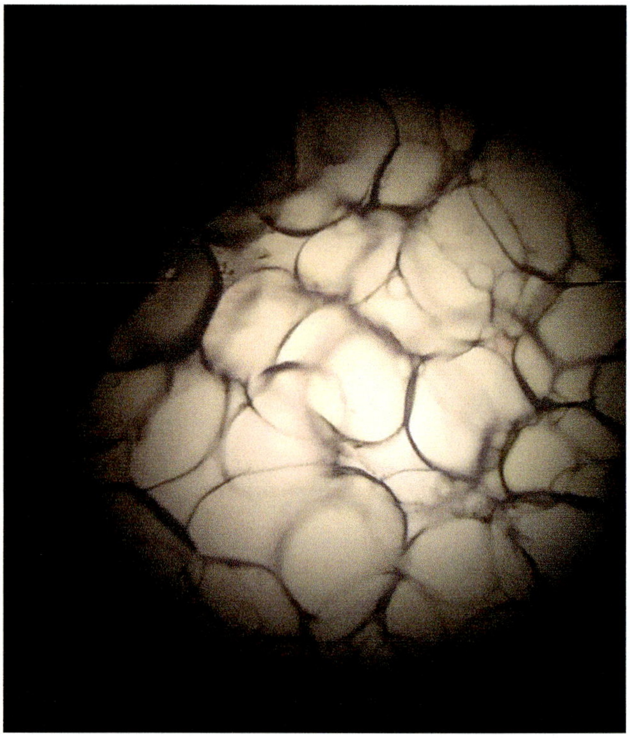

Fig. 2.8 Histological examination of fat harvested by a Goisis cannula. The adipocytes are well preserved. (Published by kind permission of ©Mario Goisis 2018. All Rights Reserved)

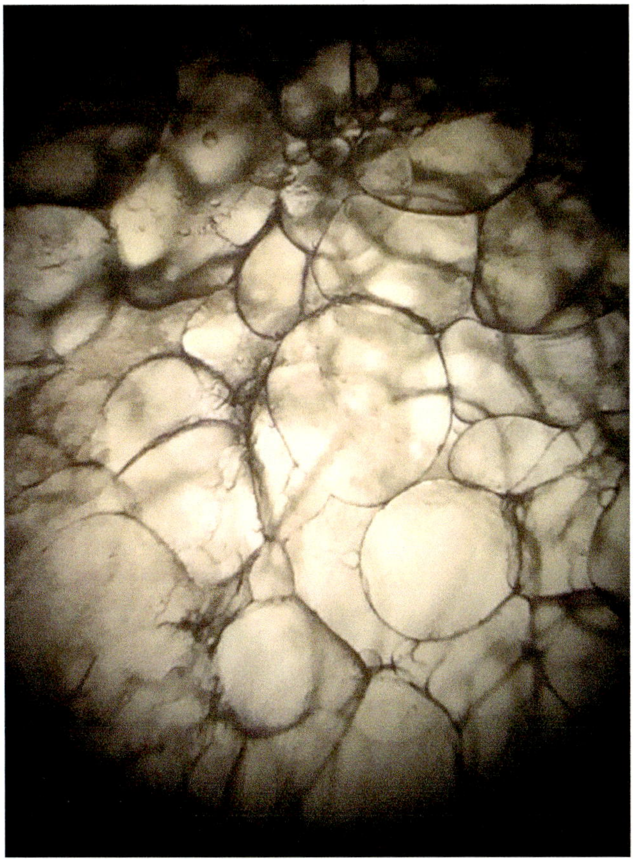

Fig. 2.9 Histological examination of fat harvested using a single-hole cannula. The adipocytes are less well preserved. (Published by kind permission of ©Mario Goisis 2018. All Rights Reserved)

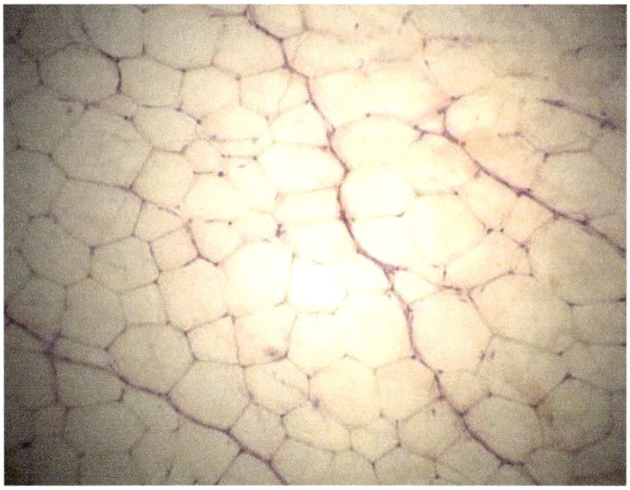

Fig. 2.10 Histological examinations of fat cells harvested using a Goisis cannula. (Published by kind permission of ©Mario Goisis 2018. All Rights Reserved)

Fig. 2.11 (**a, b**) Fat harvested with Goisis cannula is associated with a higher number of stromal and vascular components when compared with fat harvested using a single-hole cannula. (Published by kind permission of ©Mario Goisis 2018. All Rights Reserved)

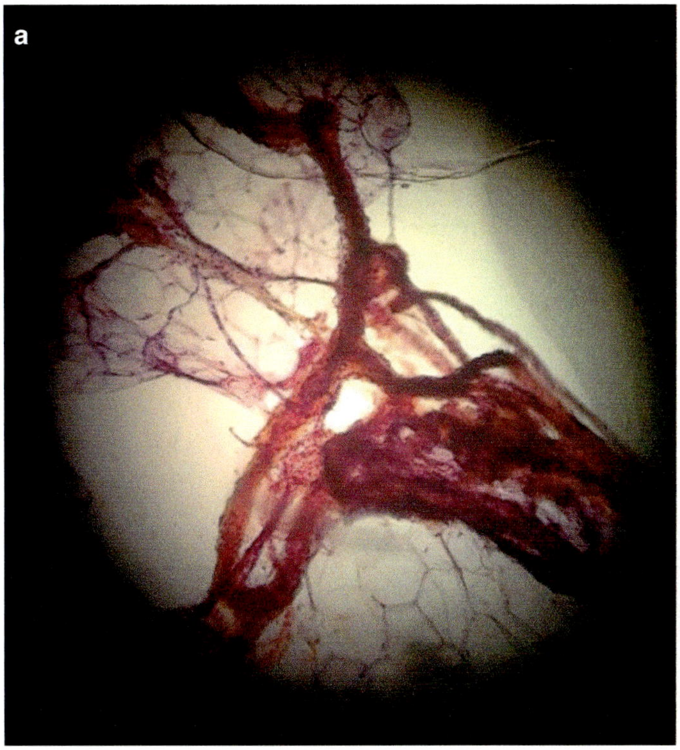

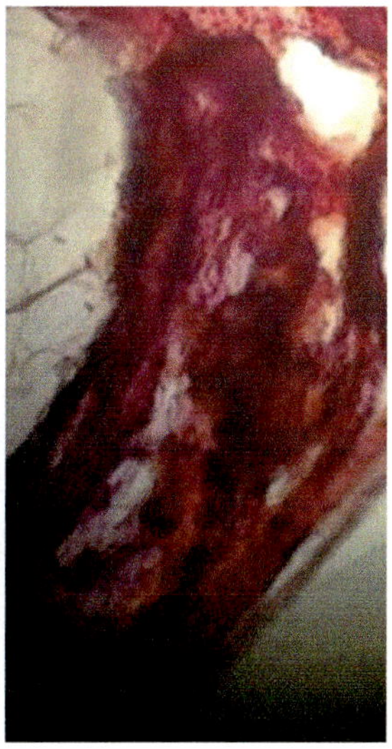

Fig. 2.11 (continued)

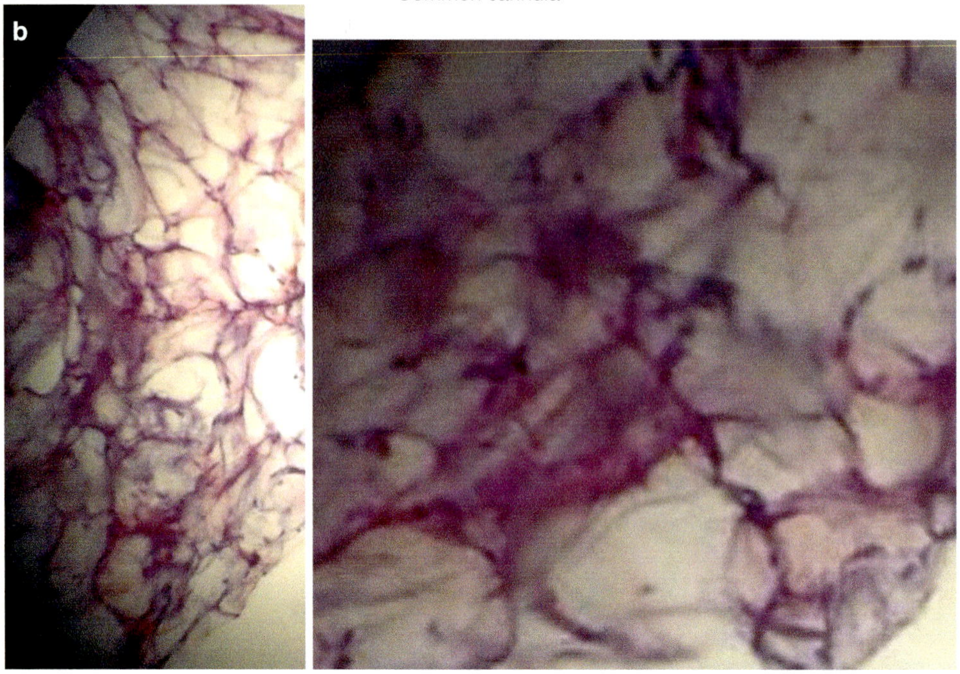

Table 2.1 The number of stem-cell of 2 different samples was measured at 72 hours, 7 days and 14 days after colture.In Blu fat harvested with Coleman canula, in orange microfat harvested with goisis cannula

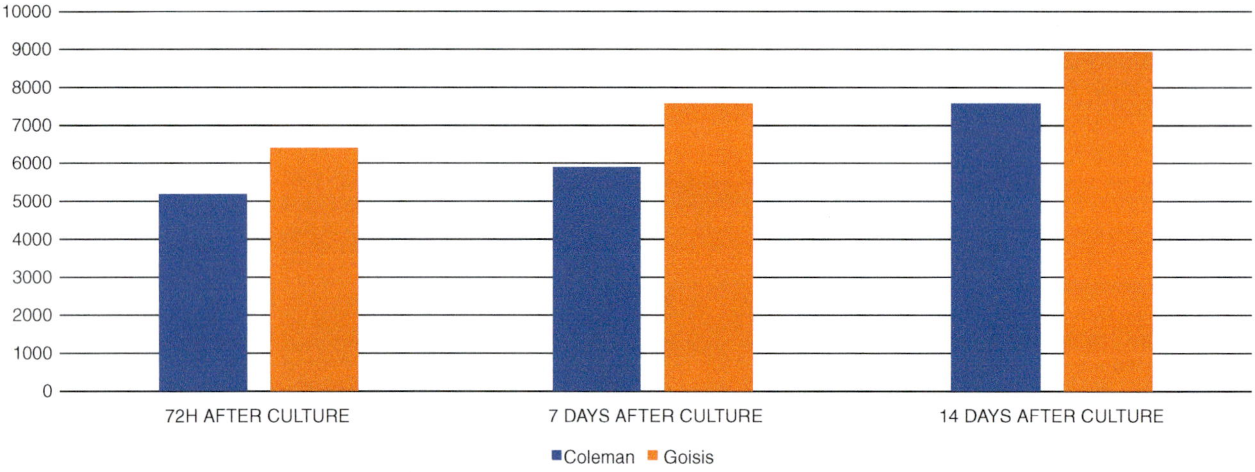

role of Goisis cannula is stem-cells viability was discussed. The number of stem-cell of 2 different samples was measured at 72 hours, 7 days and 14 days after colture. The first sample was harvested with Goisis Cannula, with high values of stem-cells. The second sample was harvested with Coleman cannula with lower levels of stem-cells (Table 2.1).

2.5 The Effect of Negative Pressure Upon Fat and Stem-Cell Viability

Shiffman and Mirrafati compared suction pressures to establish their effect on cellular survival. The significant result was that greater cellular damage corresponded with a vacuum pressure in excess of 700 mmHg [8].

In the study by Cheriyan et al., adipose viability was 47% higher after aspiration at low pressure (−250 mmHg) compared with aspiration at high negative pressure (−760 mmHg). In addition, cell survival at 7 days was significantly higher with low-pressure aspiration [13]. This observation was confirmed by Nguyen et al. who proved that only 10% of the cells survived after liposuction at 760 mmHg [14].

Mojallal et al. evaluated the effect of pressure on the harvest of stromal vascular fraction (SVF) cells. Five different harvesting techniques were tested: pump suction at −350, pump suction at −700 mmHg, and power-assisted liposuction at −350 and −700 mmHg. Cell harvest with a pressure of −350 mmHg, assisted or not, was greater than that obtained at −700 mmHg. The conclusion was that −700 mmHg decreases the number of SVF cells harvested [15].

References

1. Gause T, Kling R, Sivak W, Marra K, Rubin J, Kokai L. Particle size in fat graft retention: a review on the impact of harvesting techniques in surgical lipofilling outcomes. Adipocyte. 2014;3(4):273–9.
2. Neuber G. Fettransplantation. Chir Kongr Verhandl Dsch Gesellch Chir. 1893;22:66.
3. Gurney CE. Experimental study of the behavior of free fat transplants. Surgery. 1937;3:679–92.
4. Peer A. The neglected free fat graft. Plast Reconstr Surg. 1956;18:233–50.
5. Fournier P. Liposculpture: the syringe technique. Paris: Arnette Blackwell; 1991. p. 265–6.
6. Illouz YG. The fat cell "graft": a new technique to fill depressions. Plast Reconstr Surg. 1986;78:122–3.
7. Kato H, Mineda K, Eto H, Doi K, Kuno S, Kinoshita K, Kanayama K, Yoshimura K. Degeneration, regeneration, and cicatrization after fat grafting: dynamic total tissue remodeling during the first 3 months. Plast Reconstr Surg. 2014;133:303e–13e.
8. Shiffman MA, Mirrafati S. Fat transfer techniques: the effect of harvest and transfer methods on adipocyte viability and review of the literature. Dermatol Surg. 2001;27:819–26.
9. Leong DT, Hutmacher DW, Chew FT, Lim T-C. Viability and adipogenic potential of human adipose tissue processed cell population obtained from pump-assisted and syringe-assisted liposuction. J Dermatol Sci. 2005;37:169–76.
10. Harris LJ, Zhang P, Abdollahi H, et al. Availability of adipose-derived stem cells in patients undergoing vascular surgical procedures. J Surg Res. 2010;163:e105–12.
11. Farr ST, Trivisonno A. Differential fat harvesting. Plast Aesthet Res. 2014;1:103–7.
12. Alharbi Z, Opländer C, Almakadi S. Conventional vs. micro-fat harvesting: how fat harvesting technique affects tissue-engineering approaches using adipose tissue-derived stem/stromal cells. J Plast Reconstr Aesthet Surg. 2013;66:1271–8.
13. Cheriyan T, Kao HK, Qiao X, Guo L. Plast Reconstr Surg. 2014;133(6):1365–8.
14. Nguyen P, Desouches C, Gay A, Hautier A, Magalon G. Development of micro-injection as an innovative autologous fat graft technique: the use of adipose tissue as dermal filler. J Plast Reconstr Aesthet Surg. 2012;65:1692–9.
15. Mojallal A, Auxenfans C, Lequeux C, Braye F, Damour O. Influence of negative pressure when harvesting adipose tissue on cell yield of the stromal-vascular fraction. Biomed Mater Eng. 2008;18(4-5):193–7.

Fat Harvesting Step by Step

3

Mario Goisis and Sara Izzo

3.1 Microfat Preparation: Harvesting in the Hip-Pelvis Area

Before providing a step-by-step description of the procedure, it is useful to recall some of the basic elements of the anatomy of the hip. The pelvic skeleton is formed, to the front, by the sacrum and the coccyx bones and by a pair of hip-bones to the left and right. The two hip-bones connect the lower limbs to the spine, while the lower limbs are connected to each other anteriorly and attached to the sacrum posteriorly.

Each hip-bone comprises three sections: the ilium, the ischium, and the pubis. The name of the ilium comes from the Latin word *ile* or *ilis*, meaning "groin" or "flank". The ilium is the largest of the coxal bones (Figs. 3.1 and 3.2).

The iliac crest is the upper border of the wing of the ilium (Fig. 3.3, green points). Palpable along its entire length, the crest is situated between the anterior superior iliac spine (ASIS) (Fig. 3.3, red point) and the posterior superior iliac spine (PSIS) (Fig. 3.4). The anterior superior iliac spine (ASIS) is a bony projection of the iliac bone and an important landmark of surface anatomy. It refers to the anterior extremity of the iliac crest of the pelvis, which provides an anchor for the inguinal ligament and the sartorius muscle (Figs. 3.5, 3.6, 3.7, 3.8, 3.9, and 3.10).

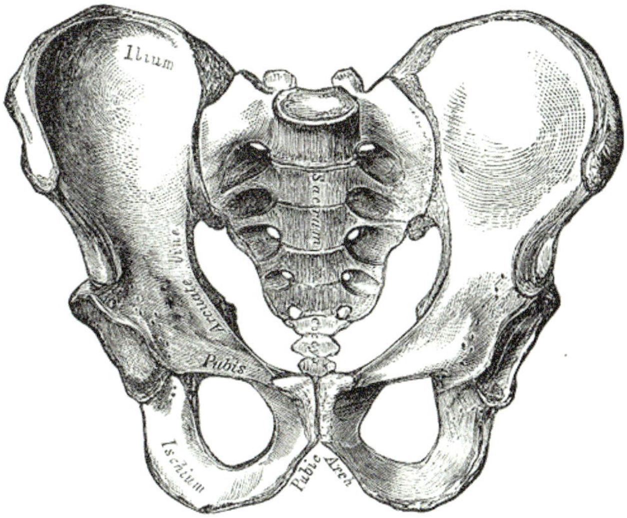

Fig. 3.1 The ilium is the largest of the coxal bones (reproduced from Gray's Anatomy, 20th edition, 1918, under public domain). (Published by kind permission of ©Mario Goisis 2018. All Rights Reserved)

3.2 Low-Pressure Microfat Aspiration: Materials and Methods

Microfat harvesting can be carried out in a small operating thetare/medical practice. Oxygen, pulse oximetry, and a crash cart/box should be present. A standard procedure microfat box is used (Courtesy of Microfat.com) (Fig. 3.11). The microfat box is composed of some single-use elements: a ramp with a closed system for washing and filtration, 4 60-cc syringes, 2 10-cc syringes, one 1-cc syringe, a 30-gauge needle, a 16-gauge needle, a 21-gauge needle, and a 22-gauge 4-cm blunt cannula.

This microfat box can be used in conjunction with some autoclavable elements, in particular the microfat tray (Fig. 3.12, Published by kind permission of ©Mario Goisis 2018. All Rights Reserved) and the autoclavable 10-cm Goisis cannula (Microfat or Tulip). The Goisis tray is composed of a plastic support for the ramp and of two trays for the Klein and

M. Goisis (✉)
Maxillo-Facial and Aesthetic Surgeon, Go Easy Clinic, Milan, Italy

S. Izzo
Department of Plastic Surgery, University of Campania "Luigi Vanvitelli", Piazza Miraglia, Milan, 80138, Italy

M. Goisis (ed.), *Outpatient Regenerative Medicine*, https://doi.org/10.1007/978-3-319-44894-7_3

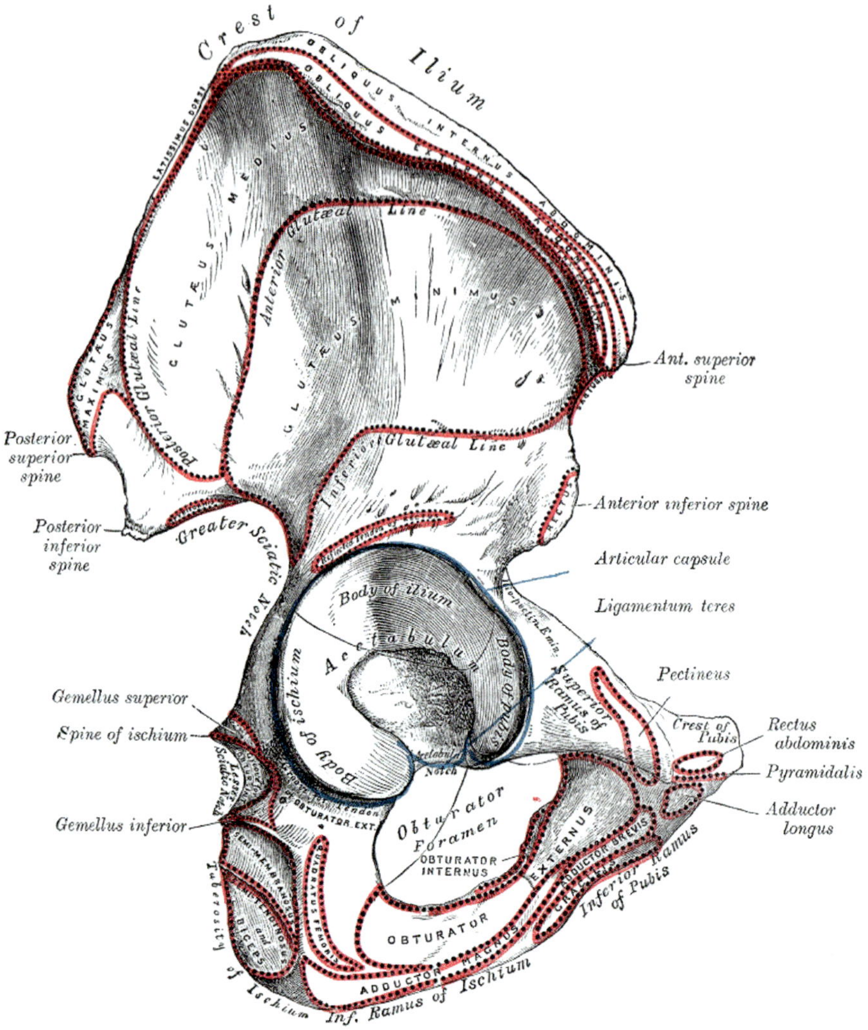

Fig. 3.2 The ilium is the largest of the coxal bones (reproduced from Gray's Anatomy, 20th edition, 1918, under public domain). (Published by kind permission of ©Mario Goisis 2018. All Rights Reserved)

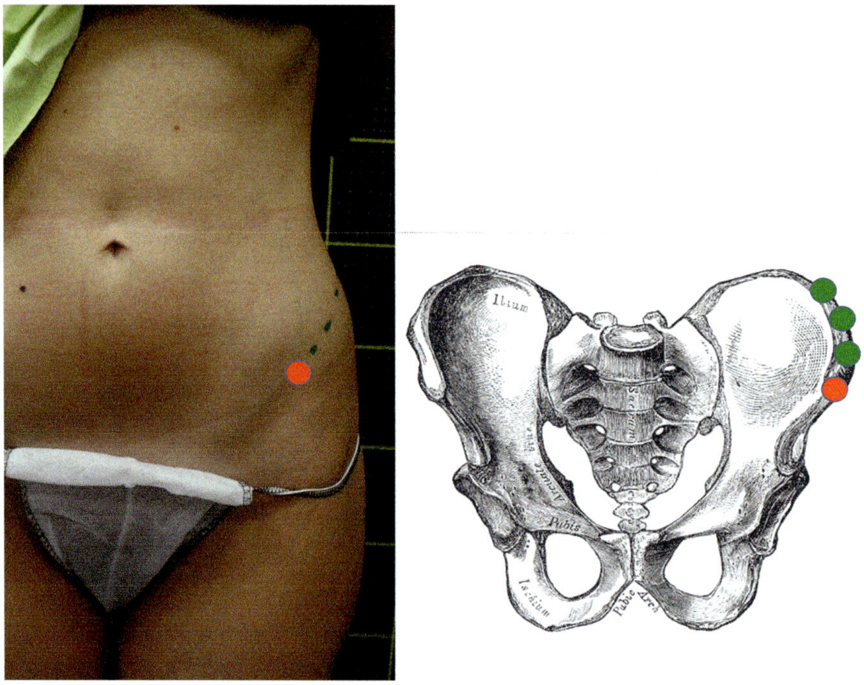

Fig. 3.3 The iliac crest is the upper border of the wing of ilium (green points). It is palpable along its entire length. The crest is situated between the anterior superior iliac spine (ASIS) (Fig. 3.3, red point) and the posterior superior iliac spine (PSIS) (Fig. 3.4). (Published by kind permission of ©Mario Goisis 2018. All Rights Reserved)

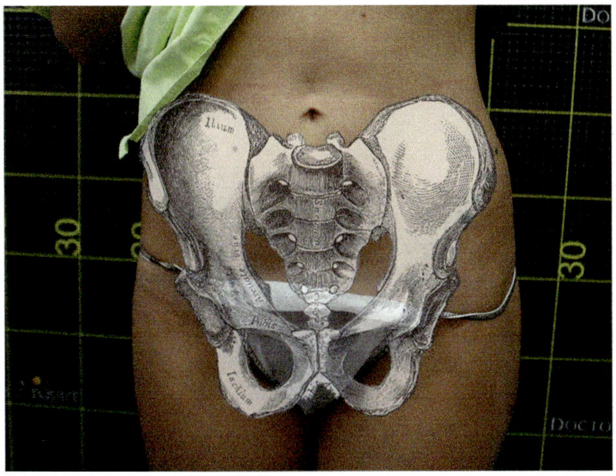

Fig. 3.4 The iliac crest is the superior border of the wing of ilium (green points). It is palpable along its entire length. The crest is included between the anterior superior iliac spine (ASIS) (Fig. 3.3, red point) and the posterior superior iliac spine (PSIS) (Fig. 3.4). (Published by kind permission of ©Mario Goisis 2018. All Rights Reserved)

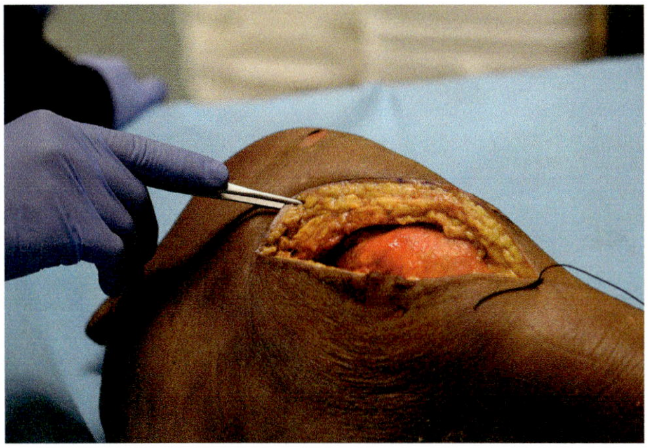

Fig. 3.5 Anatomical dissection of the harvesting area. The subcutaneous plane is exposed. (Published by kind permission of ©Mario Goisis 2018. All Rights Reserved)

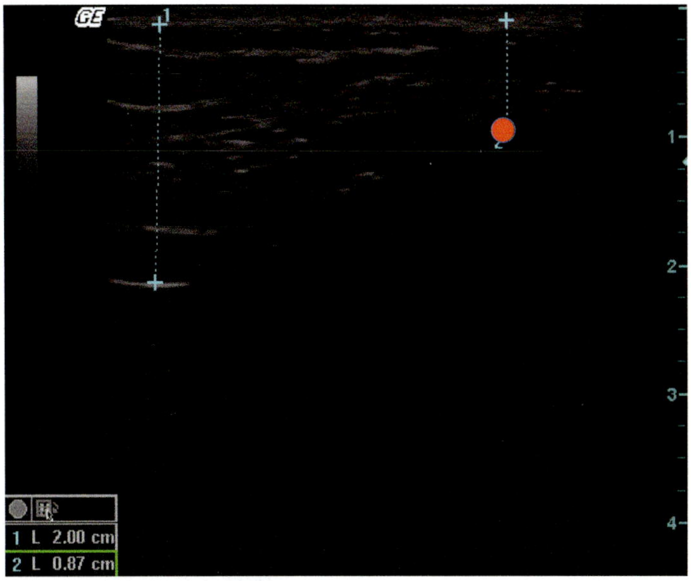

Fig. 3.6 An ultrasound image of the harvesting area. The red spot appears in correspondence to the anterior superior iliac spine. The use of ultrasound in thin patients can be supported by measuring the thickness of the adipose tissue in the aspiration site considered for harvesting and seeking the optimal position to prepare for the procedure. Ultrasound assistance may be considered for the initial learning curve or in thin patients. (Published by kind permission of ©Mario Goisis 2018. All Rights Reserved)

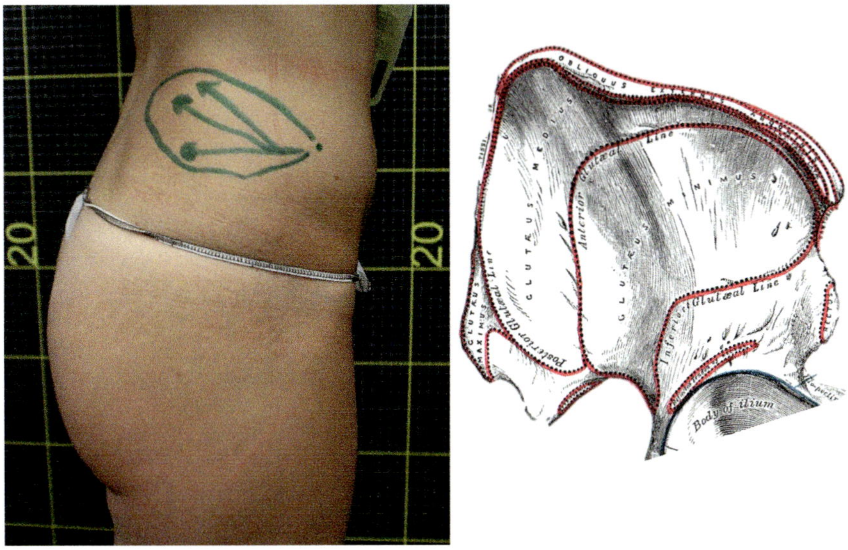

Fig. 3.7 Marking the harvesting area: the entry-point is signed in correspondence to the anterior superior iliac spine (ASIS). The flank fat pad is pinched and marked. (Published by kind permission of ©Mario Goisis 2018. All Rights Reserved)

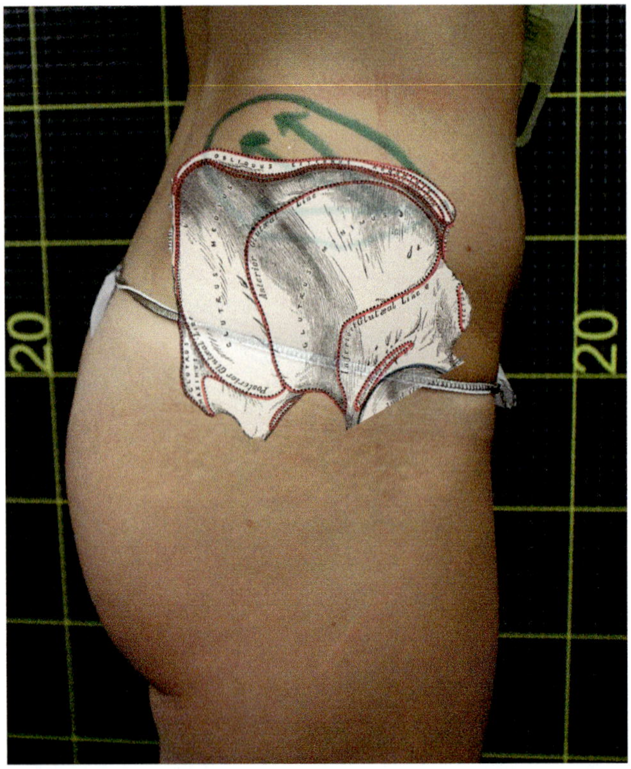

Fig. 3.8 Marking the harvesting area: the entry-point is signed in correspondence to the anterior superior iliac spine (ASIS). The flank fat pad is pinched and marked. (Published with kind permission of ©Mario Goisis 2018. All Rights Reserved)

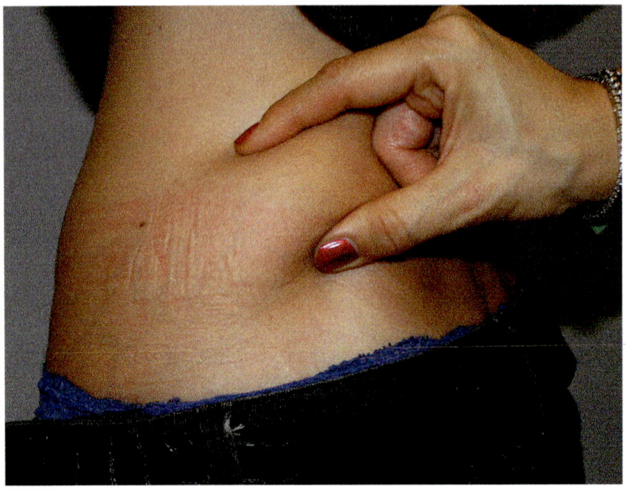

Fig. 3.9 Locating the pad of fat on the flank before harvesting. (Published by kind permission of ©Mario Goisis 2018. All Rights Reserved)

saline solutions. The autoclavable cannula is produced also in a single-use version.

Other necessary supplies are a chlorhexidine-alcohol solution (2% chlorhexidine gluconate and 70% isopropyl

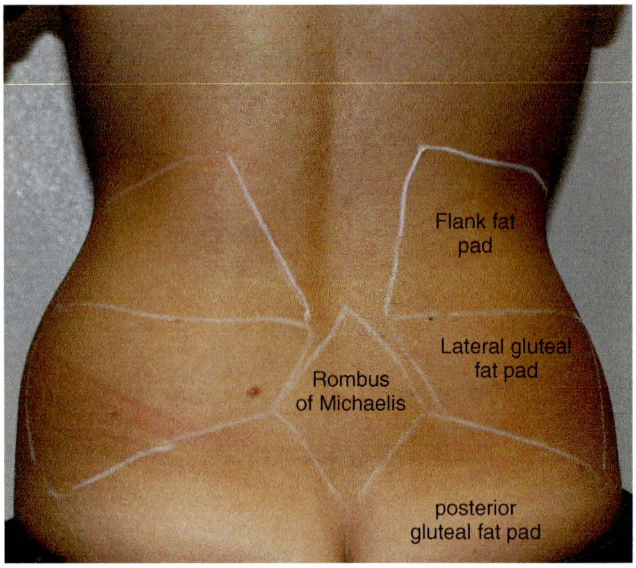

Fig. 3.10 Posterior view of areas from which fat may be harvested. (Published by kind permission of ©Mario Goisis 2018. All Rights Reserved)

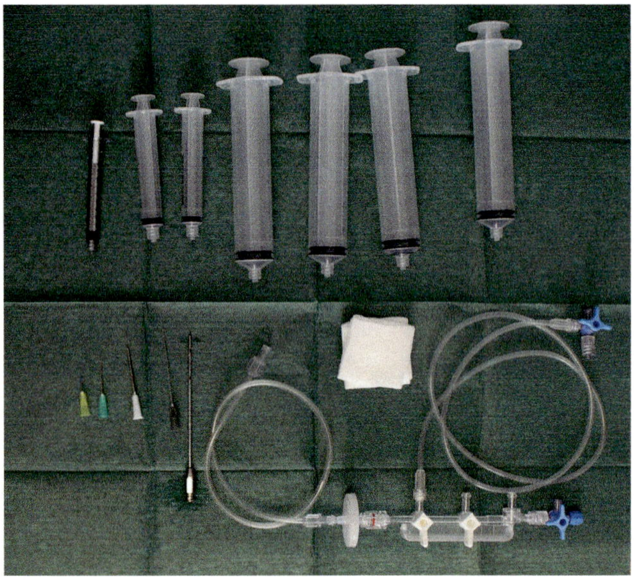

Fig. 3.11 The instruments used for harvesting using the Microfat Box. (Published by kind permission of ©Mario Goisis 2018. All Rights Reserved)

alcohol), sterile drapes or towels, ice packs, sterile 2 cm x 2 cm gauze squares, and an occlusive dressing cover.

When initially performing lipoaspiration, ultrasound guidance can be very useful, but once one's level of competence improves, it is not always needed. However, it should be included in the procedure when operating on thin patients. Ultrasound is a useful tool to determine the thickness of adipose tissue and the optimal site for harvesting. When using ultrasound, a sterile ultrasound transducer condom is required.

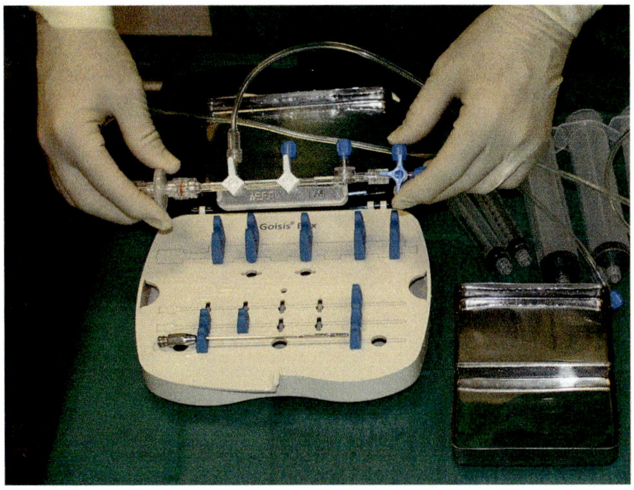

Fig. 3.12 The Microfat Tray. (Published by kind permission of ©Mario Goisis 2018. All Rights Reserved)

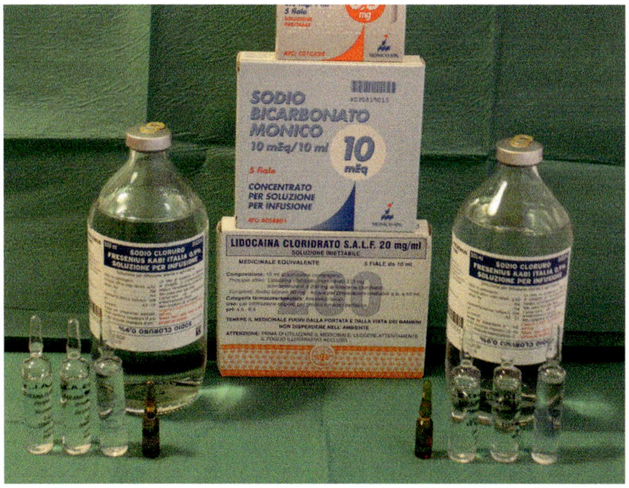

Fig. 3.13 Medications. (Published by kind permission of ©Mario Goisis 2018. All Rights Reserved)

Medications include:

- 100 cc of cold saline solution
- 120 cc of cold Klein solution

1 litre of Klein solution is composed of 800 mg of lidocaine, 1 mg of epinephrine, 40 MEq of sodium bicarbonate, and 1000 cc of saline solution. The use of an anaesthetic with epinephrine will reduce local bleeding and help speed up recovery (Fig. 3.13).

3.3 Preparation of the Klein Solution

Two 500-cc bottles of saline solution, four 200-mg bottles of lidocaine, two 0.5-mg bottles of epinephrine, and two 20-MEq bottles of sodium bicarbonate (Figs. 3.14, 3.15, 3.16, and 3.17).

Assistance: An assistant should be present to transfer items to the procedure field in a sterile manner during the first stage of the procedure, nevertheless, the complete procedure may be performed by a single doctor: careful handling is recommended.

3.3.1 The Low-Pressure Lipoaspiration Technique

The initial steps will be quite difficult, and the aspiration of the fat will be limited. The aspirate will appear transparent, usually with a large component of local anaesthesia. The later steps will be easier and run more smoothly, as the tissue is mobilised. The aspirate will appear yellow, preferably with a limited amount of blood.

The usual goal is 15–25 mL of adipose tissue. If a larger volume is desired, the use of a second site can be contemplated (Figs. 3.18, 3.19, 3.20, 3.21, 3.22, 3.23, 3.24, 3.25, 3.26, 3.27, 3.28, 3.29, 3.30, 3.31, 3.32, 3.33, 3.34, 3.35, 3.36, 3.37, 3.38, 3.39, 3.40, 3.41, 3.42, 3.43, 3.44, 3.45, 3.46, 3.47, 3.48, 3.49, 3.50, 3.51, 3.52, 3.53, 3.54, 3.55, 3.56, 3.57, 3.58, 3.59, 3.60, 3.61, 3.62, 3.63, 3.64, 3.65, 3.66, 3.67, and 3.68).

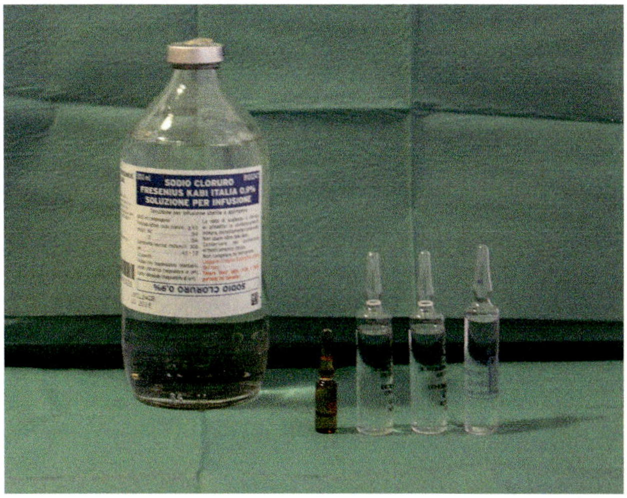

Fig. 3.14 Preparation of 500 mg of Klein solution step by step. The elements contained in 500 cc of Klein solution: one 500-cc bottle of saline solution, two 200-mg bottles of lidocaine, one 0.5-mg bottle of epinephrine, one 20-MEq bottle of sodium bicarbonate. (Published by kind permission of ©Mario Goisis 2018. All Rights Reserved)

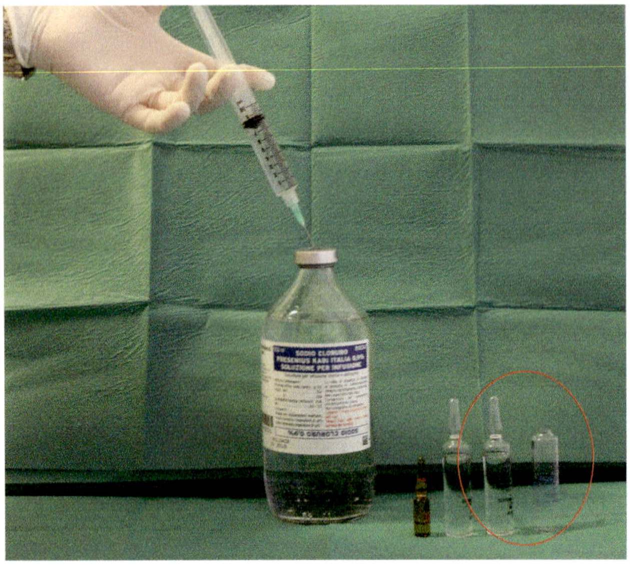

Fig. 3.15 The contents of the two 200-mg bottles of lidocaine are mixed with 500 cc of saline solution. (Published by kind permission of ©Mario Goisis 2018. All Rights Reserved)

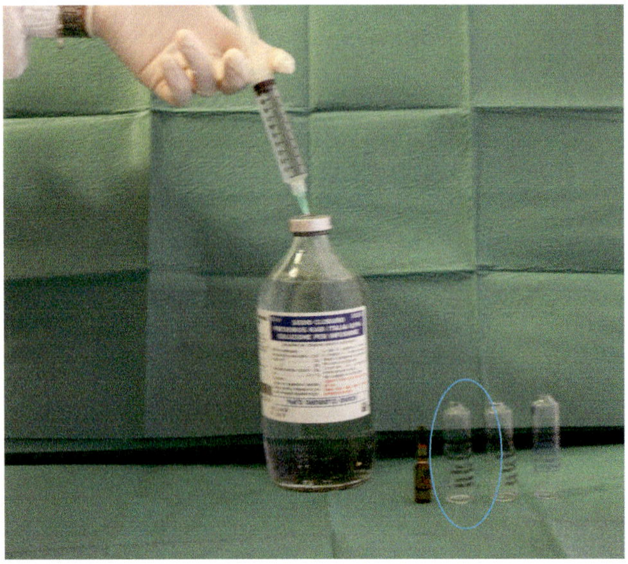

Fig. 3.16 The contents of the 20-MEq bottle of sodium bicarbonate is added. (Published by kind permission of ©Mario Goisis 2018. All Rights Reserved)

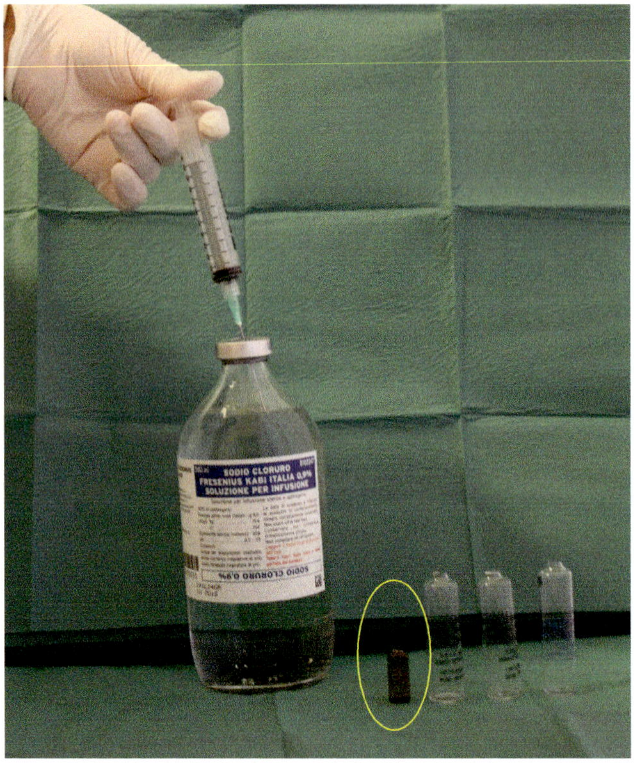

Fig. 3.17 Finally, the contents of the 0.5-mg bottle of epinephrine is added. (Published by kind permission of ©Mario Goisis 2018. All Rights Reserved)

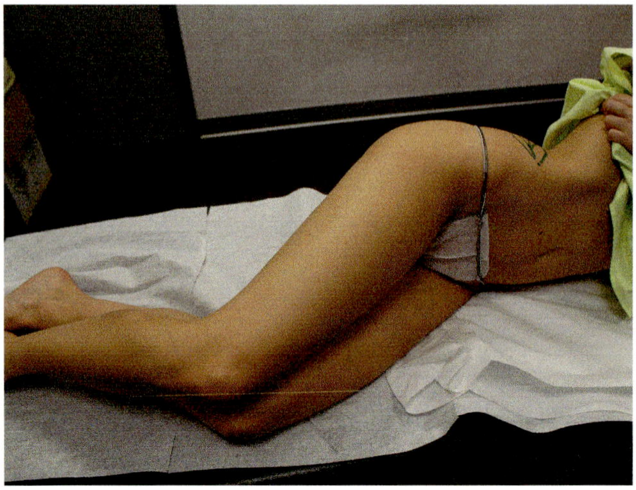

Fig. 3.18 If a patient is not too thin, the easiest sites from which to obtain lipoaspirate are those above the area of the flank. The lateral decubitus position is preferred (Fig. 3.14). (Published by kind permission of ©Mario Goisis 2018. All Rights Reserved)

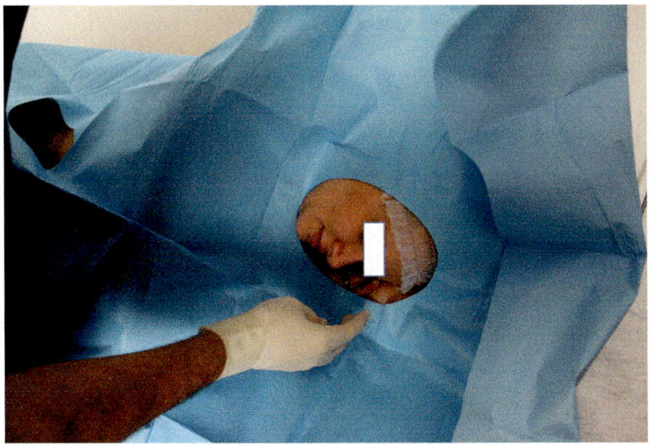

Fig. 3.19 Once the site has been chosen , it should be marked, and the area then cleansed, with a chlorhexidine-alcohol solution, and draped. (Published by kind permission of ©Mario Goisis 2018. All Rights Reserved)

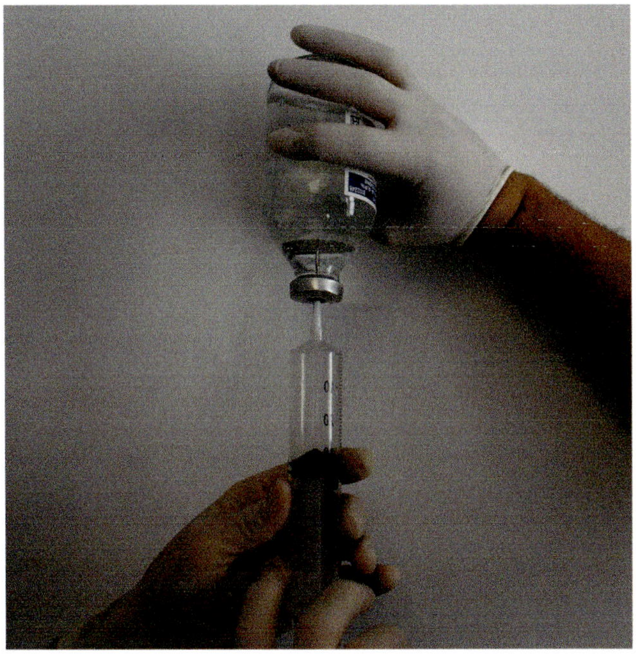

Fig. 3.20 The first syringe is filled with 60 cc of Klein solution. (Published by kind permission of ©Mario Goisis 2018. All Rights Reserved)

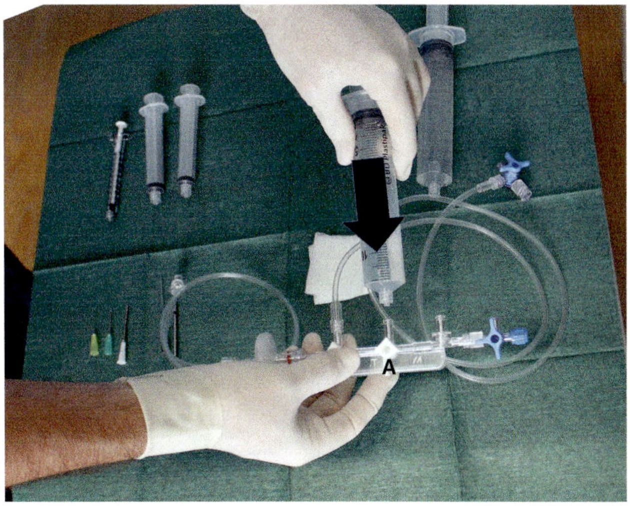

Fig. 3.21 The syringe is connected to the entry-duct marked "A" in the photograph. (Published by kind permission of ©Mario Goisis 2018. All Rights Reserved)

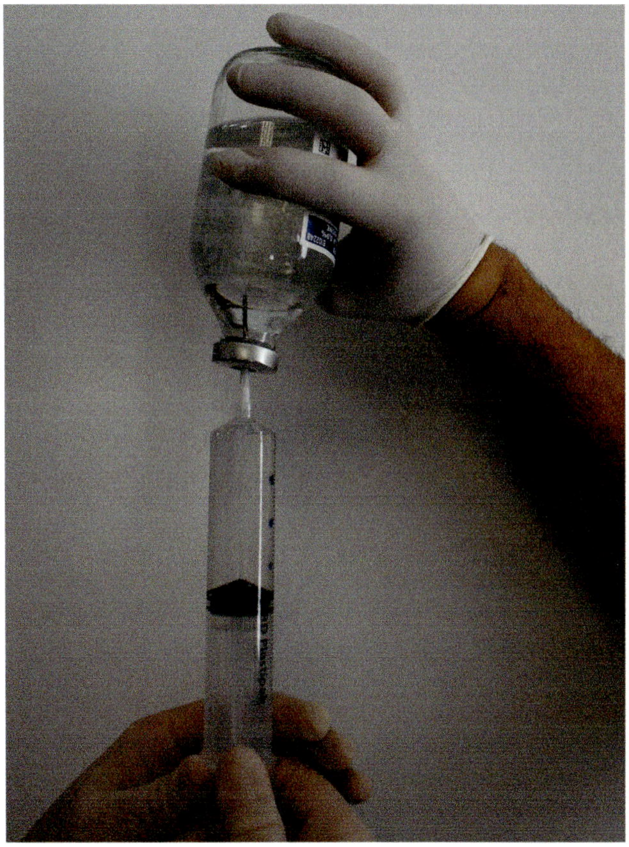

Fig. 3.22 The second syringe is filled with 60 cc of Klein solution. (Published by kind permission of ©Mario Goisis 2018. All Rights Reserved)

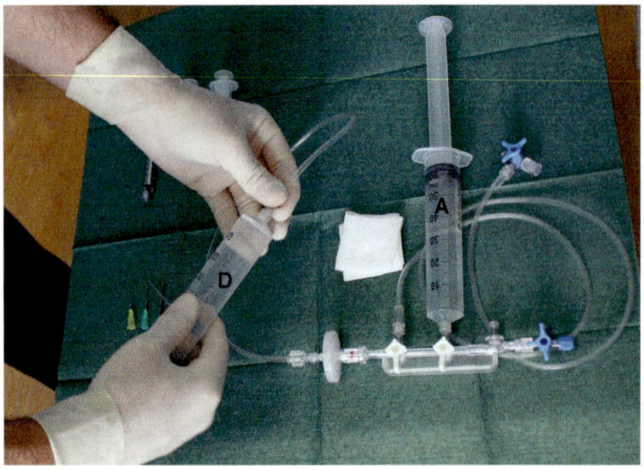

Fig. 3.23 The syringe is connected to the tube marked "D". (Published by kind permission of ©Mario Goisis 2018. All Rights Reserved)

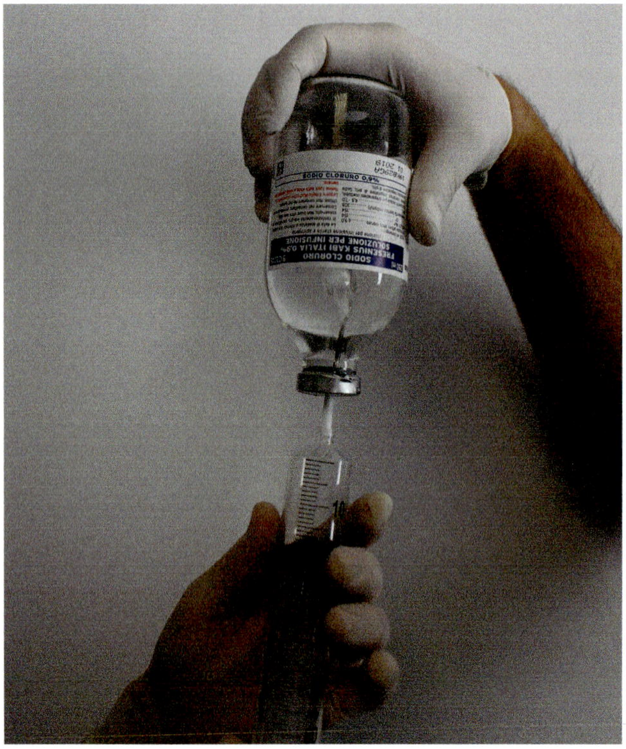

Fig. 3.24 The third syringe is filled with 60 cc of the saline solution. (Published by kind permission of ©Mario Goisis 2018. All Rights Reserved)

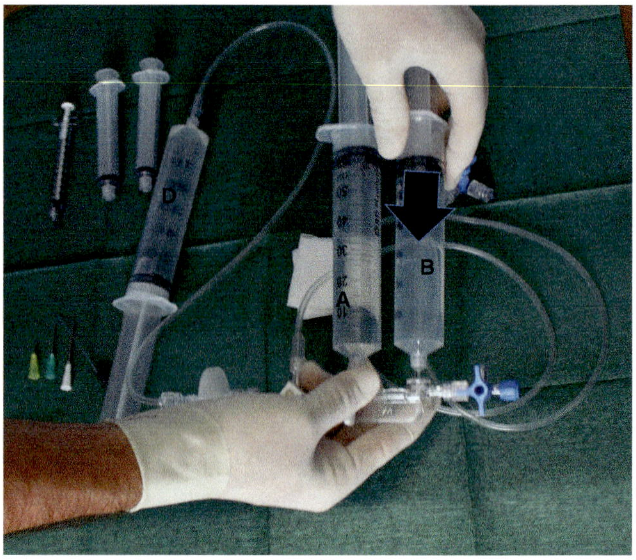

Fig. 3.25 The syringe filled with the saline solution is connected to position B (see the black arrow). (Published by kind permission of ©Mario Goisis 2018. All Rights Reserved)

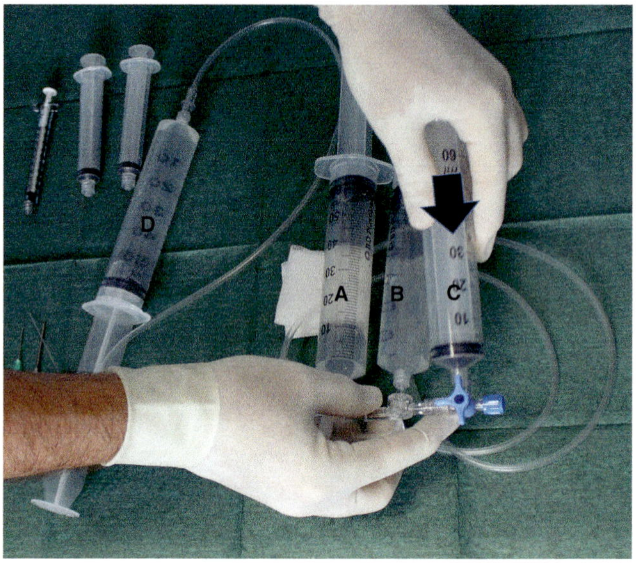

Fig. 3.26 An empty 60 cc syringe is connected to position C (see the black arrow). (Published by kind permission of ©Mario Goisis 2018. All Rights Reserved)

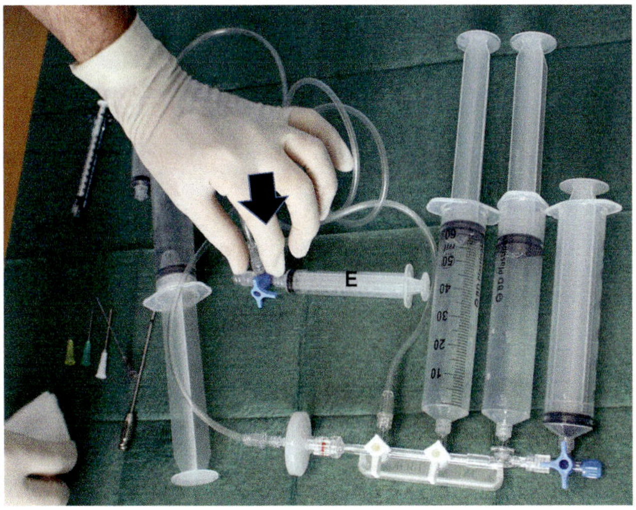

Fig. 3.27 An empty 10-cc syringe is connected to position E (see the black arrow). (Published by kind permission of ©Mario Goisis 2018. All Rights Reserved)

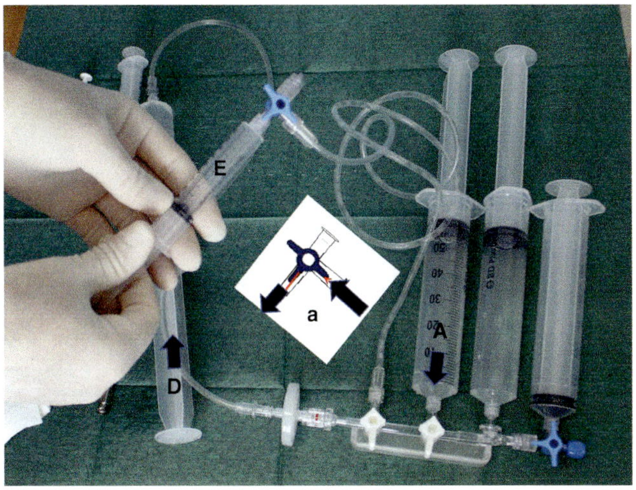

Fig. 3.28 The local anaesthetic is transferred directly from the syringes A and D to the 10-cc syringe E. In particular, when the stopcock is in position "a" by pulling the plunger, the syringe E is filled with air and anaesthetic solution. (Published by kind permission of ©Mario Goisis 2018. All Rights Reserved)

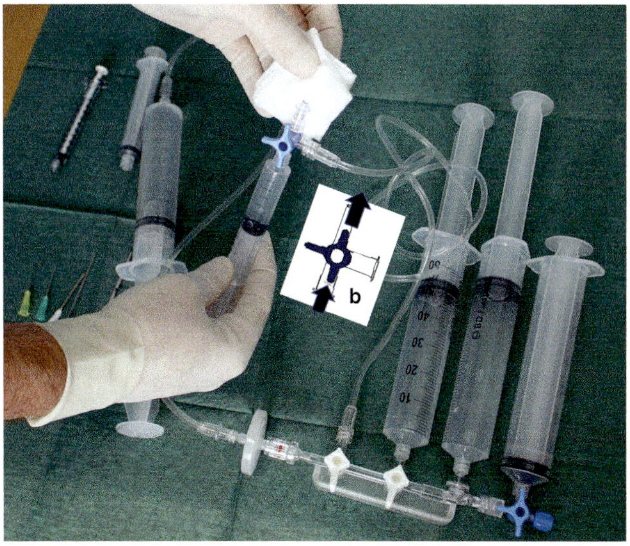

Fig. 3.29 By moving the stopcock to position "b," the air is pushed out from the syringe. (Published with kind permission of ©Mario Goisis 2018. All Rights Reserved)

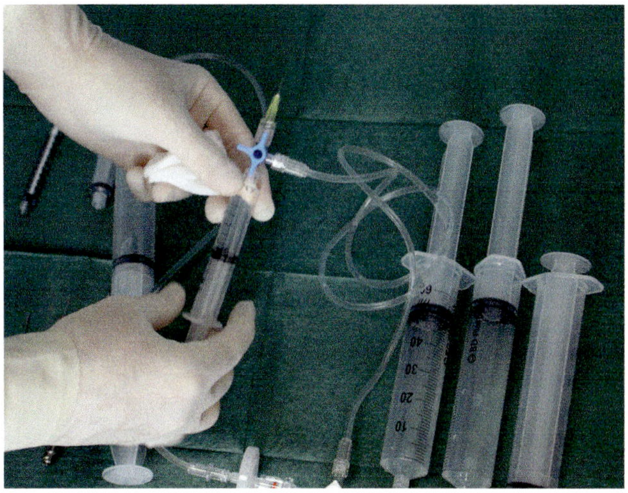

Fig. 3.30 A 30-gauge needle is connected to syringe E. (Published by kind permission of ©Mario Goisis 2018. All Rights Reserved)

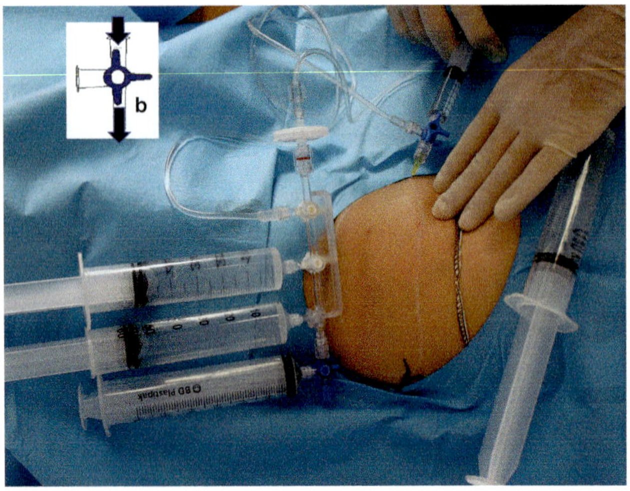

Fig. 3.31 1 cc of Klein solution is injected into the entry-point. The stopcock is in the "b" position, connecting the syringe to the needle. (Published by kind permission of ©Mario Goisis 2018. All Rights Reserved)

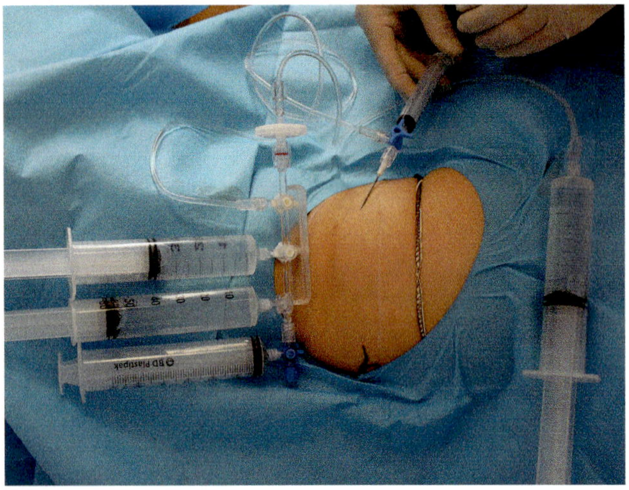

Fig. 3.32 The 30-gauge needle is exchanged for a 16-gauge needle. (Published by kind permission of ©Mario Goisis 2018. All Rights Reserved)

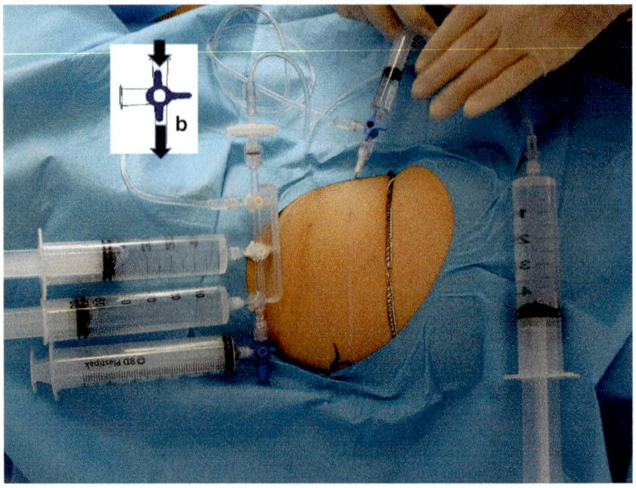

Fig. 3.33 The entire contents of the syringe is injected into the entry-point. (Published by kind permission of ©Mario Goisis 2018. All Rights Reserved)

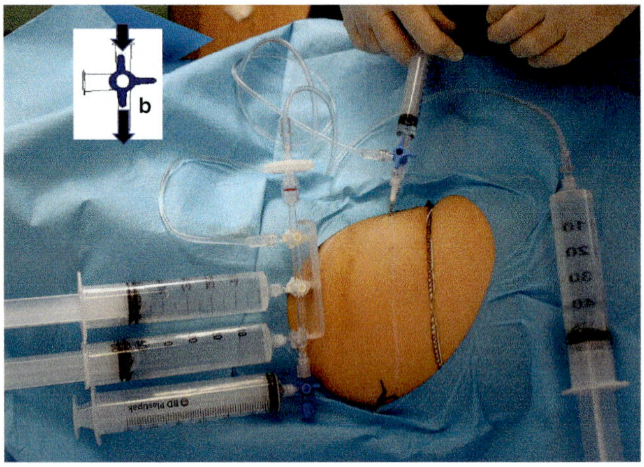

Fig. 3.34 The entire contents of the syringe is injected into the entry-point. (Published by kind permission of ©Mario Goisis 2018. All Rights Reserved)

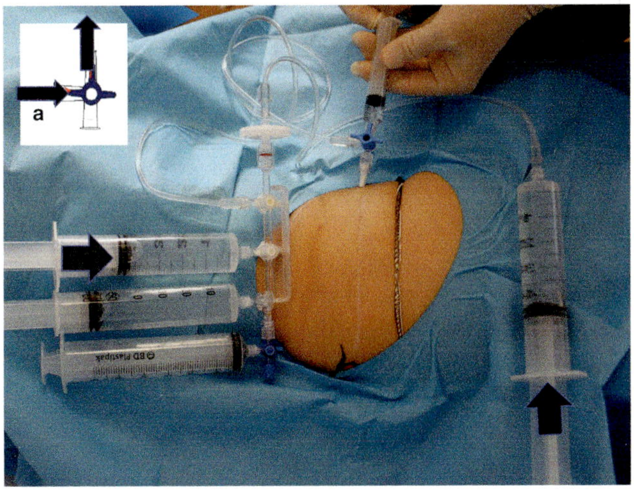

Fig. 3.35 The stopcock connected to the empty syringe is moved to position “a.” When the stopcock is in the "a" position, by pulling the plunger, syringe E is filled with Klein solution. In fact, it is aspirated directly from syringes A and D. (Published by kind permission of ©Mario Goisis 2018. All Rights Reserved)

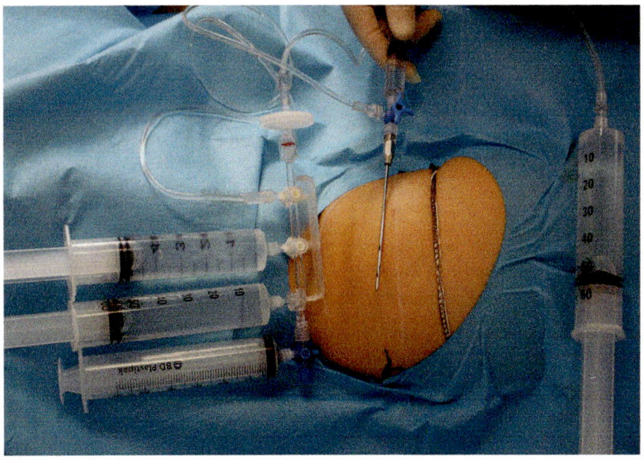

Fig. 3.37 Fan distribution of the Goisis cannula into the donor site. (Published by kind permission of ©Mario Goisis 2018. All Rights Reserved)

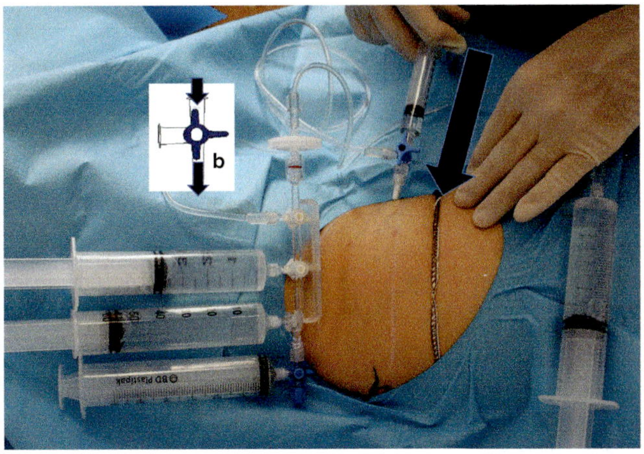

Fig. 3.36 With the stopcock in the "b" position, 10 cc of Klein solution is injected. (Published by kind permission of ©Mario Goisis 2018. All Rights Reserved)

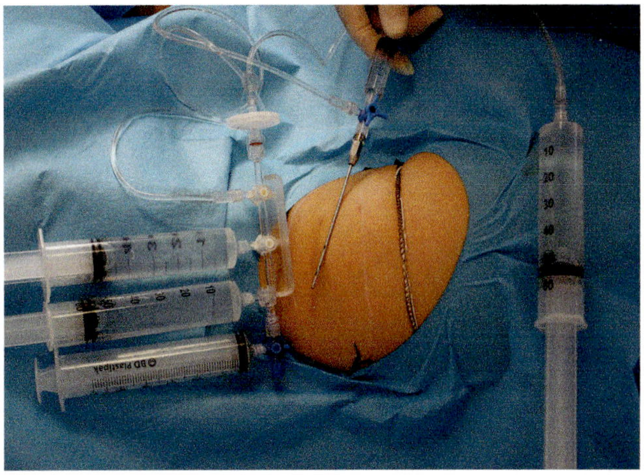

Fig. 3.38 Fan distribution of the Goisis cannula into the donor site. (Published by kind permission of ©Mario Goisis 2018. All Rights Reserved)

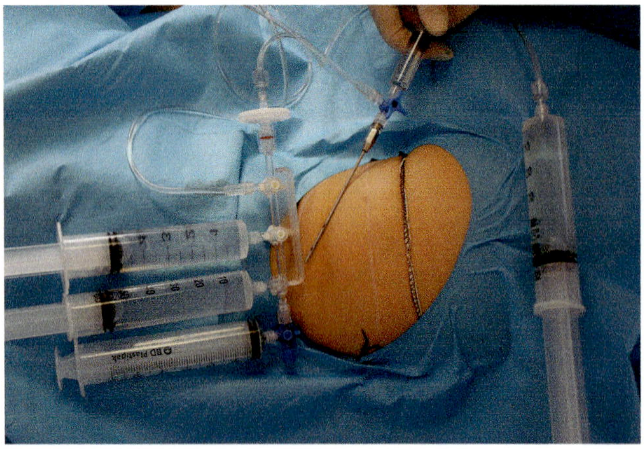

Fig. 3.39 Fan distribution of the Goisis cannula into the donor site. (Published by kind permission of ©Mario Goisis 2018. All Rights Reserved)

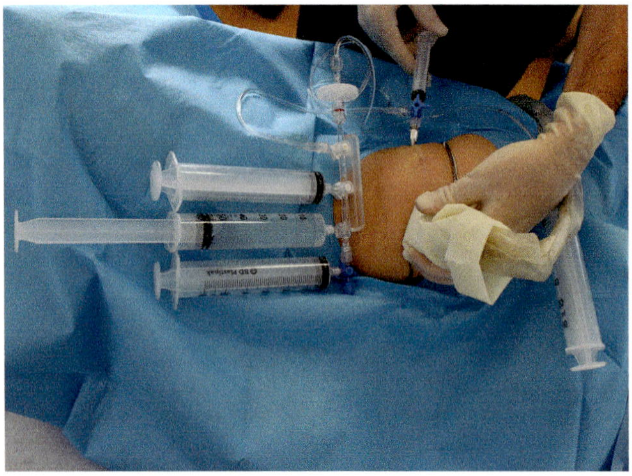

Fig. 3.40 The cannula is inserted into the area, and a few slow passes are carried out to distribute the Klein solution. (Published with kind permission of ©Mario Goisis 2018. All Rights Reserved)

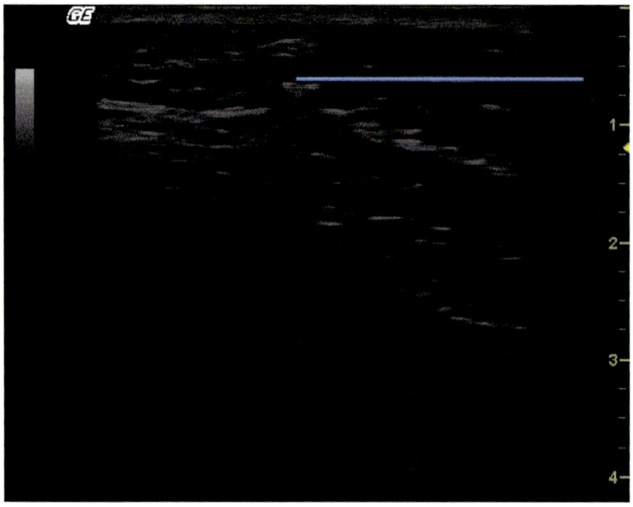

Fig. 3.41 An ultrasound image shows the relationship between the cannula and the anatomical structure of the area. The cannula is inserted into the subcutaneous tissue, at a depth of 1 cm from the cutis. (Published by kind permission of ©Mario Goisis 2018. All Rights Reserved)

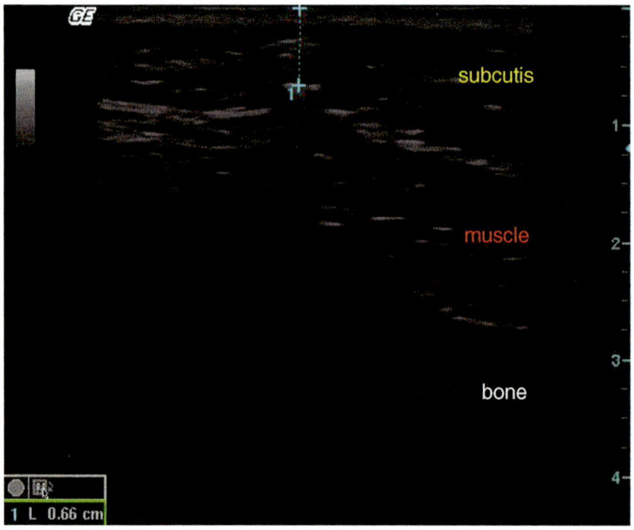

Fig. 3.42 An ultrasound image shows the relationship between the cannula and the anatomical structure of the area. The cannula is inserted into the subcutaneous tissue, at a depth of 1 cm from the cutis. (Published by kind permission of ©Mario Goisis 2018. All Rights Reserved)

Fig. 3.43 The remaining 120 cc of the Klein solution is injected in small spots of 5 cc (blue circle). The injection of anaesthesia takes 3–5 min. (Published by kind permission of ©Mario Goisis 2018. All Rights Reserved)

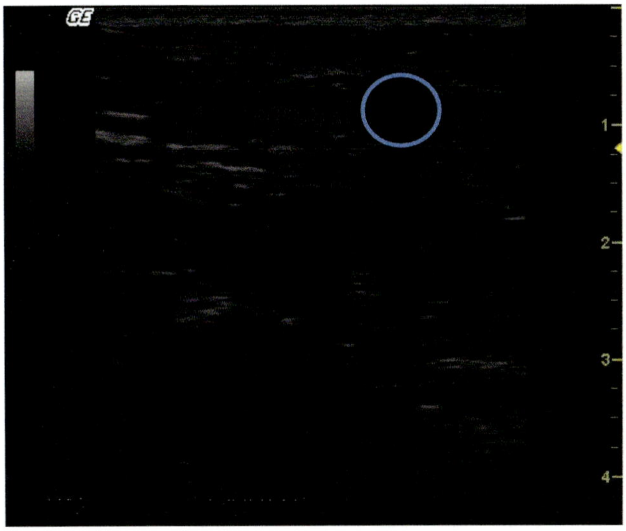

Fig. 3.44 The remaining 120 cc of Klein solution is injected into small spots of 5 cc (blue circle). The injection of anaesthesia takes 3–5 min. (Published by kind permission of ©Mario Goisis 2018. All Rights Reserved)

Fig. 3.45 The Klein solution injected begins to break down/mobilise the adipose tissue. The infiltrated area is indicated with the blue arrows. (Published with kind permission of ©Mario Goisis 2018. All Rights Reserved)

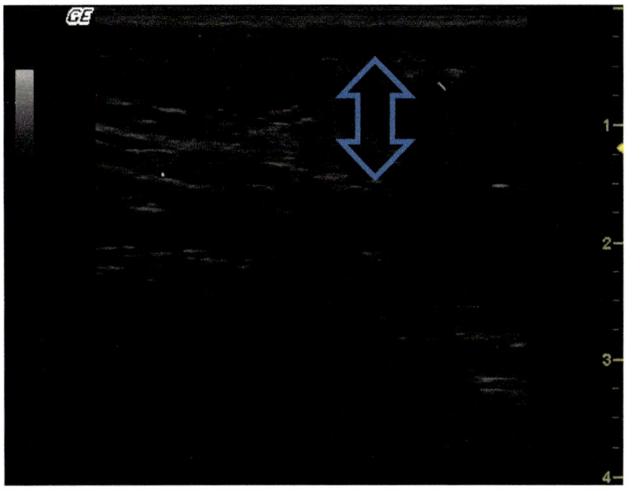

Fig. 3.46 The Klein solution injected begins to break down/mobilise the adipose tissue. The infiltrated area is indicated with the blue arrows. (Published by kind permission of ©Mario Goisis 2018. All Rights Reserved)

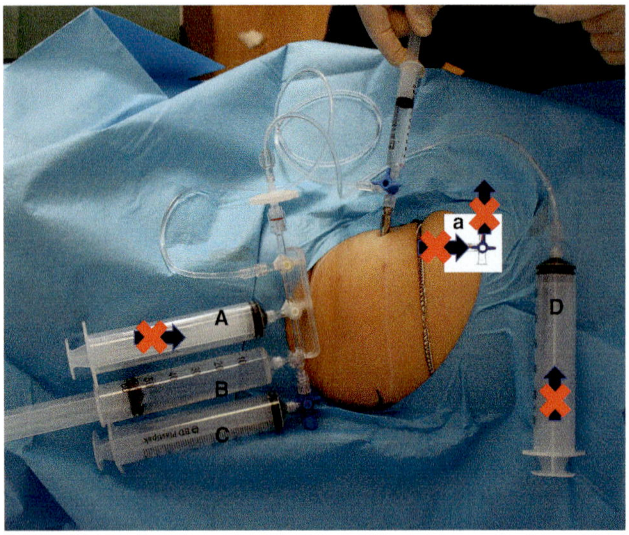

Fig. 3.47 The infiltration of the Klein solution ceases automatically when syringes A and D are empty. In fact, when all of the content of these syringes has been injected, it is impossible to fill syringe E either with the stopcock in position "a". (Published by kind permission of ©Mario Goisis 2018. All Rights Reserved)

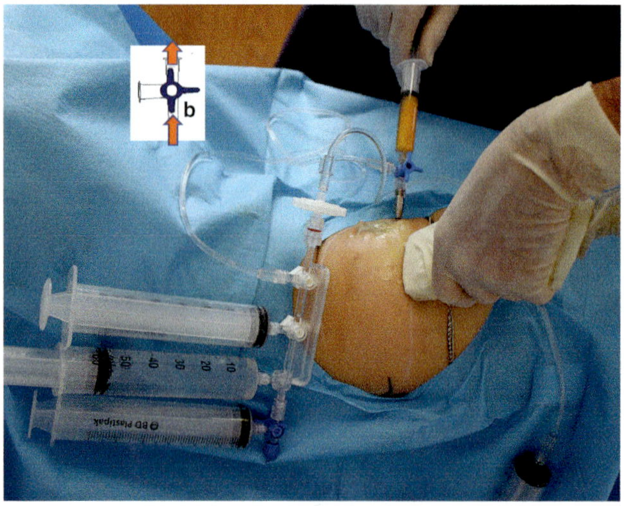

Fig. 3.48 The stopcock is moved to position "b," and the harvesting of the fat can start. It is mandatory that the aspiration holes of the cannula remain in the skin the whole time. When the plunger of the syringe is pulled back, a negative pressure is created, and the syringe is progressively filled with fat. The practitioner can then easily move the cannula back and forth inside the anaesthetized region. Pinching the tissue to raise it up often makes the process simpler. Additionally, pinching the tissue can reduce procedural pain by stimulating mechanoreceptors. (Published by kind permission of ©Mario Goisis 2018. All Rights Reserved)

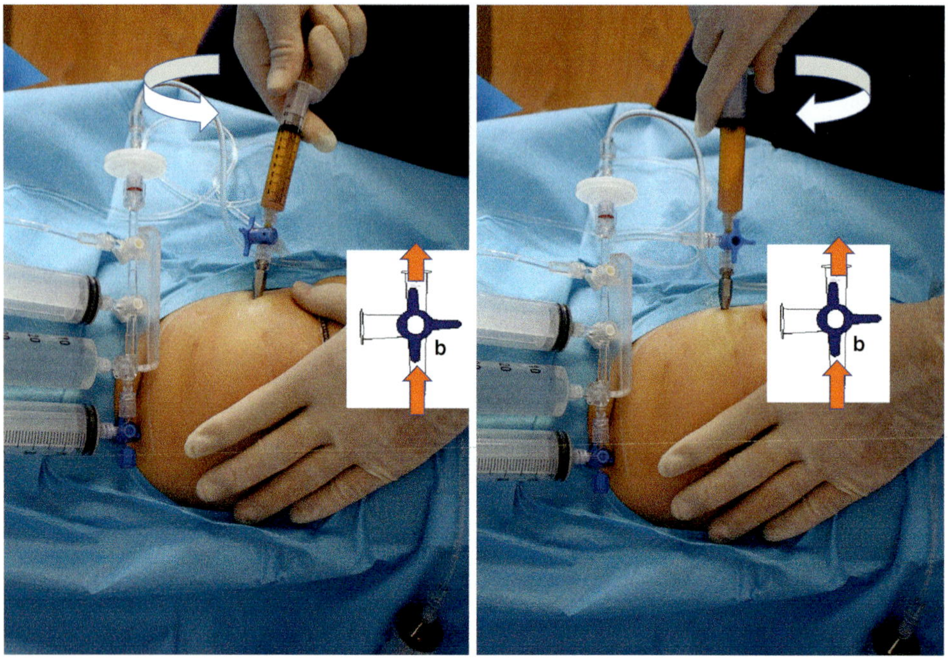

Fig. 3.49 A rotational movement is applied to the cannula by rotating the wrist. (Published by kind permission of ©Mario Goisis 2018. All Rights Reserved)

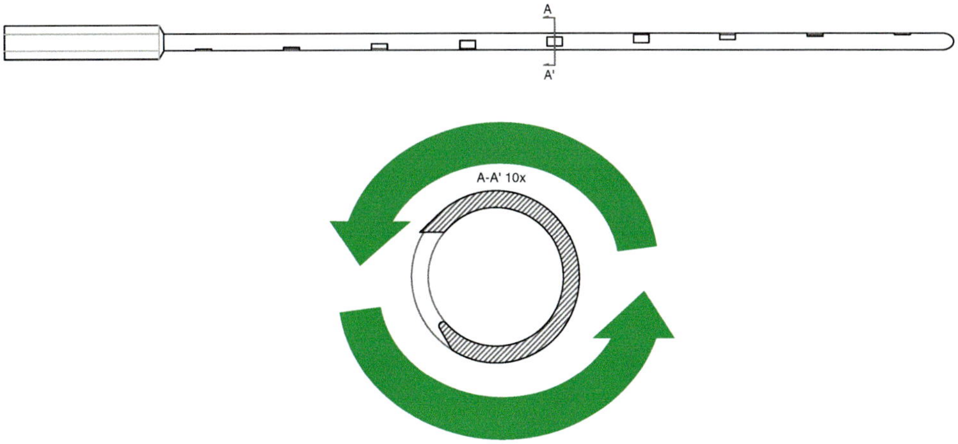

Fig. 3.50 Design of the Goisis cannula. By bring a rotational movement to bear, it is possible to increase the harvesting of the fat. In particular, the depressed edge of the holes increases the entrance of the fat into the cannula and the barbed edge favours its dissection. (Published by kind permission of ©Mario Goisis 2018. All Rights Reserved)

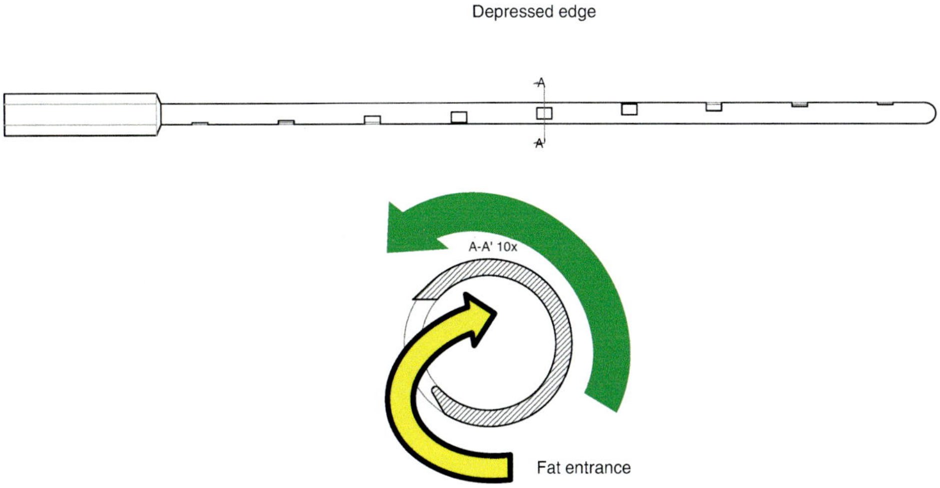

Fig. 3.51 Design of the Goisis cannula. A rotational movement makes increasing the amount of fat to be harvested possible. In particular, the depressed edge of the holes increases the entrance of the fat into the cannula and the barbed edge favours its dissection. (Published by kind permission of ©Mario Goisis 2018. All Rights Reserved)

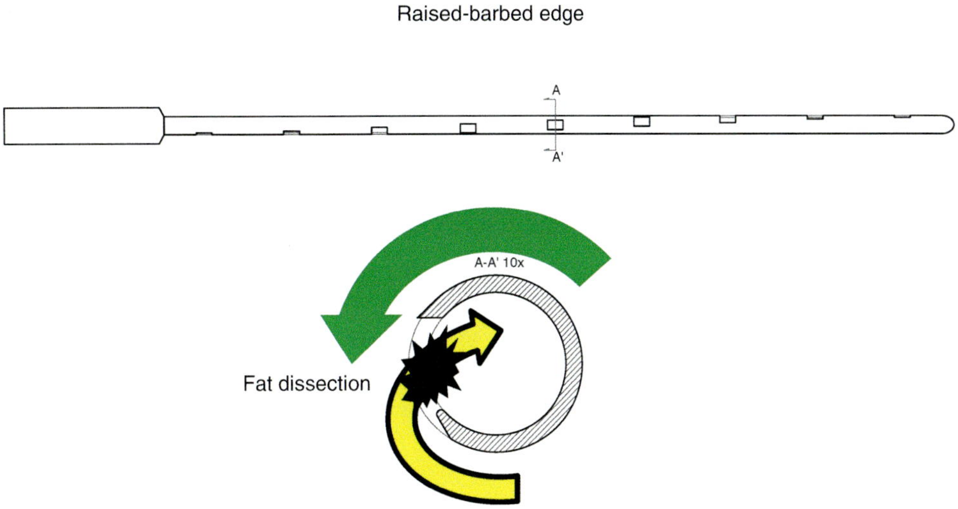

Fig. 3.52 Design of the Goisis cannula. A rotational movement makes it possible to increase the amount of fat to harvest. In particular, the depressed edge of the holes increases the entrance of the fat into the cannula and the barbed edge favours its dissection. (Published by kind permission of ©Mario Goisis 2018. All Rights Reserved)

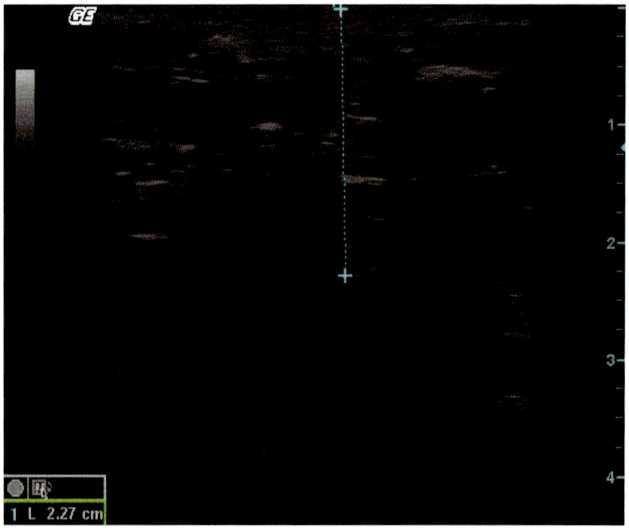

Fig. 3.53 Ultrasound image of the position of the cannula (in blue). It is important not to aspirate too large a volume close to the skin, because this can result in dimpling of the skin. The correct depth of the cannula is at least 1 cm from the dermis. It is also mandatory to minimise trauma to the underlying muscle, by avoiding entinto the muscular plane. (Published by kind permission of ©Mario Goisis 2018. All Rights Reserved)

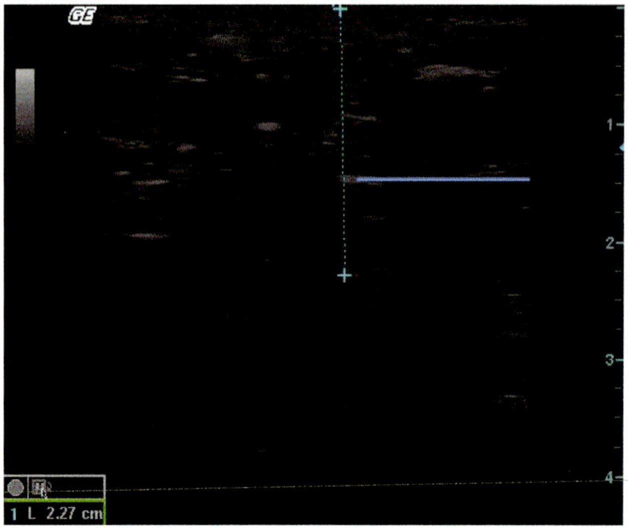

Fig. 3.54 Ultrasound image of the position of the cannula (in blue). It is important to not aspirate too large a volume close to the skin, because this can cause dimpling of the skin. The correct depth of the cannula is at least 1 cm from the dermis. It is also mandatory to minimise trauma to the underlying muscle, by avoiding to enter into the muscular plane. (Published with kind permission of ©Mario Goisis 2018. All Rights Reserved)

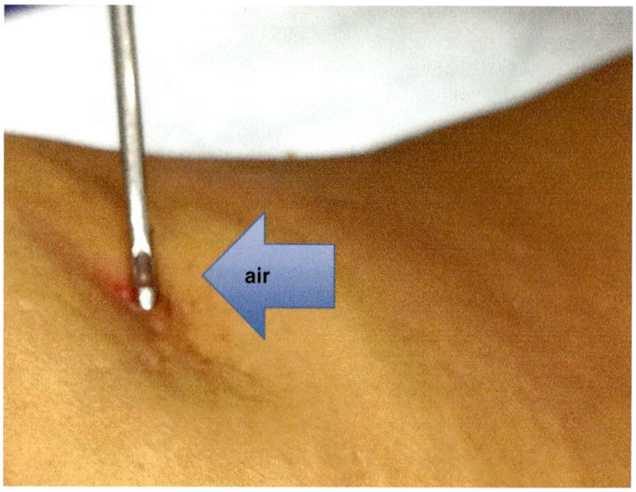

Fig. 3.55 If one of the aspiration holes is removed from the skin, the air enters the syringe, and the vacuum is lost. (Published by kind permission of ©Mario Goisis 2018. All Rights Reserved)

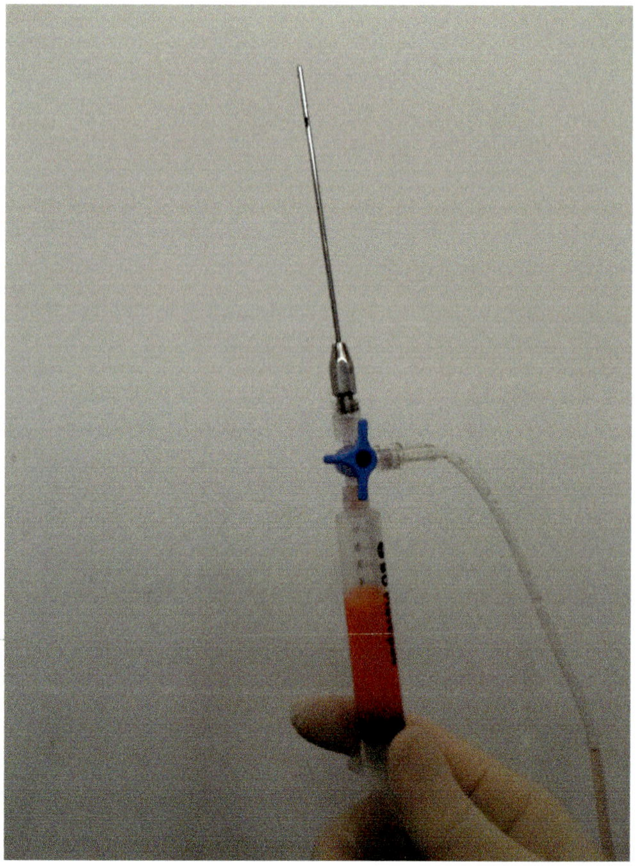

Fig. 3.56 Then it is necessary to remove the cannula, leave the plunger, hold a sterile gauze over the cannula holes, express the excess air from the syringe, and repeat the initial steps. (Published by kind permission of ©Mario Goisis 2018. All Rights Reserved)

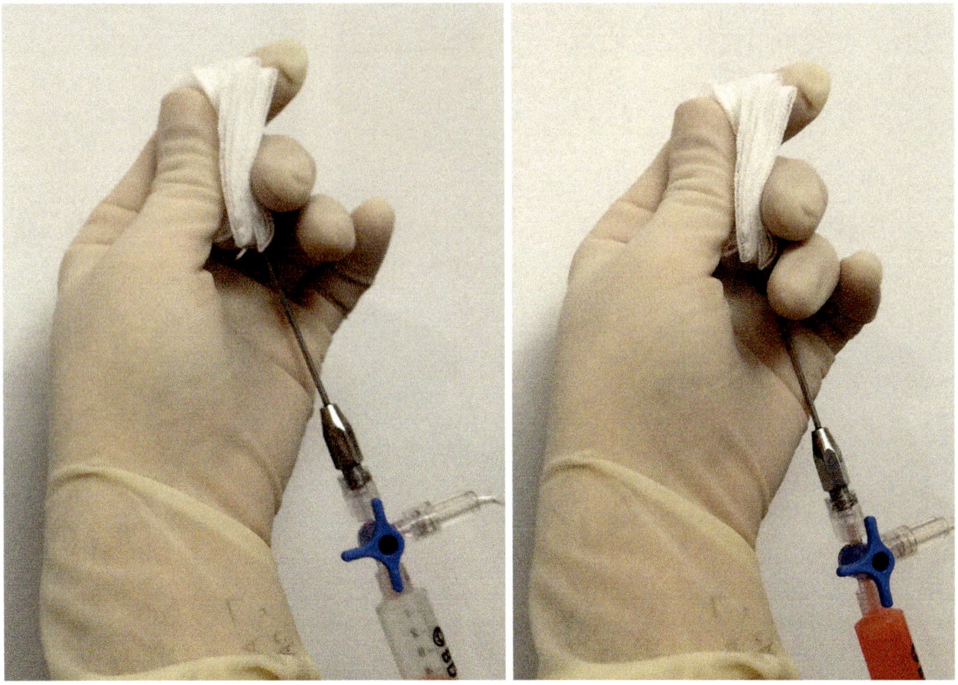

Fig. 3.57 Then it is necessary to remove the cannula, leave the plunger, hold a sterile gauze over the cannula holes, express the excess air from the syringe, and repeat the initial steps. (Published by kind permission of ©Mario Goisis 2018. All Rights Reserved)

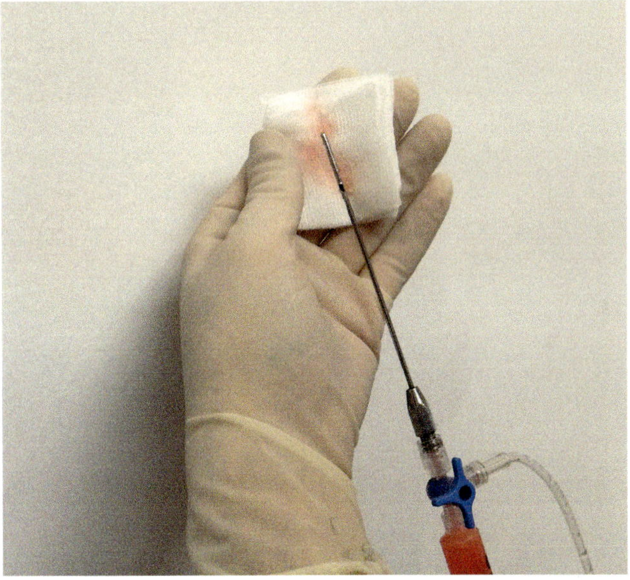

Fig. 3.58 Then it is necessary to remove the cannula, leave the plunger, hold a sterile gauze over the cannula holes, express the excess air from the syringe, and repeat the initial steps. (Published by kind permission of ©Mario Goisis 2018. All Rights Reserved)

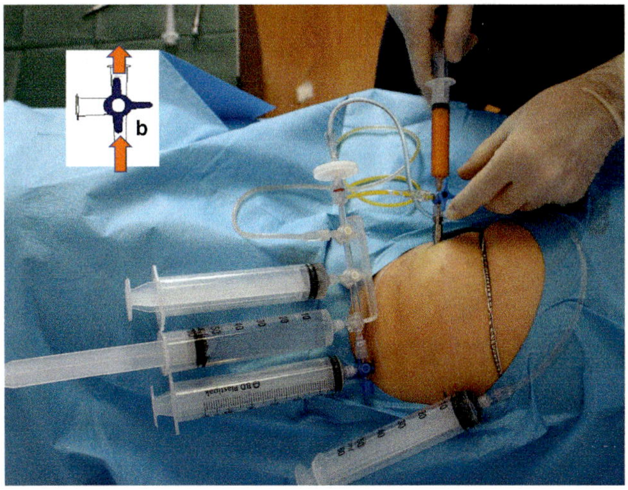

Fig. 3.59 When the syringe E is completely filled, move the stopcock into position "a". (Published by kind permission of ©Mario Goisis 2018. All Rights Reserved)

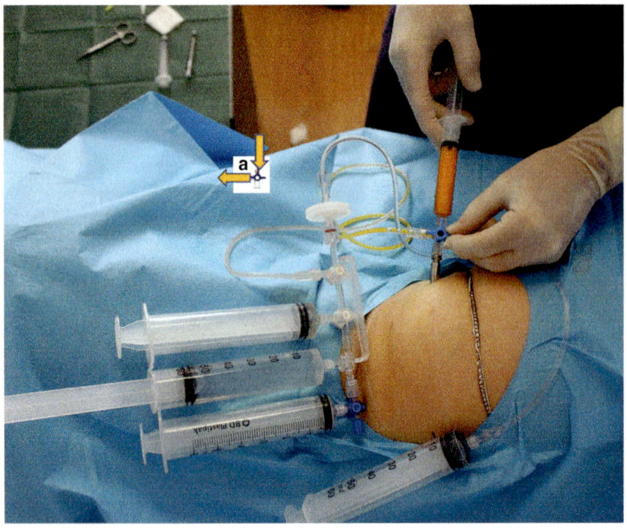

Fig. 3.60 The fat mixed with blood and anaesthesia is pushed and transferred directly from syringe E to syringe A. (Published by kind permission of ©Mario Goisis 2018. All Rights Reserved)

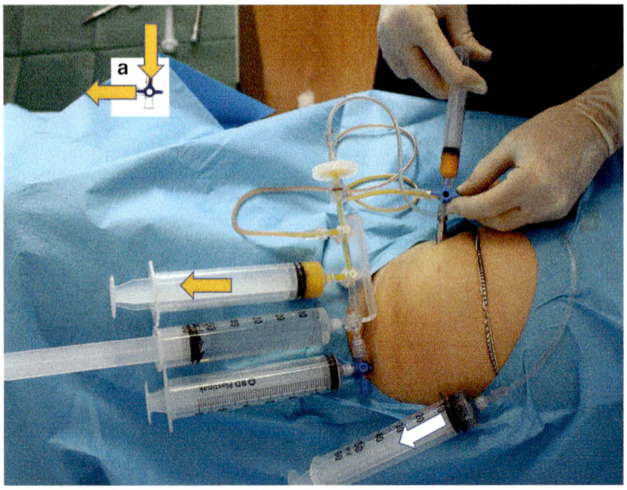

Fig. 3.61 The fat mixed with blood and anaesthesia is pushed and transferred directly from syringe E to syringe A. (Published by kind permission of ©Mario Goisis 2018. All Rights Reserved)

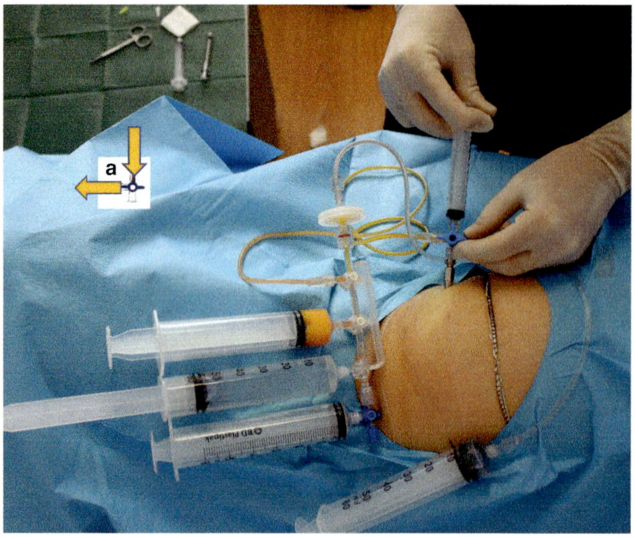

Fig. 3.62 The fat mixed with blood and anaesthesia is pushed and transferred directly from syringe E to syringe A. (Published by kind permission of ©Mario Goisis 2018. All Rights Reserved)

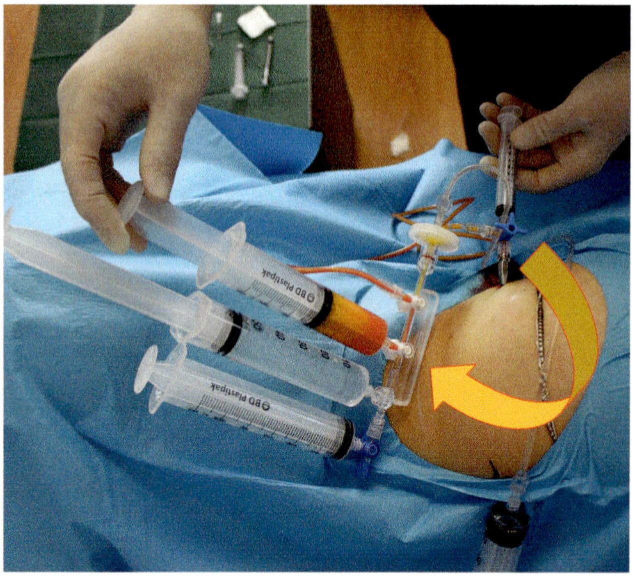

Fig. 3.63 Repeat the procedure 4–6 times in order to obtain a sufficient amount of fat. (Published by kind permission of ©Mario Goisis 2018. All Rights Reserved)

3.4 Complications

With the widespread use of micro-cannulas, few complications are now reported. A patient may be intolerant to the addition of epinephrine, which may increase anxiety. Bleeding, bruising, and post-procedure pain in the area of harvesting are commonly reported. Microfat procedure harvests a relatively low volume of aspirate, and therefore skin dimpling is uncommon.

The clear occlusive bandage (e.g., Tegaderm or similar) is removed the day after the treatment. Ice is applied to the donor site for 20 min every hour for 6 h, in order to minimize bleeding and pain and to speed recovery. Close attention and the time of application of ice should be observed, because the skin is anesthetized. After 10–15 min of observation, vital signs should be obtained, and if the patient is stable, he or she is discharged. The area should be kept clean and dry for 24 h. No soaking in a hot tub, pool, or bath is permitted for 3 days. Written instructions assist in getting compliance because the patient can refer to them. The area may be painful for several days to a week, but the soreness should not be increasing. Increased donor site soreness, erythema, sweating, or fever should prompt the patient to return, so the harvesting area can be inspected for infection. Rehydration by drinking abundantly of water for 24 h after the procedure should be encouraged. Vigorous activity or heavy lifting should be avoided for 5–6 h. A treatment with antibiotic (azithromycin 500 mg for 3 days) and pain killers (acetilsalicilic acid) is usually prescribed.

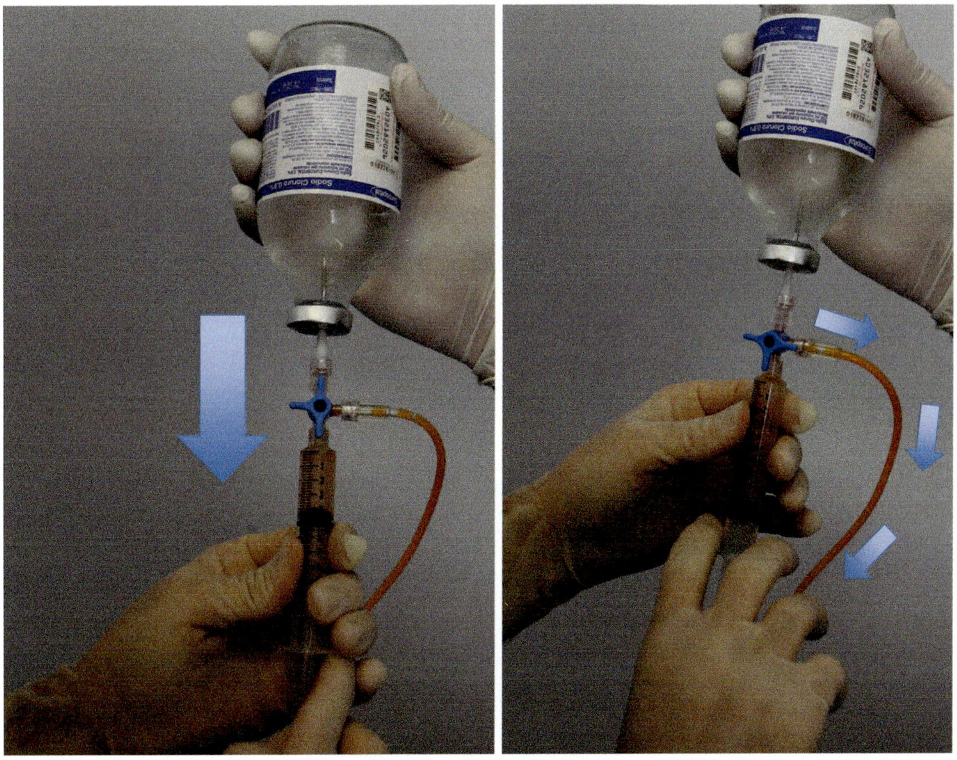

Fig. 3.64 At the end of the procedure, syringe E is filled with 10 cc of saline solution. (Published by kind permission of ©Mario Goisis 2018. All Rights Reserved)

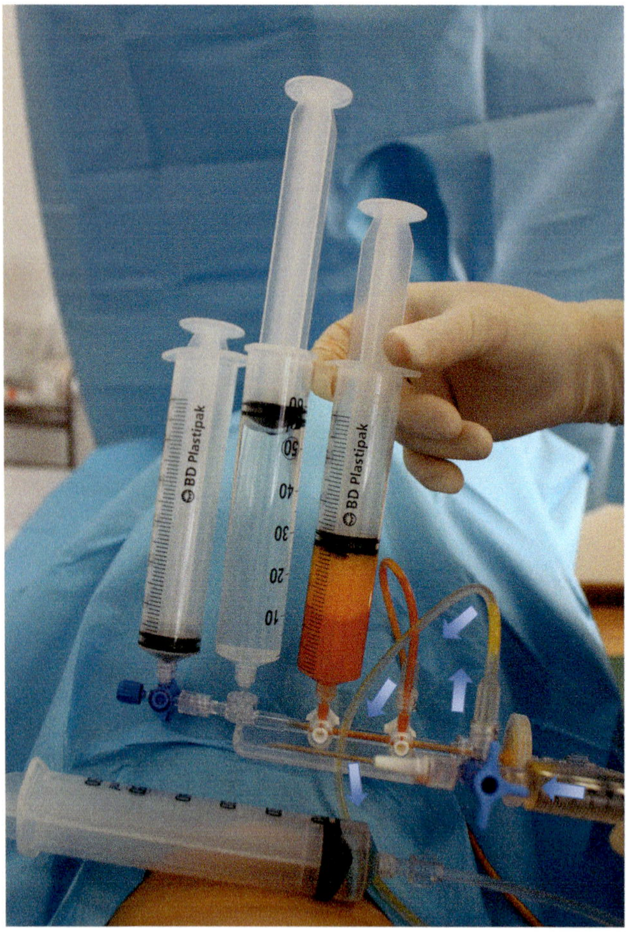

Fig. 3.65 The saline solution is transferred into the system in order to wash the tube. (Published by kind permission of ©Mario Goisis 2018. All Rights Reserved)

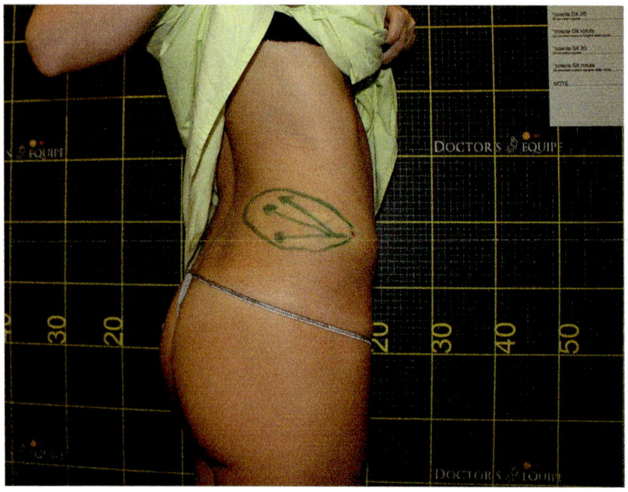

Fig. 3.66 When the cannula is removed, compression is applied to the insertion site, and the area is cleaned. (Published by kind permission of ©Mario Goisis 2018. All Rights Reserved)

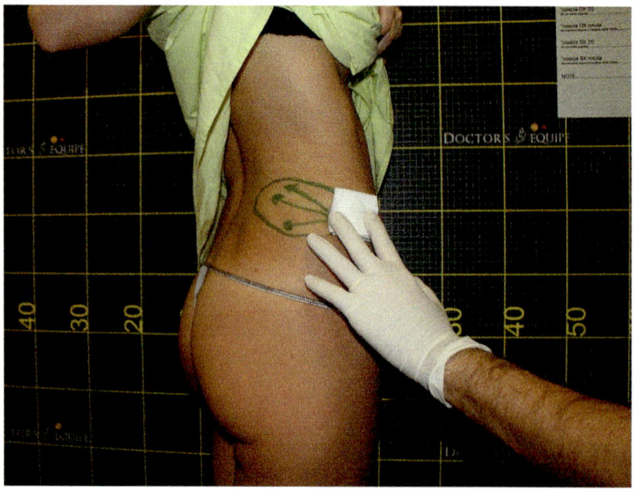

Fig. 3.67 A 2 x 2 cm gauze square, without antibiotic gel, and a clear occlusive bandage (e.g., Tegaderm) are applied. (Published by kind permission of ©Mario Goisis 2018. All Rights Reserved)

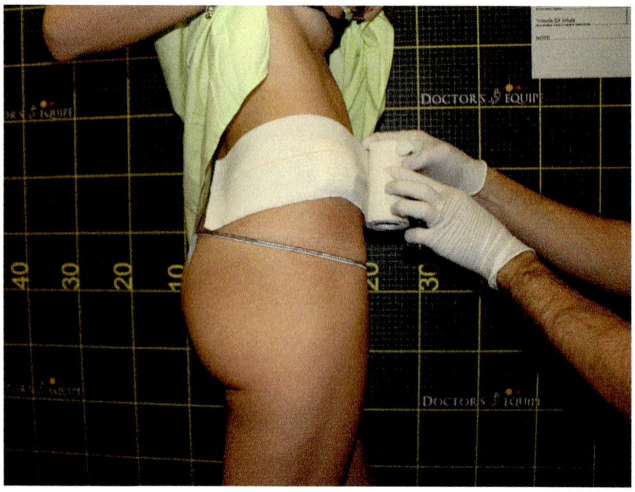

Fig. 3.68 A 2 x 2 cm gauze square, without antibiotic gel, and a clear occlusive bandage (e.g., Tegaderm) are applied. (Published by kind permission of ©Mario Goisis 2018. All Rights Reserved)

Processing Harvested Fat

4

Mario Goisis, Sara Izzo, Andrea Sbarbati, Giamaica Conti, and Giovanni Francesco Nicoletti

4.1 Reasons Behind the Processing of Harvested Fat

As it is the case of outpatient procedures, there are different methods by which to process fat. These methods produce different results, in particular those regarding the four most important aspects of the long-term durability of a graft.

The first element regarding the durability of a graft is the absence of contaminants in the tissue transferred. The aim of all of these methods is the elimination of nonviable, pro-inflammatory, and toxic components from lipoaspirate, including blood cells, local anaesthesia, fragments of ruptured fat cells including oil droplets, and cellular debris. Direct contact with air has also a negative effect on adipocytes, because it stimulates pro-inflammatory reactions and oxidative damage. All of these elements have a negative impact on the graft's ability to take. Furthermore, water mixed with fat creates a false volume which disappears immediately after grafting.

- The first aim of the graft processing and preparation method is, therefore, that of removing all contaminants and water while avoiding contact with the air.

The second element regarding long-term durability is represented, obviously, by the integrity of the fat transferred. This element was first stressed by Peer in a very important article of his, published in 1955 and known as the "cell survival theory." According to this theory, the graft with the greatest number of undamaged adipocytes was destined to have the greatest chance of long-term durability.

- The second aim of the graft preparation method is therefore that of preserving the integrity of the adipocytes.

Finally, in recent years, many studies were focused on a third element, the concentration of the adipose stem-cells (ASCs). This element is known as the "host replacement theory": it stipulates that most of the grafted adipocytes die after injection, and that the remaining extracellular matrix serves as a scaffold for replacement cells, which recreate the tissue. The ASCs play a key role in this regeneration process. Consequently, the conservation of the highest number possible of adipose stem-cells (ASCs) is shown to improve fat retention, along with the growth potential of the adipose-derived mesenchymal stem-cells quoted as a major contributing factor.

- The third aim of the graft preparation method is, therefore, to preserve and concentrate the highest number of adipose stem-cells.

Finally, a fourth element also plays a preeminent role in the election of the graft processing method: its efficiency. The efficiency of a method can be appraised in terms of how time-consuming it is, of its cost-efficiency, and the quantity of fat that is lost during the preparation. This last element is highly important in cases of mini-invasive treatments of the face, neck, and hands. In these cases, the patients usually undergo a small fat harvest, with the aim of injecting 15–20 cc of this fat into the chosen site. There exist a number of low-efficiency methods that require a harvest of 100 cc or more of fat in order to obtain 20 cc of processed fat. The other 80 cc are lost during the processing system. One needs to be kept in mind that whereas in some patients it is very simple to harvest 100 cc, in other, slimmer patients, with excess fat, this operation is more

M. Goisis (✉)
Maxillo-Facial and Aesthetic Surgeon, Go Easy Clinic, Milan, Italy

S. Izzo · G. F. Nicoletti
Department of Plastic Surgery, University of Campania "Luigi Vanvitelli", Naples, Italy
e-mail: giovannif.nicoletti@unicampania.it

A. Sbarbati · G. Conti
Department of Neuroscience, Biomedicine and Movement, Human Anatomy and Histology Section, University of Verona, Verona, Italy
e-mail: andrea.sbarbati@univr.it; giamaica.conti@univr.it

M. Goisis (ed.), *Outpatient Regenerative Medicine*, https://doi.org/10.1007/978-3-319-44894-7_4

difficult, and may require a time-consuming harvesting from different donor areas.

- The fourth aim of the graft preparation method is, therefore, to be efficient in terms of procedural costs and in terms of percentages of fat wasted during preparation.

4.2 Fat-Processing Procedures

A wide variety of methods currently used to process harvested fat, exist. The most commonly used are simple decantation, cotton gauze-rolling, centrifugation, washing, and simultaneous washing and filtration of tissue.

4.2.1 Telfa-Rolling Fat Processing

The Telfa-rolling procedure consists in pouring the aspirate from the syringe onto large (3 × 8-in.) pieces of non-adherent Telfa dressing (courtesy of Covidien, Mansfield, MA) (Fig. 4.1). The fat is then rolled and kneaded gently for 5 minutes along the gauze using a sterile scalpel handle (Fig. 4.2). The fat is then loaded using a small spatula into 10-ml syringes and transferred by Luer lock adapter into 1-ml syringes for injection. Because of the large dimension of the fat particles, it is usually necessary to inject the harvested and processed fat with a larger cannula (1.5 mm in diameter or more) (Fig. 4.3).

4.2.2 Puregraft Fat Processing

- Step 1: Preparation
- The initial phase will be devoted to arranging, opening, and arranging the contents of the box within the sterile field, while the manifold is connected as follows: First (1), the filter is connected to a tube, placed in the small tray. The tray is filled with local anaesthesia. Then (2) the tube is connected to a 20-cc VacLok© syringe. The empty 60-cc syringe (3) is then filled with saline solution (4). The empty 60-cc syringe (see 5), and the tube connected to a 10cc syringe (see 6). The manifold (see 7) then needs to be connected to the PRP syringe, while the manifold (see 8) will be connected to an empty 60-cc syringe.
- Step 2: Anaesthesia
- The local anaesthetic is transferred directly from the tray to the syringe, and as the system is completely closed, the risks of infection are reduced. In particular, when the stopcock is in the "a" position, when the plunger is pulled, the syringe is filled with anaesthetic solution. By moving the stopcock to position "b," the anaesthetic solution is injected rapidly. This way, all the infiltrations of anaesthesia take 5 min to complete.
- Step 3: Fat harvesting

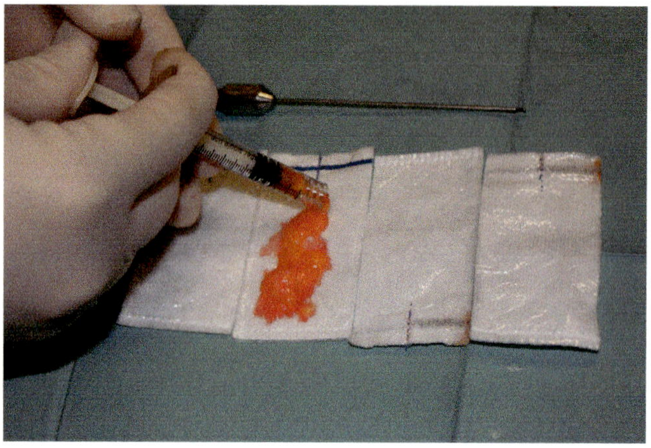

Fig. 4.1 The aspirate is poured from the syringe onto large (3 × 8-in.) pieces of non-adherent Telfa dressing. (Published by kind permission of ©Mario Goisis 2018. All Rights Reserved)

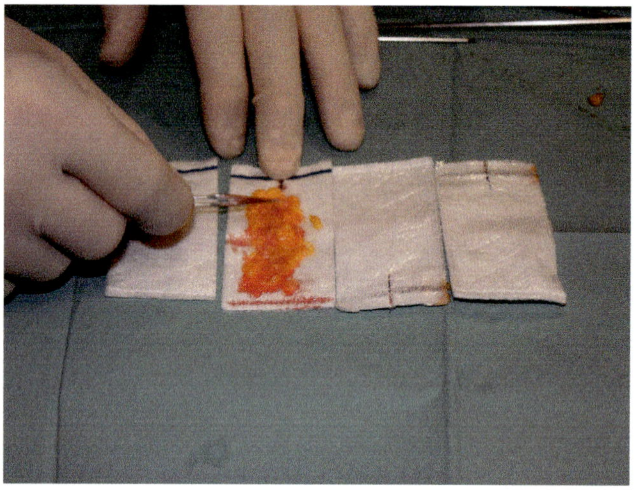

Fig. 4.2 The fat is rolled and kneaded gently for 5 minutes along the gauze using a sterile scalpel handle. (Published by kind permission of ©Mario Goisis 2018. All Rights Reserved)

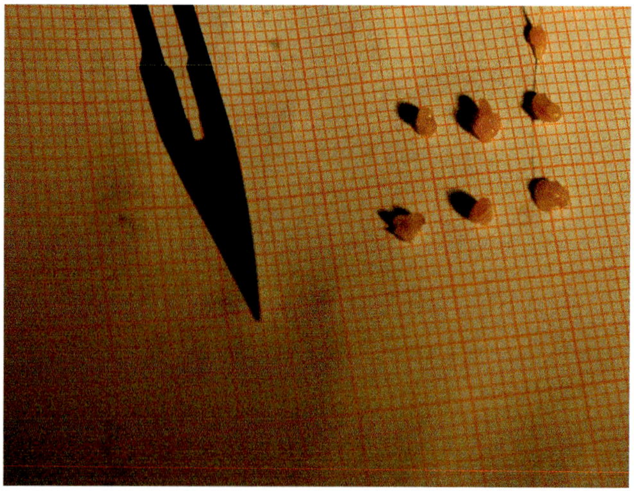

Fig. 4.3 The final dimension of the fat particles. (Published by kind permission of ©Mario Goisis 2018. All Rights Reserved)

- For fat harvesting, the VacLok© syringe is moved from the "normal sliding" to the "lock to hold vacuum" position. In particular, to lock the syringe, the plunger has to be moved completely forward or completely back and the plunger turned in order to have the locking fins engage the stop pin. This way, the VacLok syringe allows one to lock the plunger in multiple positions a negative-pressure vacuum. The negative pressure is maintained and the syringe is progressively filled with fat. The stopcock is in the "b" position (see Figs. 4.4, 4.5, 4.6, 4.7, 4.8, and 4.9 below).
- Step 4: Transfer of the fat into the system
- Once the syringe is completely filled, the stopcock needs to be moved to the "a" position. The fat, mixed with blood and anaesthesia, is then expelled and transferred directly from the syringe into the system.
- Step 5: Filtration

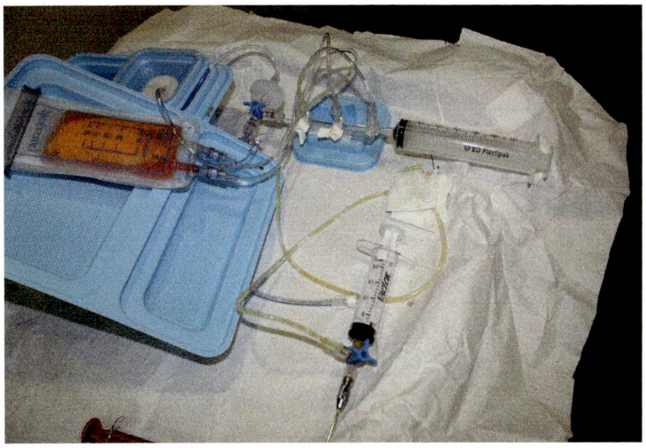

Fig. 4.6 The fat is washed twice with lactated Ringer's solution at a ratio of one volume of washing agent to two volumes of tissue. (Published by kind permission of ©Mario Goisis 2018. All Rights Reserved)

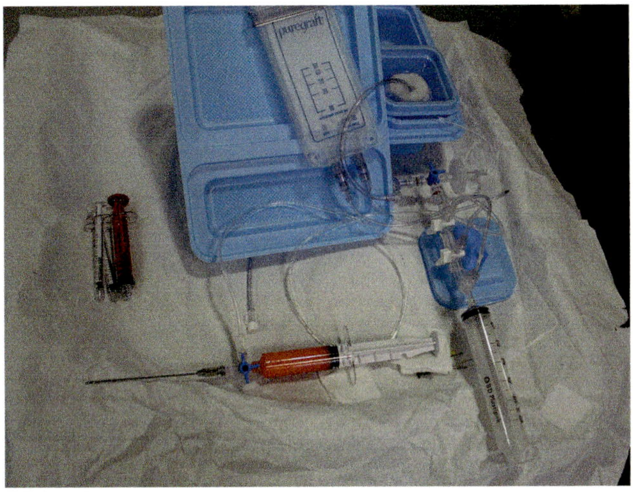

Fig. 4.4 The fat is collected by means of a 20-cc syringe connected to the Microfat kit (Courtesy of Microfat.com). (Published by kind permission of ©Mario Goisis 2018. All Rights Reserved)

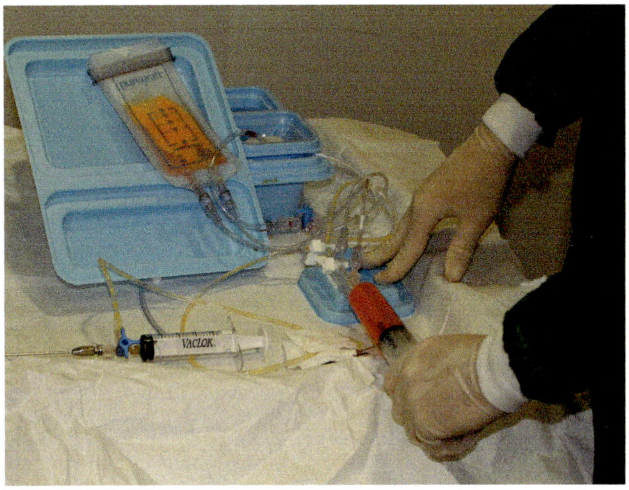

Fig. 4.7 The required draining time after each wash is approximately 3 min. (Published by kind permission of ©Mario Goisis 2018. All Rights Reserved)

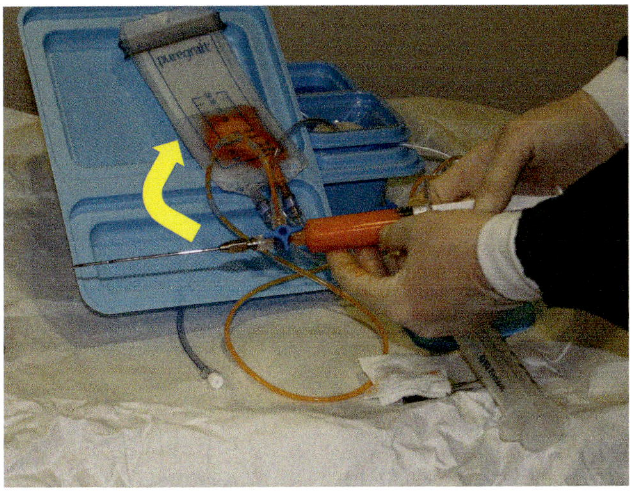

Fig. 4.5 The fat mixed with blood and local anaesthesia is transferred into the Puregraft system. (Published by kind permission of ©Mario Goisis 2018. All Rights Reserved)

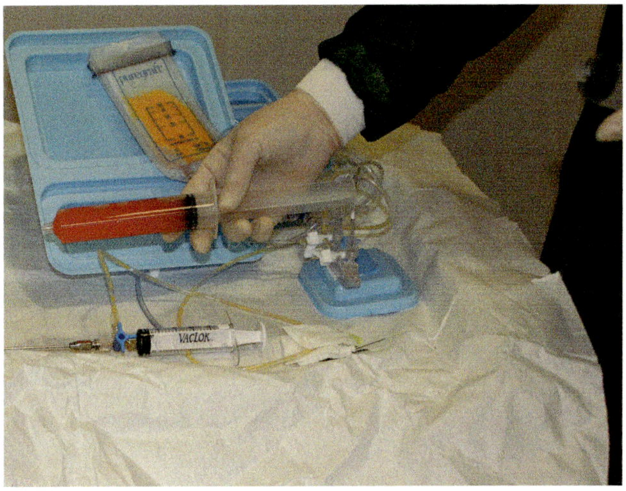

Fig. 4.8 The blood and local anaesthesia are separated from the fat. (Published by kind permission of ©Mario Goisis 2018. All Rights Reserved)

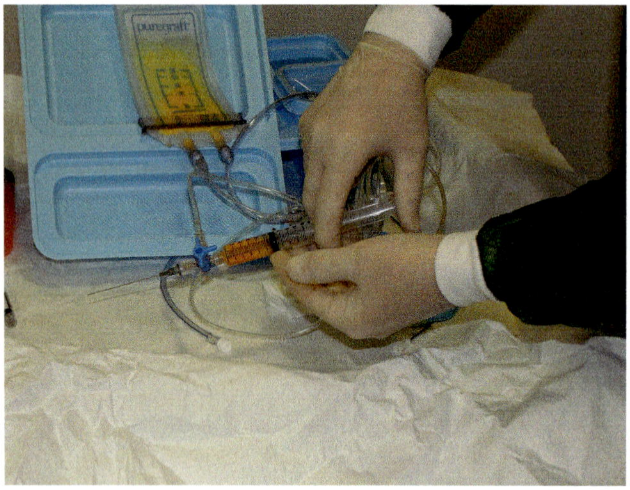

Fig. 4.9 The fat is injected using the closed system, including the related box. (Published by kind permission of ©Mario Goisis 2018. All Rights Reserved)

- The stopcock is moved to the "b" position and then the plunger of syringe 3 may be pressed down. Because the filter is in position 1, most of the blood cells and the anaesthesia fluid are directed to the tray (see red arrow). Contrariwise, the fat cells are transferred to syringe number 5 (see the yellow arrow). The procedure is entirely automatic avoiding cumbersome movements of stopcocks or valves.
- Step 6: Washing
- When the plunger of syringe 5 is pulled, it will automatically draw saline solution from syringe 4. It is then necessary to wait 60 seconds before pushing the plunger down to expel the content from the lower part of syringe 5. Due to separation caused by gravity the concentrated blood, water, and local anaesthesia will settle in the lower part of the syringe. A check valve automatically directs these elements to syringe 3 and to the filter. After 60 seconds the separation of the fat from the water is complete, and the procedure can be repeated to obtain a thorough washing: the colour of the fat changes from orange to yellow.
- Step 7: The second filtration
- The procedure now requires the removal of syringe 3. When the plunger of syringe 5 is pushed down, the residual water is squeezed out and into filter 1 (see white arrow). Contrariwise, the fat cells are automatically transferred to syringe 8 (see the yellow arrow).
- Step 8: Mixing the fat with PRP
- Mixing the fat with PRP is very simple when using the valve system; as soon as the plunger of syringe 8 is pulled back, the syringe fills with the PRP contained in syringe 7.
- Step 9: Injecting the fat with PRP
- To inject the processed fat, syringe 3 has to be removed; the stopcock of syringe 6 needs to be moved from position "b" to position "a," allowing the automatic transfer of the fat plus PRP from syringe 8 to syringe 6.
- Step 10: Waste disposal
- Once the cover is closed, the sterile field is wrapped, and the box be safely disposed of and placed in the clinical waste bin.

4.3 Considerations Regarding Fat-Processing Procedures

Different methods certainly lead to different results, in particular as far as the three most important elements involved in long-term durability of the graft, are concerned. In 2012, Gir et al. published a review, in order to evaluate the different methods of fat processing, and in the last 4 years, many other clinical and experimental studies have tried to investigate the most efficient single method for processing fat for an ideal autologous graft.

Condé-Green et al. compared decanting, centrifugation, washing, and stromal vascular-cell augmentation of washed samples on an athymic animal model. They demonstrated that decanted grafts have the poorest viability and present severe cystic changes at 11 weeks after grafting, compared to centrifuged and washed grafts. In their study, centrifugation using the Coleman technique (1200 g for 3 min) showed higher rates of calcification and fibrosis compared to those prepared by washing.

Finally Condé-Green demonstrated, experimentally, that fat washing is superior to decantation and centrifugation in terms of histologic appearance and long-term viability. This article confirmed the clinical observations previously published by Condé-Green with Pitanguy et al.

The authors compared the clinical effects of three fat-processing techniques (decantation, washing, and centrifugation) in 20 patients. A standard liposuction with a three-hole blunt cannula with a 3-mm diameter and a length of 20 cm was performed, creating light negative pressure using a 10-ml Luer-lock syringe. The aspirated adipose tissue was divided into three samples, each processed by decantation, washing, or centrifugation. After the processing, three basic layers were observed in all samples: the upper layer, composed of an oily liquid; the central layer, consisting of a firmer yellow tissue; and the lower layer, composed predominantly of blood, infiltration, or washing liquids. The latter, the pellet, can be recognised at the bottom of the centrifuged sample.

Decantation was the only method that maintained the integrity and number of adipocytes, while centrifugation destroyed the vast majority. The washing also reduced the number of intact nucleated cells, but the result was better than that obtained by centrifugation. However, washing and centrifugation reduced by over 50% the quantity of blood cells compared to the decanted sample.

The middle or central layer of the centrifuged sample showed the least quantity of adult stem-cells (or ASCs), with no in-vitro expansion after 10 days of culture. However, the pellet showed the greatest number of ASCs, concentrated at the bottom of the syringe due to centrifugal force. The conclusion of Pitanguy et al. was that the middle layer of the centrifuged sample is a compact tissue composed mostly of destroyed, nonviable adipocytes, with very few ASCs. On the other hand, the middle layer of the washed lipoaspirate contained significantly more mesenchymal stem-cells (MSCs) than the decanted and centrifuged middle-layer samples. Therefore, washed lipoaspirates represent the better graft option: they are mainly composed of intact adipocytes cleared of most peripheral blood cells, with a great number of endothelial cells and ADCs compared to the decanted samples, which contain large quantities of blood and very few ADCs.

This conclusion was in part confirmed by Kolle et al. in 2013 in their triple-blind, placebo-controlled trial, published in the Lancet. They compared the survival of non-enriched fat grafts processed using the Coleman technique versus fat enriched with autologous adipose-derived stem-cells (ASCs). The fat processed using the Coleman technique retained less than 17% of the initial volume of the bolus, compared to the 80% obtained in cases of enriched fat.

Hoareau et al. found that standard centrifugation (900 *g* for 3 min) led to high percentages of adipocyte death. In a murine model, they demonstrated a significantly high percentage of oil cysts among decanted and standard-centrifugated grafts. Pfaff et al. examined the number of adipose-derived stem-cells in lipoaspirate samples processed by means of Telfa rolling versus centrifugation for 3 minutes at 1500 rpm. They esteemed that Telfa-rolling grafts resulted in a significantly higher number of ASCs and a significantly higher number of vital cells.

Salinas et al. compared cotton-gauze rolling against centrifugation. All samples were washed with normal saline before being rolled on Telfa gauze or centrifuged. They demonstrated that standard centrifugation techniques (1200 *g* for 3 min) are equivalent to cotton gauze rolling when it comes to removing water from lipoaspirate and maintaining ADCs. In nude mice, the retention-rate was equivalent for centrifuged and gauze-rolled grafts.

Zhu et al. compared a control sample (no preparation), with processing by gravity separation, by centrifugation (as described by Coleman), and by simultaneous tissuewashing and filtration. See 6, 12. The last sample was processed using the Puregraft system. Fat was washed twice with lactated Ringer's solution at a ratio of one volume of wash solution to two volumes of tissue. Draining time after each wash was approximately 3 min.

Microscopic evaluation indicated that grafts prepared by washing associated with filtration exhibited lower red blood-cell content as well as a reduced presence of microscopic droplets of free lipid compared with grafts prepared using either unit gravity sedimentation or centrifugation. This difference was confirmed following centrifugation of the grafts to separate them into their fundamental parts. In particular, grafts prepared by gravity sedimentation presented the highest relative aqueous content, whereas grafts prepared by centrifugation presented the lowest aqueous content. Grafts prepared using the Puregraft system presented intermediate aqueous liquid levels; these levels were significantly lower than those for the control and gravity grafts.

The level of free lipid-oil in grafts prepared by washing accompanied by filtration was, statistically speaking, significantly lower than that in the control grafts, gravity grafts, and grafts prepared by centrifugation. Analysis of the cells showed that the gravity sedimentation and centrifugation techniques removed approximately 50% of the red blood-cells and 60–70% of the white blood-cells present in the original aspirate. By way of contrast, washing with filtration using the Puregraft system removed more than 95% of both blood-cell types.

In conclusion, the literature shows some consistent findings. Simple decantation has been demonstrated to preserve a large number of intact and nucleated adipocytes. The main issue is that it allows a significantly greater amount of aqueous and lipid contaminants to remain in the specimen, particularly red blood-cells and free oil, which are pro-inflammatory, and local anaesthesia, which is toxic. Recent scientific evidence confirms this, indicating lower rates of decanted graft viability compared to centrifuged and washed specimens. There are some data to indicate that cotton gauze rolling removes water, oil, and contaminants, with high rates of adipose-derived mesenchymal stem-cell content. This technique is, however, rather time-consuming and labour intensive.

Centrifugation is a key element of the standard Coleman technique. The settings used are those described by Coleman, whereby the lipoaspirate is spun at 1200 *g* (3000 rpm) for 3 min, followed by discarding the lower aqueous layer and removing the oily top layer by Telfa wrapping. The middle adipose layer is then grafted. Recent literature has demonstrated lower rates of graft viability after centrifugation relative to washing.

Washing the lipoaspirate has been proved to preserve both a large number of mesenchymal stem-cells and a large number of adipocytes. Cleveland et al., in their updated review of the literature, identified several additional articles that appear to further support the sustainability of washing as a processing technique. Several commercially-available technologies that use washing techniques together with filtration (as the Puregraft and Revolve systems) also appear promising for efficient, effective processing of lipoaspirate.

Goisis et al. (2016 imcas) recently described a method for washing accompanied by filtration, which has the advantage of being a completely closed system. The harvest, the processing and the injection of the fat are performed inside of the system, thus avoiding the contact with the air. The removal of the nonviable, pro-inflammatory, and toxic components is obtained by 2–4 washings. The integrity and the viability of the adipocytes and the preservation of the highest concentration of adipose stem-cells are guaranteed by the washing system [1–14]. The experimental data demonstrating the highter preservation of Adipose stem-cells (ASCs) of Goisis microfat system compared with Coleman procedure is reported in Table 4.1.

The method has highly efficient in terms of time saving, because it reduces the duration of the complete procedure to 15 min from harvesting to injection. In terms of efficiency and reduction of costs, the procedure can be performed by one surgeon, in a small operating theatre or medical surgery. Finally, the loss of fat during the preparation is very low in terms of percentages (15%). In particular, the harvesting of 24 cc of fat is sufficient to obtain 20 cc of processed fat (Figs. 4.10, 4.11, 4.12, 4.13, 4.14, 4.15, 4.16, 4.17, 4.18, and 4.19).

Table 4.1 The experimental data demonstrate the highter preservation of Adipose stem-cells (ASCs) after processing with Goisis microfat system compared with Coleman centrifugation

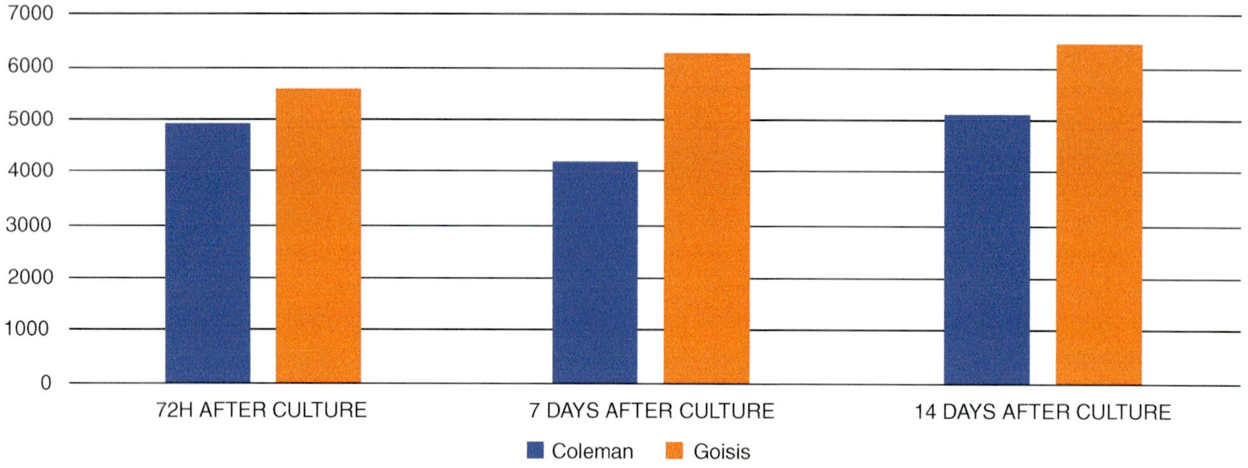

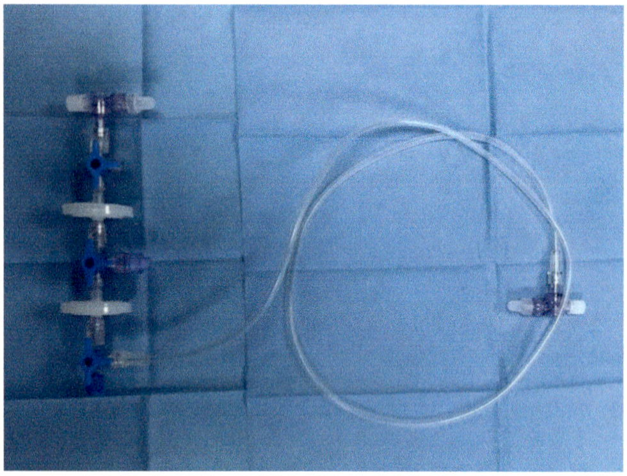

Fig. 4.10 Step 1: Preparation. Arranging the contents: Open and dispose the content of the kit onto the sterile field: the kit is composed by: 1: first filter for filtration of fluids and stem-cells, connected with a tube. The tube is one meter long. 2: second filter for filtration of fluid. 3: automatic filtration device with inbound and outbound valves. (Published by kind permission of ©Mario Goisis 2018. All Rights Reserved)

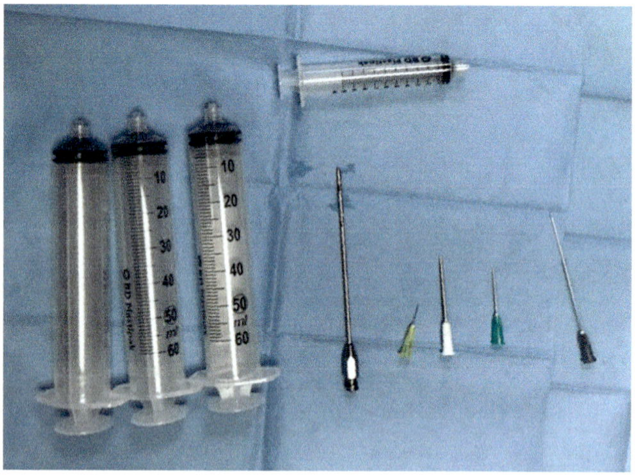

Fig. 4.11 Three 60 cc syringe, three 10 cc syringe, 2 mm diameter single use cannulas for harvesting of dermal fat, 30G needle, 16 Gauge needle, 22 gauge canula for infiltration, 21 Gauge needle. (Published by kind permission of ©Mario Goisis 2018. All Rights Reserved)

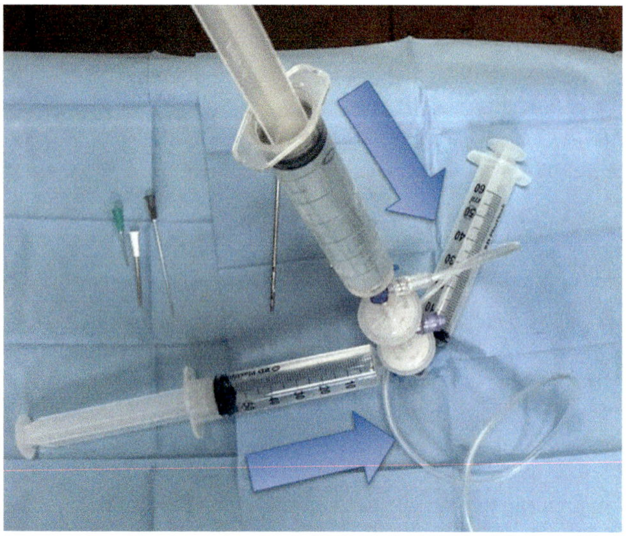

Fig. 4.12 The three 60 cc are connected to the system. One is empty, the other two are filled by Klein solution. (Published by kind permission of ©Mario Goisis 2018. All Rights Reserved)

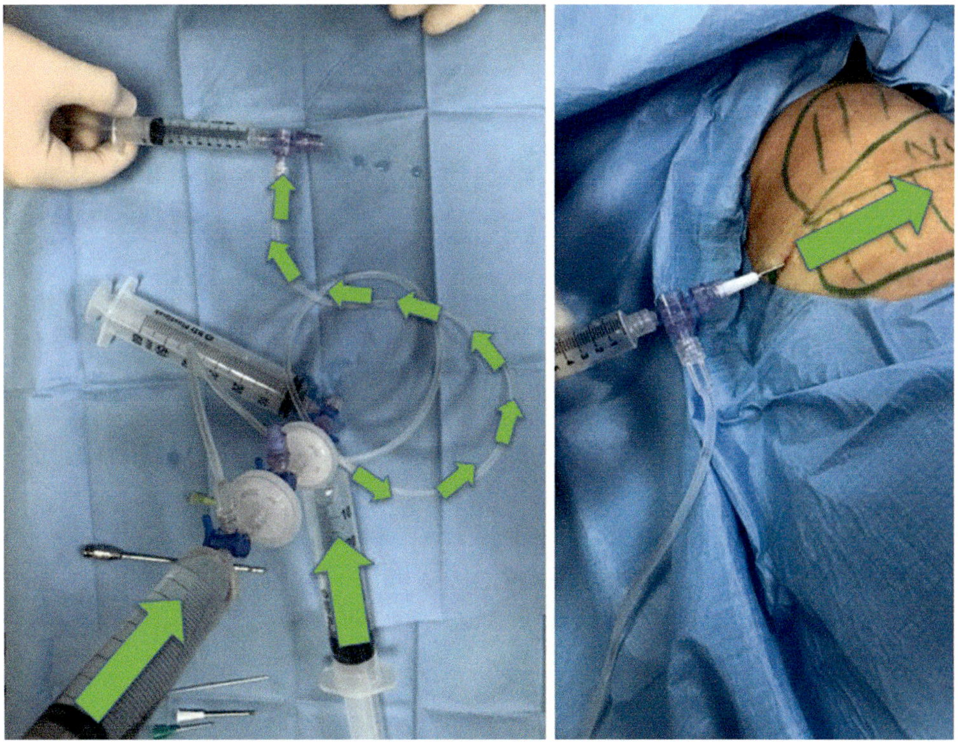

Fig. 4.13 Anesthesia. The local anesthetic is transferred directly from the system to the syringe. In this way, the infiltration of 120 cc anesthesia takes 5 min of operating time. (Published by kind permission of ©Mario Goisis 2018. All Rights Reserved)

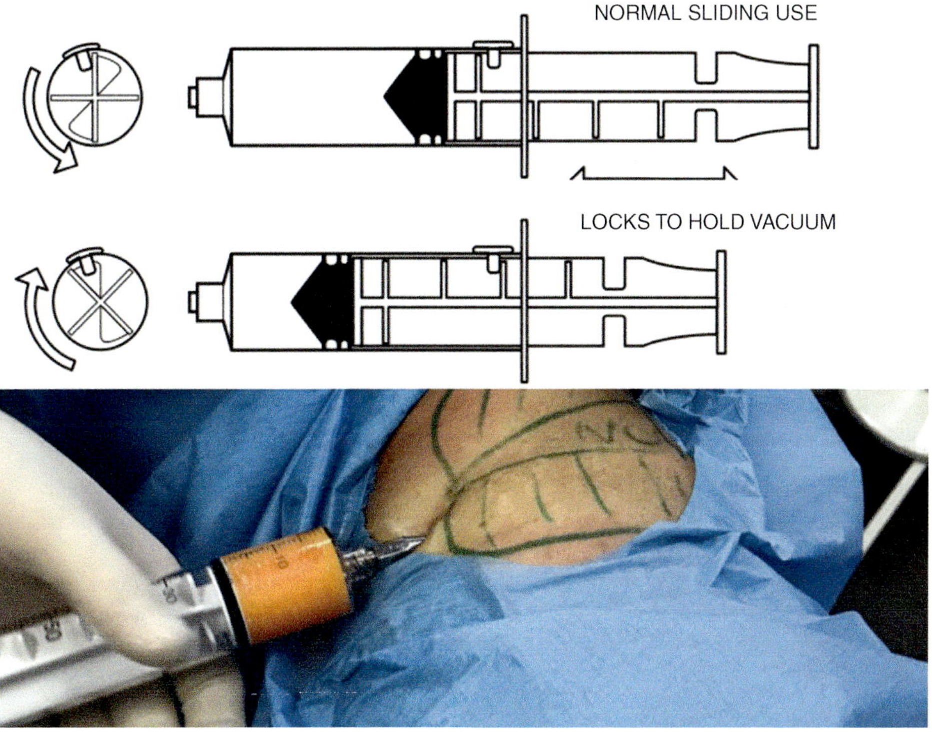

Fig. 4.14 Intradermal fat harvesting. For fat harvesting, the VacLok© syringe is moved from the way of use "normal sliding" to the "lock to hold vacuum" use. In particular, to setup the syringe to lock, move the plunger completely forward or completely back and turn the plunger so that the locking fins can engage the stop pin. In this way, the VacLok syringe allow you to lock the plunger in multiple positions for a negative pressure vacuum. The negative pressure is maintained and the syringe is progressively filled by fat. The stopcock is in position "b". (Published by kind permission of ©Mario Goisis 2018. All Rights Reserved)

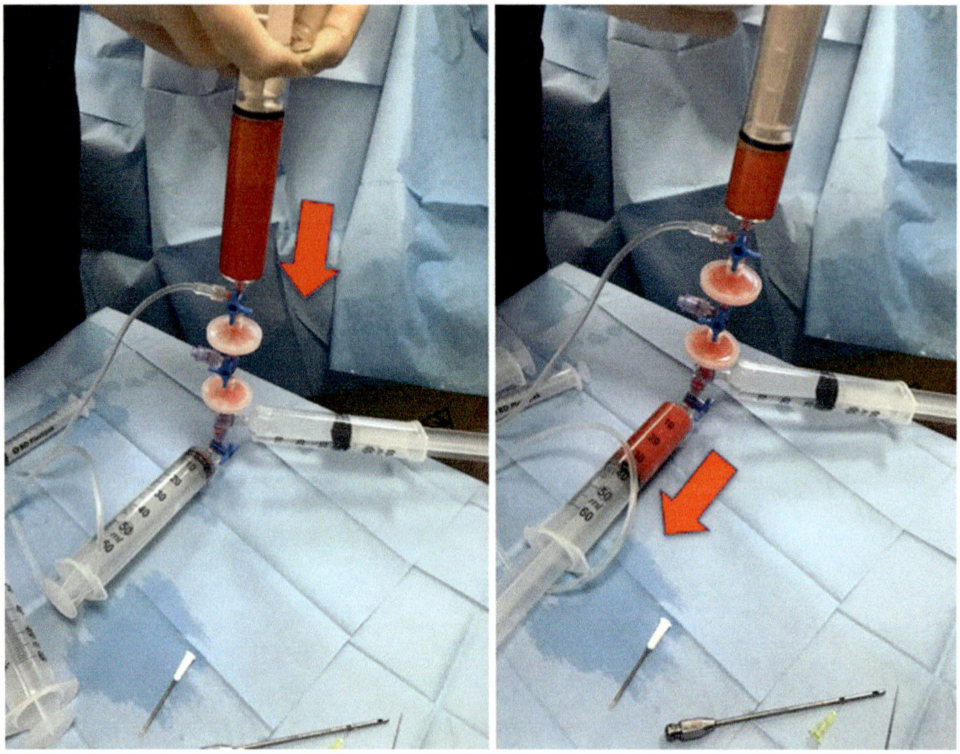

Fig. 4.15 Transferring of fat into the system and filtration. When the syringe is completely filled by fat mixed with blood and anesthesia, it is connected directly to the system. The lower content of the syringe (red cells and the Klein solution, red arrow) are pushed automatically in one direction. (Published by kind permission of ©Mario Goisis 2018. All Rights Reserved)

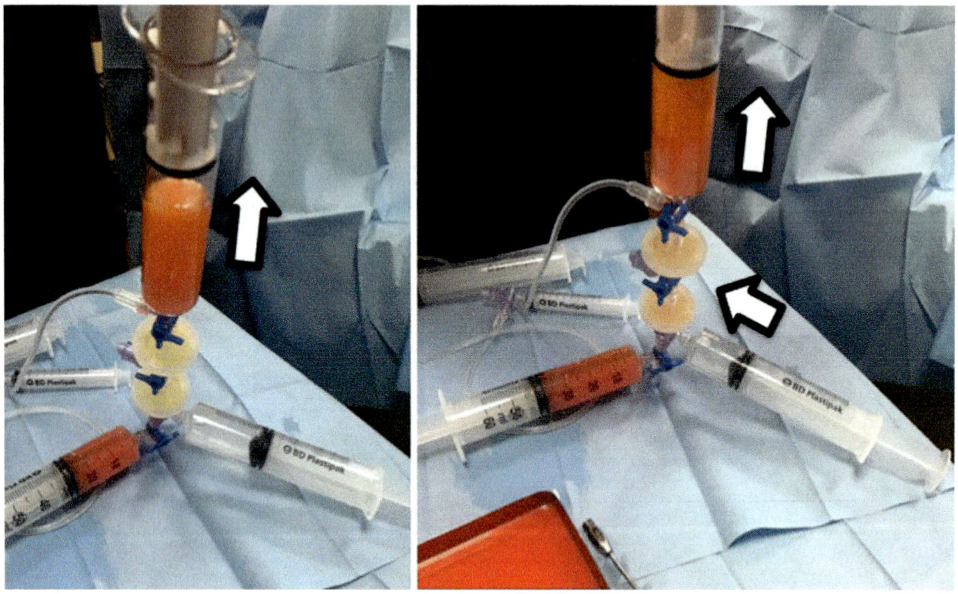

Fig. 4.16 Washing. Pull the plunger of the VacLok syringe. This will automatically draw saline solution. Wait 60 s, then push down on the plunger to move out the content of the lower part of the VacLok. In fact, because of separation by gravity, in the lower part of syringe are concentrated blood, water and local anesthesia. A check valve automatically directs these elements to waste syringe Wait for 60 s the separation between fat and water, and repeat the procedure for the third time. The color of fat move from orange to yellow. (Published by kind permission of ©Mario Goisis 2018. All Rights Reserved)

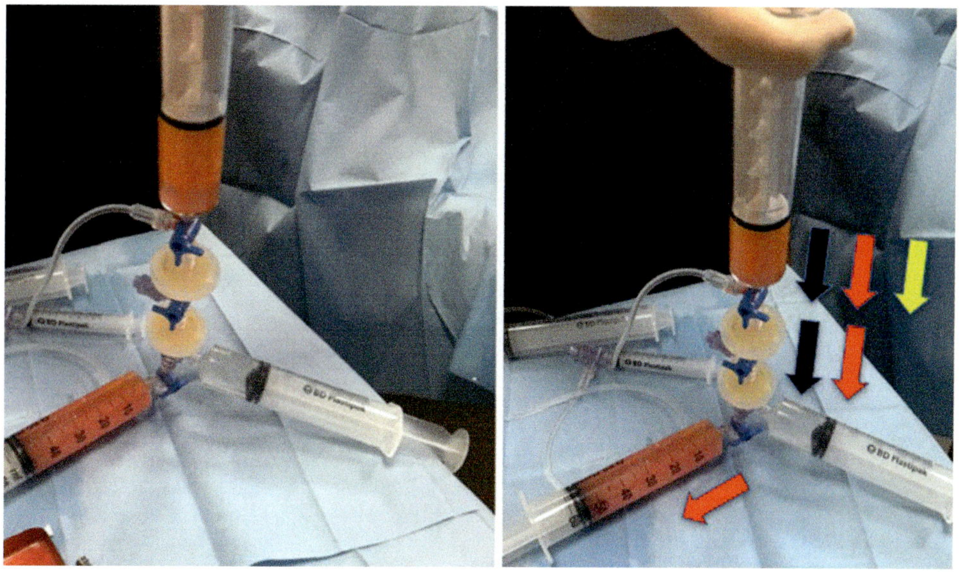

Fig. 4.17 Last filtration. Push down on the plunger of syringe for the last time. The microfat (yellow arrow) is stopped by the first filter. At the opposite, The residual water with SVF and red cells are squeezed out to the first filter. The stromal vascular fraction (black arrow) is stopped by the second filter. The red and white cells and liquids (red arrow) are pushed automatically in the waste syringe. All is automatic and there is no need to move stopcocks or valves. (Published by kind permission of ©Mario Goisis 2018. All Rights Reserved)

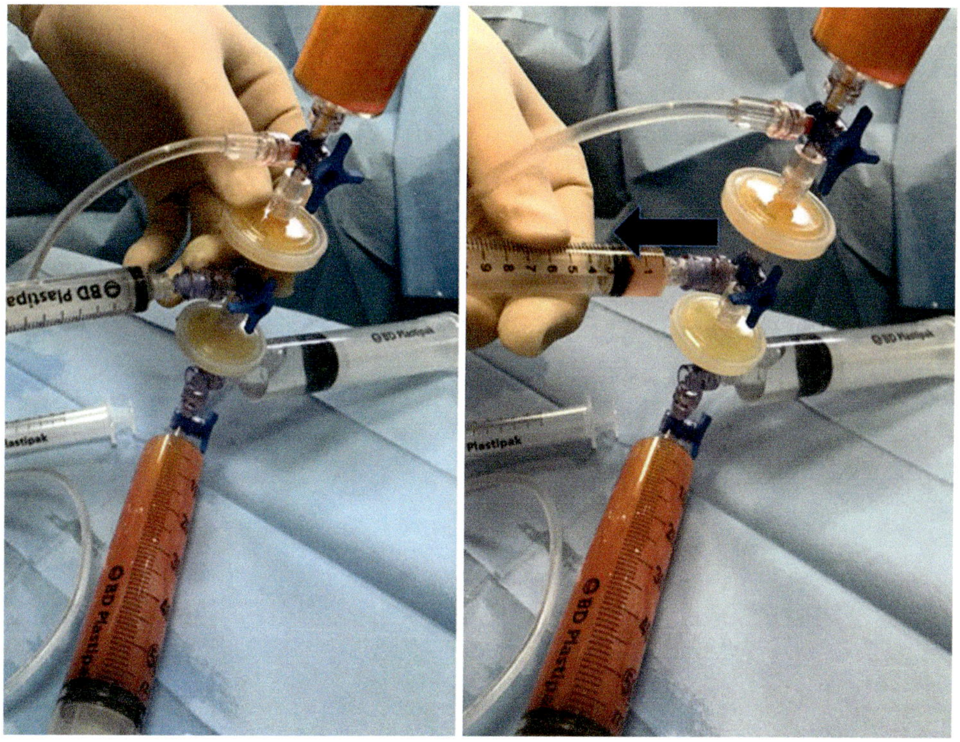

Fig. 4.18 Collection of SVF. A 10 cc syringe is connected in order to collect the SVF (stromal vascular fraction). (Published by kind permission of ©Mario Goisis 2018. All Rights Reserved)

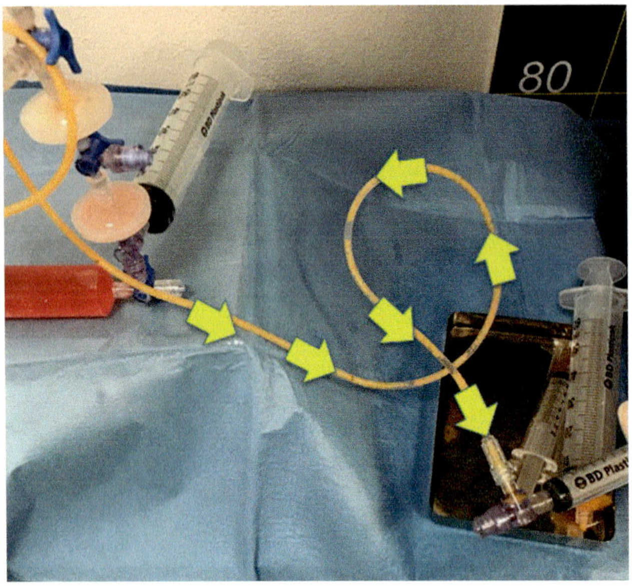

Fig. 4.19 Injection. The microfat is ready for injection. (Published by kind permission of ©Mario Goisis 2018. All Rights Reserved)

References

1. Boschert MT, Beckert BW, Puckett CL, Concannon MJ. Analysis of lipocyte viability after liposuction. Plast Reconstr Surg. 2002;109:761–5.
2. Peer LA. Cell survival theory versus replacement theory. Plast Reconstr Surg (1946). 1955;16:161–8.
3. Eto H, Kato H, Suga H, Aoi N, Doi K, Kuno S, Yoshi- mura K. The fate of adipocytes after nonvascularized fat grafting: evidence of early death and replacement of adi- pocytes. Plast Reconstr Surg. 2012;129:1081–92.
4. Zuk PA, Zhu M, Ashjian P, et al. Human adipose tis- sue is a source of multipotent stem cells. Mol Biol Cell. 2002;13:4279–95.
5. Kølle SF, Fischer-Nielsen A, Mathiasen AB, et al. Enrichment of autologous fat grafts with ex-vivo expanded adipose tissue- derived stem cells for graft survival: a randomised placebo- controlled trial. Lancet. 2013;382:1113–20.
6. Zhu M, Cohen SR, Hicok KC, Shanahan RK, Strem BM, Yu JC, Arm DM, Fraser JK. Comparison of three different fat graft preparation methods: gravity separation, centrifugation, and simultaneous washing with filtration in a closed system. Plast Reconstr Surg. 2013;131(4):873–80.
7. Cleveland EC, Albano NJ, Hazen A. Roll, spin, wash, or filter? Processing of lipoaspirate for autologous fat grafting: an updated, evidence-based review of the literature. Plast Reconstr Surg. 2015;136(4):706–13.
8. Botti G, Pascali M, Botti C, Bodog F, Cervelli V. A clinical trial in facial fat grafting: filtered and washed versus centrifuged fat. Plast Reconstr Surg. 2011;127:2464–73.
9. Gir P, Brown SA, Oni G, Kashefi N, Mojallal A, Rohrich RJ. Fat grafting: evidence-based review on autologous fat harvesting, processing, reinjection, and storage. Plast Reconstr Surg. 2012;130:249–58.
10. Hoareau L, Bencharif K, Girard AC, et al. Effect of centrifugation and washing on adipose graft viability: a new method to improve graft efficiency. J Plast Reconstr Aesthet Surg. 2013;66:712–9.
11. Condé-Green A, Wu I, Graham I, et al. Comparison of 3 techniques of fat grafting and cell-supplemented lipotransfer in athymic rats: a pilot study. Aesthet Surg J. 2013;33:713–21.
12. Pu LL, Coleman SR, Cui X, Ferguson RE Jr, Vasconez HC. Autologous fat grafts harvested and refined by the Coleman technique: a comparative study. Plast Reconstr Surg. 2008;122:932–7.
13. Conde-Green A, Gontijo de Amorim N, Pitanguy I. Influence of decantation, washing and centrifugation on adipocyte and mesenchymal stem cell content of aspirated adipose tissue: a comparative study. J Plast Reconstr Aesthet Surg. 2010;63:1375–81.
14. Pfaff M, Wu W, Zellner E, Steinbacher DM. Processing technique for lipofilling influences adipose-derived stem cell concentration and cell viability in lipoaspirate. Aesthet Plast Surg. 2014;38:224–9.

Processing Microfat Step by Step

5

Mario Goisis, Sara Izzo, Andrea Sbarbati,
Giamaica Conti, and Giovanni Francesco Nicoletti

The Method of processing with closed washing and filtration with microfat system is described (Figs. 5.1–5.29).

5.1 Materials and Methods

The microfat may be processed in a medicalsurgenry/small operating theatre.

A standard microfat box is used for the procedure (www.microfat.com) (Fig. 5.11).

The microfat box is composed of some single-use elements: a ramp with a closed system for washing and filtration (www.microfat.com), four 60-cc syringes, two 10-cc syringes, and one 1-cc syringe.

The microfat box can be used in conjunction with some autoclavable elements: in particular the microfat tray (www.microfat.com) (Fig. 5.12). The Goisis tray is composed of a plastic support for the ramp and two trays for the Klein and saline solutions.

Medications include:

100 cc of cold saline solution

Assistance: no assistant is needed when processing fat.

M. Goisis (✉)
Maxillo-Facial and Aesthetic Surgeon, Go Easy Clinic, Milan, Italy

S. Izzo · G. F. Nicoletti
Department of Plastic Surgery, University of Campania "Luigi Vanvitelli", Naples, Italy
e-mail: giovannif.nicoletti@unicampania.it

A. Sbarbati · G. Conti
Department of Neuroscience, Biomedicine and Movement, Human Anatomy and Histology Section, University of Verona, Verona, Italy
e-mail: andrea.sbarbati@univr.it; giamaica.conti@univr.it

5.2 The Procedure Step by Step

Then push down on the plunger to move the content out of the lower part of syringe C. Because of separation by gravity, blood, water, and local anaesthesia are concentrated in the lower part of the syringe. A check valve automatically directs these elements to syringe A and to the filter (orange arrow). Wait for 60 s for the separation between fat and water to occur. Repeat the procedure until the colour of the fat which in syringe C changes from orange to yellow (Figs. 5.13, 5.14, 5.15, 5.16, 5.17, 5.18, 5.19, 5.20, 5.21, 5.22).

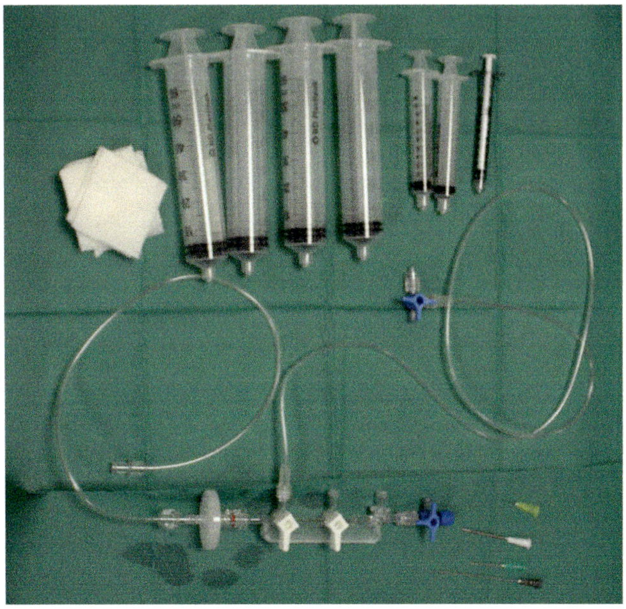

Fig. 5.1 A standard procedure microfat box is used (www.microfat.com courtesely by Doctor's Equipe). The microfat box is composed by some single use elements: a ramp with a closed a system for washing and filtration (www.microfat.com), four syringes 60 cc, two syringes 10 cc, one syringe 1 cc. (Published by kind permission of ©Mario Goisis 2018. All Rights Reserved)

M. Goisis (ed.), *Outpatient Regenerative Medicine*, https://doi.org/10.1007/978-3-319-44894-7_5

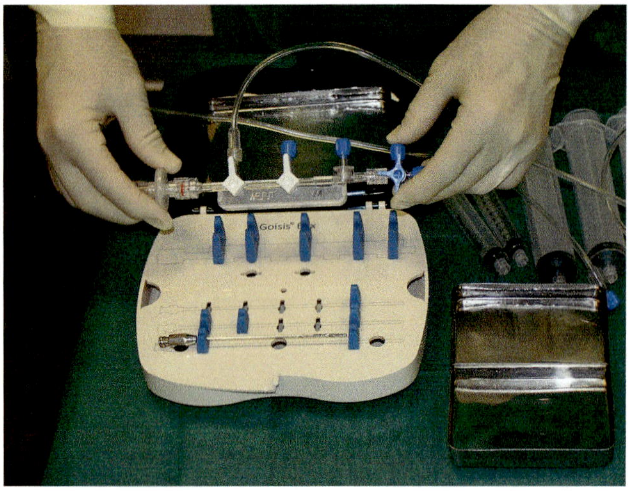

Fig. 5.2 The microfat box can be used in conjunction with some autoclavable elements: in particular the microfat tray (www.microfat.com) (Fig. 5.12). The Goisis tray is composed by a plastic support for the ramp and by two trays for Klein solution and saline solution. Medications include: 100 cc of cold saline solution. Assistants: no assistant is needed for fat processing. Procedure step by step. (Published by kind permission of ©Mario Goisis 2018. All Rights Reserved)

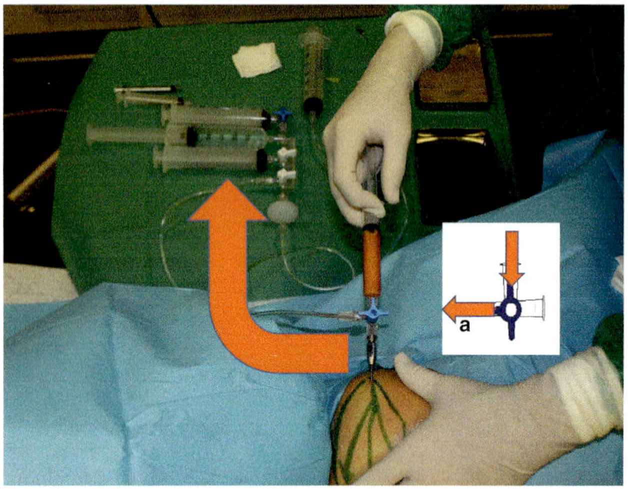

Fig. 5.3 The fat is harvested by the syringe E. When the syringe E is completely filled, move the stopcock in position "a". (Published by kind permission of ©Mario Goisis 2018. All Rights Reserved)

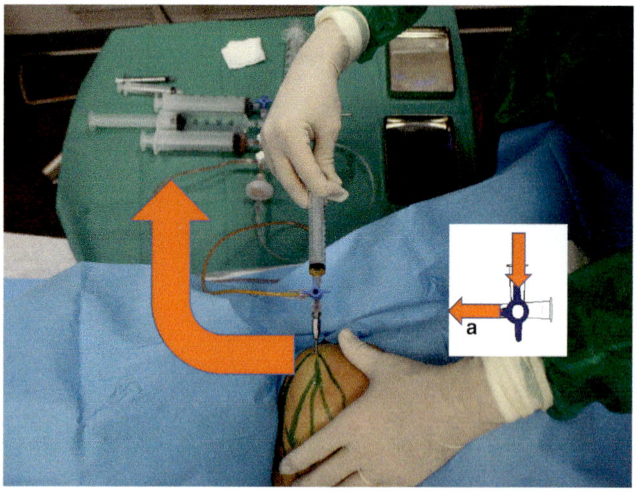

Fig. 5.4 The fat mixed with blood and anesthesia is pushed and transferred directly from the syringe E to the syringe A. (Published by kind permission of ©Mario Goisis 2018. All Rights Reserved)

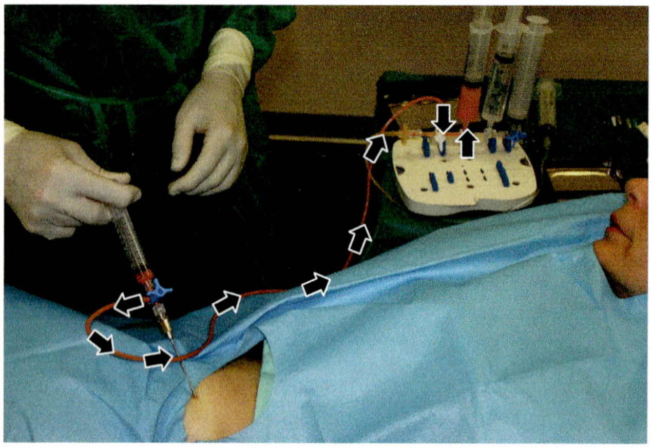

Fig. 5.5 Repeat the procedure 4–6 times in order to obtain the sufficient amount of fat. (Published by kind permission of ©Mario Goisis 2018. All Rights Reserved)

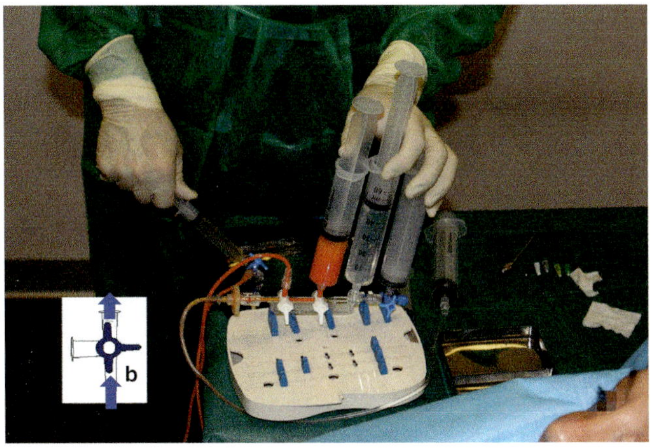

Fig. 5.6 At the end of the harvesting procedure, the syringe E is filled by saline solution. (Published by kind permission of ©Mario Goisis 2018. All Rights Reserved)

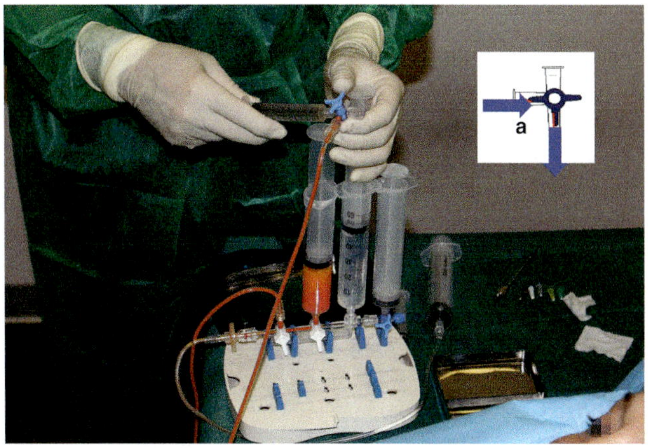

Fig. 5.7 By moving the stopcock in position "a" the saline is transferred into the system. (Published by kind permission of ©Mario Goisis 2018. All Rights Reserved)

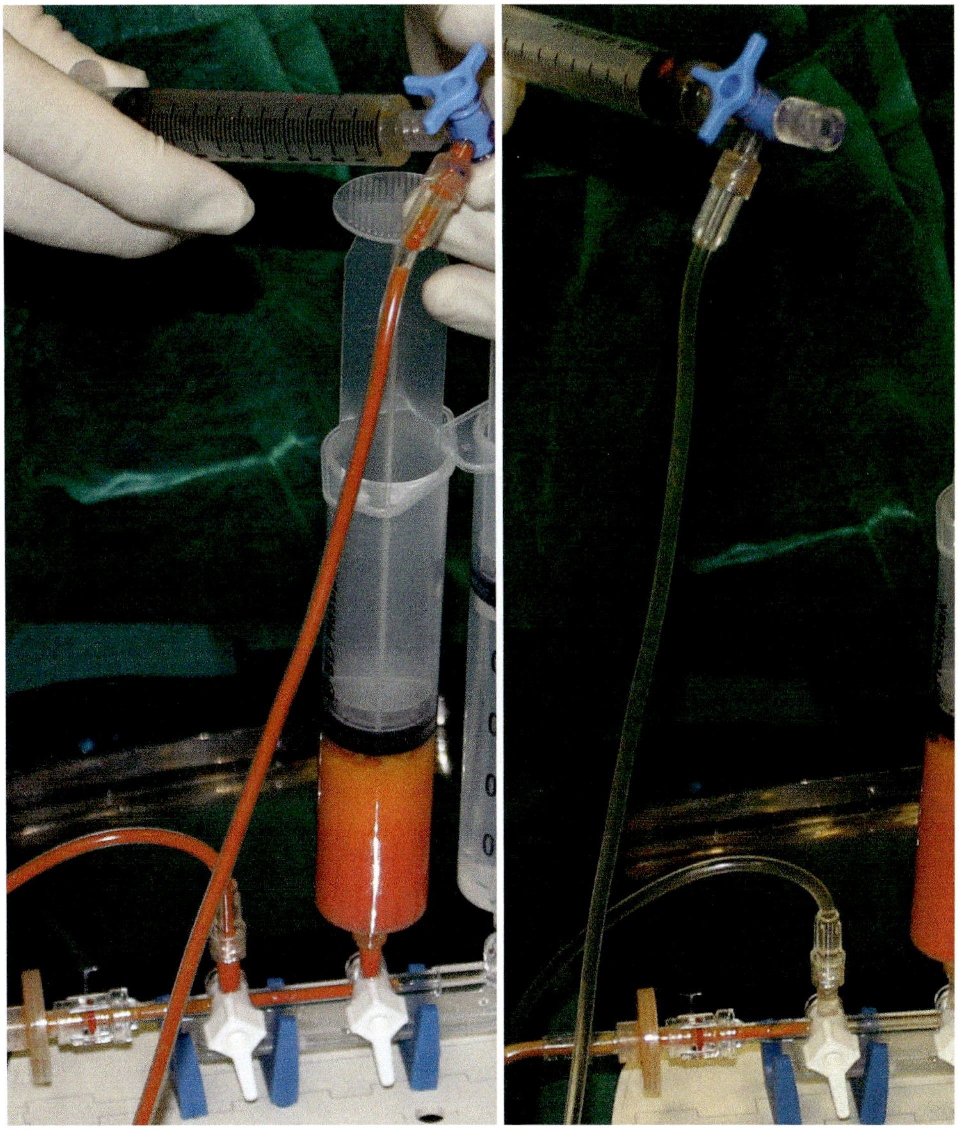

Fig. 5.8 In this way, the content of the tube which connect the syringe E to the system is washed out. On the right: the tube is filled by fat mixed with blood. On the left: the tube is filled by saline. (Published by kind permission of ©Mario Goisis 2018. All Rights Reserved)

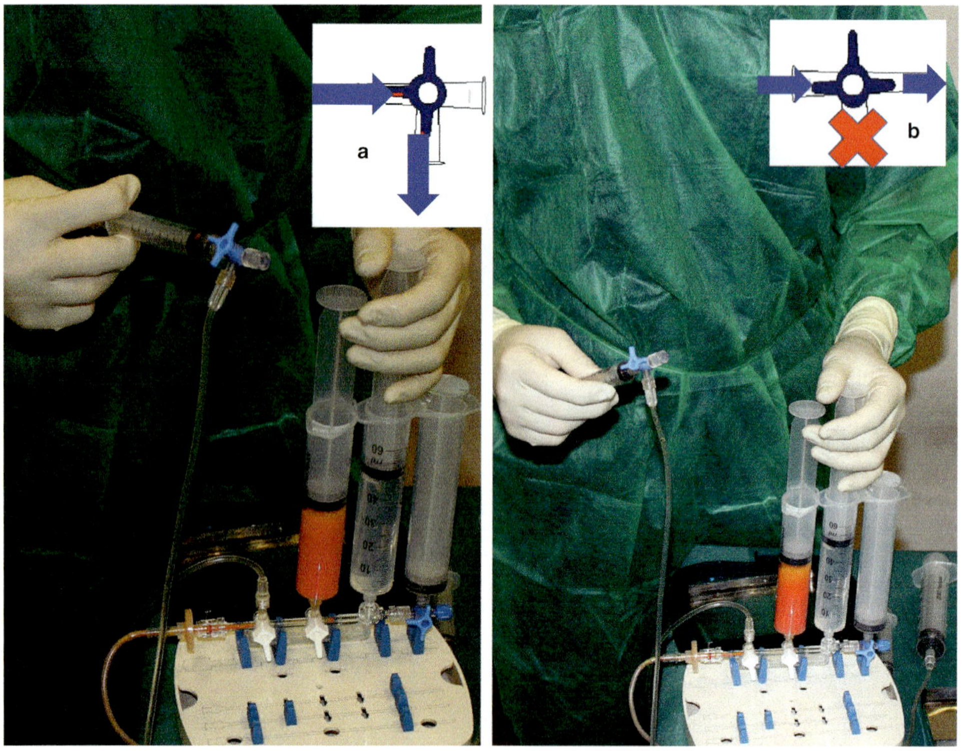

Fig. 5.9 The stopcock is moved from position "a" to position "b". (Published by kind permission of ©Mario Goisis 2018. All Rights Reserved)

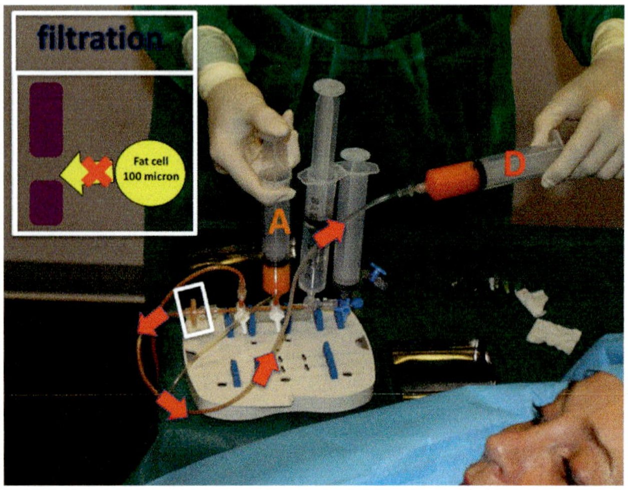

Fig. 5.10 Then, push down on the plunger of syringe A. Because of the filter, most of the blood cells and anesthesia are automatically directed to the syringe D (red arrow). At the opposite, the fat cells are maintained into the system. In fact, fat stem cells and many component of the SVF are too big to pass trough the filter

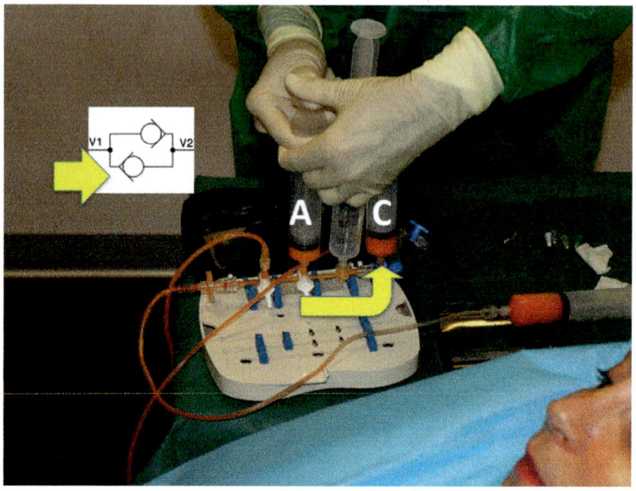

Fig. 5.11 Because of the fat and the SVF can't pass trough the filter, the pressure into included into the system will automatically open. In this way, without opening (yellow arrow)

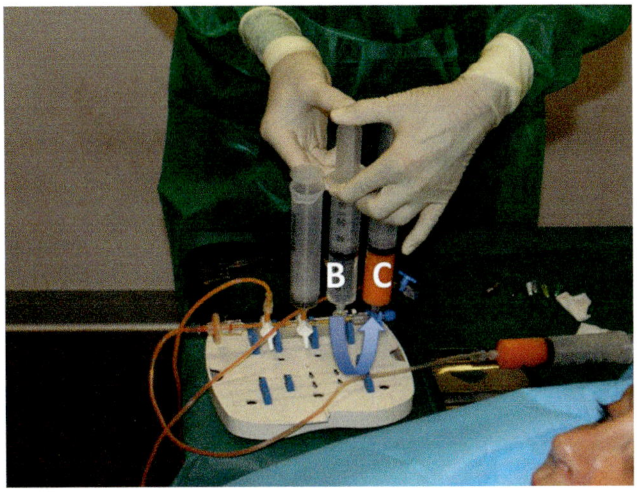

Fig. 5.12 In order to remove completely the Klein solution and the red cells, the fat has to be washed. The system has single direction valves that guarantee a very simple and fast washing of the fat. (Published by kind permission of ©Mario Goisis 2018. All Rights Reserved)

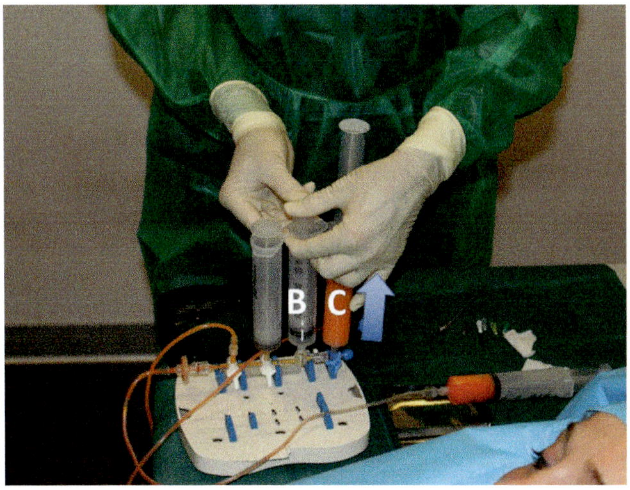

Fig. 5.13 By pushing the plunger of syringe B, the saline content of the syringe will be automatically moved into the syringe

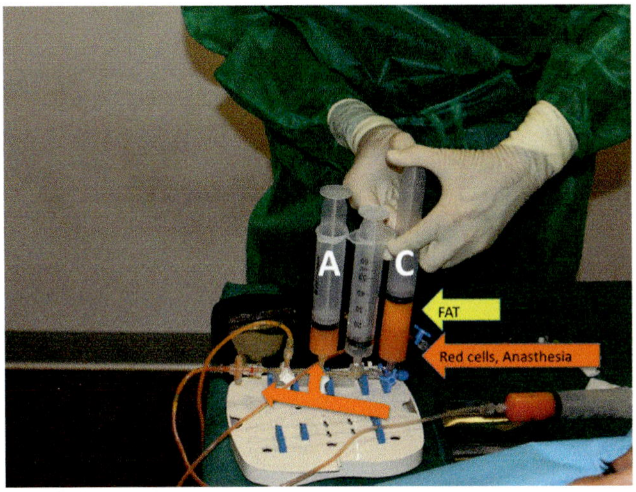

Fig. 5.14 Wait 60 seconds, in order to leave that the fat move spontaneously in the upper part of the syringe C. Then push down on the plunger to move out the content of the lower part of the syringe C. In fact, because of separation by gravity, in the lower part of syringe are concentrated blood, water and local anesthesia. A check valve automatically directs these elements to syringe A and to the filter (orange arrow). Wait for 60 seconds the separation between fat and water, and repeat the procedure. The color of fat which is in syringe C move from orange to yellow

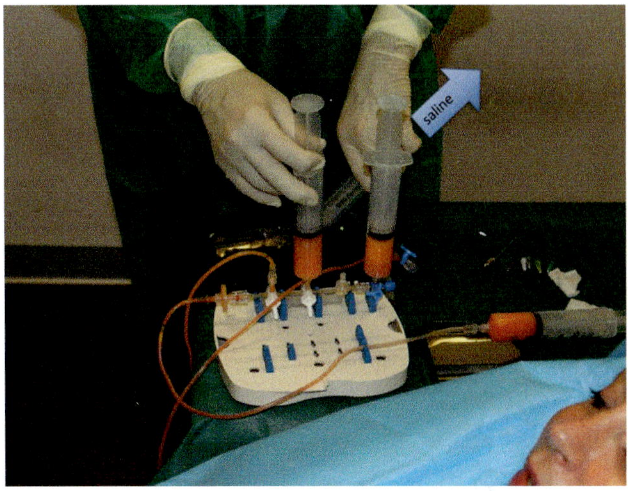

Fig. 5.15 Replace the saline solution in syringe B. (Published by kind permission of ©Mario Goisis 2018. All Rights Reserved)

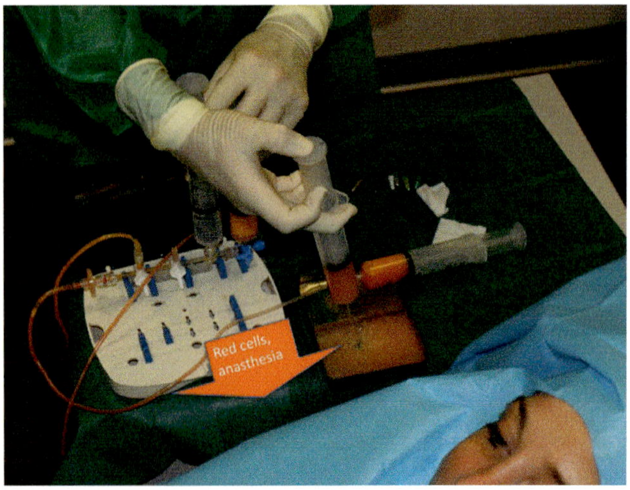

Fig. 5.16 Remove the washed solution by syringe A. (Published by kind permission of ©Mario Goisis 2018. All Rights Reserved)

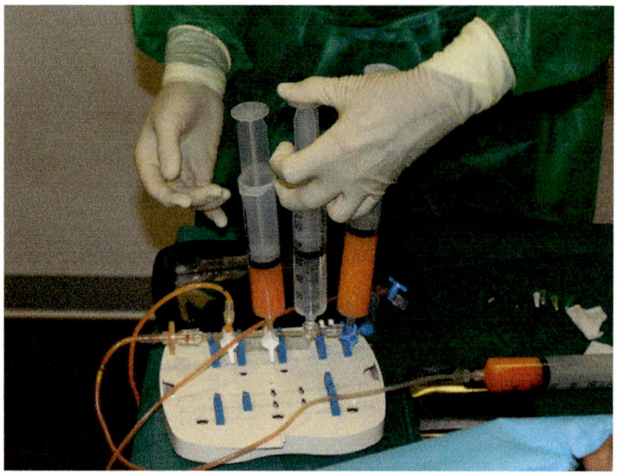

Fig. 5.17 Repeat the washing procedure one or more time inorder to obtain the change of the color of the content of the syringe C form orange to yellow (Published by kind permission of ©Mario Goisis 2018. All Rights Reserved)

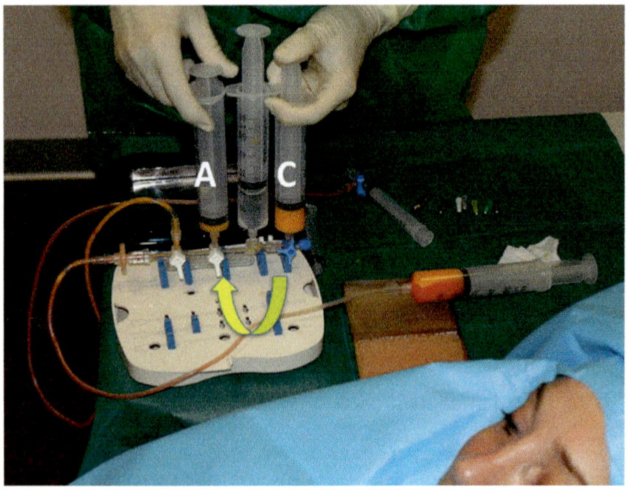

Fig. 5.18 Move the washed fat form syringe C to syringe A. The saline solution is then pushed into the tube. In this way the entire content of fat is transferred into the syringe. (Published by kind permission of ©Mario Goisis 2018. All Rights Reserved)

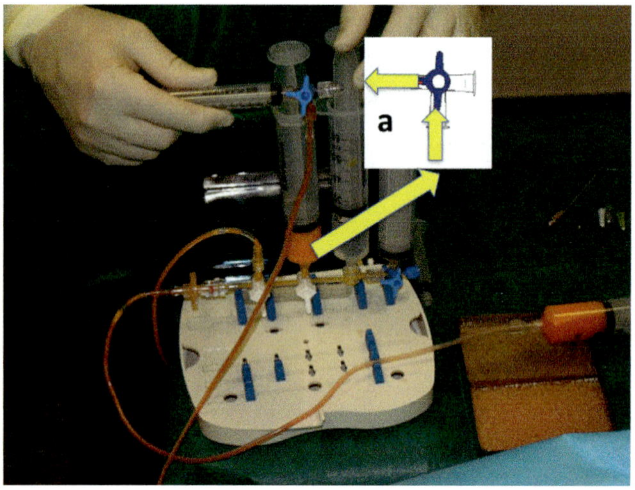

Fig. 5.19 Open the stopcock from position "b" to position "a". In this way, the syringe E is connected to the tube and to the system. In this way, by pushing the plunger of syringe A, the syringe E is directly filled from the ramp. And because of the tube was previously filled by saline solution, the syringe E will be initially filled by saline. (Published by kind permission of ©Mario Goisis 2018. All Rights Reserved)

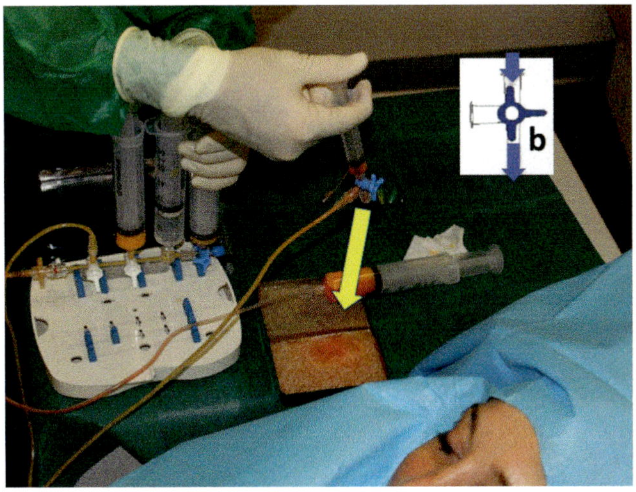

Fig. 5.20 The saline solution is pushed put form syringe E. The stopcock is in position “b”. (Published by kind permission of ©Mario Goisis 2018. All Rights Reserved)

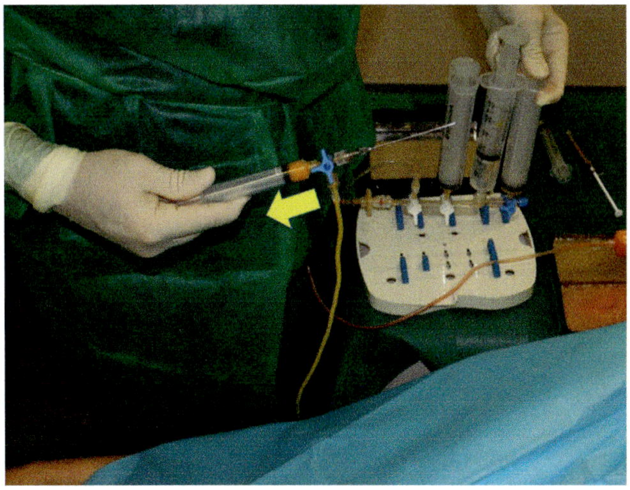

Fig. 5.21 The syringe E is filled by microfat. (Published by kind permission of ©Mario Goisis 2018. All Rights Reserved)

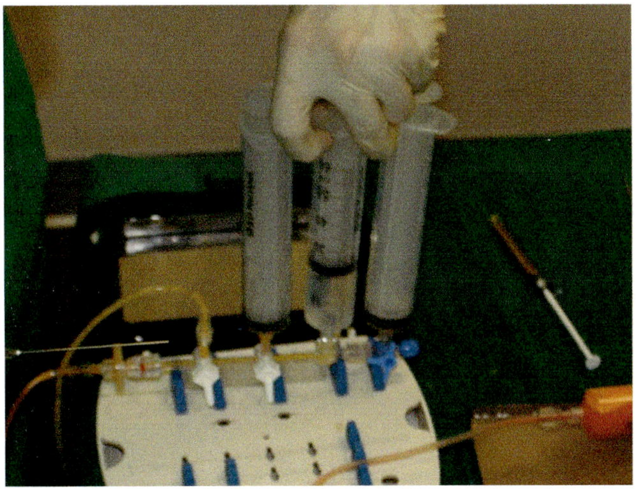

Fig. 5.22 In order to increase the efficiency of the procedure, it is important to use the fat contained into the tube: in fact it is around 6-8cc. (Published by kind permission of ©Mario Goisis 2018. All Rights Reserved)

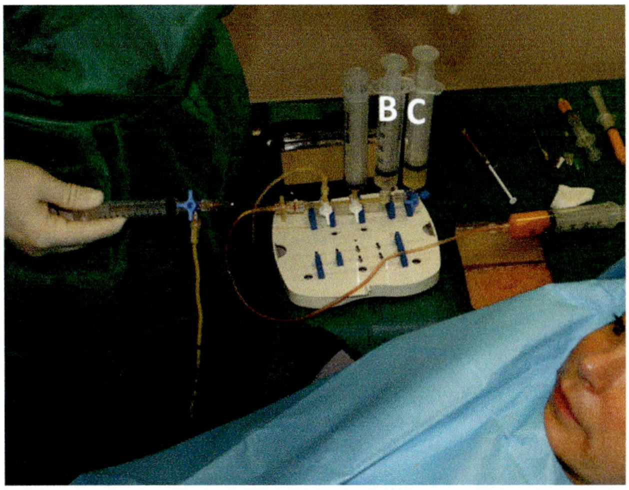

Fig. 5.23 To do that, the content of saline solution of syringe B is moved in syringe C

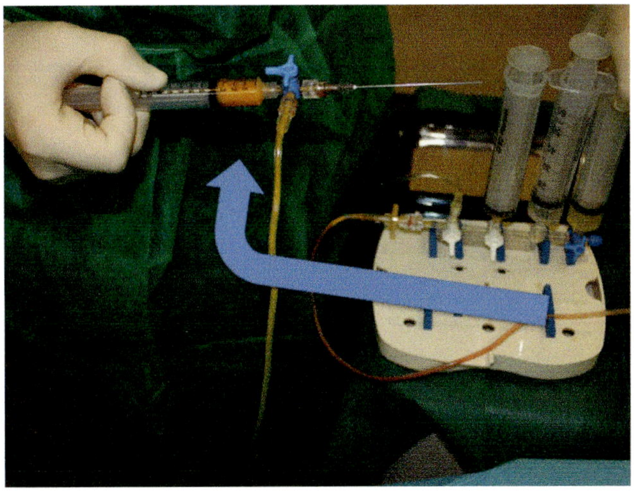

Fig. 5.24 The saline is then pushed into the tube

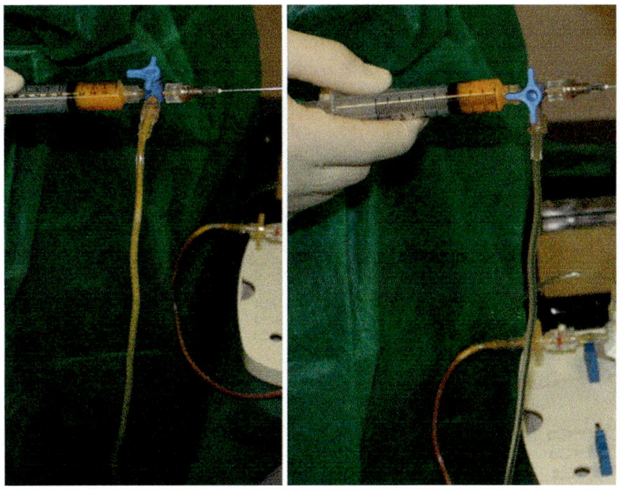

Fig. 5.25 In this way the entire content on the right: the tube filled by fat. On the left: the tube washed by saline

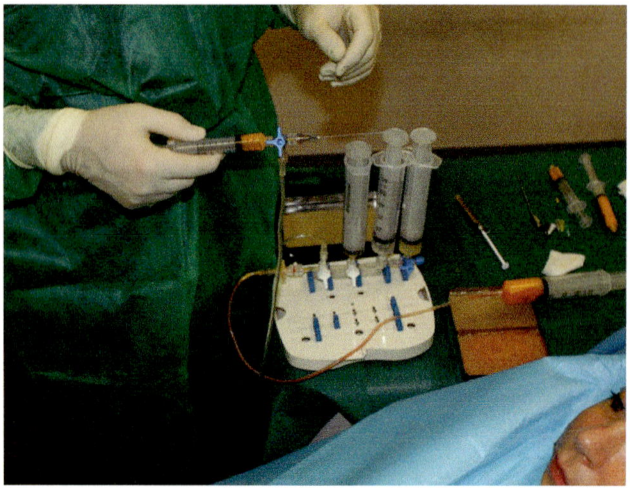

Fig. 5.26 It is important to keep attention at the level of saline: when the saline is close to syringe E, the stopcock is changed form position "a" to position "b"

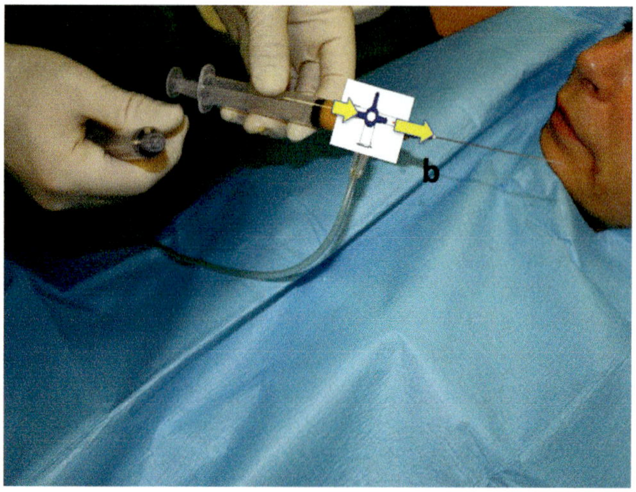

Fig. 5.27 The syringe E is ready for injection

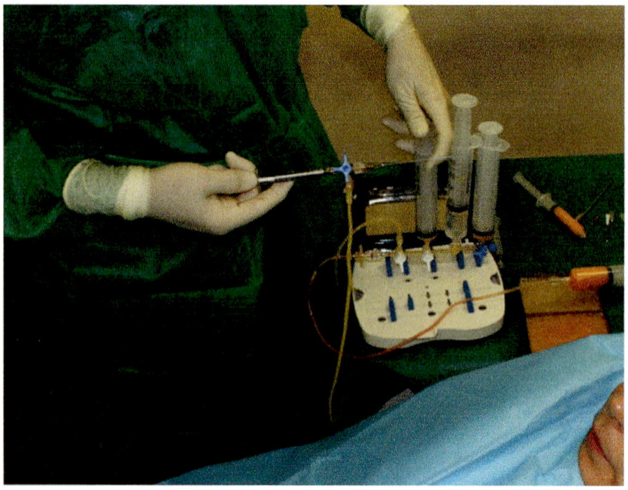

Fig. 5.28 In order to inject the fat more easily, a 1 cc syringe can be connected to the system

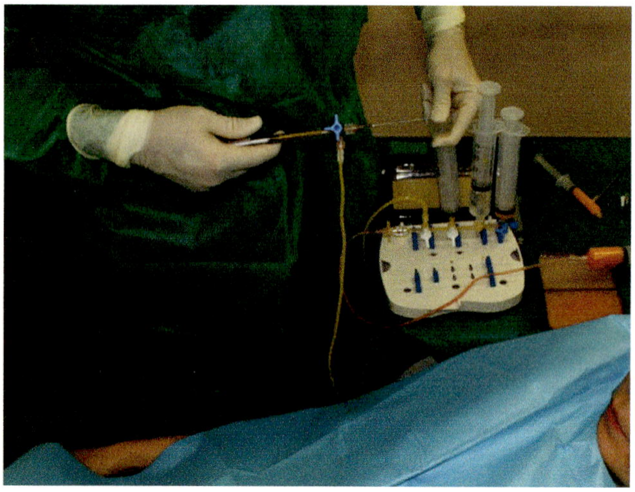

Fig. 5.29 By moving the stopcock alternatively from position "a" to Position "b" is it possible to fill many time this small syringe

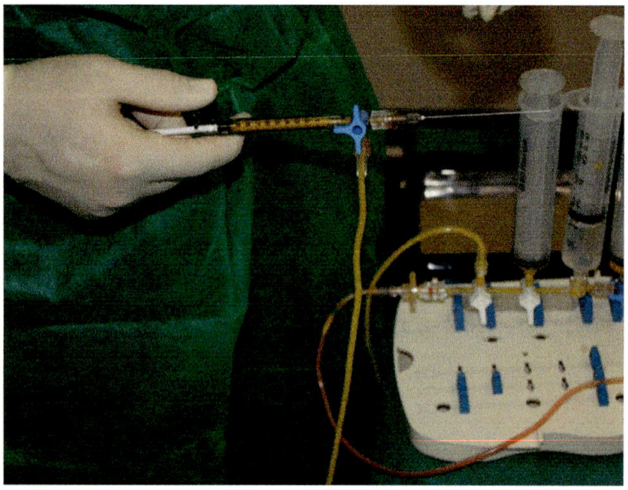

Injection Techniques

6

Mario Goisis, Giuseppe A. Ferraro, and Sara Izzo

Many scientific articles have been published concerning the harvesting and processing of fat; on the contrary, there very few EBM articles regarding reinjection of fat are available in literature.

By examining the mechanical properties of fat, schemes may be devised for the preservation of fat during injection. Given this principle, it is convenient to evaluate each element of injection techniques carefully and to comprehend the physical biomechanics and the rheology involved.

One of the most significant physical measurements of fat is its viscosity.

Viscosity *is a measure of a fluid's resistance to flow*. It defines the internal friction of a moving fluid.

For example, if we put honey into a funnel, we will that the funnel drains very slowly (Fig. 6.1).

This is because the viscosity of honey is high compared to that of other liquids. In fact, if we fill the same funnel with water, the funnel drains much more rapidly.

A fluid with a high viscosity rate repels motion because its molecular structure gives it a lot of inner friction. A fluid with low viscosity, flows easily because its molecular structure causes very little friction when it is in motion.

When the fluid is forced through a tube or through a cannula, the particles which compose the fluid generally move more quickly at the centre of the cannula and more slowly near its walls: therefore, some stress (such as the difference between the pressure in the two ends of the cannula) is needed to overcome the friction existing between particle layers and keep the fluid moving. The stress required is proportional to the fluid's viscosity, for the same pattern of velocity. When velocity increases, the stress, too, increases (Fig. 6.2).

A fluid that has no resistance to shear stress is known as an *ideal* or *inviscid* fluid. Zero viscosity is found only in superfluids at very low temperatures. So, all fluids have some degree of viscosity. Generally, a liquid is assumed to be viscous if its viscosity is greater than that of water; it is considered mobile if its viscosity is less than that of water.

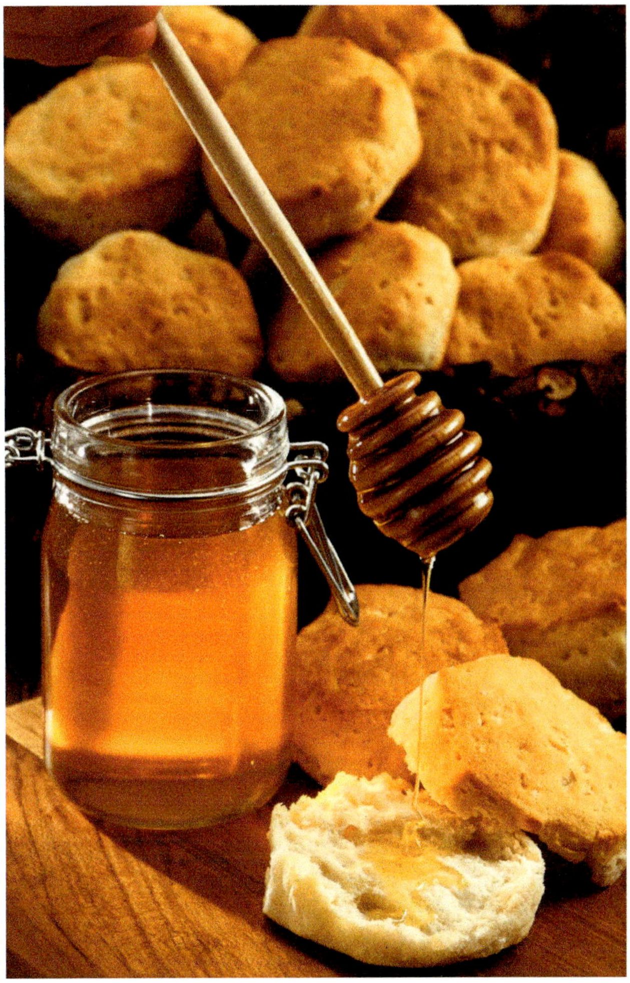

Fig. 6.1 Honey has a high viscosity rate. (Published by kind permission of ©Mario Goisis 2018. All Rights Reserved)

Rheology is the study of the flow of materials. It is particularly advantageous when analysing viscoelastic materials, which display properties somewhere between *elastic*

M. Goisis (✉)
Maxillo-Facial and Aesthetic Surgeon, Go Easy Clinic, Milan, Italy

G. A. Ferraro · S. Izzo
Doctor's Equipe, Milan, Italy

M. Goisis (ed.), *Outpatient Regenerative Medicine*, https://doi.org/10.1007/978-3-319-44894-7_6

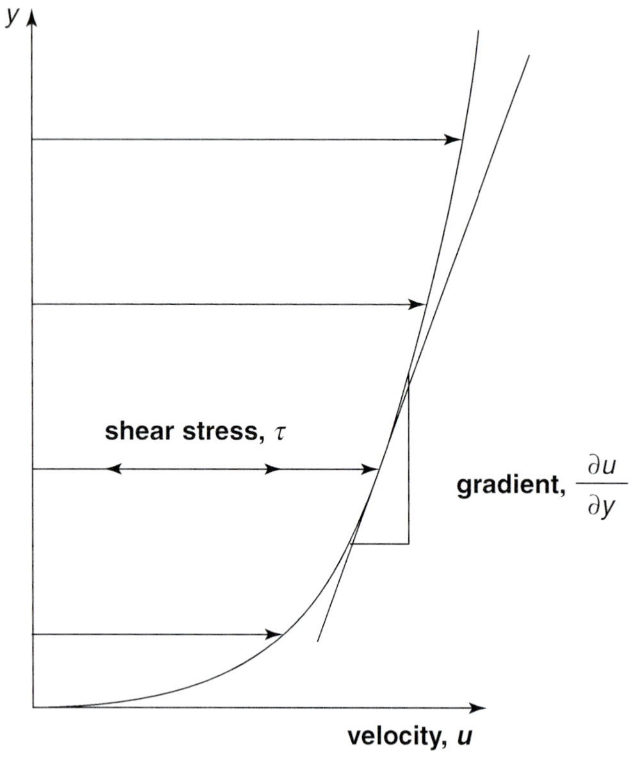

Fig. 6.2 When the fluid is forced through a tube or through a cannula, the shear stress is proportional to the gradient of the velocity. (Published by kind permission of ©Mario Goisis 2018. All Rights Reserved)

solids and *viscous* liquids. Elastic solids are termed by their instantaneous deformation in response to an applied force followed by instantaneous return to their original shape when that force is removed. On the contrary, viscous liquids are subject time-dependent (permanent) deformation. Viscoelastic materials display both instantaneous and time-dependent deformation with regard to applied forces. *Fat is a biological viscoelastic tissue*, as are ligaments, tendons, and cartilage [3, 4].

The rheology of fat is interrelated to shear stress. Shear stress appears when a force acts parallel to a surface, despite the force perpendicular to it. For example, rubbing one's hands together induces shear stress, while pressing one's palms into each other does not.

For lipofilling, shear stress is applied on the fat as it is pushed through a tube, such as a cannula. At the same rate of velocity, the shear stress is proportional to the viscosity of the fat. When viscosity is high, a high degree of shear stress will be produced.

At the same time, because fat is a viscoelastic material, it is subjected to shear thinning. This simply means that as shear stress increases, the viscosity of the material decreases.

Some shear-thinning materials can "self-heal," meaning that they can recover their original viscosity fully after being exposed to high shear rates.

Fat is not a "self-heal" material. *It [was] has been demonstrated by rheology tests that exposing fat to high shear rates will result in irreversible damage, and the mechanical integrity of the fat cannot fully [retrieve] recover from this damage.*

6.1 Flow Rate and Fat Viability

Atashroo et al. using rheology tests proved that the exposure of fat to high shear rates results in irreversible damage [1]. In particular, they harvested and processed fat applying the Coleman technique, and injected it using a 2-mm-diameter Coleman cannula. During the first set of tests, the fat was injected through an automatic device; during the second set, it was injected by means of syringes following the standard Coleman technique. Interestingly, the viscosity of the fat injected using the automatic device was similar to that of the fat before injection, while it was significantly greater than the viscosity for the fat injected using a classical 1-cc Coleman syringe.

This was related to the lower flow-rate guaranteed by the automated device.

H[h]igh flow rates have been shown, in fact, to be damaging to fat inducing more shear stress. For example, flow rates in the order of 0.5–1 cc/s have been recommended, therefore, by Lee et al. to optimise the viability of fat [5].

In the same article, the authors, validating the work of Shiffman and Mirrafati, used histology to demonstrate that high flow-rate damages fat significantly [6].

Goisis et al. at the Face conference presented a study about shear stress which occurs during the washing, filtration, and injection of fat comparing the Goisis system with the Coleman and Lipogems techniques.

The reduction of the viscosity of the fat when using the Goisis system (injection with a 22-gauge cannula) was significantly lower compared to the reduction obtained with the Lipogems system (injection using a 25-gauge cannula) or the Coleman system (injection with a 22-gauge cannula [7] (Figs. 6.3 and 6.4). In an other study presented by Goisis et al. Imcas 2018 (Goisis et al., comparing protocols, IMCAS 2018) the importance of shear stress in preservation of stem-cells was discussed. The number of stem-cell of 6 different samples was measured at 72 hours, 7 days and 14 days after colture. Three samples were related to Goisis technique, with high values of stem-cells immediately after harvesting with Goisis Cannula (6443, 7596, 8950), after processing with Goisis System (5601, 6300, 6500) and after passing through a 22G cannula (3976, 5950, 6460). The last 3 samples were related with Coleman technique with a very significant modification: the Coleman fat was passed through a 22G cannula. The value of stem-cells after harvesting with Coleman cannula were 5180, 5930 and 7410. The value after Coleman processing (centrifugation) were 4940, 4210 and 5140. But after passage throught the 22G cannula the stem-cells were destroyed by high level of shear stress, with no survival of stem-cells.

Key Point

- High flow rates damage fat, because they indice greater shear stress.
- Inject slowly!

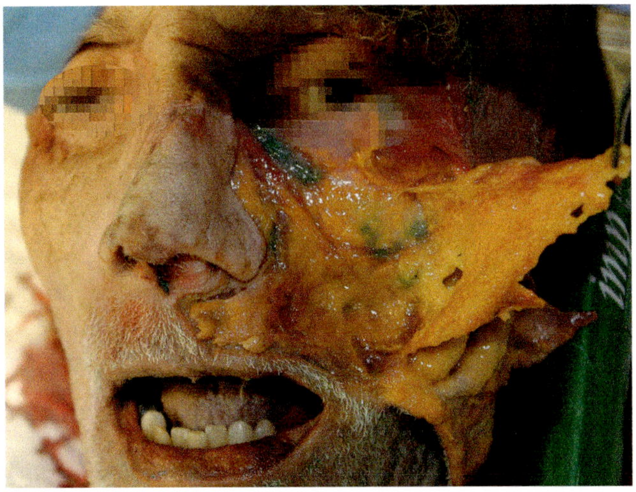

Fig. 6.3 Anatomical dissection demonstrating a deep, intramuscular injection of fat. The fat was coloured green before injection (courtesy of the Doctor's Equipe). (Published by kind permission of ©Mario Goisis 2018. All Rights Reserved)

6.2 Viscosity

The size of a cannula's ports affects the viscosity of the graft adipocytes direcly. In particular, the use of larger port sizes increases the viscosity of the graft [8–10].

In case of high viscosity, the fat that is pushed through a small cannula will produce a high shear-stress rate. This shear stress will result in irreversible damage, and the mechanical integrity of the fat cannot fully recover from this damage.

Key Point

- The use of larger port sizes during fat harvesting increases the risk of damage to the graft during injection.
- Use harvesting cannulas with smaller port sizes.

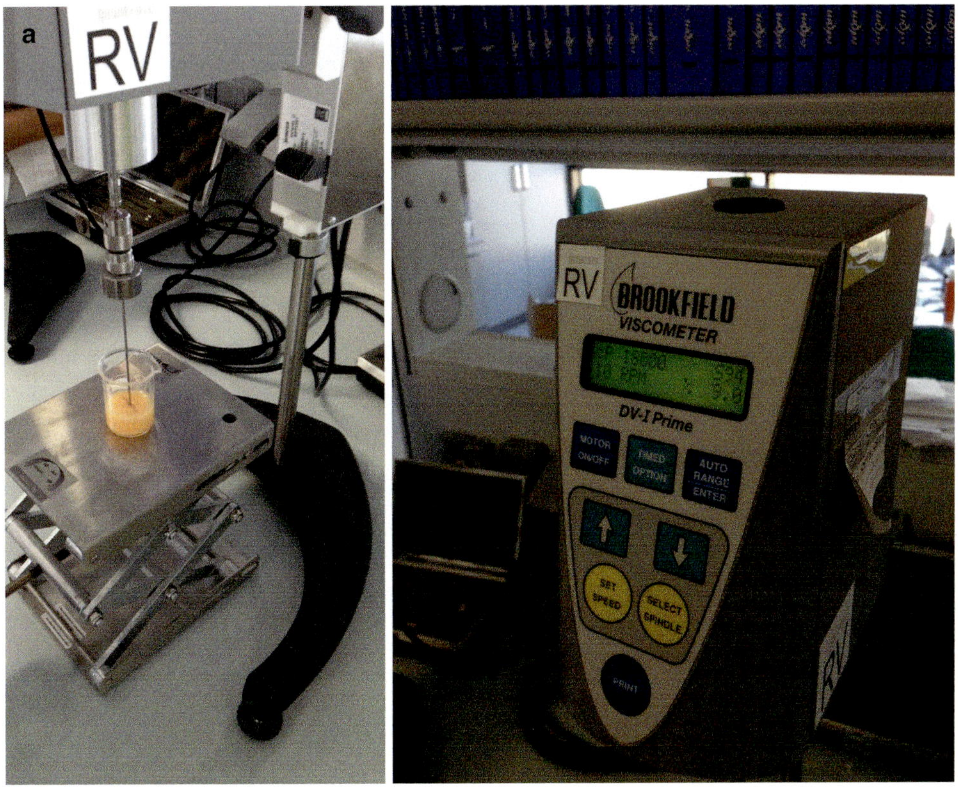

Fig. 6.4 (a–c)Viscosimeter and slide glass test: comparison between the viscosity of harvested fat and that of processed fat when passed through an injection cannula. (courtesely Istituto Ganassini, Milano). (Published by kind permission of ©Mario Goisis 2018. All Rights Reserved)

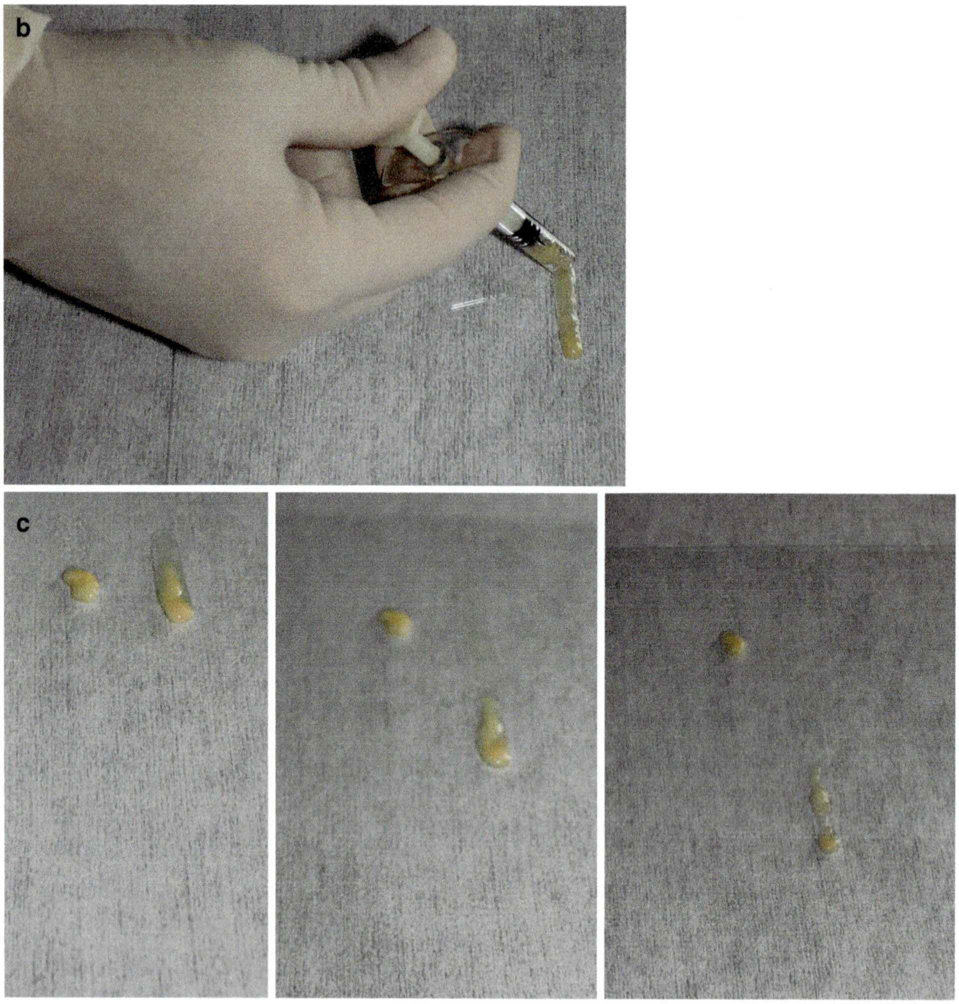

Fig. 6.4 (continued)

6.3 Cannulas or Needles for Injection

A work by Smith et al. indicates that using needles for injection may be more destructive to fat than using cannulas because of potentially greater shear stress induced [11].

Key Point

- The of use of needle increases damages to the fat.
- Do not use needles to inject fat.

6.4 Where to Inject

Amar et al. described the FAMI technique, a technique for facial rejuvenation using fat grafting that targets specific anatomic structures and tissue beds [12].

They called it FAMI, an acronym meaning "facial autologous muscular injection." In their opinion, it is possible to increase the survival-rate of the adipocyte by injecting the fat in close proximity or even within the facial-expression muscles. Fat is transferred into one or more 1-cc syringe and attached to one or more of the nine different cannulas. These cannulas are shaped to match musculoskeletal shapes. The group of muscles is injected, retrograde fashion, with 1–3 cc of fat, from the insertion to the source or vice versa, in one to three administrations. The only exception is the infraorbital area, where no more than 0.5 cc can be grafted because of reported risks of nodules and cysts. The rationale of the FAMI technique is that the fat will live optimally when grafted into a rich muscular vascular plexus [13–15].

FAMI's postoperative suggestions are based on the opinion that "The fewer movements there are, the more successful the graft will ultimately be." For this reason, patients should avoid not only laughing or abrupt, sudden facial movements but also talking. They should also avoid public occasions demanding vocal interaction, as well as talking on the phone.

This avoidance of stress to the facial muscle also extends to a patient's diet, which not contain hard foods like apples or tough breads. Instead, patients should eat softer foods, such as bananas, taking pains to avoid any food items requiring undue stress to the jaws (http://www.drrogeramar.com/fami_step_step.php).

Goisis et al. described the injection of fat into the deep intramuscular plane using a 22-gauge cannula. In particular, by using an elastic cannula and one injection-point it is possible to inject fat into this deep plane of the middle and lower third of the face. The injection technique was demonstrated using anatomical dissections [16] (Fig. 6.3).

Key Point

- The injection of fat into rich muscular vascular plexuses increases the survival of cells.
- Inject fat into a deep plane, in close proximity or into the muscular plane.

6.4.1 Diameter of the Cannula Used for Injection

In the classical Coleman technique, fat injection is performed using Coleman cannulas (diameters 1–2 mm) with which droplets are injected into a tri-dimensional space. Between 10 and 25 cc of fat are injected into the superficial and deeper planes on each side of the face. Usually, superficial injection is performed in the temporal region (above the superficial temporal fascia for reasons of vascularisation), the crow's feet area, and the anterior part of the cheek (to allow for direct support of the skin in the latter two zones). Injection into deeper planes is performed on the malar eminence, suborbicularis oculi fat (SOOF), tear trough, the central part of the midface, the nasolabial and the marionette folds.

The big diameter of the cannulas, combined with the multiplane technique, is usually associated with oedemata and haematomas. Willemsen et al. reported that patients who underwent lipofilling using the Coleman technique took 18.9 days to resume their social activities, a time span reduced to 13.2 days when the fat was combined with PRP [17].

Despite this, the dead space is increased when larger cannulas are used. This space will be filled with serum on the scarring tissue, and reduce cell integration.

Goisis et al. [16] suggested thin deep-layer injection using a 22-gauge cannula.

In particular, the fat harvested using a Goisis microcannula has a low viscosity rate. Because of that, it is possible to inject it using a small cannula thus creating a low shear-stress rate. Goisis et al. compared viscosity before and after injection, demonstrating that the variation was slight. The preservation of viscosity is a demonstration of the preservation of the integrity of fat.

The use of small cannulas creates a small dead space, reducing the scarring tissue interfering with cell integration.

Injection into the deep plane takes place in close proximity to rich muscular vascular plexuses. The technique is very simple, and is based on four key entry-points. Through these points it is possible to inject the malar area, cheeks, nasolabial folds, lips, chin, and lacrimal sulcus.

Key Point

- The use of larger-guage cannulas increases the dead space, and reduces the survival of cells.
- The use of large-guage cannulas increases the incidence of oedemata and hematomas.
- Use smaller cannulas to inject fat!

6.4.2 Vascularisation of the Recipient Site

The success of fat-grafting is increased when the recipient site is well-vascularised [18].

Despite this, fat grafting has been described by many authors with reference to scarred surgical fields and clearly ischemic irradiated tissues [19, 20].

Garza et al. examined the result of fat grafting on the irradiated skin of a nude mouse. Fat grafting caused decreased dermal thickness, augmented vascular density, and decreased collagen content. CT analysis demonstrated significantly decreased graft survival rates in the irradiated group when related to the non-irradiated group [21].

This observation can be related to the results of a study by Eto et al. These authors have proven that transferred fat demonstrates three zones of healing: the central necrotic area, the peripheral surviving area, and intermediate regenerating area. The regeneration of the intermediate area is due to vascularisation. Because irradiated tissue provides a poorer vascularized bed during early fat-graft incorporation, this probably causes lower ultimate retention rates, that affect final surviving graft volume.

Key Point

- The survival of fat is reduced in cases of irradiated skin.
- After the injection of fat, skin amelioration associated with adipose stem-cells can be observed.

- It has been suggested that fat may also be injected into irradiated area, but it is mandatory to inform the patient about the risk of high resorption rates and about the need for multiple touch-up sessions.

6.4.3 How Much to Inject

Kato et al. recently published an interesting study, emphasising the importance of the size of fat particles in grafting [22]. As previously discussed, the particle structure of fat does not occur in the native tissue but rather is created during harvesting and processing procedures.

At the same time, it is important to note that injection is the final step/element of a unique treatment/chain. To obtain small particles of fat harvesting and processing are not sufficient. In fact, the small particle is injected very close to other particles and a single big bolus is created. In particular, the adipocytes most likely to survive are located closer to the surface of the bolus. Based on histological findings, this bolus may be divided into three sections: the layer closest to the surface where all the adipocytes survive, the middle layer where the adipocytes die but are replaced by proliferating stem-cells, and a central core dominated by necrosis, oil cysts, and fibrosis. Demarcation of the outer survival zone and the middle regenerational occurs at 1–300 um and 600–1200 um from the surface, respectively. Prior to the reestablishment of the blood supply, fat particles depend largely on the simple diffusion for nutrients. As the diameter of adipose lobules becomes larger, the central zone of necrosis will expand according to its diffusional limitations.

Therefore, one can see that the size of the injected bolus may ultimately influence how much of the grafted material survives.

Key Point

- To increase fat survival, it is mandatory not to inject the particles of fat very close to other particles.
- It is suggested to inject a small amount of fat using a small cannula, by moving the cannula in the recipient bed, avoiding injection of the particle very close to other particles.

References

1. Atashroo D, Raphel J, Chung MT, Paik KJ, Parisi-Amon A, McArdle A, Senarath-Yapa K, Zielins ER, Tevlin R, Duldulao C, Walmsley GG, Hu MS, Momeni A, Domecus B, Rimsa JR, Greenberg L, Gurtner GC, Longaker MT, Wan DC. Studies in fat grafting: part II. Effects of injection mechanics on material properties of fat. Plast Reconstr Surg. 2014;134(1):39–46.
2. Chung MT, Paik KJ, Atashroo DA, Hyun JS, McArdle A, Senarath-Yapa K, Zielins ER, Tevlin R, Duldulao C, Hu MS, Walmsley GG, Parisi-Amon A, Momeni A, Rimsa JR, Commons GW, Gurtner GC, Wan DC, Longaker MT. Studies in fat grafting: part I. Effects of injection technique on in vitro fat viability and in vivo volume retention. Plast Reconstr Surg. 2014;134(1):29–38.
3. Pearson B, Espino DM. Effect of hydration on the frequency-dependent viscoelastic properties of articular cartilage. Proc Inst Mech Eng H. 2013;227:1246.
4. Davis FM, De Vita R. A nonlinear constitutive model for stress relaxation in ligaments and tendons. Ann Biomed Eng. 2012;40:2541–50.
5. Lee JH, Kirkham JC, McCormack MC, Nicholls AM, Randolph MA, Austen WG Jr. The effect of pressure and shear on autologous fat grafting. Plast Reconstr Surg. 2013;131:1125–36.
6. Shiffman MA, Mirrafati S. Fat transfer techniques: the effect of harvest and transfer methods on adipocyte viability and review of the literature. Dermatol Surg. 2001;27:819–26.
7. Goisis M. Comparison between different techniques. Face congress, London; 2016.
8. Farr ST, Trivisonno A. Differential fat harvesting. Plast Aesthet Res. 2014;1:103–7.
9. Kirkham JC, Lee JH, Medina MA 3rd, McCormack MC, Randolph MA, Austen WG Jr. The impact of liposuction cannula size on adipocyte viability. Ann Plast Surg. 2012;69:479–81.
10. Erdim M, Tezel E, Numanoglu A, Sav A. The effects of the size of liposuction cannula on adipocyte survival and the optimum temperature for fat graft storage: an experimental study. J Plast Reconstr Aesthet Surg. 2009;62:1210–4.
11. Smith P, Adams WP Jr, Lipschitz AH, et al. Autologous human fat grafting: effect of harvesting and preparation techniques on adipocyte graft survival. Plast Reconstr Surg. 2006;117:1836–44.
12. Amar RE, Fox DM. The facial autologous muscular injection (FAMI) procedure: an anatomically targeted deep multiplane autologous fat-grafting technique using principles of facial fat injection. Aesthet Plast Surg. 2011;35(4):502–10.
13. Amar RE, Fox DM, Balin A. Cannulation and injection of the muscles of facial expression: a cadaver study. Dermatol Surg. 2010;36(3):331–8. https://doi.org/10.1111/j.1524-4725.2009.01438.x. Epub 2010 Jan 19
14. Butterwick KJ. Fat autograft muscle injection (FAMI): new technique for facial volume restoration. Dermatol Surg. 2005;31(11 Pt 2):1487–95.
15. Butterwick KJ. Enhancement of the results of neck liposuction with the FAMI technique. J Drugs Dermatol. 2003;2(5):487–93.
16. Goisis M. Anatomy of fat injection, a cadaveric dissection demonstration. 5CC congress, Barcellona; 2016.
17. Willemsen JP, van der Lei B, Stevens HP. The effects of platelet-rich plasma on recovery time and aesthetic outcome in facial rejuvenation: preliminary retrospective observations. Aesthet Plast Surg. 2014;38:1057–63.
18. Coleman SR. Facial recontouring with lipostructure. Clin Plast Surg. 1997;24:347–67.
19. Panettiere P, Accorsi D, Marchetti L, Sgro F, Sbarbati A. Large-breast reconstruction using fat graft only after prosthetic reconstruction failure. Aesthet Plast Surg. 2011;35:703–8.
20. Rigotti G, Marchi A, Galie M, et al. Clinical treatment of radiotherapy tissue damage by lipoaspirate transplant: a healing process mediated by adipose-derived adult stem cells. Plast Reconstr Surg. 2007;119:1409–22. discussion 1423–1404
21. Garza RM, Paik KJ, Chung MT, Duscher D, Gurtner GC, Longaker MT, Wan DC. Studies in fat grafting: part III. Fat grafting irradiated tissue—improved skin quality and decreased fat graft retention. Plast Reconstr Surg. 2014;134(2):249–57.
22. Eto H, Kato H, Suga H, et al. The fate of adipocytes after nonvascularized fat grafting: evidence of early death and replacement of adipocytes. Plast Reconstr Surg. 2012;129:1081–92.

Injection of Fat Step by Step

7

Mario Goisis and Sara Izzo

A full face treatment with microfat is described.

7.1 Materials

- *6–12 cc of microfat for injection on both sides:*
  - *A 21-gauge needle*
  - *A 22-gauge, 4-cm blunt cannula*

To harvest and process microfat, a standard system is used, in particular:

- A microfat box (www.microfat.com), composed of a ramp with a closed a system for washing and filtration
- 4 60-cc syringes
- 2 10-cc syringes
- One 1-cc syringe 1 cc
- A 30-gauge needle
- A 16-gauge needle
- A 2-mm-diameter, 10-cm-long Goisis cannula for fat harvesting
- A chlorhexidine-alcohol solution (2% chlorhexidine gluconate and 70% isopropyl alcohol), sterile drapes, or towels
- Ice packs
- Sterile 2 cm × 2 cm gauze squares
- Occlusive dressing cover

Medications include:

100 cc of cold saline solution
120 cc of cold Klein solution

M. Goisis (✉)
Maxillo-Facial and Aesthetic Surgeon, Go Easy Clinic, Milan, Italy

S. Izzo
Department of Plastic Surgery, University of Campania "Luigi Vanvitelli", Naples, Italy

One litre of Klein solution is composed by 800 mg of lidocaine, 1 mg of epinephrine, 40 MEq of sodium bicarbonate, and 1000 cc of saline solution

Location: The microfat may be harvested in a small operating theatre/medical surgery. The oxygen, pulse oximetry, and a crash cart/box should be present.

Assistants: An assistant is useful to transfer items to the procedure field in a sterile manner during the first part of the procedure. Nevertheless, a single doctor can easily carry out the entire procedure unaided.

7.2 Complications and Management

Immediate complications (within 72 h after injection) include transient erythema, oedema, induration, pruritus, and ecchymosis.

Early complications (days to weeks after injection) include hypercorrection, local infection, necrosis of the skin, reactivation of herpes, discoloration, and persistent local symptoms (erythema, oedema, induration, pruritus, and hyperpigmentation).

Later or delayed complications include high rates of fat resorption and cysts (Figs. 7.1, 7.2, 7.3, 7.4, 7.5, 7.6, 7.7, 7.8, 7.9, 7.10, 7.11, 7.12, 7.13, and 7.14).

M. Goisis (ed.), *Outpatient Regenerative Medicine*, https://doi.org/10.1007/978-3-319-44894-7_7

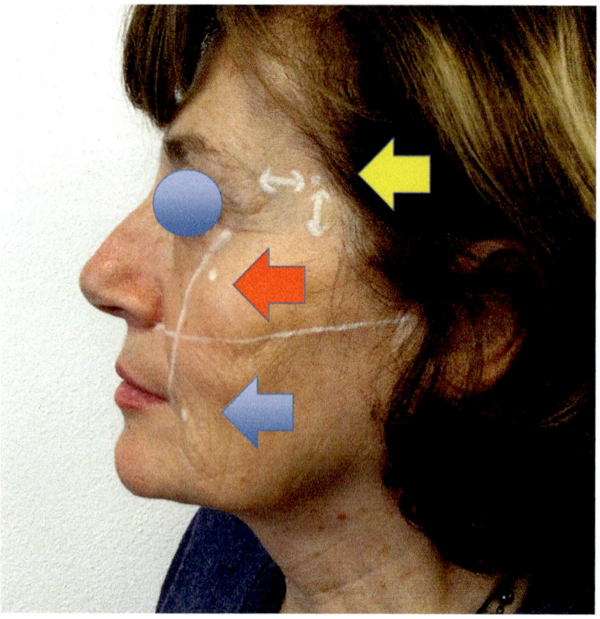

Fig. 7.1 The standard three safe-injection points are marked on the patient's skin. The blue arrow indicates the modiolus. The red arrow indicates the safe-point for injection into the lacrimal area. It is located in the upper lateral quadrant between the Hinderer lines: one joining the external cantus of the eye to the lateral rim of the mouth, the other going from the nasal wing to the tragus. The yellow arrow indicates the safe point of injection into the temporal area which is located 2 cm to the side of the lateral margin of the orbital cavity and 2 cm above the upper border of the zygomatic arch. (Published by kind permission of ©Mario Goisis 2018. All Rights Reserved)

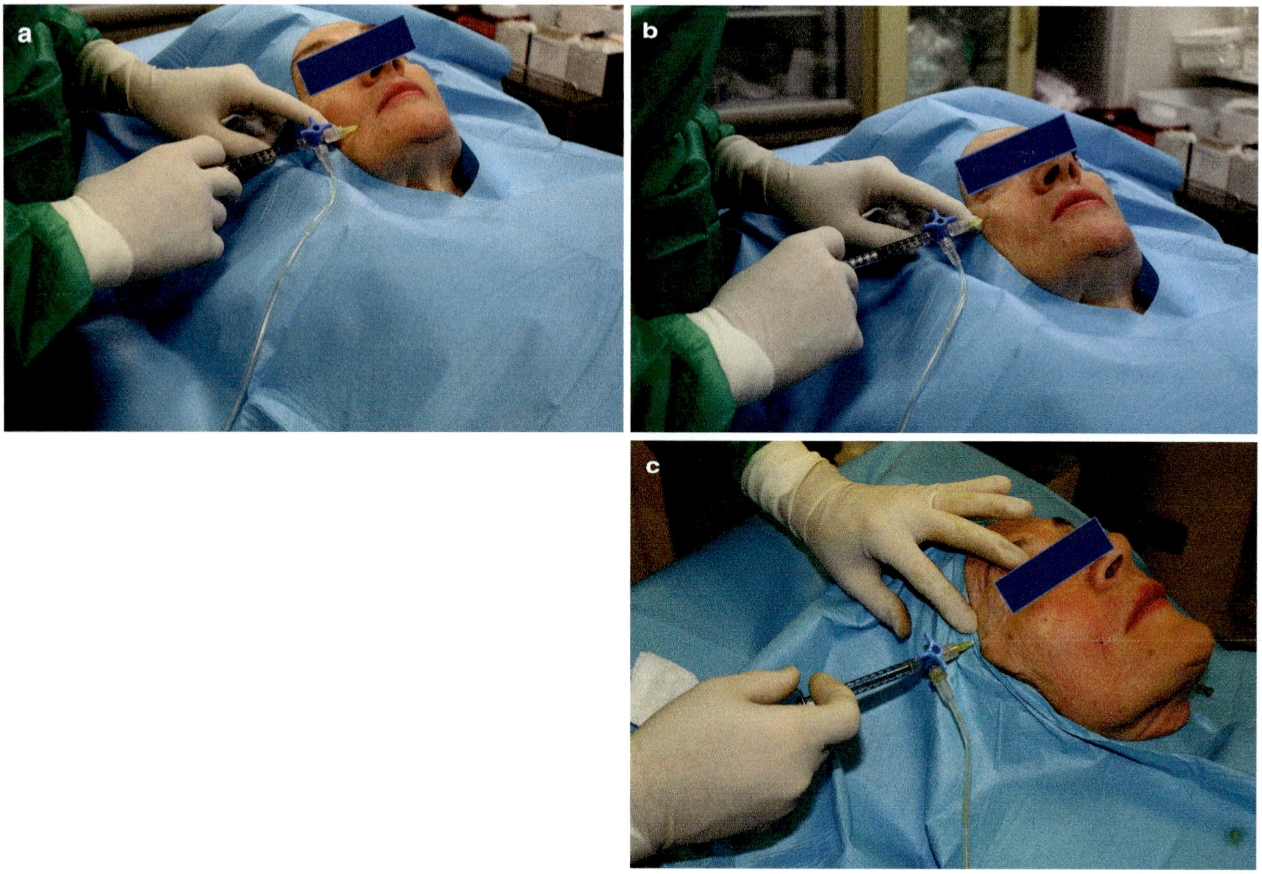

Fig. 7.2 (**a**–**c**) 0.2 cc of anaesthesia (Klein solution) is injected into each of the safe points. (Published by kind permission of ©Mario Goisis 2018. All Rights Reserved)

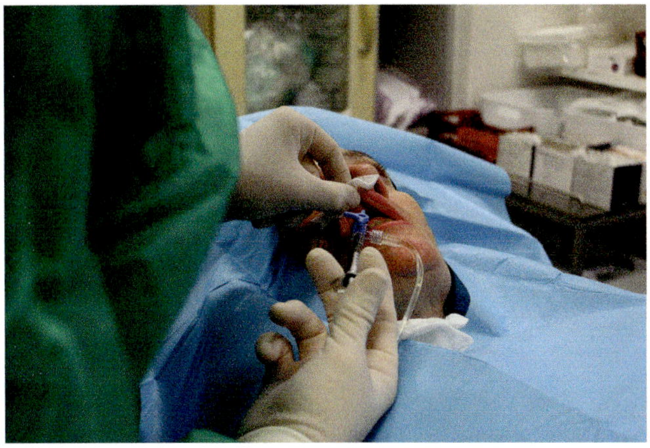

Fig. 7.3 Troncular anaesthesia is injected into the upper and lower lips. (Published by kind permission of ©Mario Goisis 2018. All Rights Reserved)

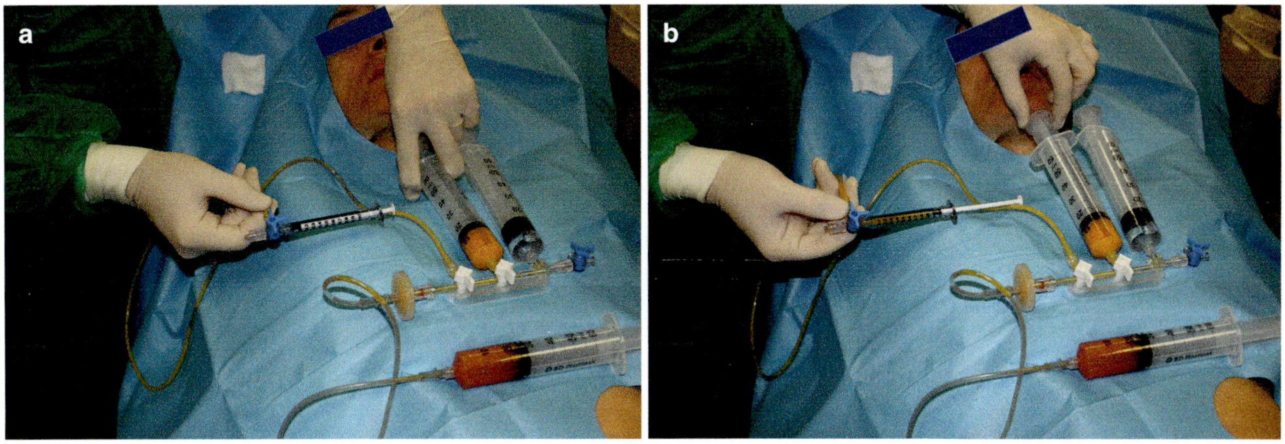

Fig. 7.4 (**a**, **b**) The fat is transferred directly from the Goisis microfat kit to the 1 cc syringe. (Published by kind permission of ©Mario Goisis 2018. All Rights Reserved)

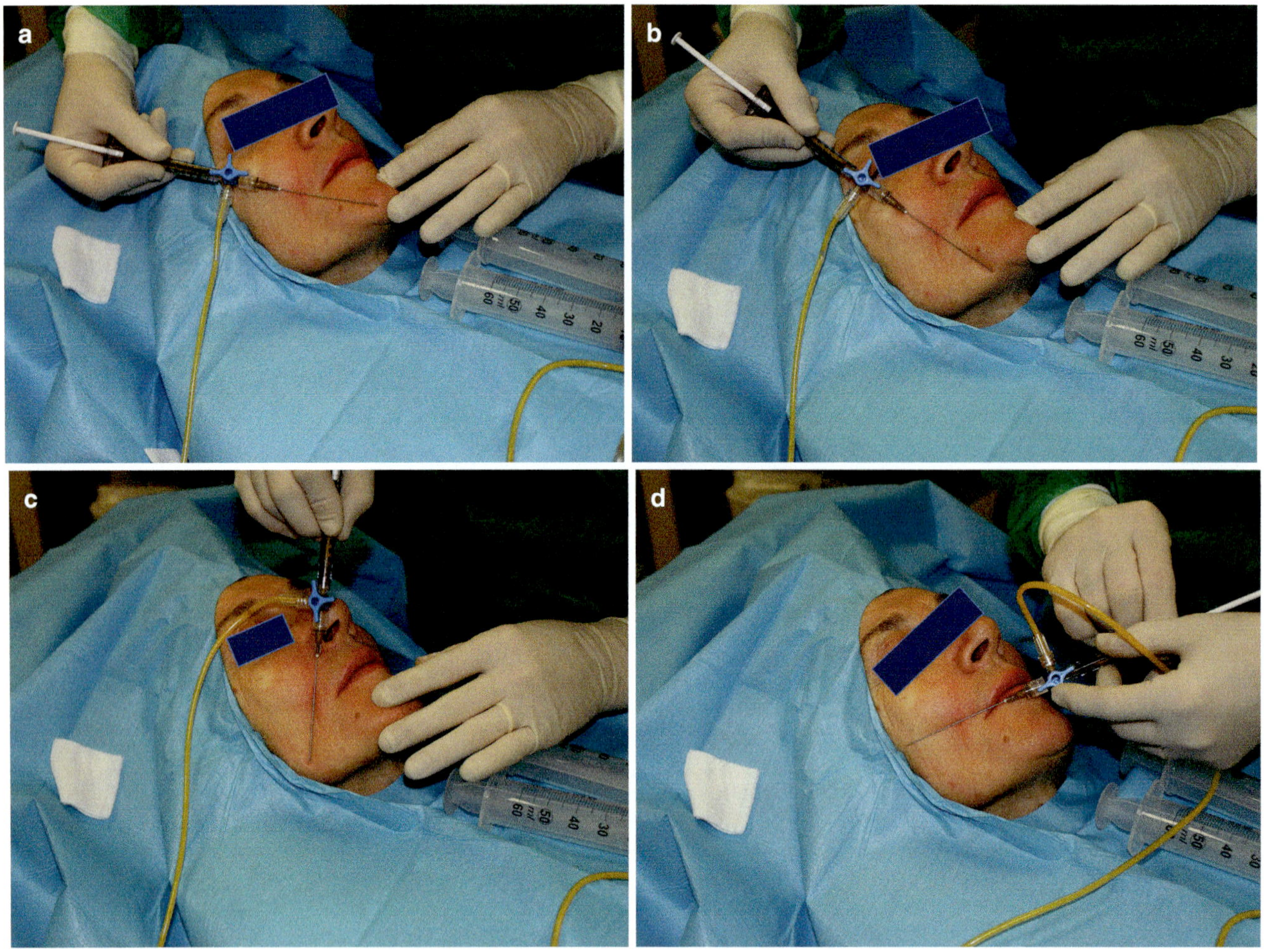

Fig. 7.5 (**a**–**j**) The route of the cannula, starting from the modiolus, is demonstrated here. (Published by kind permission of ©Mario Goisis 2018. All Rights Reserved)

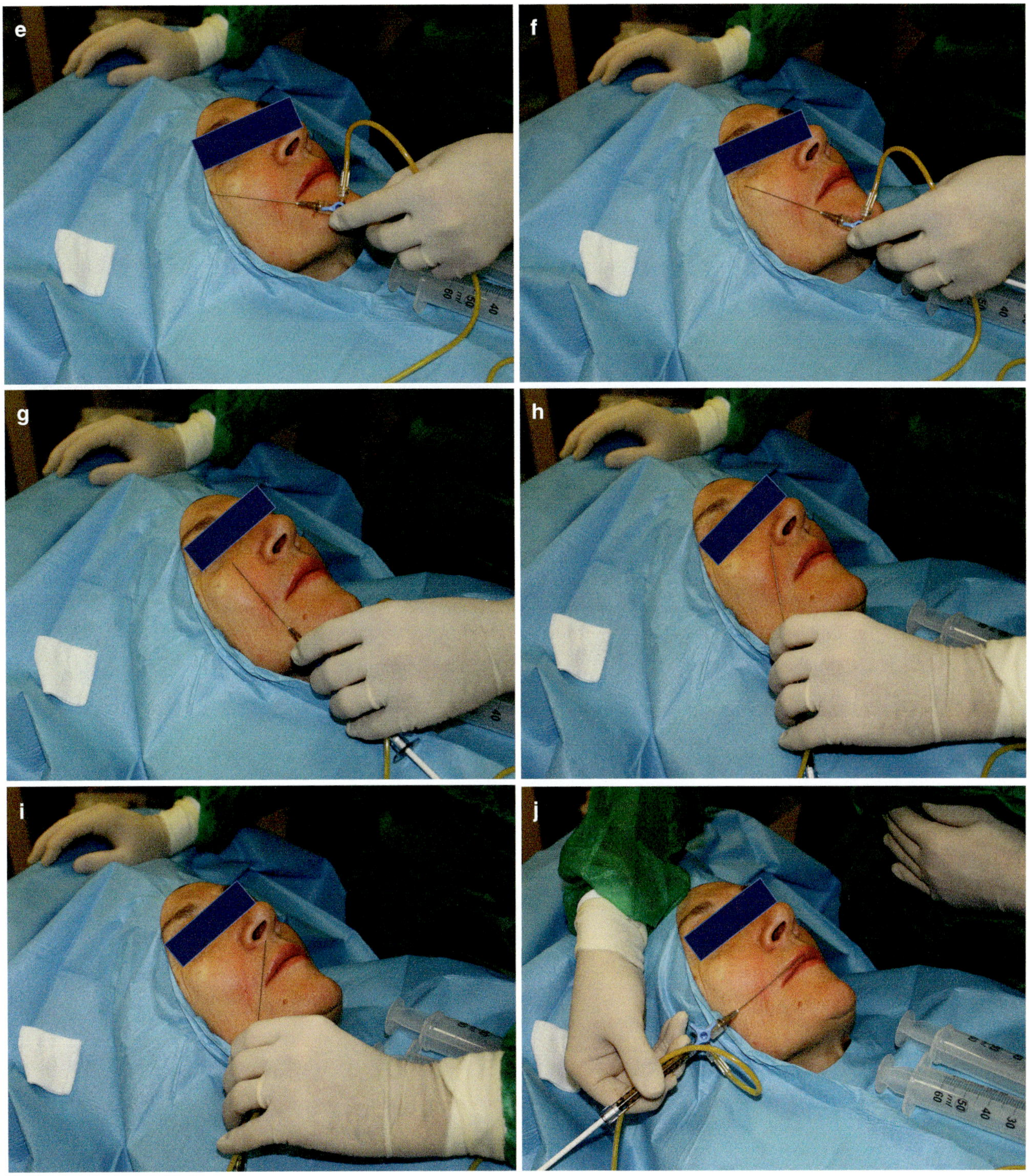

Fig. 7.5 (continued)

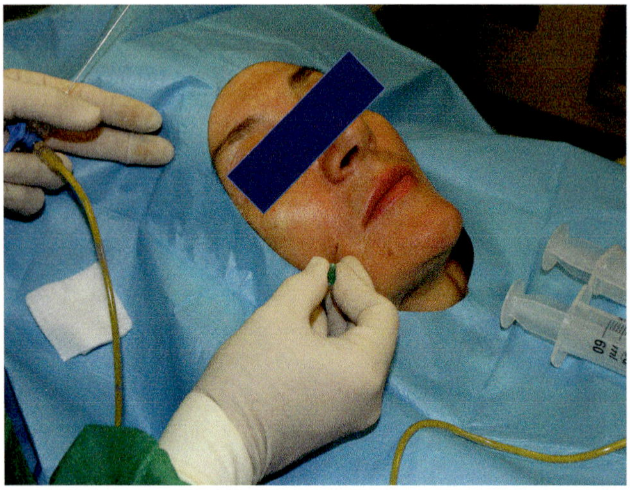

Fig. 7.6 An entrance hole is created using a sharp 21G needle. (Published by kind permission of ©Mario Goisis 2018. All Rights Reserved)

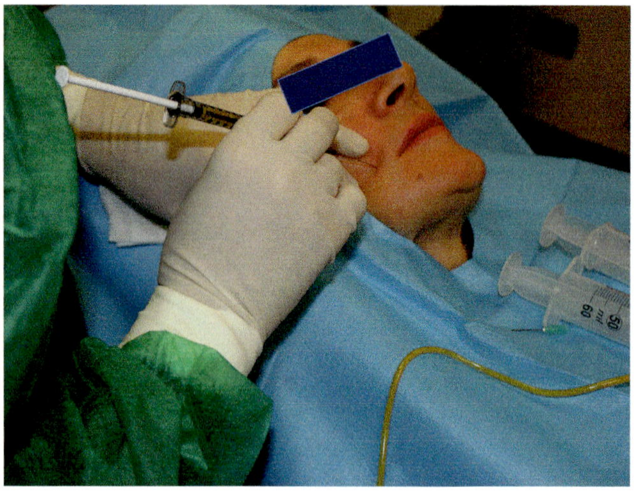

Fig. 7.7 The cannula is inserted perpendicularly into the skin. (Published by kind permission of ©Mario Goisis 2018. All Rights Reserved)

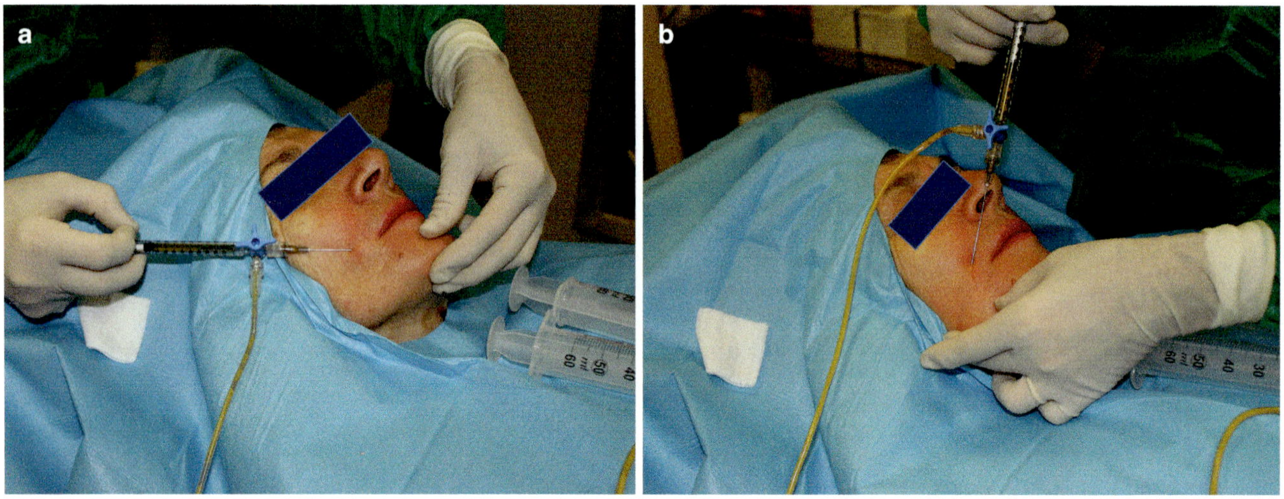

Fig. 7.8 (**a**–**e**) The fat is injected into the middle and lower thirds of the face. (Published by kind permission of ©Mario Goisis 2018. All Rights Reserved)

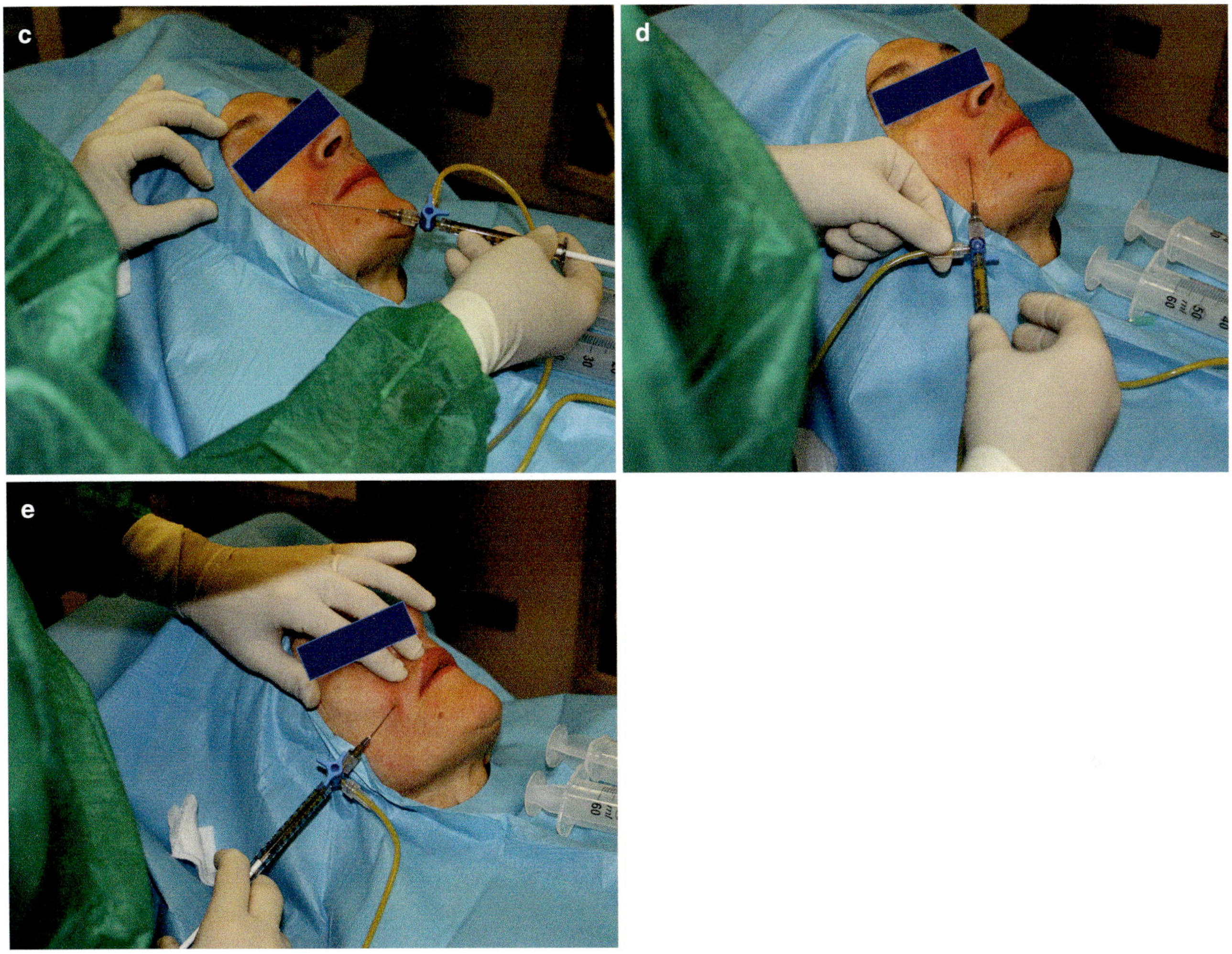

Fig. 7.8 (continued)

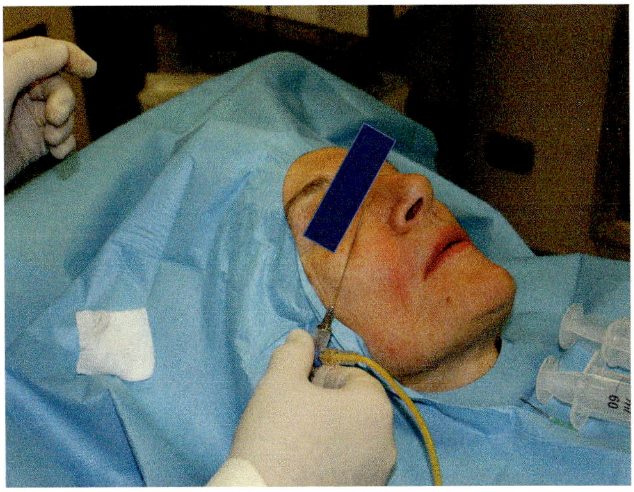

Fig. 7.9 The route of the cannula in the lachrymal area. (Published by kind permission of ©Mario Goisis 2018. All Rights Reserved)

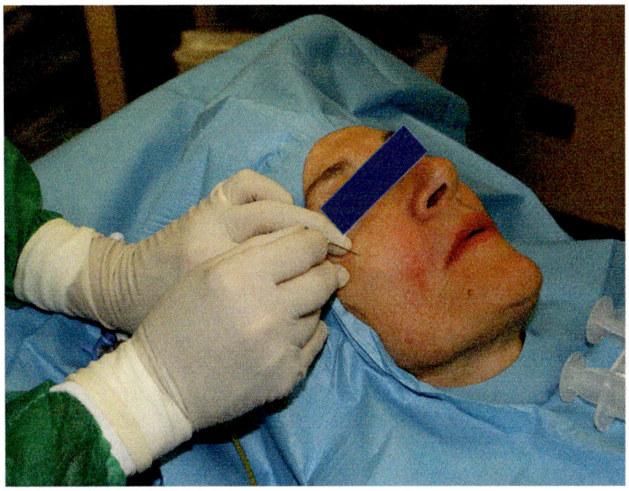

Fig. 7.10 An entrance hole is created using a sharp 21G needle. (Published by kind permission of ©Mario Goisis 2018. All Rights Reserved)

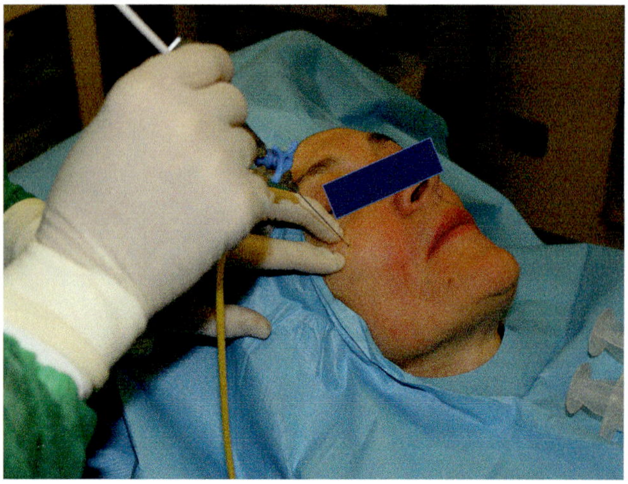

Fig. 7.11 The cannula is inserted perpendicularly into the skin. (Published by kind permission of ©Mario Goisis 2018. All Rights Reserved)

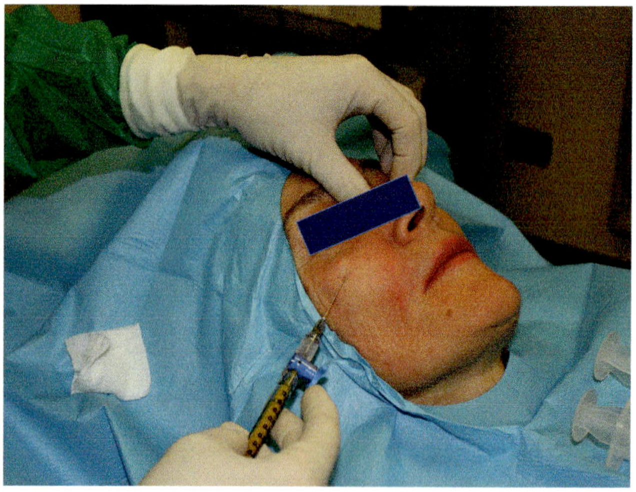

Fig. 7.12 Injection of microfat into the lachrymal area. (Published kind permission of ©Mario Goisis 2018. All Rights Reserved)

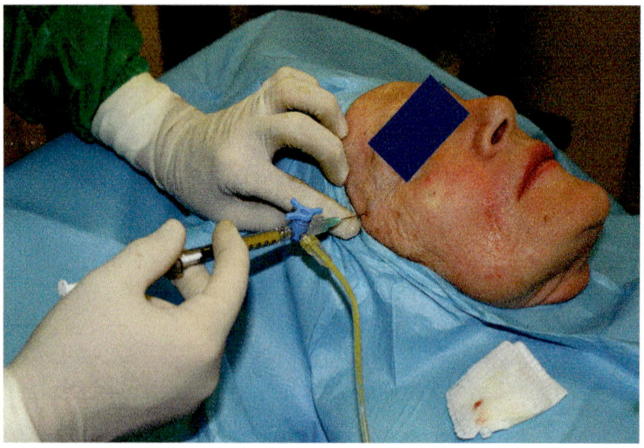

Fig. 7.13 Injection of fat into the temporal area. (Published by kind permission of ©Mario Goisis 2018. All Rights Reserved)

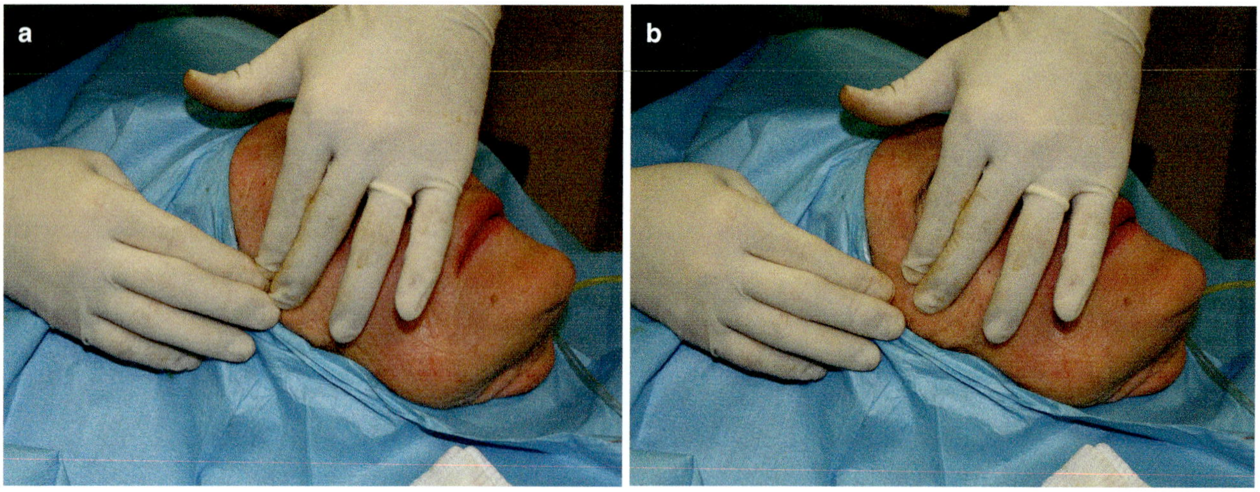

Fig. 7.14 (**a**–**j**) A strong massage is applied to the area treated. (Published by kind permission of ©Mario Goisis 2018. All Rights Reserved)

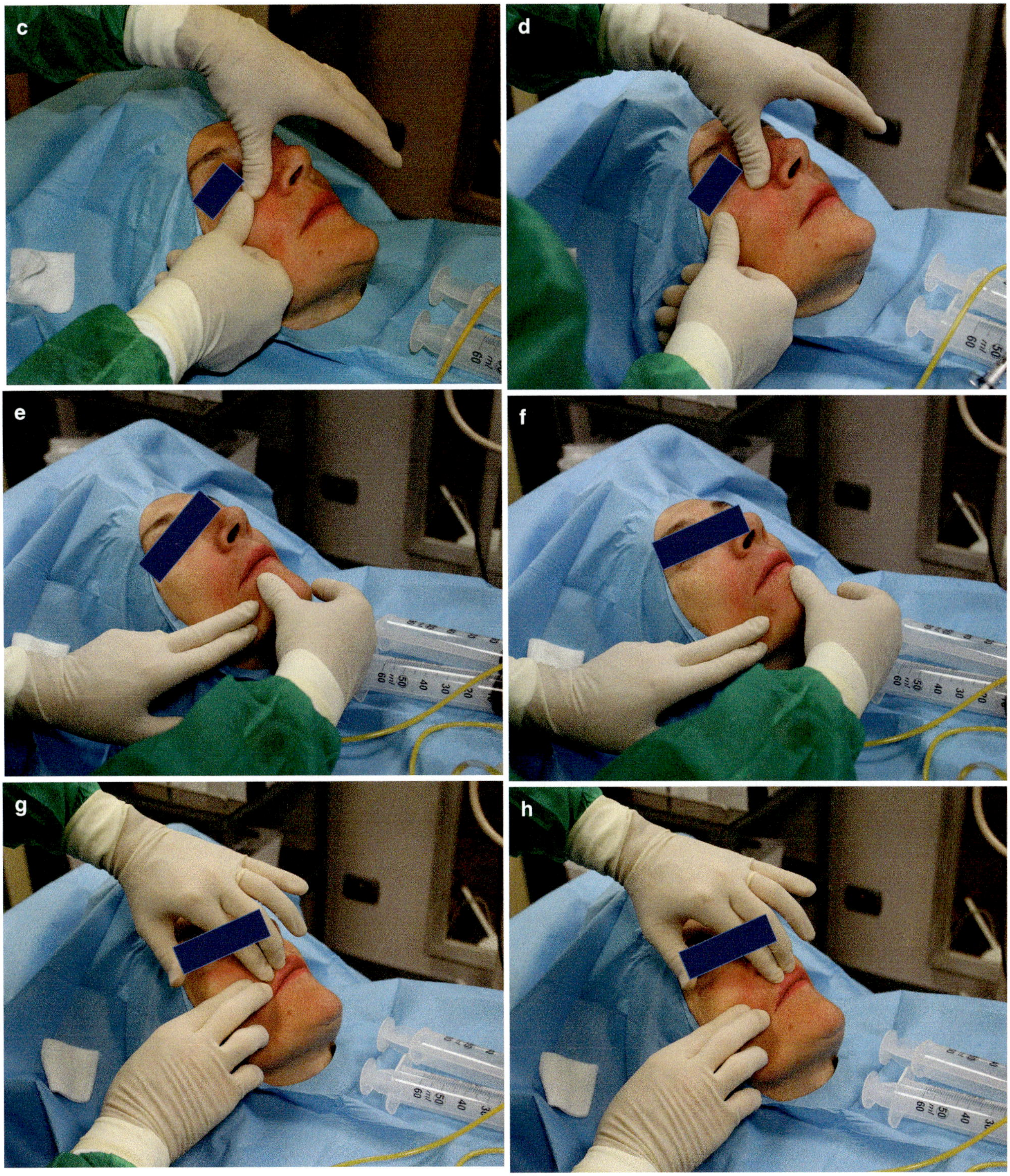

Fig. 7.14 (continued)

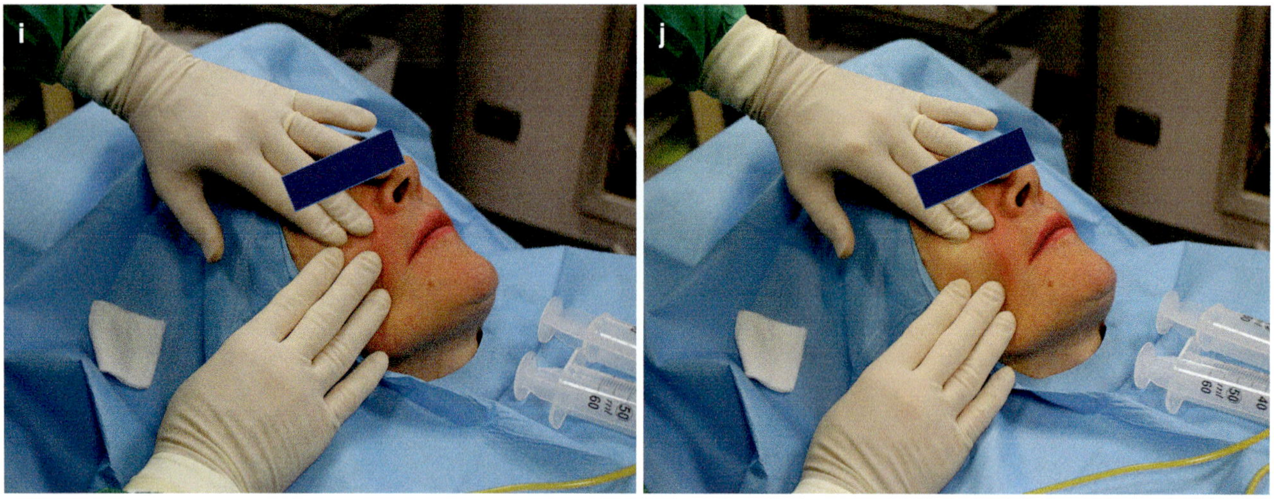

Fig. 7.14 (continued)

The Chain and the Fat Killers

8

Mario Goisis, Sara Izzo and Giovanni Francesco Nicoletti

The microfat procedure consists in a number of different steps. For example, we have to harvest the fat, process it, mix it with prp, and, finally, inject it into recipient sites. These four steps may be considered the four different links of a chain, as it were.

Because a chain is only as strong as its weakest link, it is mandatory to construct an optimal procedure from start to finish.

In fact, if one the links of the chain is weak, then the entire procedure will be compromised.

8.1 The Large Dimensions of the Fat Particle

Fat particles are intact globules of adipocytes linked together in a mesenchymal network. It should be noted that fat particles do not exist naturally within the native tissue, but are created during a harvesting procedure.

Kato et al. recently published a landmark study, underlining the importance of the size of fat particles in grafting. He reported that within a particle, the adipocytes most likely to survive were located closest to the surface of the lobule (Fig. 8.1).

Prior to the reestablishment of a blood supply, fat particles depend largely on the simple diffusion for nutrients. As the diameter of adipose lobules become larger, the central zone of necrosis will theoretically expand according to diffusional limitations (Figs. 8.1, 8.2, and 8.3).

Therefore, one may conclude that the size of fat particles may ultimately influence how much of the grafted material survives [1].

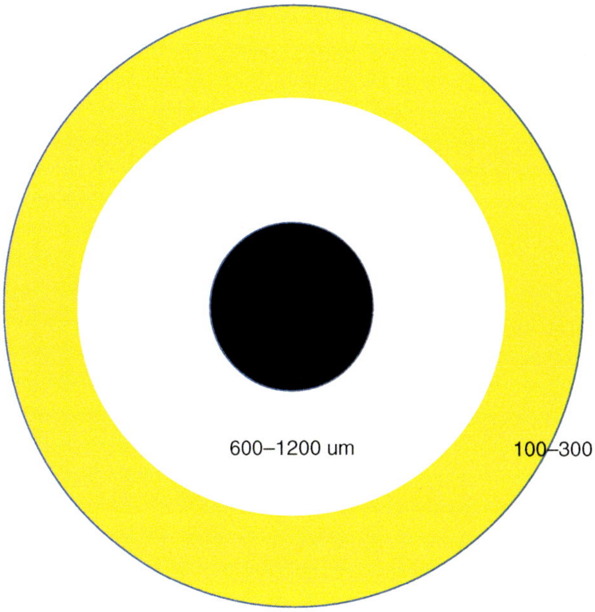

Fig. 8.1 The relationship between the diameter of a fat particle and the survival of fat. Anatomical dissection demonstrating the intramuscular and deep injection of fat. The fat was colored green before injection. (Published by kind permission of ©Mario Goisis 2018. All Rights Reserved)

Key Point

- To increase the survival of fat, it is mandatory to obtain small particles of fat.

Solution

- To use harvesting cannulas with a small port size

M. Goisis (✉)
Maxillo-Facial and Aesthetic Surgeon, Go Easy Clinic, Milan, Italy

S. Izzo · G. F. Nicoletti
Department of Plastic Surgery, University of Campania "Luigi Vanvitelli", Naples, Italy
e-mail: giovannif.nicoletti@unicampania.it

M. Goisis (ed.), *Outpatient Regenerative Medicine*, https://doi.org/10.1007/978-3-319-44894-7_8

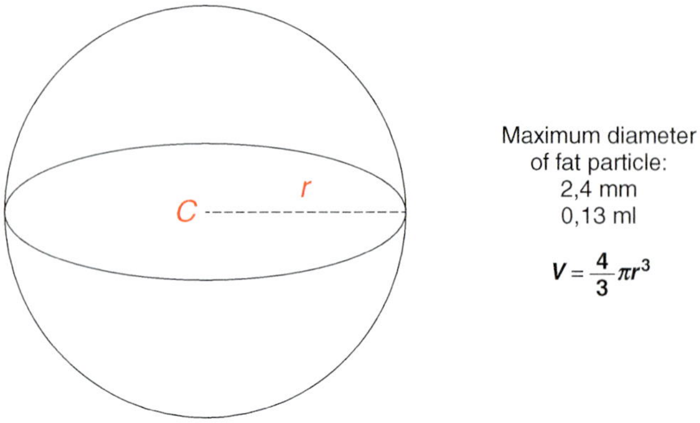

Fig. 8.2 The relationship between the diameter of the fat particle and the survival of fat. Fat injected using cannulas having a large diamenter. (Published by kind permission of ©Mario Goisis 2018. All Rights Reserved)

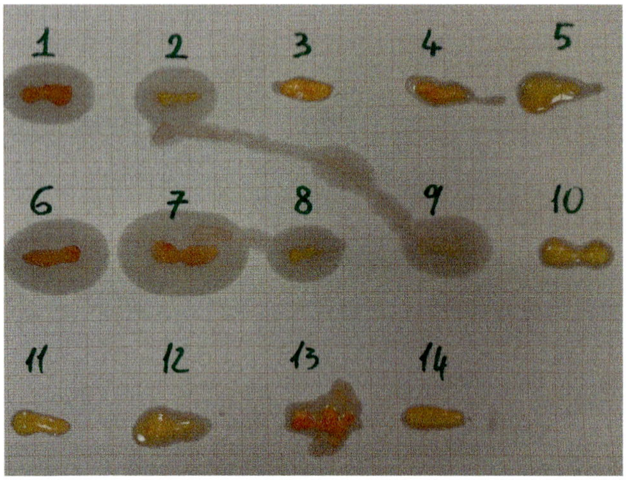

Fig. 8.3 Different sizes of fat particles. (Published by kind permission of ©Mario Goisis 2018. All Rights Reserved)

8.2 Negative Pressure

Shiffman and Mirrafati demonstrated that cellular damage was caused by vacuum pressure in excess of 700 mmHg [2].

Cheriyan et al. investigated the effect of harvest pressure on adipose survival and on the viability of the surviving cells [3].

Lipoaspiration was performed at high levels of pressure (−760 mmHg) and low levels of pressure (−250 mmHg). Adipocyte survival and cell viability were subsequently measured. Adipose viability after harvest was 47% higher when aspirated at low pressure that at higher levels of pressure. In addition, cell viability at 7 days was significantly higher when low-pressure aspiration had been applied.

This observation was confirmed by the work of Nguyen et al. that demonstrated that only 10% of the adipose particles survived after liposuction at 760 mmHg [4].

Mojallal et al. evaluated the influence of pressure on the yield of stromal vascular fraction (SVF) cells in relation to the aspiration technique. Six different harvesting conditions were tested: manual aspiration using a 10 mL syringe, wall suction, pump suction at −350, pump suction at −700 mmHg, and power-assisted liposuction at −350 and −700 mmHg. Cell yield with a pressure of −350 mmHg, assisted or not, was greater than that obtained at −700 mmHg and significantly superior to aspiration with a syringe ($p < 0.05$). The conclusion was that −350 mmHg increases the number of SVF cells harvested [5].

Lee et al. examined the effect of pressure on a nude mouse model. Positive pressure was applied to lipoaspirate up to 6 atm for up to 3 min and then injected into the flanks of mice. The application of positive pressure levels did not produce a significant difference in graft weight or histology at 4 weeks.

Key Point

- An excess of vacuum pressure destroys fat cells and ADSC.

Solution

- To use low pressure during suction, in particular by availing oneself of small or specific syringes (VacLok syringes)

8.3 Lipid

Extracellular free lipid is released from ruptured adipocytes. This material is scavenged by tissue phagocytes, and can induce an inflammatory response. Lipid cysts can be induced by inflammatory cells during foreign body response. To avoid these problems, lipid is regularly removed from grafts prepared by means of centrifugation [6].

Zhu et al. showed that extracellular lipid accounts for approximately 12% of the total graft volume in grafts prepared by centrifugation and approximately 8% of grafts prepared by gravitational sedimentation, with significant retention of lipid within the graft as demonstrated by examination at the microscope, Contrarywise, retention of oil is reduced to less than 1% in grafts prepared by washing and filtering [7].

Key Point

- Lipids induce inflammation and foreign -body response.

Solution

- Removal of the lipids. The most effective system is by washing and filtering.

8.4 Extravasated Blood Cells

Once grafted, extravasated blood cells are cleansed by means of an inflammatory process that can lead to collateral damage and loss of graft volume (Fig. 8.4). Zhu et al. showed that centrifugation and gravitational sedimentation remove approximately 50–60% of red and white blood cells [7]. Similar data were reported by Rohrich et al. and Kurita et al. [8, 9].

By comparison, washing accompanied by filtration removes more than 95% of both blood-cell types.

Key Point

- Extravasated blood cells are cleansed by means of an inflammatory process that can lead to collateral damage and loss of graft volume.

Solution

- To remove extravasated blood cells the most effective system consists in centrifugation along with washing and filtration.

8.5 Free Haemoglobin

The levels of free haemoglobin said to promote inflammation and mediate different pathways that lead to nitric oxide depletion and reactive oxidative species generation. Villaboa et al. demonstrated that after washing with an isotonic saline solution, the adipose tissue was restored to optimal physiological conditions suitable for reimplantation [10] (Fig. 8.5).

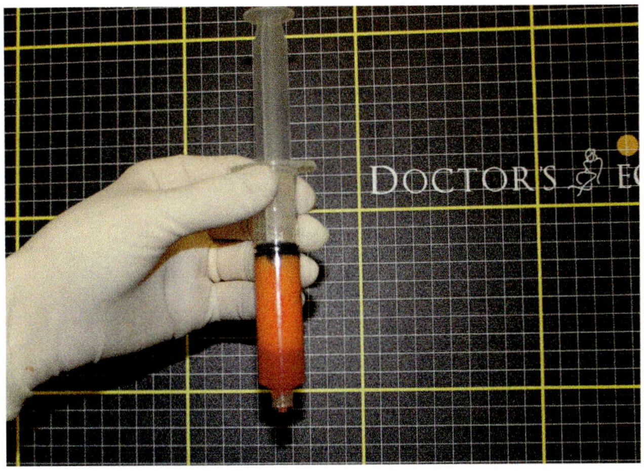

Fig. 8.4 Fat after harvesting: the extravasated blood-cell component is visible in the lower part of the syringe. (Published by kind permission of ©Mario Goisis 2018. All Rights Reserved)

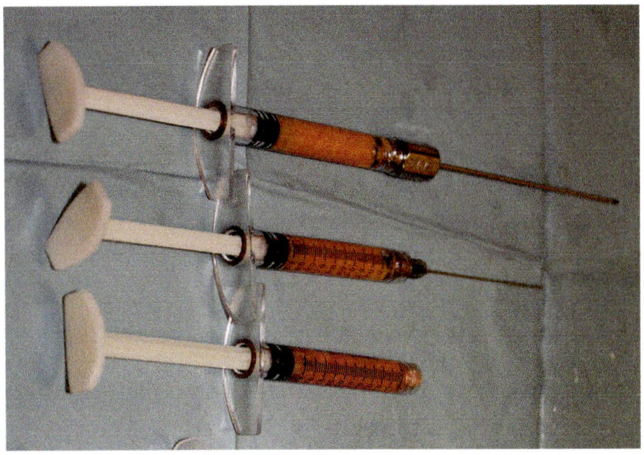

Fig. 8.5 Different sizes of fat particles

Key Point

- Free haemoglobin mediates different pathways leading to nitric oxide depletion and the generation of reactive oxidative species.

Solution

To remove free haemoglobin, washing accompanied by filtration proves to be a very effective method.

8.6 Bacteria

Infections are possible complications of fat grafting. Closed processing methods avoid exposure of fat, reducing the risks of contact with bacteria [11].

Key Point

- Bacteria can create infection.

Solution

- To reduce exposure to bacteria, use closed methods of harvesting, processing, and injection.

8.7 Local Anaesthesia

Girard et al. evaluated the role of lidocaine. In particular, infiltration was performed on the same patient with two different tumescent solutions: one side of the abdomen was infiltrated with a solution containing 1 mg/L of adenaline per 1 L of Ringer's lactate (RL), but without lidocaine; the other side was infiltrated with 0.8 mg/mL lidocaine (40 mL lidocaine 2% and adrenalin 1 mg/L per 1 L of RL).

The *adipose tissue was then processed by decantation, washing, and centrifugation* [12].

Each of the two types of adipose tissue was then injected into immunodeficient mice. Grafts were collected after 1 month and analysed histologically using a detailed scoring method. After use of lidocaine, the decantation protocol produced popr-quality adipose grafts with high resorption rates and formation of oil vacuole. On the other hand, it was demonstrated that by simply washing the adipose tissue once and using decantation without centrifugation, it was possible to obtain a graft efficiency equivalent to that of centrifugation alone. This work confirms the deleterious effects of local anesthetics in vivo (previously demonstrated in vitro).

Key Point

- The contact of fat with local anaesthesia for many hours leads to poor-quality adipose grafts with high resorption rates and formation of oil vacuole.

Solution

- Not to use local anaesthesia in the harvesting site.
- To remove local anaesthesia from the graft. The most effective system is washing accompanied by filtration.
- To inject only a small amount of local anaesthesia into the recipient site.

8.8 Irregular Distribution of Water

The amount of aqueous fluid present in a fat graft jeopardises graft retention, as the water is rapidly resorbed by the body following implantation. Surgeons routinely compensate for this phenomenon by overfilling the site of the graft. This can create problems in cases of volume limitations at the implantation site. Despite this, it is mandatory to be able to avail oneself of a system which standardises the percentage of the amount of aqueous fluid. In fact, it is obvious that the use of a graft with a low percentage of water on one side of the face and of one with a high percentage of water on the other side, will lead clearly to asymmetry.

Zhu et al. showed that centrifugation and processing by washing accompanied by filtration using the Puregraft system were the most effective ways of reducing the amount of aqueous liquid in the graft. This is coherent with data from Kurita et al., who showed that centrifugation condenses the tissue, thereby reducing the aqueous liquid content [7, 8].

Key Point

- The amount of aqueous fluid resent in a fat graft compromises graft retention, as the water is rapidly resorbed. Irregular distribution of water can lead to asymmetry in the grafted area.

Solution

- To use a system that guarantees uniform removal of the fraction of aqueous fluid from a fat graft. Washing accompanied by filtration is a very effective method by which to achieve removal.

8.9 Shear Stress

For lipofilling, shear stress is brought to bear on the fat as it is pushed through some kind of tube, such as a cannula. As to velocity that of shear stress is proportional to the viscosity of the fat. When viscosity is high, a high level of shear stress will also be produced. *Exposing fat to high shear rates will result in irreversible damage, and the mechanical integrity of the fat cannot fully recover from this damage.*

Key Point

- Exposing fat to high shear rates will result in irreversible damage.

Solution

- To use a system that guarantees low viscosity and low shear stress

8.10 High Speed During Injection

High flow rates have been shown to be harmful to fat because they induce [inducing] [more] greater shear stress. In particular, flow rates in the order of 0.5–1 cc/s have thus been recommended by Lee et al. to optimize fat viability [13].

In the same article, the authors, validating the work of Shiffman and Mirrafati, demonstrated that high flow rates significantly damage fat when evaluated by histology [2].

At the FACE conference, Goisis et al. presented a study on shear stress during the washing, filtration, and injection of fat using the Goisis system and comparing it with Coleman technique and Lipogems technology.

The reduction in terms of viscosity of the fat using the Goisis system (injection with a 22-gauge cannula) was significantly lower compared with the reduction obtained aplly-ing the Lipogems (injection with the 25-gauge cannula) and Coleman (injection with the 22-gauge cannula systems [14].

Key Point

- High flow rates damage fat, inducing more shear stress.

Solution

- Inject slowly!

8.11 Size of the Ports of the Harvesting Cannula

The size of the port of a cannula affects the viscosity of the graft adipocytes direcly. In particular, the use of larger port sizes increases the viscosity of the graft [15–17].

In cases of high viscosity, the fat that is pushed through a small cannula will produce a high level of shear stress. This shear stress will result in irreversible damage, and the mechanical integrity of the fat cannot fully recover from this damage.

Key Point

- Use of larger port sizes during fat harvesting increases the risk of damage to the graft during injection.

Solution

- Use harvesting cannulas with smaller port sizes.

8.12 Sharp Needle Used to Inject the Fat

A work by Smith et al. indicates that using needles for injection may be more harmful to fat than using cannulas because of potentially greater shear stress induced [18].

Key Point

- Use of needle increases damage to fat.

Solution

- Reduce the use of sharp needles to inject fat.

8.13 Injecting Fat Too Close to the Surface

Amar et al. described a technique for fat grafting rejuvenation that targets specific anatomic structures and tissue beds [19].

They called it the "facial autologous muscular injection" (FAMI) technique. In their opinion, it is possible to maximize the survival of the adipocyte by placing it within close proximity to or ever within the facial -expression muscles. Fat is transferred to 1 cc syringes and attached to one of nine different cannulas shaped to conform to the musculoskeletal contours. The groups of muscles is injected with 1–3 cc of fat, retrograde fashion, from the insertion to the origin or vice versa. Each syringe is emptied in one to three passes. The only exception is the infraorbital area, where no more than 0.5 cc can be grafted because of the risk of nodules and cysts. The rationale of the FAMI technique is that fat will survive optimally when grafted into a rich muscular vascular plexus.

Postoperative suggestions are based on the principle that "The less movement there is, the more successful the graft will ultimately be." For this reason, patients should avoid, not only laughing or brusque, marked facial movements but also talking of any kind. Patients should avoid public appearances that demand vocal interaction, as well as talking on the phone.

This limitation of facial -muscle stress also extends to a patient's diet, which should excluse hard foods like apples or harder breads. Instead, patients should eat softer foods, such as bananas, take pains to avoid food items requiring e undue stress to their jaws [20] (http://www.drrogeramar.com/fami_step_step.php).

Goisis et al. described the injection of fat with a 22-gauge cannula into an intramuscular deep plane. In particular, by using a flexible cannula and a sole injection point it is possible to inject fat into this deep plane in the middle and lower third of the face. The injection technique was demonstrated by anatomical dissection [21].

Key Point

- The injection of fat into a rich muscular vascular plexus increases the survival of cells.

Solution

- Inject fat into a deep plane, in close proximity to, or into the muscular plane.

8.14 Injecting Fat with Cannulas with a Large Diameter

In the classical Coleman technique, injection of fat is performed using Coleman cannulas (diameter 1–1.5 mm) with which droplets are injected into a three-dimensional space.

Between 10 and 25 cc of the fat is injected into the superficial and deeper planes on each side of the face. Generally, superficial injection is performed in the temporal region (above the superficial temporal fascia for reasons of vascularization), the crow's -feet area, and the anterior part of the cheek (to allow for direct support of the skin in the latter two zones). Injection into deeper planes is performed in the case of malar eminence, suborbicularis oculi fat (SOOF), tear trough, the central part of the midface, the nasolabial folds, and the marionette folds.

The large diameter of the cannulas, combined with the multiplane technique, is usually associated with the production of oedema and hematomas. Willemsen et al. reported that patients who underwent lipofilling using the Coleman technique took 18.9 days to resume their social activities, which was reduced to 13.2 days when the fat was combined with PRP (Fig. 8.2).

Despite this, the dead space in the healing phase increases when large cannulas are used. This space will fill the scarring tissue with serum and reduce cell integration [22].

Goisis et al. [21] suggested a thin deep layer injection with a 22-gauge cannula. In particular, the fat harvested using the Goisis microcannula has a low level of viscosity. Because of this, it is possible to inject it with a small cannula creating a low level of shear stress. Goisis et al. compared preinjection and postinjection viscosity; the variation proved to be minimal. The preservation of viscosity is a demonstration of the preservation of the integrity of the fat.

The use of a small cannula creates a small dead space, reducing the scarring tissue interfering with cell integration.

Injection into the deep plane takes place in close proximity to a rich muscular vascular plexus. The technique is very simple, and is based on four key points of entry. These points make it possible to inject the malar area, the cheeks, the nasolabial folds, lips, chin and lacrimal sulcus.

Key Points

- Disposing of large adipose parcel sizes during harvesting means having to use large cannulas to inject the fat.
- The use of big cannulas increases death space, and reduces the survival of the cells.
- The use of big cannulas increases oedema and haematomas.

Solution

- Harvest small-sized adipose particles and inject these with small cannulas.

8.15 Injecing Fat in Areas with Reduced Vascularization

The success of fat grafting increases in the presence of well-vascularised recipient sites [23].

Despite this, many authors report fat grafting in scarred surgical fields and in irradiated tissues that are clearly ischemic [24].

In these settings, many reports demonstrated improved quality of skin following fat grafting [25].

Garza et al. investigated the effect of fat grafting on irradiated skin in a nude mouse. Fat grafting resulted in increased vascular density, decreased dermal thickness, and decreased collagen content. Histological evaluation of grafts demonstrated no difference in quality between the irradiated and non-irradiated groups. Despite this, CT analysis demonstrated significantly decreased graft retention rates in the irradiated group when compared to the nonirradiated group [26].

Key Point

- The survival of fat is reduced in cases of irradiated skin.
- After injection of fat, improvemnet of the skin linked to adipose stem-cells can be observed.
- It is suggested that fat be injected also into irradiated area but it is mandatory to inform the patient about high resorption rates and the need for multiple touch-ups.

8.16 Injection of an Over-Large Bolus of Fat

Kato et al. recently published a landmark study, underlining the importance of the size of fat particles in grafting. As previously discussed, the particle structure of fat does not occur in the native tissue, but is created, rather, during the harvesting and processing procedure [1].

At the same time, it is important to note that injection is the third link in a single chain. It is not sufficient to obtain small particles of fat by harvesting and processing. The small particle is actually injected very close to the other particles, thus producing a single large bolus. In particular, the adipocytes most likely to survive were located closer to the surface of the bolus. Based on histological findings, this bolus may be divided into three sections: the layer closest to the surface where all the adipocytes survived, the middle layer where the adipocytes die but are replaced by proliferating stem-cells, and a central core dominated by necrosis, oil cysts, and fibrosis. Demarcation of the surviving outer zone and the regenerating middle occurred at 1–300 um and 600–1200 um from the surface, respectively. Prior to the reestablishment of a blood supply, fat particles largely depend on simple diffusion for nutrients. As the diameter of the adipose lobules become larger, the central necrotic area will expand according to its diffusional limitations.

Therefore, one can see that the size of the injected bolus may ultimately influence how much of the grafted material survives.

Key Point

- To increase the survival of fat, it is mandatory not to inject the particles of fat very close to the other particles.

Solution

- Use a small cannula to inject a small amount of fat, by moving the cannula in the recipient bed and avoid injecting particles very close to each other.

References

1. Eto H, Kato H, Suga H, Aoi N, Doi K, Kuno S, Yoshi- mura K. The fate of adipocytes after nonvascularized fat grafting: evidence of early death and replacement of adipocytes. Plast Reconstr Surg. 2012;129:1081–92.
2. Shiffman MA, Mirrafati S. Fat transfer techniques: the effect of harvest and transfer methods on adipocyte viability and review of the literature. Dermatol Surg. 2001;27:819–26.
3. Cheriyan T, Kao HK, Qiao X, Guo L. The effect of harvest pressure on adipose survival. Plast Reconstr Surg. 2014;133(6):1365–8.
4. Nguyen P, Desouches C, Gay A, Hautier A, Magalon G. Development of micro-injection as an innovative autologous fat graft technique: the use of adipose tissue as dermal filler. J Plast Reconstr Aesthet Surg. 2012;65:1692–9.
5. Mojallal A, Auxenfans C, Lequeux C, Braye F, Damour O. Influence of negative pressure when harvesting adipose tissue on cell yield of the stromal-vascular fraction. Biomed Mater Eng. 2008;18(4-5):193–7.
6. Pu LL, Coleman SR, Cui X, Ferguson RE Jr, Vasconez HC. Autologous fat grafts harvested and refined by the Coleman technique: a comparative study. Plast Reconstr Surg. 2008;122:932–7.
7. Zhu M, Cohen SR, Hicok KC, Shanahan RK, Strem BM, Yu JC, Arm DM, Fraser JK. Comparison of three different fat graft preparation methods: gravity separation, centrifugation, and simultaneous washing with filtration in a closed system. Plast Reconstr Surg. 2013 Apr;131(4):873–80.
8. Kurita M, Matsumoto D, Shigeura T, et al. Influences of centrifugation on cells and tissues in liposuction aspirates: optimized centrifugation for lipotransfer and cell isolation. Plast Reconstr Surg. 2008;121:1033–41.
9. Rohrich RJ, Sorokin ES, Brown SA. In search of improved fat transfer viability: a quantitative analysis of the role of centrifugation and harvest site. Plast Reconstr Surg. 2004;113:391–5.
10. Dos-Anjos Vilaboa S, Llull R, Mendel TA. Returning fat grafts to physiologic conditions using washing. Plast Reconstr Surg. 2013 Aug;132(2):323e–6e.
11. Yoshimura K, Coleman SR. Complications of fat grafting: how they occur and how to find, avoid, and treat them. Clin Plast Surg. 2015;42(3):383–8.
12. Girard AC, Mirbeau S, Gence L. Effect of washes and centrifugation on the efficacy of lipofilling with or without local anesthetic. Plast Reconstr Surg Glob Open. 2015;3(8):e496.
13. Lee JH, Kirkham JC, McCormack MC, Nicholls AM, Randolph MA, Austen WG Jr. The effect of pressure and shear on autologous fat grafting. Plast Reconstr Surg. 2013;131:1125–36.
14. Goisis M. Comparison between different techniques. Face congress, London; 2016.
15. Farr ST, Trivisonno A. Differential fat harvesting. Plast Aesthet Res. 2014;1:103–7.
16. Kirkham JC, et al. The impact of liposuction cannula size on adipocyte viability. Ann Plast Surg. 2012;69:479–81.
17. Erdim M, Tezel E, Numanoglu A, Sav A. The effects of the size of liposuction cannula on adipocyte survival and the optimum temperature for fat graft storage: an experimental study. J Plast Reconstr Aesthet Surg. 2009;62:1210–4.
18. Smith P, Adams WP Jr, Lipschitz AH, et al. Autologous human fat grafting: effect of harvesting and preparation techniques on adipocyte graft survival. Plastic Reconstr Surg. 2006;117:1836–44.
19. Amar RE, Fox DM. The facial autologous muscular injection (FAMI) procedure: an anatomically targeted deep multiplane autologous fat-grafting technique using principles of facial fat injection. Aesthet Plast Surg. 2011;35(4):502–10.
20. Amar RE, Fox DM, Balin A. Cannulation and injection of the muscles of facial expression: a cadaver study. Dermatol Surg. 2010;36(3):331–8. https://doi.org/10.1111/j.1524-4725.2009.
21. Goisis M. Anatomy of fat injection, a cadaveric dissection demonstration. 5cc congress, Barcellona, 2016.
22. Willemsen J, van der Lei B, Vermeulen K, Stevens H. The effects of platelet-rich plasma on recovery time and aesthetic outcome in facial rejuvenation: preliminary retrospective observations. Aesthetic Plast Surg. 2014;38:1057–63.
23. Del Vecchio D, Rohrich RJ. A classification of clinical fat grafting: different problems, different solutions. Plast Reconstr Surg. 2012;130:511–22.
24. Salgarello M, Visconti G, Farallo E. Autologous fat graft in radiated tissue prior to alloplastic reconstruction of the breast: report of two cases. Aesthet Plast Surg. 2010;34:5–10.
25. Phulpin B, Gangloff P, Tran N, Bravetti P, Merlin JL, Dolivet G. Rehabilitation of irradiated head and neck tissues by autologous fat transplantation. Plast Reconstr Surg. 2009;123:1187–97.
26. Garza RM, Paik KJ, Chung MT, Duscher D, Gurtner GC, Longaker MT, Wan DC. Studies in fat grafting: part III. Fat grafting irradiated tissue—improved skin quality and decreased fat graft retention. Plast Reconstr Surg. 2014;134(2):249–57.

Comparison of Different Techniques of Fat Grafting

9

Mario Goisis, Sara Izzo, Andrea Sbarbati, Giamaica Conti, and Giovanni Francesco Nicoletti

A chain is only as strong as its weakest link.

The famous Pala di Brera (also known as the Montefeltro Altarpiece or Brera Altarpiece), tempera on wood, was painted in 1472–1474 by the Italian Renaissance master Piero della Francesca (Figs. 9.1 and 9.2).

At the centre of the painting, hanging by a chain from the shell-shaped ceiling of the apse, is an egg, emblem of the promise of immortality and regeneration. We like to think of fat grafting as if it were the chain portrayed in the Pala. In fact, during the transfer of fat, we have four different steps: fat harvesting, fat processing, mixing of fat with PRP and/or stem-cells, and the injection of the fat into recipient sites. These four steps might be compared to four different links of a chain (Fig. 9.3).

Therefore, it is mandatory to design an optimal procedure from start to finish, because a chain is only as strong as its weakest link.

If one of the chain's links is weak, then the entire sequence will be compromised. In the case of the Piero's chain, the egg will fall. In the case of fat transfer, the fat cells will not survive and will not regenerate in the recipient site (Fig. 9.4).

9.1 The Integrity of Adipocytes

The graft with the greatest number of intact adipocytes will have the greatest chance of long-term durability.

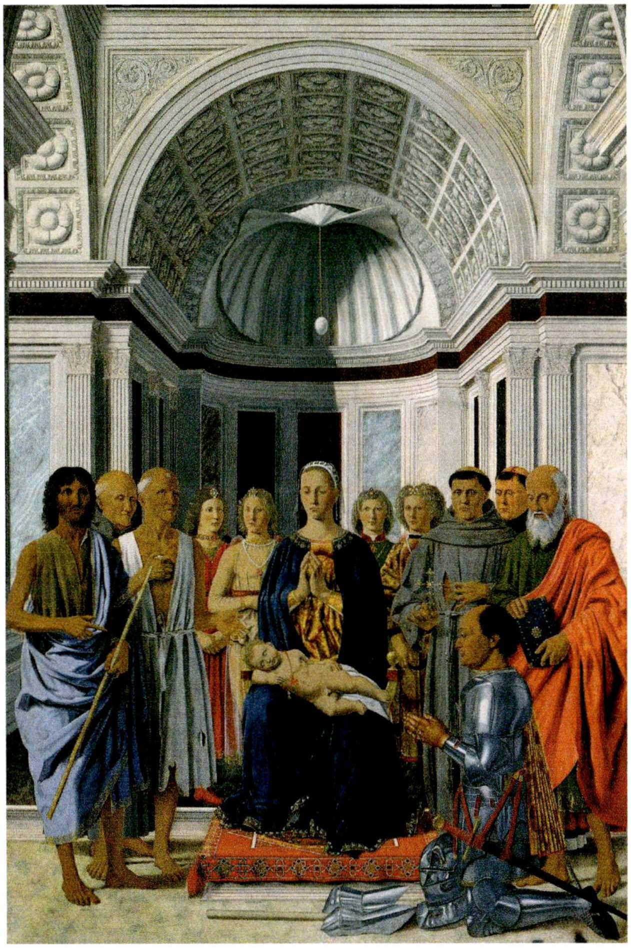

Fig. 9.1 The famous Pala di Brera. (Published by kind permission of ©Mario Goisis 2018. All Rights Reserved)

The quality of grafting procedures can be evaluated from many points of view.

The first point is that of guaranteeing the preservation of the integrity and viability of adipocytes being transferred. This element was first stressed by Peer in his landmark article of 1955, and his theory is known as "the cell survival theory." According to this theory, the graft with the greatest

M. Goisis (✉)
Maxillo-Facial and Aesthetic Surgeon, Go Easy Clinic, Milan, Italy

S. Izzo · G. F. Nicoletti
Department of Plastic Surgery, University of Campania "Luigi Vanvitelli", Naples, Italy
e-mail: giovannif.nicoletti@unicampania.it

A. Sbarbati · G. Conti
Department of Neuroscience, Biomedicine and Movement, Human Anatomy and Histology Section, University of Verona, Verona, Italy
e-mail: andrea.sbarbati@univr.it; giamaica.conti@univr.it

M. Goisis (ed.), *Outpatient Regenerative Medicine*, https://doi.org/10.1007/978-3-319-44894-7_9

number of intact adipocytes will have the greatest chance of long-term durability [1].

Many events occurring during fat harvesting, processing, and injection can disrupt adipocytes.

For example, it is mandatory to avoid an excess of negative pressure.

As regards the effects of this on fat graft, in particular, many authors reported that a great amount of cellular damage took place when a vacuum pressure of 700 mmHg was exceeded [2–4].

Despite this, to preserve adipocytes it is important to apply a low degree of shear stress.

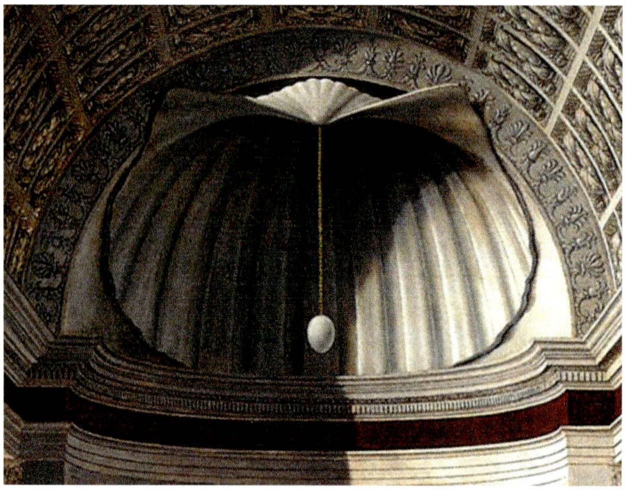

Fig. 9.2 The famous Pala di Brera or Brera Altarpiece, detail. (Published by kind permission of ©Mario Goisis 2018. All Rights Reserved)

Shear stress occurs when a force acts parallel to a surface, despite the perpendicular force brought to bear on it. For example, rubbing one's hands together induces shear stress, while pressing one's palms against each other does not.

For lipofilling, shear stress is applied to the fat as it is pushed through tubes, like cannulas used for harvesting or for injecting. As a viscoelastic material, fat undergoes shear-thinning. This simply means that as shear stress increases, the viscosity of the material decreases.

Some shear-thinning materials can "self-heal," meaning that they recover their original viscosity fully after being exposed to forces like shear stress or negative pressure.

This is not the case of fat. In fact, the exposure of fat to high shear or negative pressure rates will result in irreversible damage, and the mechanical integrity of the fat cannot fully recover from this damage.

In order to evaluate the shear stress applied by the different methods, we measured the viscosity of tissue after harvesting, after processing, and after injection.

The aim of different procedures is cause as little reduction of viscosity as possible during all the steps of fat grafting.

Here, a rheometer was used to measure the storage modulus and shear rate at which tissues began to lose their solid-like properties (Fig. 9.5). Viscosity was also measured and the gross properties of treatment groups were qualitatively evaluated by means of a glass slide test (Figs. 9.6 and 9.7).

Despite this, adipose tissue samples collected from each method were prepared for microscopic evaluation by spreading the tissue onto microscope slides. Samples were observed for the presence of free lipid and blood cells. Demonstrative

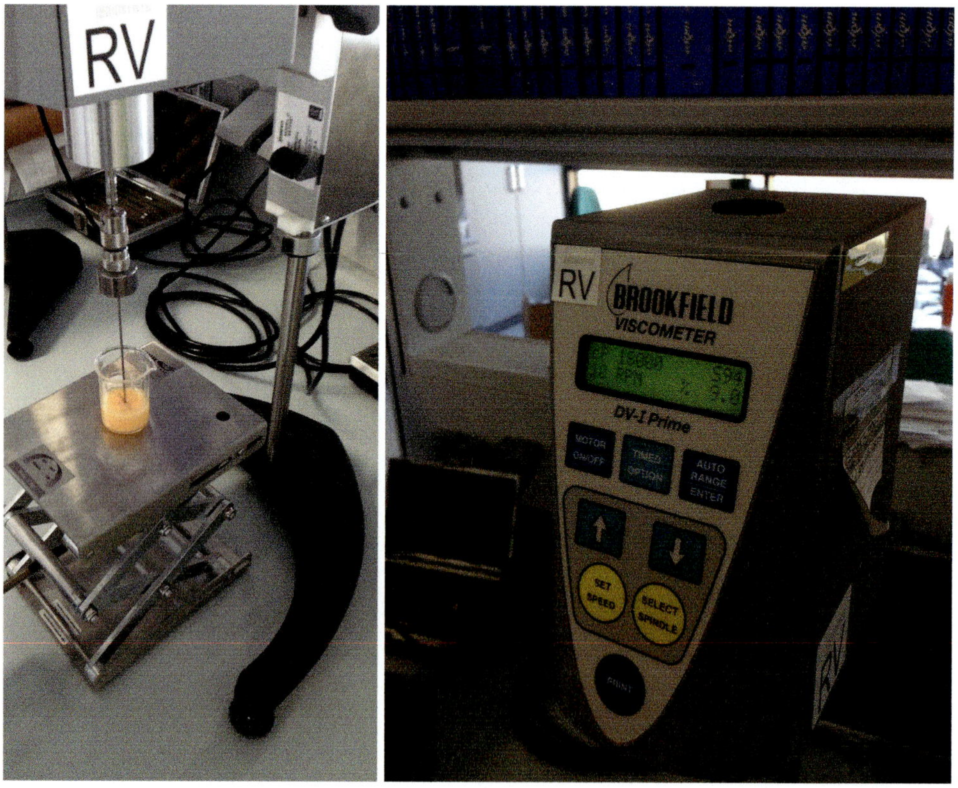

Fig. 9.3 A viscometer (also called viscosimeter) is an instrument used to measure the viscosity of a fluid. Rotational viscometers are based on the idea that the torque required to turn an object in a fluid is a function of the viscosity of that fluid. They measure the torque required to rotate a bob in a fluid at a known speed. (courtesely by Istituto Ganassini, Milano). (Published by kind permission of ©Mario Goisis 2018. All Rights Reserved)

images were captured at 100 magnification using a digital camera (Figs. 9.8, 9.9, and 9.10)

9.1.1 Methods

Lipoaspirate samples were obtained from 10 healthy donors following informed consent, in accordance with AeQ guidelines (www.microfat.com). Lipoaspirate samples were obtained using different techniques.

The viscosity of fat harvested using different techniques was measured.

The lipoaspirate was then processed applying different techniques. After processing, the viscosity of fat, harvested and processed by different techniques, was measured.

Finally, the processed lipoaspirate was passed through the cannula for injection. After passage into this cannula, the viscosity of fat harvested, processed, and injected using different techniques was measured.

In particular, a viscometer was used to measure the storage modulus and shear rate at which the tissues analysed began to lose their solid-like properties (Fig. 9.11). Viscosity was also measured and the gross properties of treatment groups were qualitatively evaluated by means of a glass slide test (Figs. 9.12 and 9.13).

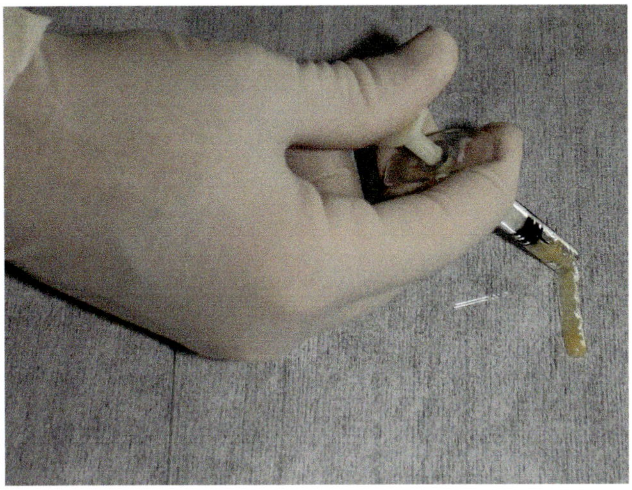

Fig. 9.4 Glass Slide Testing. (Published by kind permission of ©Mario Goisis 2018. All Rights Reserved)

A small aliquot of each sample is placed on a flat sheet of glass. The glass sheet is then quickly turned by 60 degrees and different samples are observed by standard pictures obtained using a digital Canon camera.

9.1.2 Results

9.1.2.1 Harvesting

Cannulas port sizes affect the viscosity of graft adipocytes direcly. In particular, the use of larger port sizes increases the viscosity of the graft.

High level of negative pressure disrupts adipocytes: it is better to use 10 cc or VacLok syringes to avoid an excess of negative pressure.

The Goisis cannula is associated with better preservation of fat compared with the 3 mm rounded-tip cannula with a single elliptic suction port on the side near its distal end (port diameter: 3 × 9 mm) (Figs. 9.14 and 9.15).

9.1.2.2 Processing

After decantation (Figs. 9.16, 9.17, and 9.18) the lower layer of the decanted sample is a low-viscosity liquid tissue, but its colour is red-orange because it is very rich in red cells (Figs. 9.19, 9.20, 9.21, 9.22, 9.23 and 9.24).

After centrifugation, the middle layer of the centrifuged sample is a high-viscosity compact tissue, which is, however, is very rich in destroyed, nonviable adipocytes (Fig. 9.25).

After washing and filtering, the fat has a very lowrate of viscosity and the colour is yellow (Fig. 9.26).

9.1.2.3 Injection

Injecting high or medium viscosity fat using a small cannula (22 Gauge) decreases viscosity because of high shear stress.

Sums these considerations up.

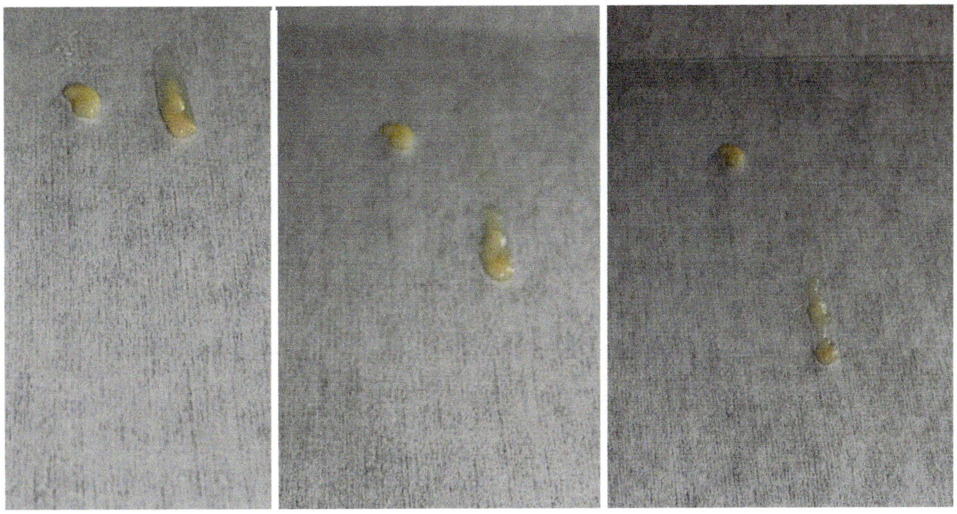

Fig. 9.5 Glass Slide Testing. (Published by kind permission of ©Mario Goisis 2018. All Rights Reserved)

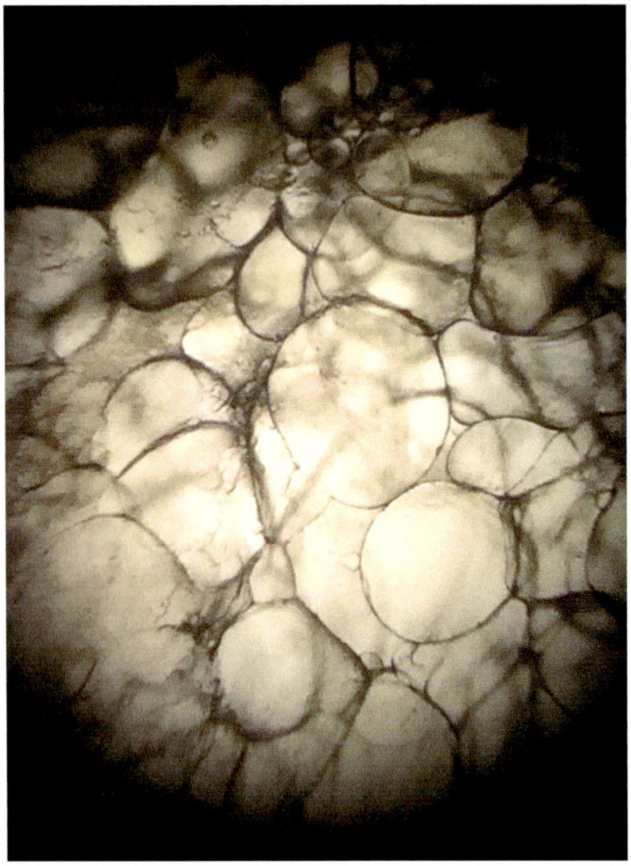

Fig. 9.6 Fat sample after harvesting (and before processing) with a 3 mm rounded-tip cannula with a single elliptic suction port on the side near its distal end (port diameter: 3 × 9 mm). A great damage of cells is demonstrated. (Published by kind permission of ©Mario Goisis 2018. All Rights Reserved)

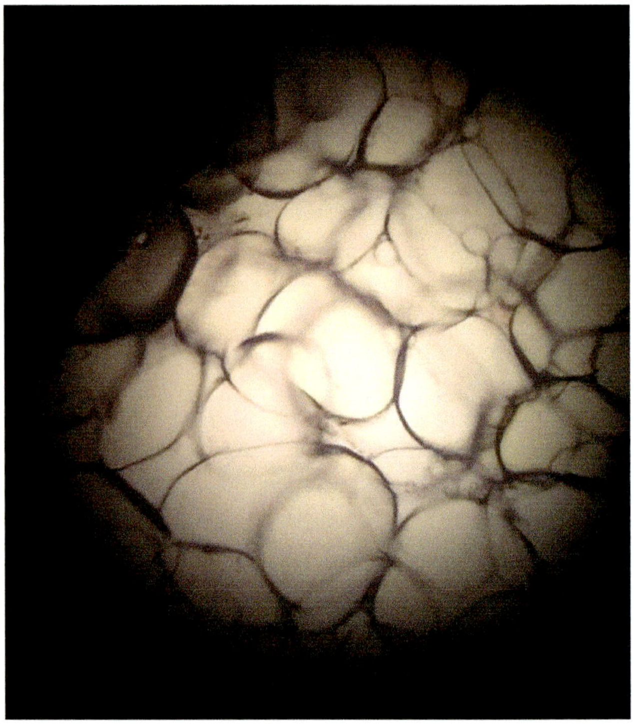

Fig. 9.7 Fat after harvesting with Goisis Cannula and before processing. A good preservation and integrity of fat cells is demonstrated. (Published by kind permission of ©Mario Goisis 2018. All Rights Reserved)

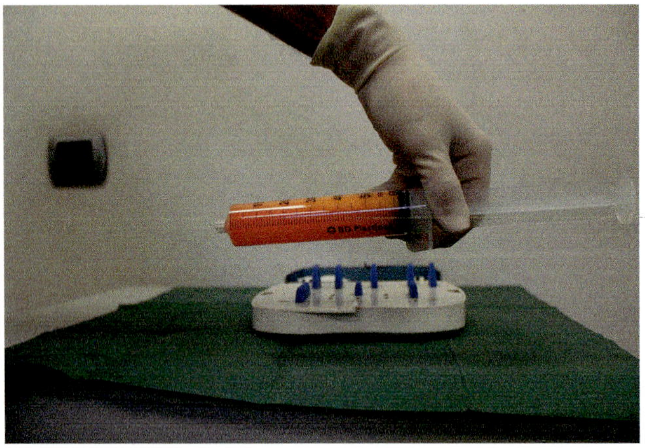

Fig. 9.8 The 60cc sirynge is filled by fat mixed with local anesthesia and blood cells. (Published by kind permission of ©Mario Goisis 2018. All Rights Reserved)

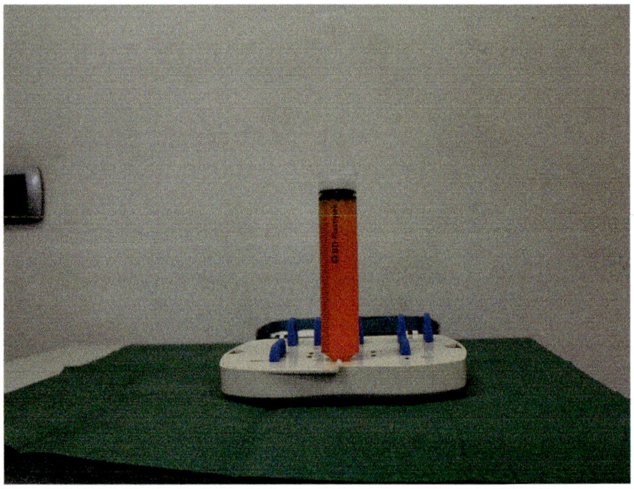

Fig. 9.9 The syringe is placed in vertical position into the Microfat Tray (www.microfat.com). (Courtesy by of the Istituto Ganassini, Milano). (Published with by kind permission of ©Mario Goisis 2018. All Rights Reserved)

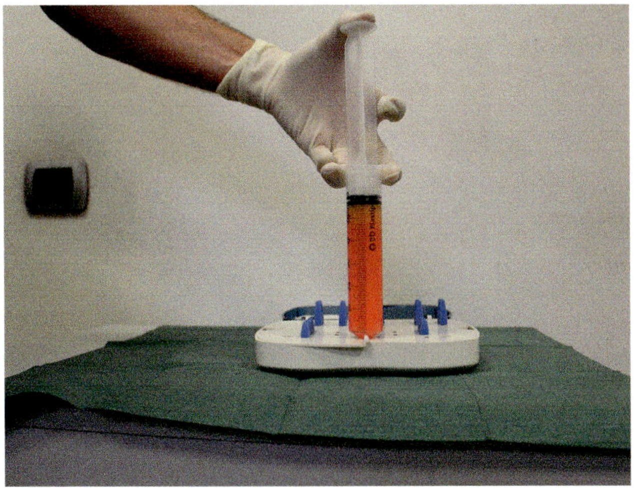

Fig. 9.10 After 10 minutes, the lower content of the syringe is pushed out. (Published by kind permission of ©Mario Goisis 2018. All Rights Reserved)

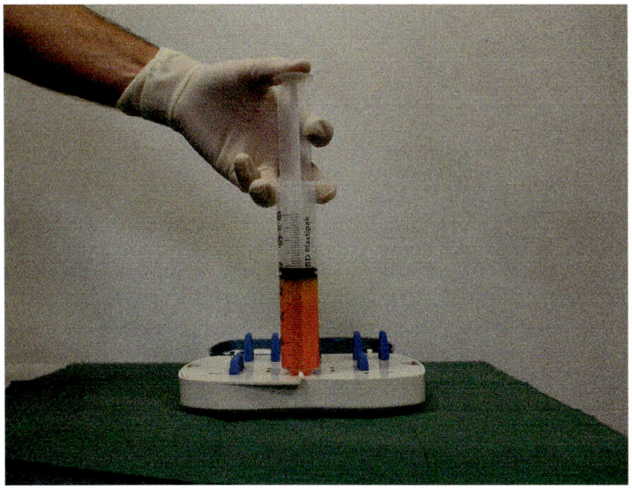

Fig. 9.11 Removal of the lower content of the syringe (Published by kind permission of ©Mario Goisis 2018. All Rights Reserved)

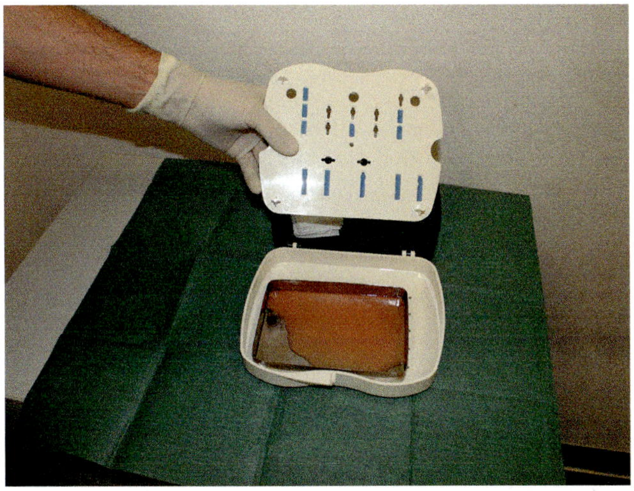

Fig. 9.12 The iron container into the Microfat tray stores the lower content of the syringe. (Published by kind permission of ©Mario Goisis 2018. All Rights Reserved)

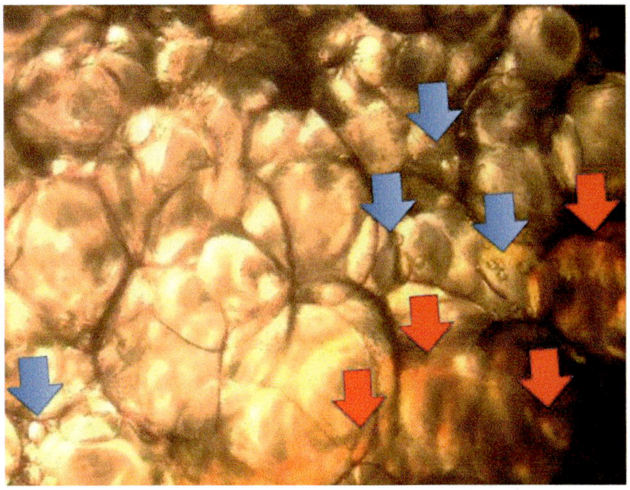

Fig. 9.13 Microscopic evaluation of fat graft tissue processed with unit gravity sedimentation. Red arrows indicate concentrated regions of red blood cells. Blue arrows identify droplets of free lipid. (Published by kind permission of ©Mario Goisis 2018. All Rights Reserved)

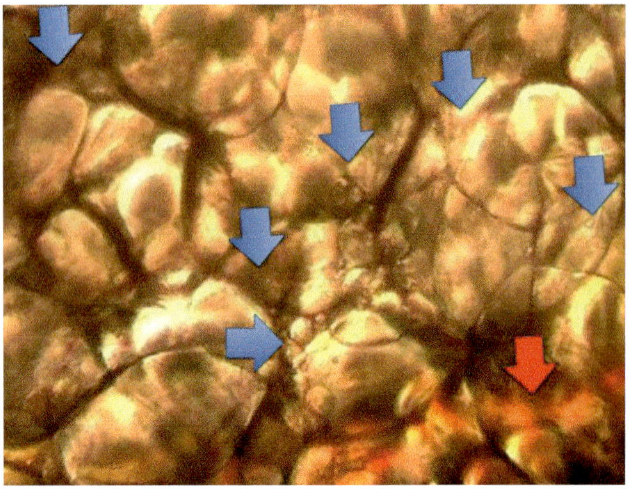

Fig. 9.14 Microscopic evaluation of fat graft tissue processed with unit gravity sedimentation. red arrows indicate concentrated regions of red blood cells. blue arrows identify droplets of free lipid. (Published by kind permission of ©Mario Goisis 2018. All Rights Reserved)

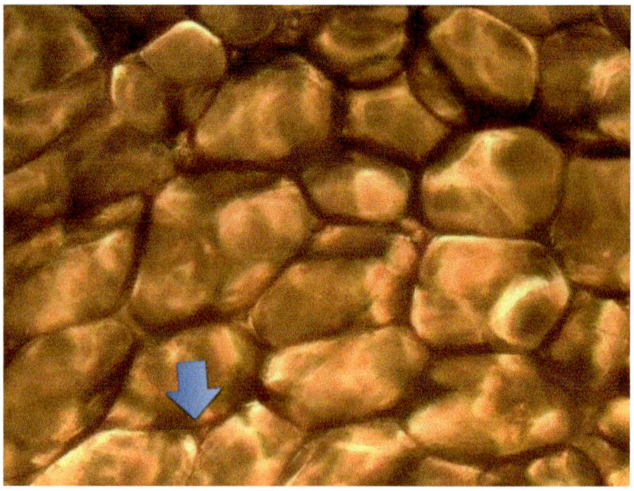

Fig. 9.15 Microscopic evaluation indicated that grafts prepared by washing with filtration with the Goisis system exhibited lower red blood cell content as well as the reduced presence of microscopic droplets of free lipid compared with grafts prepared by either gravity centrifugation or sedimentation. (Published by kind permission of ©Mario Goisis 2018. All Rights Reserved)

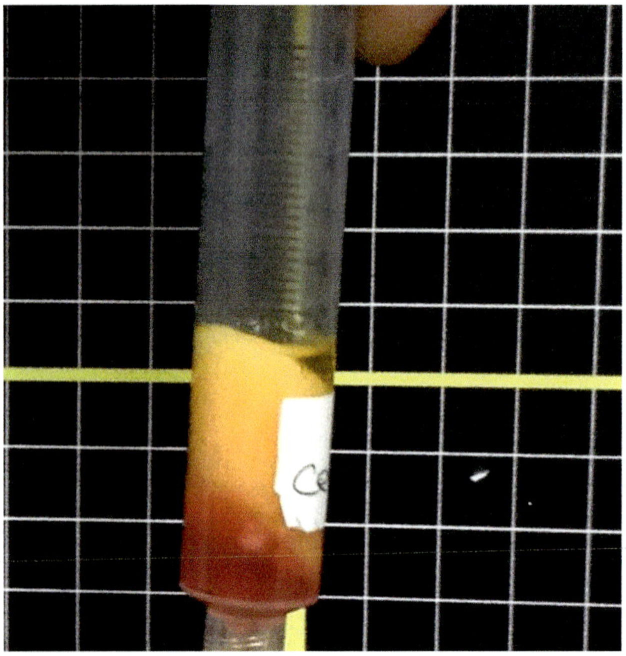

Fig. 9.16 Sample after decantation (Published by kind permission of ©Mario Goisis 2018. All Rights Reserved)

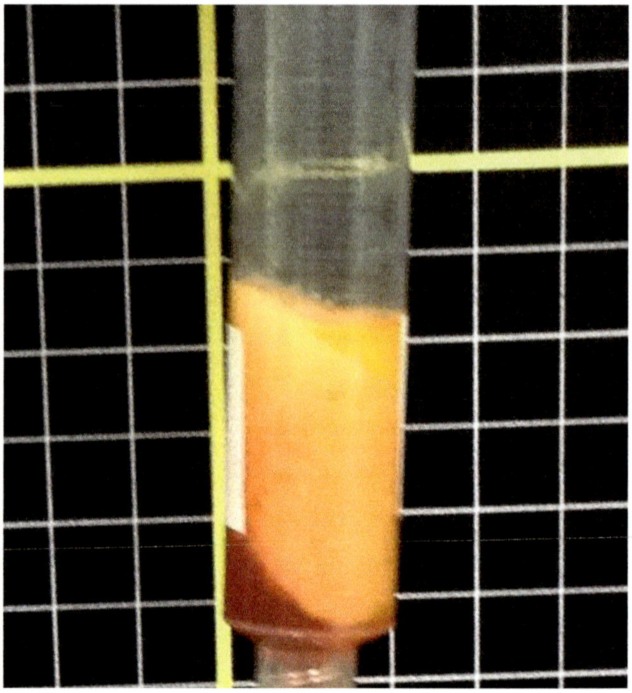

Fig. 9.17 Sample after centrifugation (Published kind permission of ©Mario Goisis 2018. All Rights Reserved)

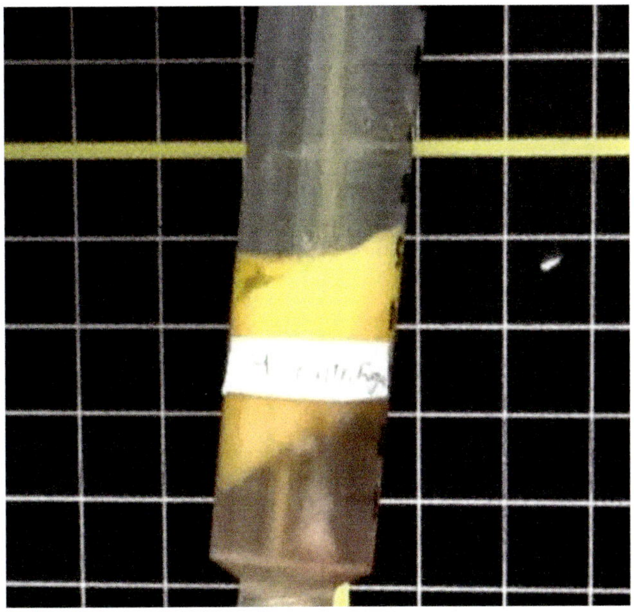

Fig. 9.18 Sample after washing with filtration. (Published by kind permission of ©Mario Goisis 2018. All Rights Reserved)

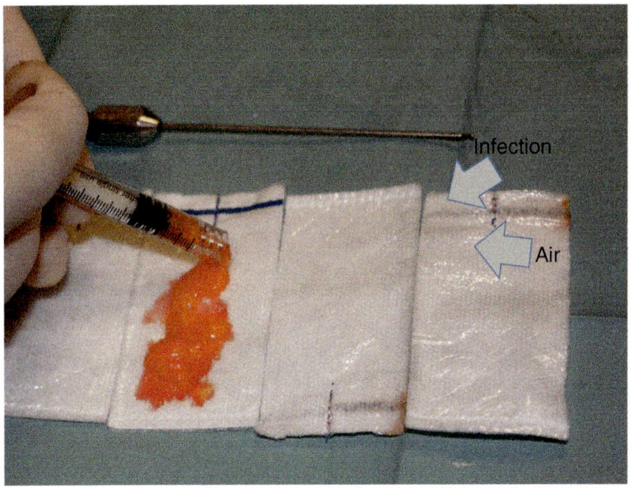

Fig. 9.19 The aspirate is poured from syringe onto large (3 × 8-inch) pieces of Telfa nonadherent dressing (Covidien, Mans eld, Mass.). All the procedure is exposed to air and potential contamination. (Published by kind permission of ©Mario Goisis 2018. All Rights Reserved)

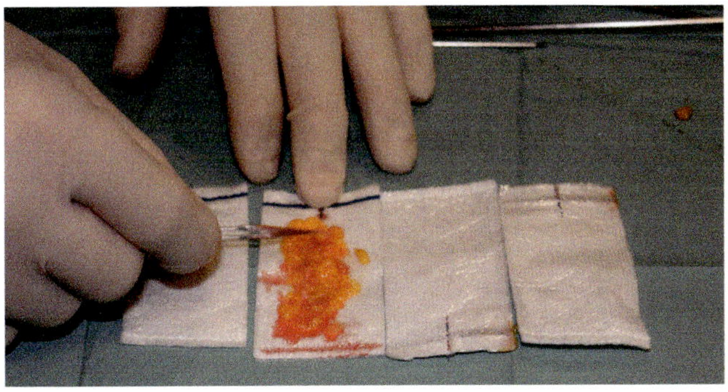

Fig. 9.20 The fat is gently rolled and kneaded along the gauze using a sterile scalpel handle. The procedure is very long and time consuming. (Published by kind permission of ©Mario Goisis 2018. All Rights Reserved)

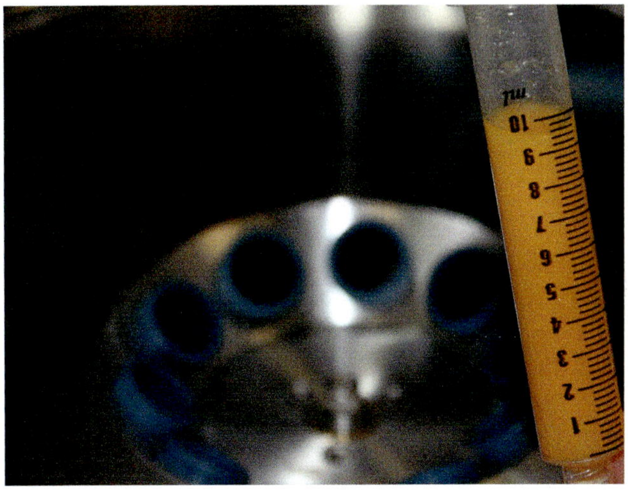

Fig. 9.21 Centrifugation: the centrifugal force damages fat cells. The greatest number of ASCs are concentrated at the bottom of the syringe by the centrifugal force and are eliminated-graft tissue processed by. The red regions of concentrated red blood cells. The blue arrows identify. (Published by kind permission of ©Mario Goisis 2018. All Rights Reserved)

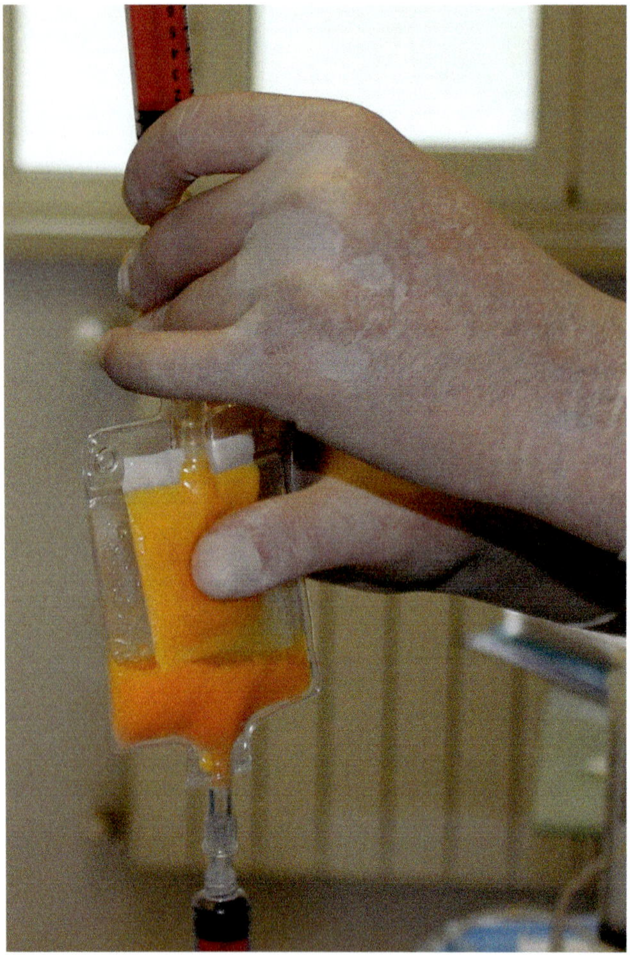

Fig. 9.22 Filtration with fastkit/PRL: damage because of compression (operator dependent), lack of filtration of blood cells and local anesthesia. (Published by kind permission of ©Mario Goisis 2018. All Rights Reserved)

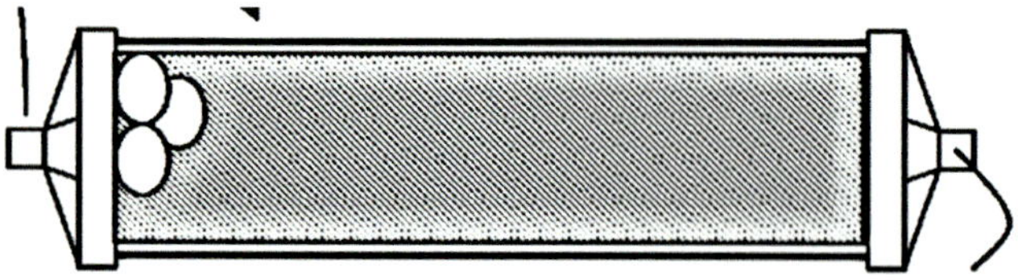

Fig. 9.23 Lipogem system: damage of fat cells by mechanical disruption. (Published by kind permission of ©Mario Goisis 2018. All Rights Reserved)

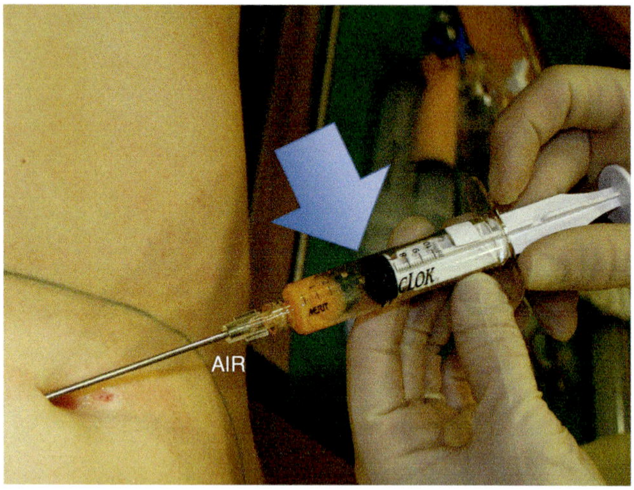

Fig. 9.25 During harvesting, because of the attachment of the cannula, the vacuum is poor. The risk of contamination is high and the time of harvesting is long (poor efficiency). (Published by kind permission of ©Mario Goisis 2018. All Rights Reserved)

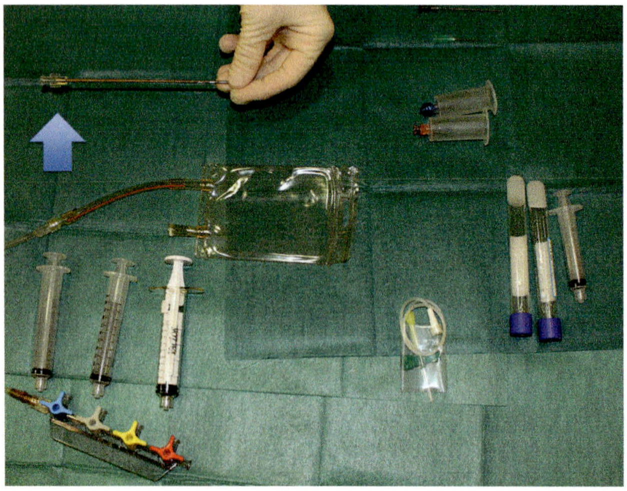

Fig. 9.24 Regenlab system. The blu arrow show the attachment of the cannula. (Published by kind permission of ©Mario Goisis 2018. All Rights Reserved)

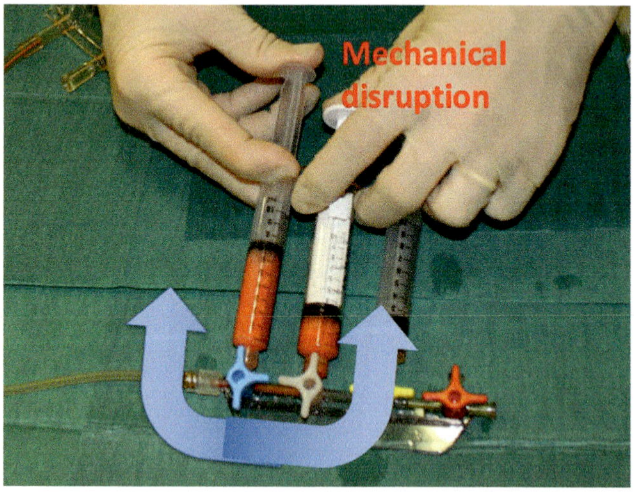

Fig. 9.26 According to the instruction provided by the producer, the fat is moved 20 times between the 2 syringes in order to mix it with saline solution. This way, the fat cells are damaged. (Published by kind permission of ©Mario Goisis 2018. All Rights Reserved)

9.2 Removal of Contaminants and Water

The removal of contaminants and water is important in order to evaluate the quality of grafting procedures.

In fact, the aim of all fat-processing procedures is the removal from lipoaspirate of nonviable, proinflammatory, and toxic components, including blood cells, the local anaesthesia used for infiltration, the remnants of ruptured fat cells, including oil droplets and cellular debris. All of these components damage fat cells.

Furthermore, it is important to remove the water component from the fat. Water mixed with fat actually creates false volume, which disappears immediately after grafting.

In order to evaluate the removal of contaminants and water in the different methods, we measured the the different densities of the components after centrifugation.

9.2.1 Methods

Lipoaspirate samples were obtained from 10 healthy donors following informed consent, in accordance with AeQ guidelines. All the lipoaspirate samples were harvested using standard techniques (Coleman cannula, 10 cc syringe).

The lipoaspirate was then processed using different techniques.

After processing, samples from each graft processing method were centrifuged at 400 g for 6 min at room temperature. After centrifugation, components with different densitieswere measured. From bottom to top: a pellet composed of stem-cells and stromal vascular fraction, microvasculature and extracellular matrix fragments, an aqueous liquid layer composed of residual anaesthetic solution or washing solution, adipose tissue, oil and free lipid layer. Volumetric measurements of different layers were recorded and reported as relative ratios of their total pre-centrifugation volume.

9.2.2 Results

Grafts prepared by gravity sedimentation had the highest relative aqueous content, whereas grafts prepared by centrifugation had the lowest aqueous content. Grafts prepared using the Puregraft and Goisis systems had intermediate aqueous liquid levels; these levels were significantly lower than those for control and gravity grafts.

The level of free lipid-oil in grafts prepared by washing and filtration was statistically significantly lower than that in the control grafts, gravity grafts, and grafts prepared by centrifugation. Analysis of the cells showed that gravity sedimentation and centrifugation techniques removed approximately 50% of the red and 60–70% of the white blood cells present in the original aspirate. By way of contrast, washing with filtration using the Goisis and Puregraft systems removed more than 95% of both blood-cell types. Telfa rolling removes water, oil, and contaminants. This technique is, however, quite long and labour intensive.

The results are shown in Figs. 9.16–9.18.

The results of our evaluations are reported in Table 9.1.

Table 9.1 The percentage of different components is classified as high, medium and low percentage

	Oil	Local anaesthesia	Washing solution	Blood cells
Telfa rolling	Low	Low	Absent	Low
Coleman	Low	Low	Absent	Medium
Sedimentation	High	High	Absent	High
Lipogems	Low	Low	High	Low
Puregraft	Low	Low	Medium	Low
PRL	High	High	Absent	High
Microfat kit	Low	Low	Medium	Low
Microfat box	Low	Low	Medium	Low

Table 9.2 Sums up the exposure of the different systems to air and infection

	The system avoids exposure to the air	Closed methods
Telfa rolling	No	No
Coleman	No	No
Sedimentation	Yes	No
Lipogems	Yes	No
Puregraft	Yes	No
PRL	Yes	No
Micrograft kit	Yes	Yes
Micrograft box	Yes	Yes

9.3 To Avoid Direct Contact between the Fat and Air and Reduce the Risk of Contamination

Air has a negative effect on adipocytes, because of the proinflammatory components and oxidative damages it activates. It is important to avoid contact with air [5].

Infections are possible complications of fat grafting. Closed methods used for processing avoid exposure of fat, reducing the risks of contact with bacteria (Table 9.2).

9.4 Preservation of the Highest Number of Viable Adipose Stem-Cells (ASCs)

For the preservation and the concentration of the highest number of viable adipose stem-cells (ASCs) it is important to evaluate the quality of the fat graft. precaution is informed by the "host replacement theory."

Table 9.3 The number of stem-cell of 6 different samples was measured . Three samples were related to Goisis technique, with high values immediately after harvesting after processing and after passing through a 22G cannula The last 3 samples were related with Coleman technique with a very signi cant modi cation: the Coleman fat was passed through a 22G cannula

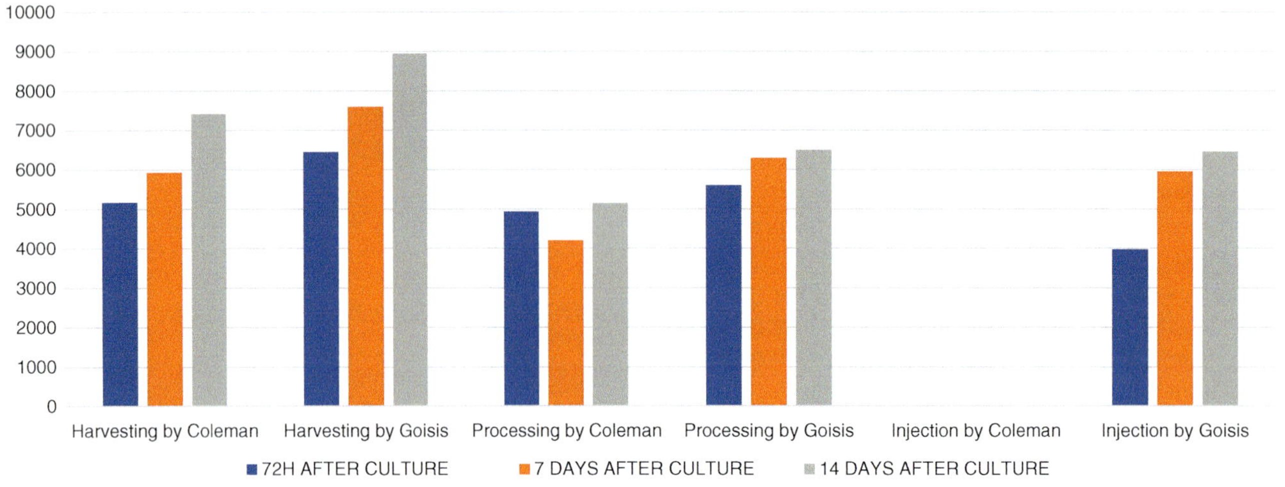

This theory stipulates that most grafted adipocytes die after injection, and the remaining extracellular matrix serves as a scaffold for donor and recipient replacement cells, which regenerate the tissue.

In this regeneration ASCs play a key role. Consequently, the preservation of the highest concentration of adipose stem-cells (ASCs) is demonstrated to improve fat retention, with the growth potential of the adipose-derived mesenchymal stem-cells cited as a major contributing factor [6, 7].

According to the results of Trevisonno et al., the reduced size of the microcannula could give an advantage in reducing the harvest of well-organized fat, which is mostly composed of mature adipocytes, and improving the collection of more superficial layers of adipose tissue, which are associated with a higher percentage of ADSC [8].

In particular, they observed more than a 2-fold increase in recovery yield of stem-cells in fat harvested using a 2 mm microcannula (port diameter 1 mm) than in fat harvested with a 3 mm diameter cannula (port diameter: 3 × 9 mm). The importance of every step (harvesting, processing and injection) in the preservation of the highest number of viable Adipose stem-cells (ASCs) was discussed by Goisis et al Imcas 2019 (Goisis et AL, comparing protocols, IMCAS 2019) The number of stem-cell of 6 different samples was measured at 72hours, 7 days and 14 days after colture. Three samples were related to Goisis technique, with high values of stem-cells immediately after harvesting with Goisis Cannula (6443, 7596, 8950), after processing with Goisis System (5601, 6300, 6500) and after passing through a 22G cannula (3976, 5950, 6460). The last 3 samples were related with Coleman technique with a very significant modification: the Coleman fat was passed through a 22G cannula. The value of stem-cells after harvesting with Coleman cannula were 5180, 5930 and 7410. The value after Coleman processing (centrifugation) were 4940, 4210 and 5140. But after passage throught the 22G cannula the stem-cells were destroyed by high level of shear stress, with levels around zero. (see Table 9.3).

9.5 Obtaining a Good Level of Efficiency

The efficiency of the method can be evaluated in terms of time consumption, of the cost of procedure, and loss of fat during the preparation.

In terms of time consumption, the choice of the harvesting cannula is very important. Usually, the use of small cannulas with small ports reduces the viscosity of the harvested fat but increases the time of the procedure. An exception is the Goisis cannula. In fact, aspiration of fat using the Goisis cannula is performed with a rotational movement. The depressed edge of the ports promotes the entrance of fat into the hole. The raised edge facilitates the dissection of the fat particles. This way, the shape of the multiple ports yields a large volume of aspirated tissue with each rotation. The use of the Goisis cannula is, therefore, several times more efficient compared to the Coleman harvesting cannula (approximately twice as fast compared to the Coleman 3-mm cannula).

Efficiency in terms of fat loss is very important in cases of mini-invasive treatment of the face, neck, and hands. In these cases, the patients usually undergo the the harvesting of small amounts of fat, with a view to injecting 15–20 cc of fat. Some low-efficiency methods require harvesting of 100 cc or more of fat to obtain 20 cc of processed fat. The other 80 cc is are lost during processing. In some patients it is very simple to harvest 100 cc, but in many many others it is more difficult, and may require a long time andharvesting from a number of different donor areas.

9.5.1 Harvesting

Technique	Harvesting	Dimension of the harvesting cannula	Dimension of the fat particles	Number of stromal and vascular components	Negative pressure control	Preservation of intact adipocyte during harvesting
Telfa rolling	Coleman cannula, 10 cc	5	4	4	1	1
	syringe	a	f	m	q	
Coleman	Coleman cannula, 10 cc	5	4	4	1	1
	syringe	a	f	m	q	
Lipogems	13G special cannula,	3	3	3	1	1
	VacLok syringe	b	g	n		
Coleman	Coleman cannula, 10 cc	5	4	4		1
	syringe, 22 G cannula	a	f	m	q	
Puregraft	Coleman harvesting cannula, 10 cc syringe for harvesting	5	4	4	1	1
Regenlab	Regenlab cannula	a	f	m	q	
		5	1	1	5	1
		aaa	lll	ppp	S	
Sedimentation with low aspiration pressure	A 3 mm rounded-tip cannula with a single elliptic suction port on the side near its distal end (port diameter: 3 × 9 mm	4	4	4	1	3
	10 cc syringe for aspiration	c		m		
			h		q	
Sedimentation with height pressure	A 3 mm rounded-tip cannula with a single elliptic suction port on the side near its distal end (port diameter: 3 × 9 mm	4	4	5	5	5
	Lipoaspiration at high			m, o	r	R
	pressure (−760 mmHg)	c	h			
prl	3.5 mm cannula, big holes,	5	4	4	1	3
	VacLok syringe	d	i	m	s	
Goisis dermal graft	2.1 mm Goisis cannula with	1	1	1	1	1
	VacLok syringe	e	L	p	s	
Goisis microfat kit	2.1 mm Goisis cannula with	1	1	1	1	1
	10 cc syringe	e	L	p	q	

Valuation of the method in terms of: (1, optimal, 2 very good, 3 good, 4 sufficient, 5 inadequate)

Dimension of the harvesting cannula

Big dimension of the harvesting cannula is related with bigger scar in the insertion point and generally in more important pain and edema in the donor site

Notes

a: The Coleman cannula has a relative big diameter, which creates more scar in the insertion points. The ports on the tip of the cannula increase the risk of vascular injury

b: 13 Gauge Cannula of Lipogem is a quite big cannula with multiple ports

c: a 3 mm rounded-tip cannula with a single elliptic suction port on the side near its distal end (port diameter: 3 × 9 mm) is a quite big cannula. The high pressure and force necessary for fat harvesting creates many damages to fat cells

d: 3.5 mm cannula used for this system is a quite big cannula

e: The Goisis microcannula reduces the incidences of patient trauma, discomfort, skin irregularities and minimizes the risk of vascular injury due to multiple reduced-size ports. Because the insertion requires less force and is more precise, the microcannula affords superior manual control

aaa: during harvesting, because of the attachment of the cannula, the vacuum is poor. The risk of contamination is high and the time of harvesting is long

Dimension of the fat particles

Fat particles are defined as intact globules of adipocytes interconnected by mesenchymal tissue

As the diameter of fat particles becomes larger, the central zone of necrosis will expand according to diffusional limitations

f: Coleman Cannula has big suction ports. The dimensions of fat particles are consequently quite big

g: Lipogem Cannula has suction port of medium dimensions. The dimensions of fat particles are consequently intermediate

h: a 3 mm rounded-tip cannula with a single elliptic suction port on the side near its distal end has big port (port diameter: 3 × 9 mm). The dimensions of fat particles are consequently quite big
i: Gentile Cannula has suction port of medium dimensions. The dimensions of fat particles are consequently intermediate
l: Goisis cannula has small suction port. The dimensions of fat particles are consequently small
lll: Regenlab cannula has small suction port. The dimensions of fat particles are consequently small

Quantity of stromal and vascular components

The small size of the cannula gives an advantage in reducing the harvest of well-organized fat, which is mostly composed of mature adipocytes, and improves the collection of more superficial layers of adipose tissue, which are associated with a higher percentage of ADSC
m: the big size of the cannula increases the harvest of well-organized fat, which is mostly composed of mature adipocytes, and reduces the collection of more superficial layers of adipose tissue, which are associated with a higher percentage of ADSC
n: the medium size of the cannula increases the harvest of well-organized fat, which is mostly composed of mature adipocytes, and reduces the collection of more superficial layers of adipose tissue, which are associated with a higher percentage of ADSC
o: high level of negative pressure destroys stem cells
p: the reduced size of the Goisis cannula reduces the harvest of well-organized fat, which is mostly composed of mature adipocytes, and improves the collection of more superficial layers of adipose tissue, which are associated with a higher percentage of ADSC

Negative pressure control

High level of negative pressure disrupt adipocytes
q: the use of 10 cc syringe avoids excess negative pressure
r: high level of negative pressure disrupts adipocytes
s: the use of VackLok syringe maintains a good control of negative pressure

Preservation of adipocytes during fat harvesting

The choice of cannula and of the suction device can preserve adipocytes
r: high level of negative pressure disrupts adipocytes
t: harvesting fat with the 3 mm rounded-tip cannula with a single elliptic need to apply a great force with disruption of adipocytes
u: Because the insertion of the cannula with rotational movement requires less force, the preservation of fat cells is improved

9.5.2 Processing

Technique	Processing	Presence of contaminants: blood cells	Presence of contaminants: oil	Presence of anaesthesia	Presence of washing solution	Risk of infection	Air exposure	Concentration of ADSC	Preservation of intact adipocyte during processing
Telfa rolling	Telfa rolling	1	1	1	1	5	5	2	1
		a1	f1	o1	u1	x1	x1	A2	f2
Coleman	centrifugation	2	3	1	0	5	5	4	4
		b1	g1	p1	u1	k1	k1	b2	g2
Lipogems	The action of the microspheres emulsified the adipose tissue	1	1	1	4	2	2	1	5
			n1	q1	v1	w1		c2	h2
Coleman	Centrifugation	2	2	2	0	5	5	4	4
		b1	f1	p1	u1	k1	k1	b2	g2
Puregraft	Washing and filtration	2	1	1	3	2	2	1	2
Regenlab	Washing	d1	h1	q1	z1	w1	w1	c2	I2
		3	5	1	2	5	5	1	5
Decantation with low pressure	Sedimentation	4	5	4	0	3	2	2	1
		c1		r1					L2
			L1		u1	w1	w1	e2	
Decantation with height pressure	Sedimentation	4	5	4	0	3	2	2	1
				r1	u1	w1	w1	e2	L2
		c1	L1						
prl	Filtration	5	5	5	0	2	2	1	2
			M1	t1	u1	w1	w1	d2	I2
Goisis dermal graft	Washing and filtration	1	1	1	3	1	1	1	1
		d1	h1	q1	z1	y1	y1	c2	M2
Goisis Microfat	Washing and filtration	1	1	1	3	1	1	1	1
		d1	h1	q1	z1	y1	y1	c2	

Valuation of the method in terms of: (1: optimal, 2 very good, 3 good, 4 sufficient, 5 inadequate)

Presence of contaminants: blood cells

Once grafted, extravasated blood cells are cleared by an inflammatory process that can lead to collateral damage and loss of graft volume

a1: Telfa rolling removes approximately 80–90% of red and white blood cells
b1: centrifugation removes approximately 60–80% of red and white blood cells
c1: gravity sedimentation removes approximately 50–60% of red and white blood cells
d1: washing with filtration removes more than 95% of red and white blood cells
e1: no removal of blood cells is done

Presence of Contaminants: oil

Extracellular free lipids are released from ruptured adipocytes. This material is scavenged by tissue phagocytes and it can induce an inflammatory response. Lipid cysts can be induced by inflammatory cells in a foreign body response

f1: Telfa rolling removes completely oil
g1: centrifugation plus Telfa removes approximately 90% of oil
h1: retention of oil is reduced to less than 1% in grafts prepared by washing with filtration
L1: gravity sedimentation does not remove oil
M1: Prl technique does not remove oil
n1: Lipogems is associated with complete removal of oil

Presence of local anesthesia

o1: Tefa rolling technique is very effective in removing liquids from lipoaspirate
p1: centrifugation condenses the tissue, thereby reducing aqueous liquid content, with efficient removal of local anesthesia
q1: the washing procedure removes completely the local anesthesia, which is substituted by washing solution
r1: grafts prepared by gravity sedimentation have a higher content of anesthesia compared with centrifugation
t1: anesthesia is totally left into the solution

Presence of washing solution

Water mixed with fat creates false volume which disappears immediately after grafting

u1: no washing is performed during the processing, consequently no presence of washing solution
v1: high percentage of washing solution
z1: medium percentage of washing solution

Presence of bacteria, risk of infection

x1: totally open system
k1: partially open system: the syringes are open during centrifugation
w1: system closed during processing
y1: it is a completely closed system. The harvest, the processing, and the injection of the fat are performed into the system, reducing the risk of infection

Contact with air

The direct contact with air has a negative effect on adipocytes, because of activation of proinflammatory components and oxidative damages

x1: totally open system
k1: partially open system: the syringes are open during centrifugation
w1: system closed during processing
y1: it is a completely closed system. The harvest, the processing, and the injection of the fat are performed into the system, reducing the risk of infection

Concentration of the adipose stem cells (ASCs)

The preservation of the highest concentration of adipose stem cells (ASCs) is demonstrated to improve fat retention

A2: Telfa rolling maintains the integrity and number of ADSC
b2: the greatest number of ASCs are concentrated at the bottom of the syringe by the centrifugal force and are eliminated
c2: the stem cells are preserved with washing with filtration
d2: the stem cells are preserved and concentrated by filtration
e2: a percentage of ADSC are loose with the liquid component during decantation

Integrity and the viability of the adipocytes after processing

The graft with the greatest number of intact adipocytes will have the greatest chance of long-term durability

f2: Telfa rolling maintains the integrity and number of adipocytes
g2: centrifugation destroys a great number of intact nucleated cells
h2: Lipogem system includes active disruption of a great number of intact nucleated cells
I2: pressure on the bag can destroy adipocytes
L2: Decantation maintains the integrity and number of adipocytes
M2: safety check valves preserve adipocytes from excess of positive pressure Goisis [2]

9.5.3 Injection

Injection	Injection	Preservation of adipocytes during injection	Comfort during injection
Telfa rolling	22 gauge cannula	5	2
		n2	q2
Coleman	Coleman infiltrating	1	5
	17 gauge cannula	o2	q2
Lipogems	25 gauge cannula	1	1
		p2	r2
Coleman	22 gauge cannula	5	2
		n2	s2
Puregraft	22 gauge cannula	5	2
Regenlab		n2	s2
		2	1
Decantation with	Coleman infiltrating	1	5
low pressure	17 gauge cannula	o2	q2
Decantation with	Coleman infiltrating	1	5
height pressure	17 gauge cannula	o2	q2
prl	17 gauge Coleman	1	5
	cannula	o2	q2
Goisis dermal	22 gauge cannula	1	2
graft		p2	s2
Goisis microfat	22 gauge cannula	1	2
		p2	s2

Preservation of adipocytes during injection

n2: big dimension of fat particles after processing, small cannula for injection

o2: big dimension of fat particles after processing, big cannula for injection

p2: small dimension of fat particles after processing, small cannula for injection

Comfort during injection

q2: the use of big cannula for injection reduce the comfort

r2: the use of very small cannula increases the comfort and precision of injection

s2: the use of small cannula increases the comfort and precision of injection

9.5.4 Efficiency

Technique: efficiency	Efficiency: time consuming	Efficiently: loose of fat	Efficiency: cost in term of surgical rooms and staff
Telfa rolling	5	5	2
	t2	a3	f3
Coleman	4	4	5
	u2	b3	g3
Lipogems	4	4	5
	v2	c3	g3
Coleman	4	4	5
	u2	b3	g3
Puregraft	3	4	2
Regenlab	z2	c3	f3
	5	5	2
	zzz2	ccc3	f3
Decantation with	2	1	2
low pressure	w2	d3	f3
Decantation with	2	1	2
height pressure	w2	d3	f3
prl	3	4	2
	x2	c3	f3
Goisis dermal	1	2	1
graft	k2	e3	h3
Goisis microfat	1	2	1
			h3

Efficiency: time consuming

t2: Telfa procedure is very long and laborious

u2: Coleman procedure requires many steps, with time for transfer and centrifugation

v2: Lipogem procedure requires a quite long time for setting the system and for the multiple washing of the fat

z2: despite its quite relative simplicity, puregraft processing requires different steps

zzz2: the procedure is very complex, in case of error it has to be repeated

w2: the decantation is one of the faster systems for processing

x2: the PRL procedure involves different steps and different bags, with many transfer from syringe to syringe

k2: Goisis system is the faster one because it is a totally closed procedure. The time from injection of anesthesia to injection of fat is 25 min

Efficiency: loosing of fat during the preparation

a3: 70%

b3: 40%

c3: 30–40%

ccc3: 80–90%

d3: 10%

e3: 15%

Efficiency: cost in terms of surgical rooms and staff

f3: small surgical room, 2 persons

g3: major surgical room, 3 persons

h3: small surgical room, 1 person

References

1. Peer LA. Cell survival theory versus replacement theory. Plast Reconstr Surg. 1955;16:161–8.
2. Shiffman MA, Mirrafati S. Fat transfer techniques: the effect of harvest and transfer methods on adipocyte via- bility and review of the literature. Dermatol Surg. 2001;27:819–26.
3. Cheriyan T, Kao HK, Qiao X, Guo L. The effect of harvest pressure on adipose survival. Plast Reconstr Surg. 2014;133(6):1365–8.
4. Nguyen P, Desouches C, Gay A, Hautier A, Magalon G. Development of micro-injection as an innovative autolo- gous fat graft technique: the use of adipose tissue as dermal filler. J Plast Reconstr Aesthet Surg. 2012;65:1692–9.
5. Boschert MT, Beckert BW, Puckett CL, Concannon MJ. Analysis of lipocyte viability after liposuction. Plast Reconstr Surg. 2002;109:761–5. discussion 766
6. Eto H, Kato H, Suga H, Aoi N, Doi K, Kuno S, Yoshimura K. The fate of adipocytes after nonvascularized fat grafting: evidence of early death and replacement of adipocytes. Plast Reconstr Surg. 2012;129:1081–92.
7. Kølle SF, Fischer-Nielsen A, Mathiasen AB, et al. Enrichment of autologous fat grafts with ex-vivo expanded adipose tissue- derived stem cells for graft survival: a randomised placebo-controlled trial. Lancet. 2013;382:1113–20.
8. Farr ST, Trivisonno A. Differential fat harvesting. Plast Aesthet Res. 2014;1:103–7.
9. Kirkham JC, Lee JH, Medina MA 3rd, McCormack MC, Randolph MA, Austen WG Jr. The impact of liposuction cannula size on adipocyte viability. Ann Plast Surg. 2012;69:479–81.

Fat and Stem-Cells

10

Mario Goisis, Ribó Planas, Muñoz del Olmo, Sara Izzo, Andrea Sbarbati, and Giamaica Conti

10.1 The Role of Stem-Cells

Human mesenchymal stem-cells (hMSCs) have multipotent differentiation properties. These cells can be obtained from different areas including bone marrow (hBMSCs), dental pulp, umbilical-cord blood, synovial membrane, placenta, the skin, the umbilical cord, skeletal muscle, Wharton's jelly, the meniscus, mother's milk, cartilage, ligament, and adipose tissue (ASCs). A great number of applications of hMSCs have been described in literature.

For example, hMSCs were used for myocardial repair in the infarcted hearts of rats [1, 2], for improving graft revascularisation in cotransplantation with islet in diabetic rats [3], and for the treatment of enteric neuropathy associated with intestinal inflammation [4].

MSCs are known to have the potential to regenerate articular cartilage and are suggested for the treatment of osteoarthritis (OA), a chronic degenerative joint disorder characterised by destruction of articular cartilage. In fact, hMSCs can modulate the immune response by effect of immunosuppressive and anti-inflammatory paracrine. Regeneration of articular cartilage in a rabbit OA model after intra-articular injection of xenogeneic hMSCs was demonstrated [5–7].

Jo et al. assessed the safety and efficacy of intra-articular injection of autologous adipose tissue-derived MSCs (AD-MSCs) for osteoarthritis of the knee. They demonstrated that intra-articular injection of AD-MSCs into an osteoarthritic knee improved the function and reduced pain in the knee joint and repaired damages to its cartilage, by regeneration of hyaline-like articular cartilage, without causing adverse events [8].

The Role of ASC in Aesthetic and Regenerative Medicine

ASC enrichment of fat grafts improves the survival of grafts significantly.

The efficacy of ASC in reducing resorption rates of fat grafts was demonstrated by Kolle et al. in 2013 in a significant scientific article published in the Lancet [9].

The authors reported the results of a triple-blind, placebo-controlled trial used to compare the survival of non-enriched fat grafts versus fat-enriched grafts with autologous adipose-derived stem-cells (ASCs).

Thirteen healthy patients underwent two fat-harvestings taken 14 days apart from each other: one for ASC isolation and ex-vivo expansion with cell manipulation and another for the preparation of fat grafts. Two purified fat grafts (30 mL each) taken from the second liposuction were prepared for each participant. One graft was enriched with ASCs (20 × 10(6) cells per mL fat) expanded in the laboratory and another graft without ASC enrichment. The latter graft was used as a control. The fat grafts were injected subcutaneously as a bolus in randomised sequence.

MRI tests measured the volumes of injected fat-grafts immediately after injection and after 121 days.

Compared with the control grafts, the ASC-enriched fat-grafts revealed a higher volume of adipose tissue and newly-made connective tissue. The newly-made connective tissue was cogitated as a product of the ASCs, because this tissue-type is not usually detected in subcutaneous adipose tissue. These conclusions are in accordance with the differentiation capabilities of ASCs, particularly, in their fibroblast-like form [10].

The ASC-enriched fat-grafts preserved more than 80% of their initial bolus volume 4 months after grafting, compared with 16% in the case of the non-enriched fat [9].

M. Goisis (✉)
Maxillo-Facial and Aesthetic Surgeon, Go Easy Clinic, Milan, Italy

R. Planas · M. del Olmo
Clínica Planas, Barcelona, Spain

S. Izzo
Department of Plastic Surgery, University of Campania "Luigi Vanvitelli", Naples, Piazza Miraglia, Naples, Italy

A. Sbarbati · G. Conti
Department of Neuroscience, Biomedicine and Movement, Human Anatomy and Histology Section, University of Verona, Strada Le Grazie 8, Verona, Italy
e-mail: andrea.sbarbati@univr.it; giamaica.conti@univr.it

M. Goisis (ed.), *Outpatient Regenerative Medicine*, https://doi.org/10.1007/978-3-319-44894-7_10

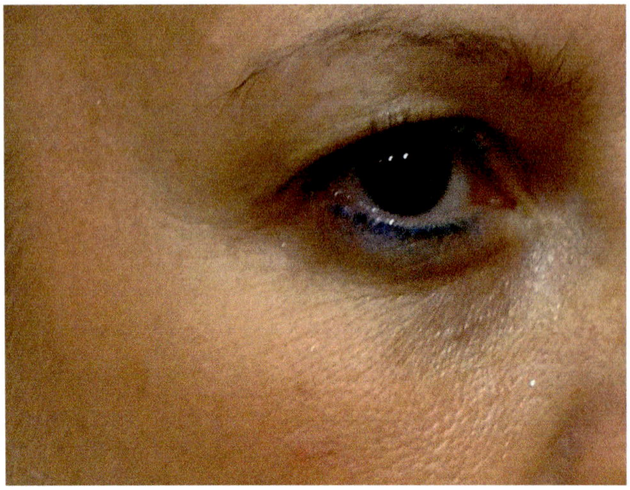

Fig. 10.1 An image of a dark circle before treatment with nanofat (Courtesy of www.microfat.com). (Published by kind permission of ©Mario Goisis 2018. All Rights Reserved)

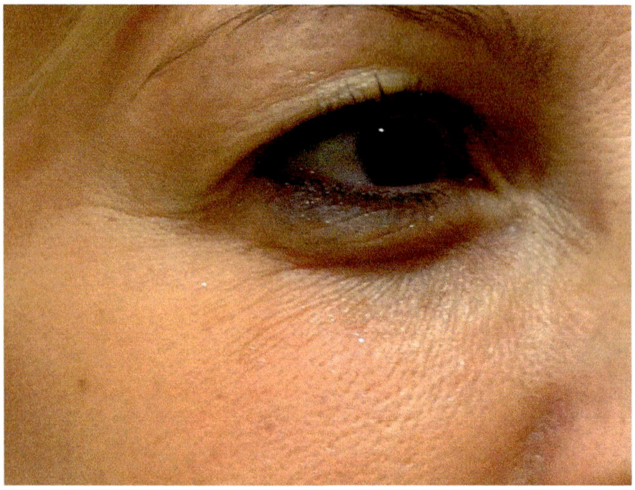

Fig. 10.2 The same patient 6 months after injection of nanofat (Courtesy of www.microfat.com). (Published by kind permission of ©Mario Goisis 2018. All Rights Reserved)

10.1.1 The Whitening Effect of Adipose-Derived Stem-Cells

The effect of adipose-derived stem-cells (ASCs) in reduced melanin synthesis was demonstrated experimentally in vitro and in vivo on animal models [11, 12].

In actual fact, ASCs have a whitening effect *via* a paracrine mechanism. In particular, tyrosinase activity, which plays a key role in the synthesis of melanin, was inhibited by the ASCs. To clarify the mechanisms of the whitening action of ADSCs, levels of expression of melanogenic proteins were evaluated. In particular, expressions of tyrosinase and TRP1 were downregulated [13].

ASCs are free radical scavengers and are endowed with potent antioxidant activity, which may result in the inhibition of the synthesis of melanin [12].

However, not only antioxidant action but also secretion of specific cytokines by ASCs may contribute to the whitening effect. TGF-b plays an inhibitory role in pigment formation, because it interferes with tyrosinase activity.

A high level of this growth-factor was detected in ASCs, which might be responsible for the inhibition of the synthesis of melanin by ADSC-CM [12].

Although further clinical studies are needed, administration of ADSC and their secretory factors suggest great promise for application in hyperpigmented skin disorders (Figs. 10.1 and 10.2).

10.1.2 The Hair-Growth-Promote Effects of ADSC

Several reports have demonstrated that growth factors like PDGF, HGF, VEGF, and fibronectin stimulate hair growth in animal and clinical models [12, 14].

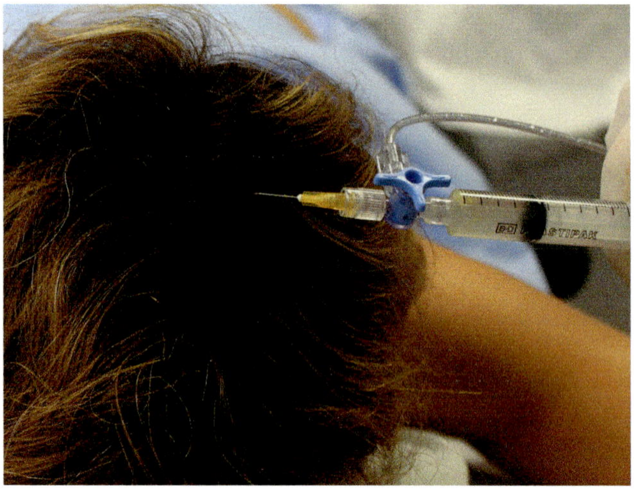

Fig. 10.3 Injection of ADSCs after separation by vibration (Courtesy of www.microfat.com). (Published by kind permission of ©Mario Goisis 2018. All Rights Reserved)

To determine whether these paracrine effects of ADSCs can promote hair growth, Won et al. investigated the effects of ADSCs on cultured human dermal papilla cells (hDPCs). ADSC treatment significantly augmented proliferation of hDPCs up to 130% at 48 h. The animal study on nude mice confirmed these results [14]. In particular, histologically, the back skin of ADSC-CM-treated mice showed increased amount of hair follicles. This study indicates that ADSCs promote hair growth by increasing the proliferation of DPCs and activating the anagen phase of hair cycles (Fig. 10.3).

Recently, it was reported that treatment with conditioned media of ADSCs (ADSC-CM) is effective for female pattern hair-loss (FPHL). A retrospective, observational study of outcomes in 27 patients presenting with FPHL and treated using ADSC-CM was carried out. The authors used microneedles to allow the ASC-CM to penetrate the human skin. To evaluate the efficacy of the treatment, patients' medical records and photo trichographic images were analysed. ASC-CM showed efficacy in treating FPHL after 12 weeks of therapy (Shin et al., 2015). For example, hair thickness and hair density increased significantly, and none of the patients reported adverse reactions [15].

Fukuoka and Suga also reported the effect of a commercial product containing a protein solution of adipose-derived stem-cell-conditioned medium in hair restoration. The product was injected intradermally in 22 patients with alopecia [16]. These patients received treatment every 3–5 weeks for a total of six sessions, and their hair was significantly increased in both male and female patients.

10.2 Sources of Stem-Cells

Clinically, the two most commonly exploited sources of human mesenchymal stem-cells (hMSCs) are bone marrow (hBMSCs) and fat (hASCs).

De Ugarte et al. demonstrated no significant differences in yield between adherent stromal cells, growth kinetics, cell senescence, multi-lineage differentiation capacity, and gene transduction efficiency between hBMSCs and hASCs.

The extraction of bone marrow is a relatively painful and invasive treatment. And with ageing the quantity and viability of hMSC obtained by marrow aspiration decline.

On the contrary, hMSC can be found in abundant amounts in fat. hASCs retain a good viability and differentiating potential even in older patients, with a lower senescence ratio and higher proliferative capacity [17, 18].

10.2.1 Stem-Cells and Local Anaesthesia

It is reported that lidocaine can have a negative effect on ASCs. In fact, a concentration of 0.03% or more of lidocaine can be toxic for stem-cells [19].

Goldman et al. conducted liposuction under general anaesthesia on one area under standard tumescent with lidocaine [20]. On the contralateral side, liposuction was carried out under the tumescent without lidocaine. Five milliliters of lipoaspirate were processed for the isolation of SVF. The adherent ASCs were counted after 24 h of culture.

The removal of lidocaine from tumescent reduced SVF and ASC apoptosis in the lipoaspirate significantly [20].

For this reason, it is very important to remove lidocaine or other anaesthetics injected during fat harvesting. Washing is an effective procedure by which to do this.

At the same time, at the moment of injection of stem-cells, anaesthetic should only be used outside the desired treatment region, and/or a regional nerve block should be used, in order to avoid the contact between stem-cells and local anaesthesia [19, 21].

10.2.1.1 Stem-Cells and Drugs

Recently, Bowen carried out a review of pharmaceutical drugs and supplements that might have an unfavourable effect on healing of ASC. In particular, the use of nonsteroidal anti-inflammatory drugs should be stopped at least 5 days prior to the procedure because of their negative impact on healing.

Because corticosteroids have a negative impact on regeneration, the procedure should be delayed for at least 8 weeks after a steroid injection. The use of inhaled steroids should be discontinued, if possible, prior to the procedure.

Some alarm has been raised regarding the effect of 3-hydroxy-3-methyl-glutaryl-coenzyme A (HMG-CoA) reductase inhibitors (e.g., atorvastatin [Lipitor]) and proton pump inhibitors (omeprazole) on stem-cell growth in vitro. In particular, HMG-CoA reductase inhibitors reduce angiogenesis. For persons who are or have been taking an HMG-CoA reductase inhibitor, supplementation with coenzyme Q-10 should be considered [22].

10.3 Different Protocols for Adipose-Derived Stem-Cell (ASCs) Isolation

10.3.1 Enzymatic Digestion

Most of the procedures for adipose-derived stem-cell isolation use enzymatic digestion with collagenase and then grow in an animal-derived medium (Table 10.1). In these protocols stem-cells are subjected to extensive manipulation (Fig. 10.4). The extensive manipulation and, in general, ex-vivo expansion is very difficult perform because of the requirements for compliance with "cell manufacturing" in accordance with current Good Manufacturing Practice (cGMP) Guidelines [23].

Moreover, enzymatic digestion takes approximately 3–27 h. Despite this, it requires animal-derived reagents (collagenase). Residual collagenase is potentially toxic and

Table 10.1 Standard isolation protocol

Standard isolation
Aspirate off saline and oil phases
Wash 250 ml fat 3–5 times for 5 min each in phosphate-buffered saline (PBS), discarding lower phase until clear
Add 0.075% collagenase in PBS and incubate on a shaker at 37 °C for 1 h
Add Dulbecco's Modified Eagle Medium (DMEM) containing 10% foetal bovine serum (FBS) to neutralise collagenase
Centrifuge digested fat in 50 ml tubes at 1200 × g for 10 min
Resuspend pellet in 160 mM redcell lysing solution (ammonium chloride-NH_4 CI) and incubate for 10 min
Centrifuge at 1,200 × g for 10 min
Wash cells 2× in PBS
Resuspend pellet and pass cells through 100 μm nylon mesh
Duration: about 3–27 h. Materials: centrifuge, heated shaker, NH_4CI, DMEM, FBS, PBS, 100-μm nylon mesh

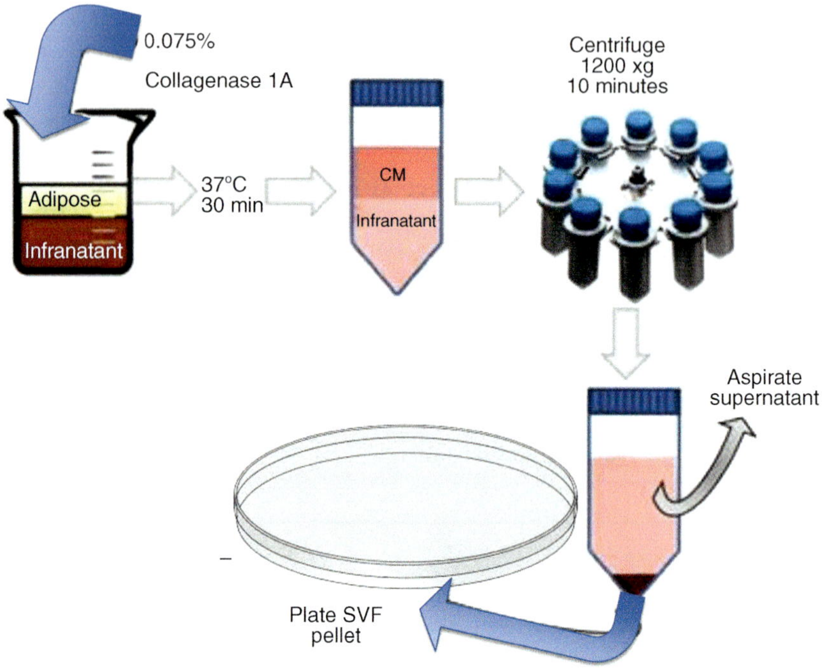

Fig. 10.4 Standard isolation protocol. (Published by kind permission of ©Mario Goisis 2018. All Rights Reserved)

is associated with the risk of serious side effects, such as allergic reactions, but also cutaneous ulcers, nerve injury, and tendon or ligament damage [23].

Furthermore, enzymatic digestion is a very expensive protocol. Collagenase costs approximately $20 or about €18 per 100 g of adipose tissue digestion, whereas the other elements involved (foetal bovine serum, Dulbecco's Modified Eagle Medium, and phosphate-buffered saline) cost about $15 or €13 per procedure [23].

10.3.2 Mechanical Isolation using a Vibrating Shaker

Raposio et al. presented a novel and effective strategy for isolating adipose-derived stem-cells from a conventional fat harvest [23].

The entire procedure takes approximately 15 min; no collagenase, serum, or animal-derived reagents are used.

In particular, the operating theatre or surgery is equipped with a vibrating shaker and a centrifuge, both placed on a laminar airflow bench. The isolation procedure is performed step by step under the laminar airflow cabinet, thus minimising the risks of contamination.

In the work of Raposio et al., adipose tissue was harvested by standard liposuction procedures using the usual blunt-tipped cannulas attached to 10-ml Luer-Lok syringes. The contents of each syringe, approximately 10 mL, were transferred under the laminar flow cabinet into 10-ml plastic test tubes. The tubes were then positioned in the vibrating shaker at 6,000 vibrations/min for 6 min and, immediately afterwards, centrifuged at 1,600 rpm for 6 min. Then, under the same laminar flow cabinet, the pellet at the bottom of each tube was collected by means of an automated pipetting system and poured into a 10-ml Luer-Lok syringe.

Raposio et al. demonstrated that this procedure leads to a stem-cell population 12% more abundant compared to that isolated using the standard enzymatic procedure.

It does not require stem-cell expansion or manipulation, and therefore, it is not subjected to the regulatory restrictions imposed by cGMP Guidelines.

10.3.3 Microfat SVF Kit: Mechanical Isolation in a Closed System

In 2016 (FACE congress, London), Goisis et al. presented the prototype of a novel kit for isolating adipose-derived stem-cells from fat.

No collagenase, serum, or animal-derived reagents are used. Because microfat SVF kit does not require stem-cell expansion or manipulation, therefore, it is not subjected to the regulatory restrictions imposed by cGMP Guidelines.

The cannula used for fat harvesting is called the Goisis cannula. On the basis of similar results obtained using small cannulas, fat harvested using Goisis cannula presented a higher percentage of stromal and vascular components (resulting in improved yields of isolated ADSC).

In particular, histological examinations performed on 247 samples demonstrated that fat cells harvested using the Goisis cannula were associated with a high percentage of stromal and vascular components when compared with fat harvested using singleport cannulas [24].

The treatment room is equipped with a vibrating shaker and a centrifuge, both placed close to the patient. The isolation procedure is performed entirely in a closed system, thus minimising the risks of contamination (Figs. 10.5, 10.6a, b, 10.7a, b, 10.8, 10.9, 10.10, 10.11a, b, 10.12a, b, 10.13a, b, 10.14, 10.15, 10.16a, b, 10.17, 10.18, 10.19, 10.20a, b, 10.21, 10.22, 10.23, and 10.24). In a study presented by Goisis et al. Imcas 2019 (Goisis et al. comparing protocols, IMCAS 2019) the role of Microfat SVF Kit

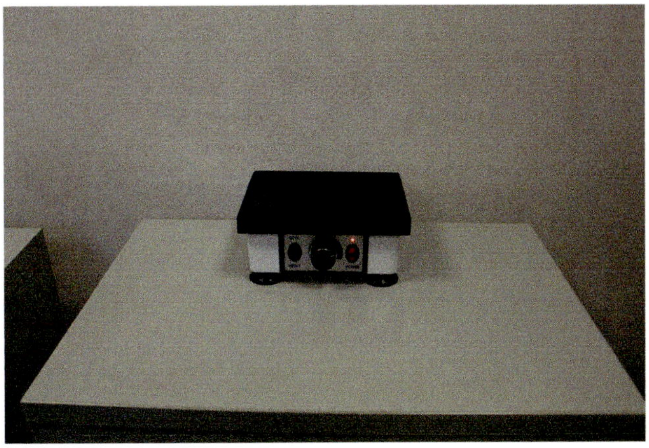

Fig. 10.5 The vibrating shaker is placed on the operating table. (Published by kind permission of ©Mario Goisis 2018. All Rights Reserved)

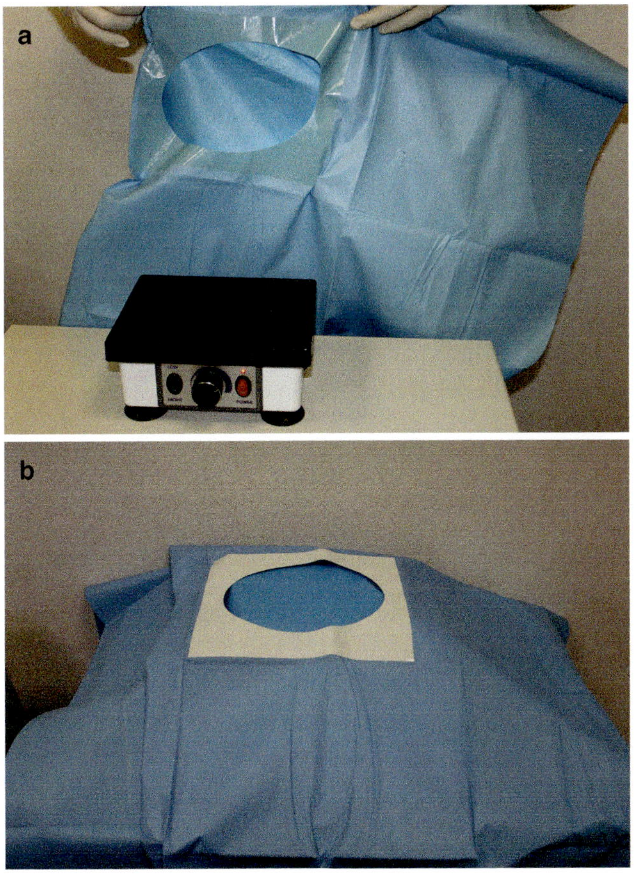

Fig. 10.6 (**a**, **b**) The shaker is covered with a bi-adhesive drape (Deltamed, Italy www.microfat.com). One side of the drape is attached to the vibrating plane. (Published by kind permission of ©Mario Goisis 2018. All Rights Reserved)

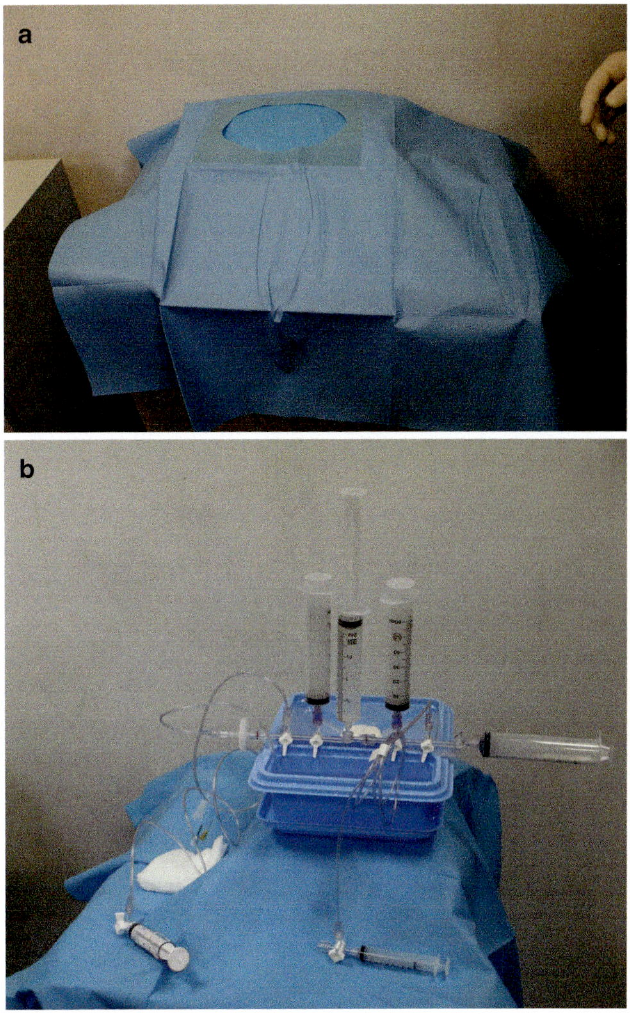

Fig. 10.7 (**a**, **b**) The upper side of the drape is attached to the microfat kit (www.microfat.com). (Published by kind permission of ©Mario Goisis 2018. All Rights Reserved)

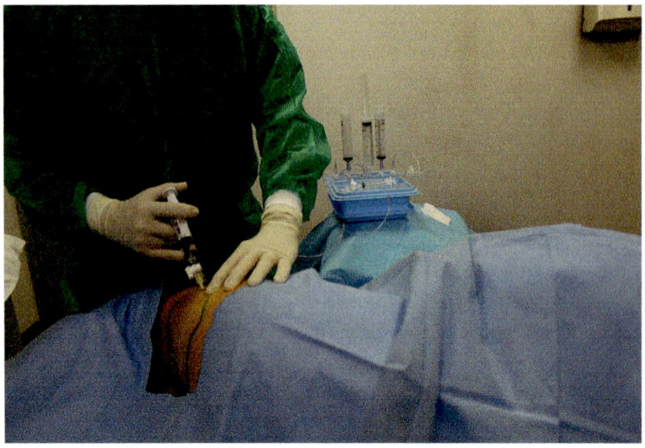

Fig. 10.8 Infiltration of local anaesthesia using the microfat kit. (Published by kind permission of ©Mario Goisis 2018. All Rights Reserved)

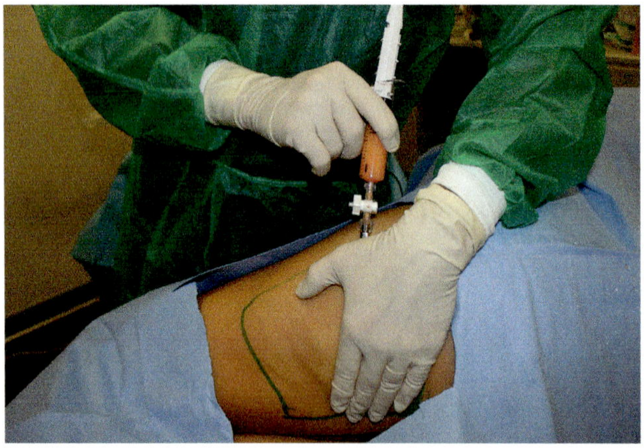

Fig. 10.9 Harvesting of 20 cc of fat using a Goisis cannula. (Published by kind permission of ©Mario Goisis 2018. All Rights Reserved)

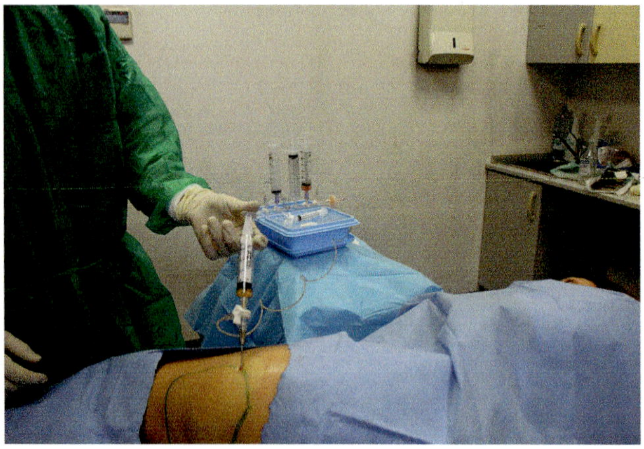

Fig. 10.10 The fat is transferred in a closed fashion into the kit. (Published by kind permission of ©Mario Goisis 2018. All Rights Reserved)

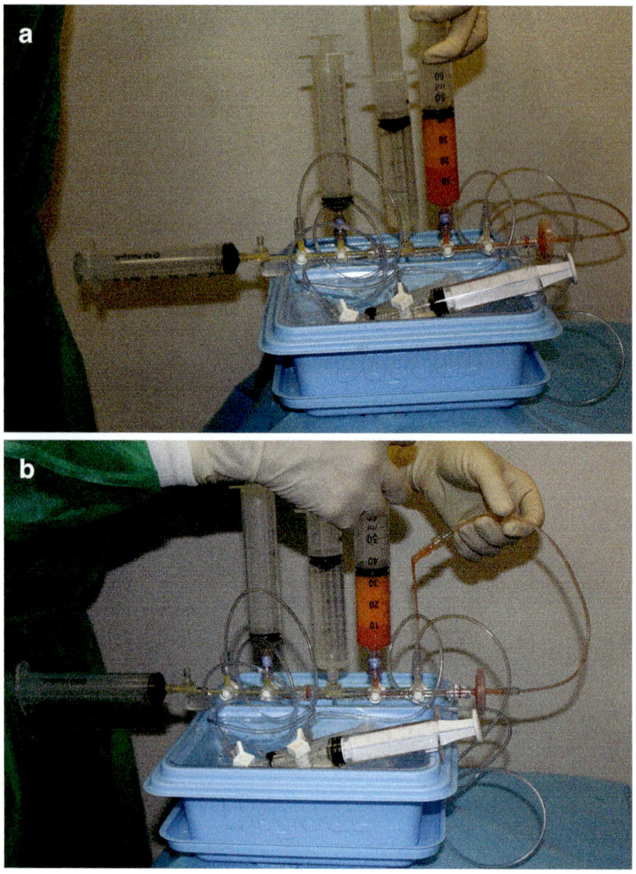

Fig. 10.11 (**a**, **b**) The filtration removes blood cells and Klein solution from the syringe. (Published by kind permission of ©Mario Goisis 2018. All Rights Reserved)

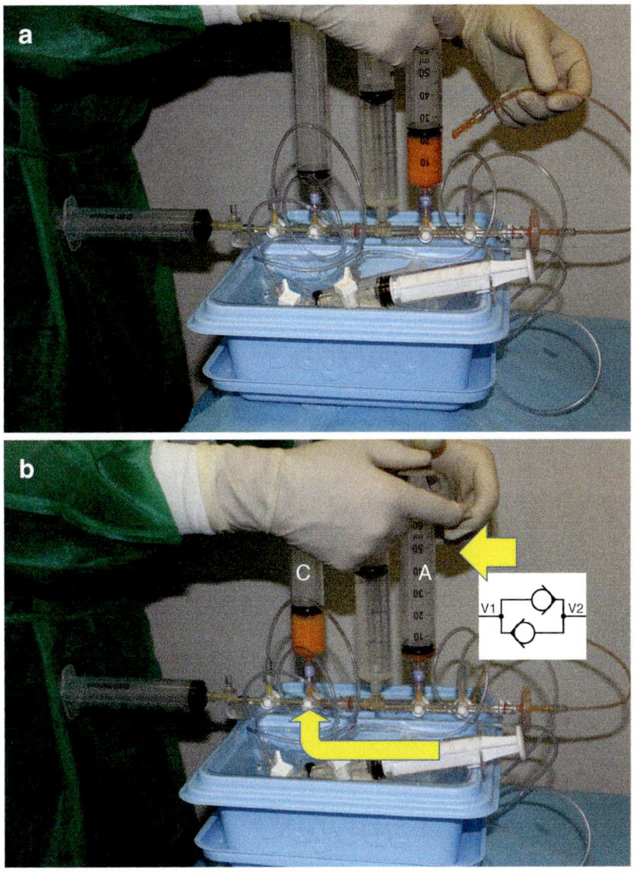

Fig. 10.12 (**a**, **b**) Because the fat and SVF cannot pass through the filtre, the pressure in syringe A increases. At a pressure of 1.5 m of water the check valves included in the system open automatically. This way, without opening the stopcocks, the content of syringe A is automatically transferred into syringe C (see the yellow arrow). (Published by kind permission of ©Mario Goisis 2018. All Rights Reserved)

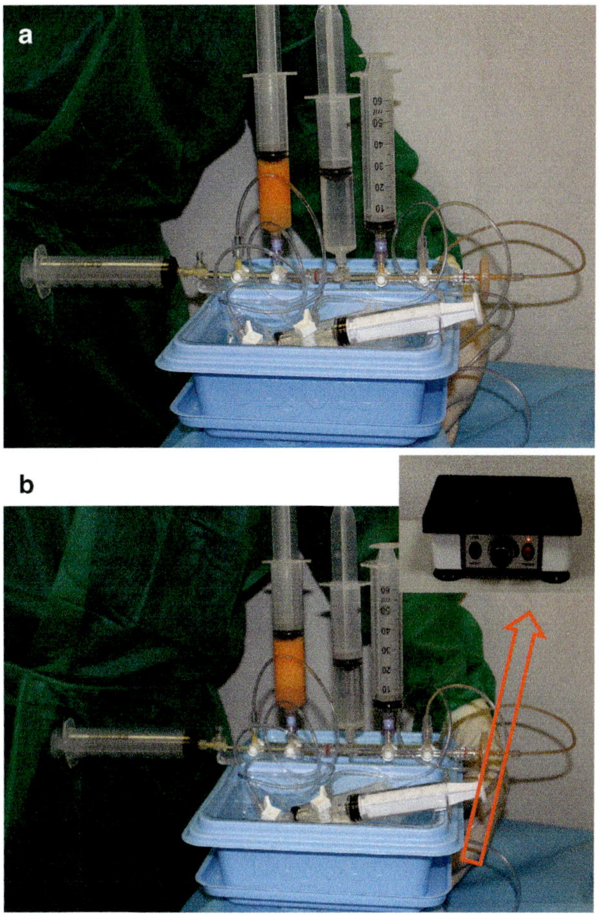

Fig. 10.13 (**a**, **b**) Vibration is then applied for 6 min at 6000 vibrations/min. (Published by kind permission of ©Mario Goisis 2018. All Rights Reserved)

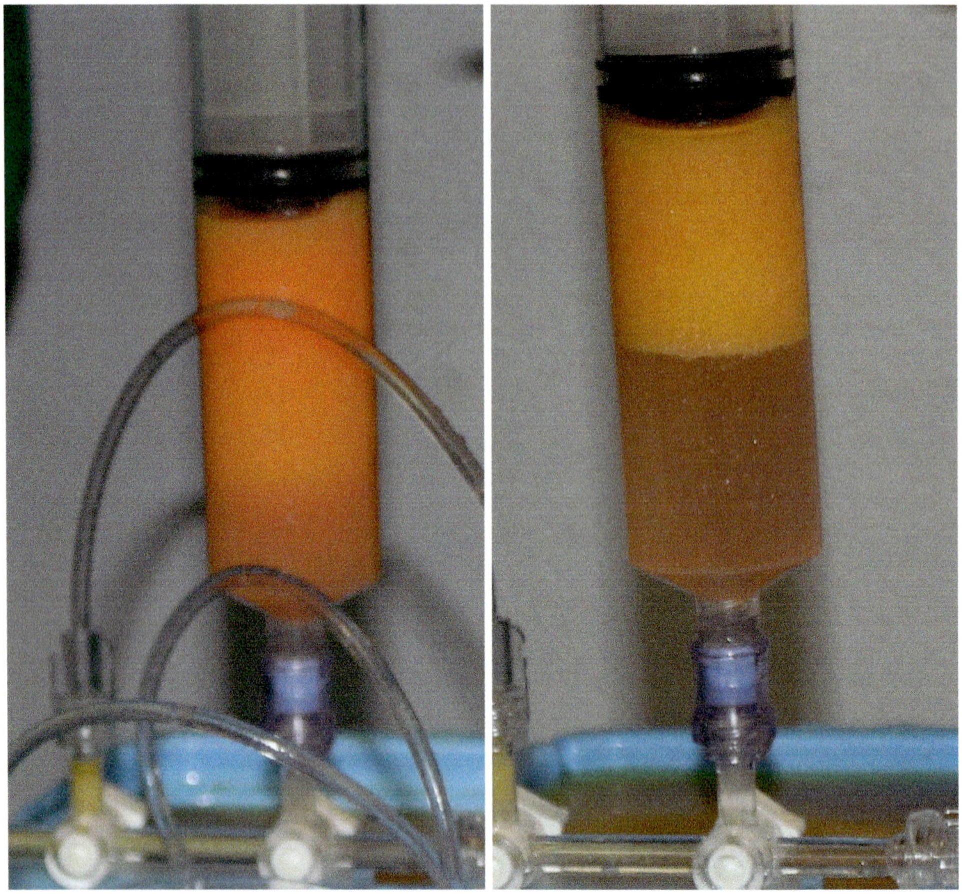

Fig. 10.14 Separation of fat and liquid parts before (image on the left) and after vibration (image on the right). (Published by kind permission of ©Mario Goisis 2018. All Rights Reserved)

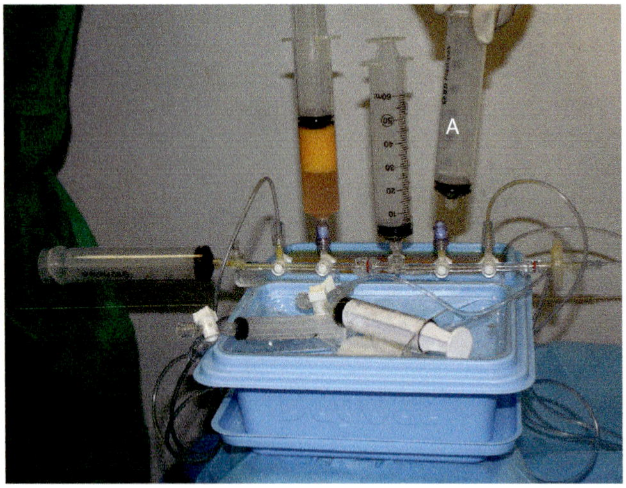

Fig. 10.15 The empty syringe, A, is removed. (Published by kind permission of ©Mario Goisis 2018. All Rights Reserved)

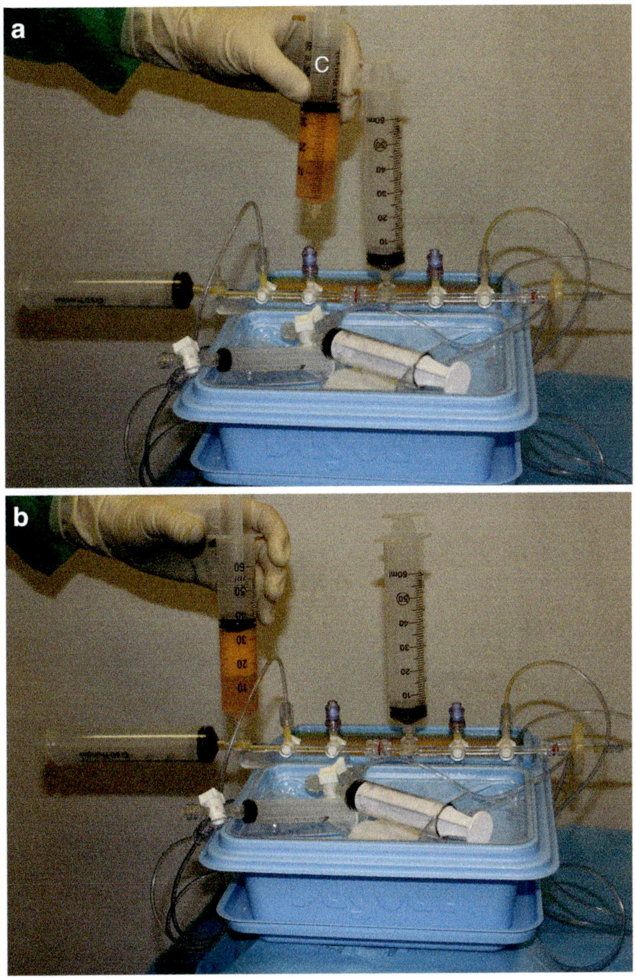

Fig. 10.16 (**a**, **b**) The position of syringe C is changed. (Published by kind permission of ©Mario Goisis 2018. All Rights Reserved)

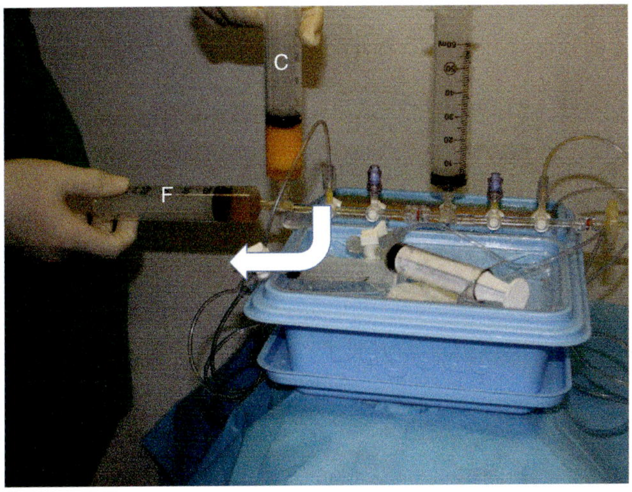

Fig. 10.17 By means of a one-way valve, the lower content of syringe C is transferred into syringe F only. This syringe contains SVF, stem-cells, and saline solution. (Published by kind permission of ©Mario Goisis 2018. All Rights Reserved)

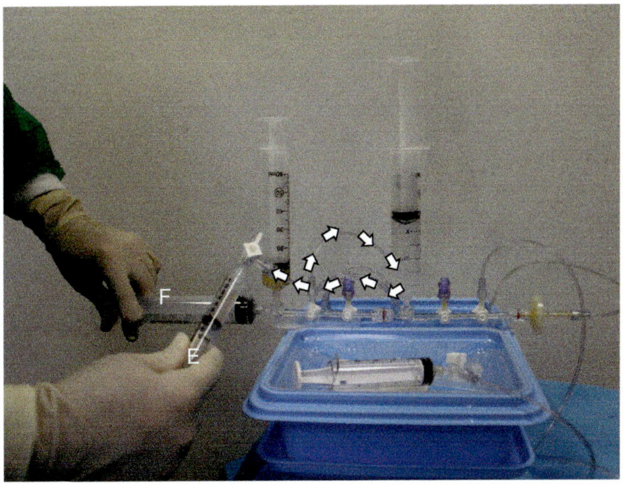

Fig. 10.18 The stopcock of syringe E is opened. This way, syringe E is connected to the tube and the system. Through the one-way valve, the content of syringe F is transferred into syringe E only. (Published by kind permission of ©Mario Goisis 2018. All Rights Reserved)

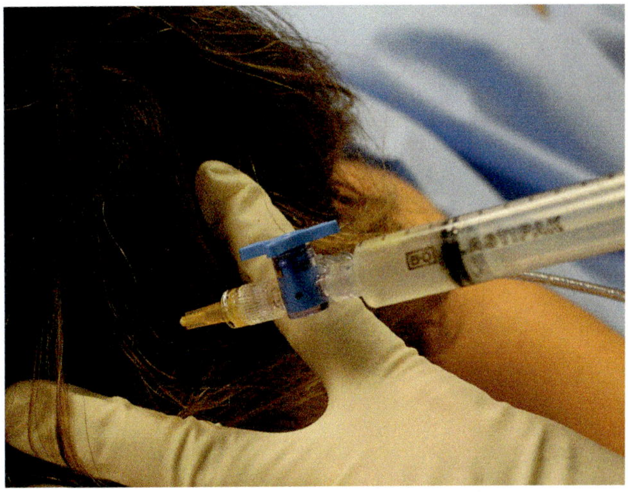

Fig. 10.19 The SVF and the stem-cells are injected into the recipient area. (Published by kind permission of ©Mario Goisis 2018. All Rights Reserved)

and stem-cells viability was discussed. The number of stem-cell of 2 different samples was measured at 72 hours, 7 days and 14 days after colture. The first sample was the microfat harvested with Goisis Cannula and processed with Goisis System, with high values of stem-cells (5600, 6300, 6500). The second sample was the ultrafiltration, with quite significant levels of stem-cells (2478, 3500 and 3900). some images of stem-cells are reported in images 10.23a, 10.23b, 10.23c and 10.23d Light microscopy of cultured ADSc after Goisis processing of lipoaspirate. Mesenchymal

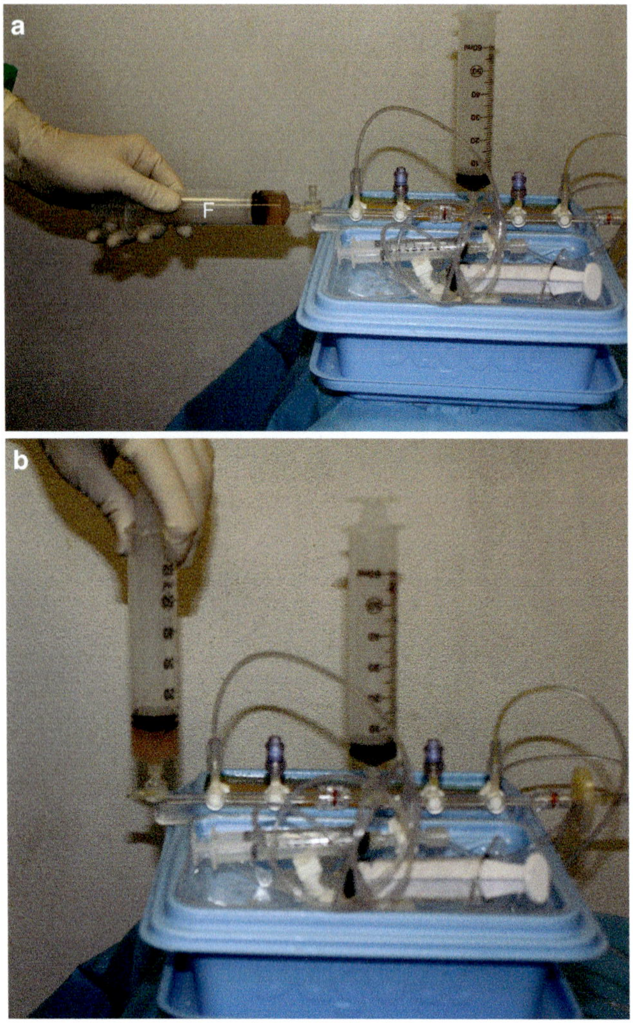

Fig. 10.20 (**a**, **b**) An alternative option is to use the SVF and stem-cells in order to enrich the fat. In this case, the position of syringe F is changed. (Published by kind permission of ©Mario Goisis 2018. All Rights Reserved)

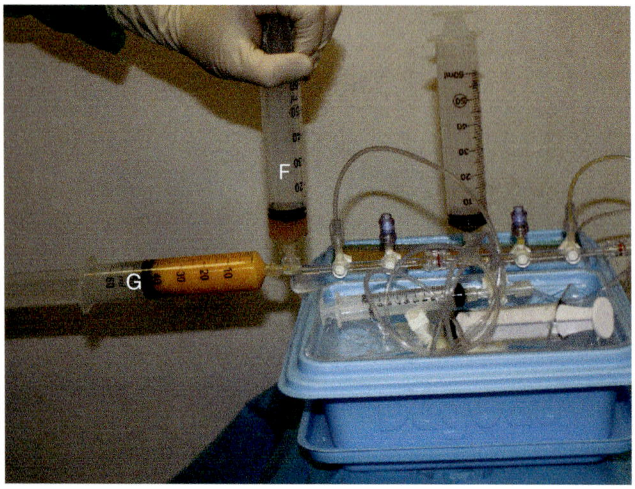

Fig. 10.21 A syringe filled with microfat (syringe G) is connected to the system. Thanks to a one-way valve, the content of syringe F is transferred into syringe G only. In particular, syringe F contains SVF, stem-cells, and saline solution. (Published by kind permission of ©Mario Goisis 2018. All Rights Reserved)

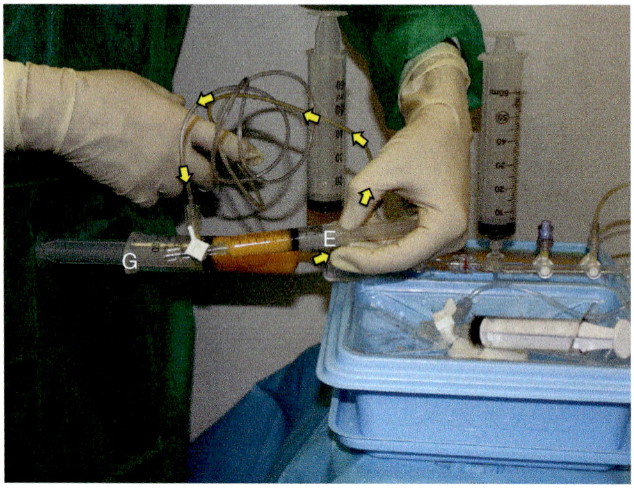

Fig. 10.22 The stopcock of syringe E is opened. In this way, syringe E is connected to the tube and to the system. Thanks to the one-direction valve, the fat enriched with stem-cells is transferred into syringe E only. (Published by kind permission of ©Mario Goisis 2018. All Rights Reserved)

stem-cells were characterized by abundant cytoplasm and central nucleus. After seven days of culture cells are quite confluent in culture flasks. 23b Scanning electron microscopy of mesenchymal stem-cells cultured for seven days. Panel A lower magnification evidenced the confluent status of cells. Panel B showed a magnification of cells and the very long cytoplasm branches protruding from cells. 23c Confocal microscopy of mesenchymal stem-cells expressing SEEA3 and CD105 markers simultaneously. The expression of these two marker allowed to identify a sub population of mesenchymal stem-cells characterized by

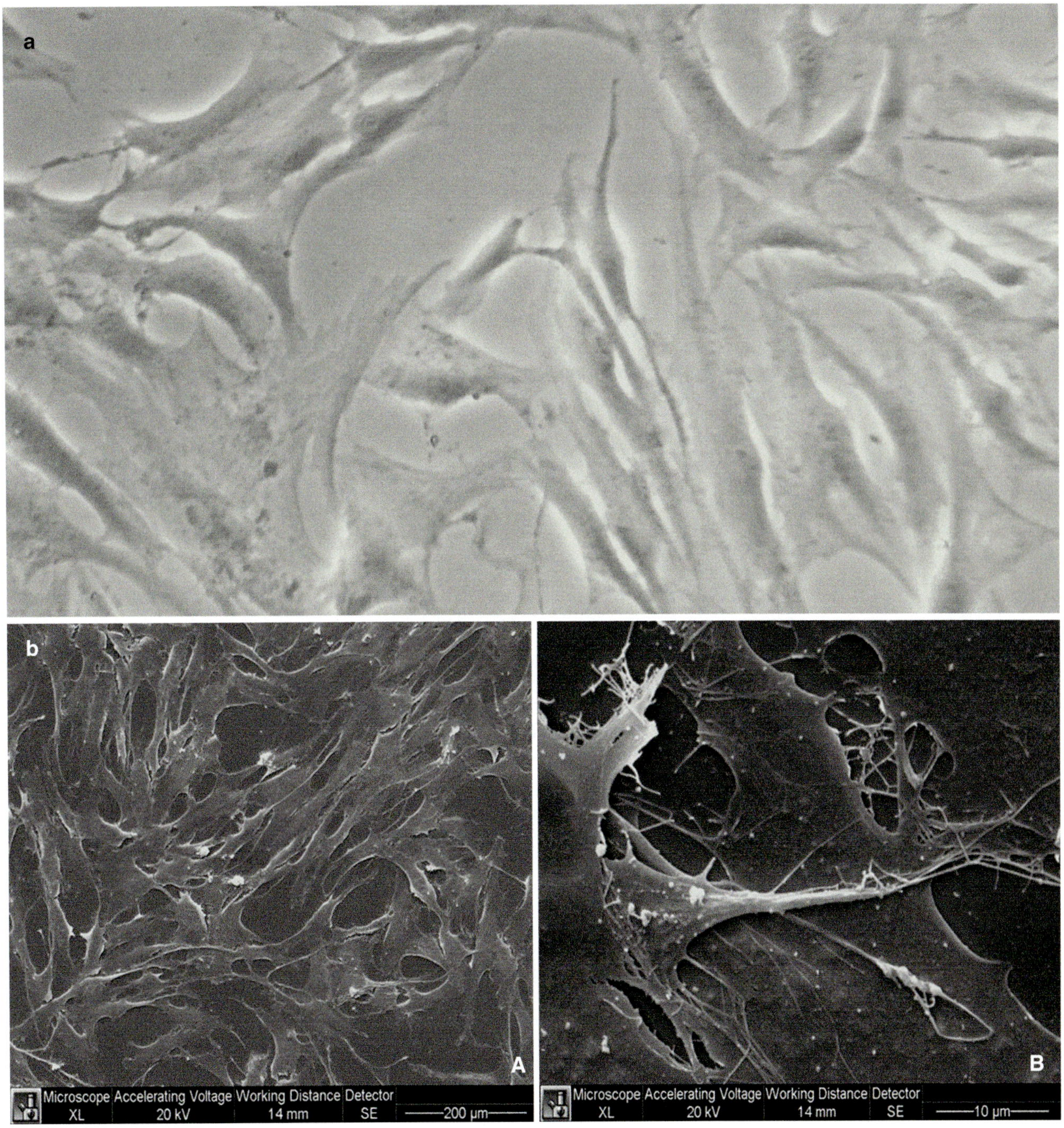

Fig. 10.23 (**a**) Light microscopy of cultured ADSc after Goisis processing of lipoaspirate. Mesenchymal stem cells were characterized by abundant cytoplasm and central nucleus. After 7 days of culture cells are quite confluent in culture flasks. (**b**) Scanning electron microscopy of mesenchymal stem cells cultured for 7 days. Panel A lower magnification evidenced the confluent status of cells. Panel B showed a magnification of cells and the very long cytoplasm branches protruding from cells. (**c**) Confocal microscopy of mesenchymal stem cells expressing SEEA3 and CD105 markers simultaneously. The expression of these two markers allowed to identify a subpopulation of mesenchymal stem cells characterized by pluripotency and able to differentiate in different adult cells. Panel A showed the subpopulation in a patient of 35 years old, while panel B showed the subpopulation of a patient of 28 years old. In younger one the expression of two markers, so the pluripotent population is higher than in older patient. (**d**) Adipogenic induction of pluripotent mesenchymal stem cells. These cells are capable to differentiate in different types of mature and adult cells, but they have the capability to differentiate into mature adipocytes in shorter time in comparison with multipotent stem cells

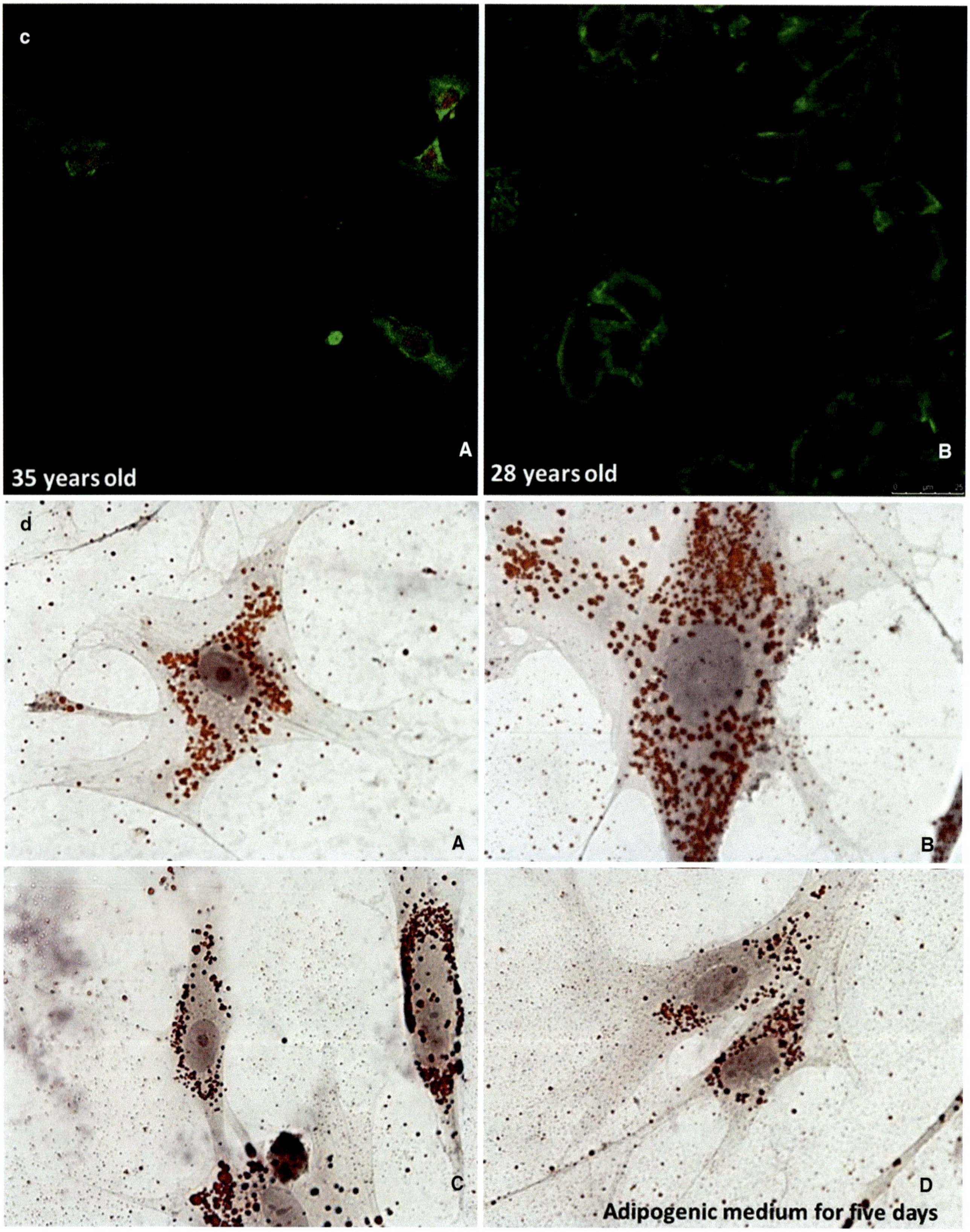

Fig. 10.23 (continued)

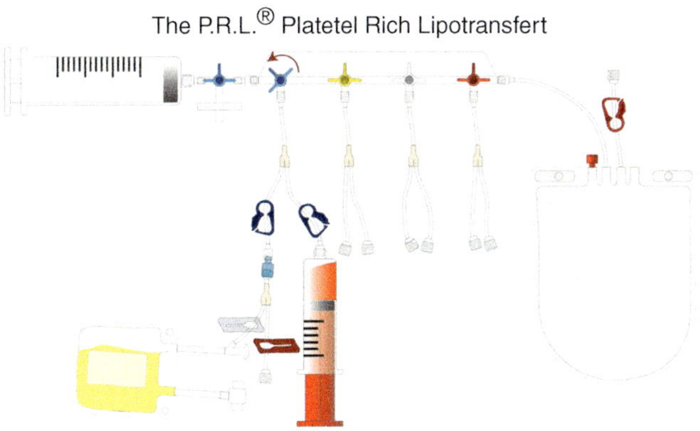

Fig. 10.24 P.R.L. protocol. (Published by kind permission of ©Mario Goisis 2018. All Rights Reserved)

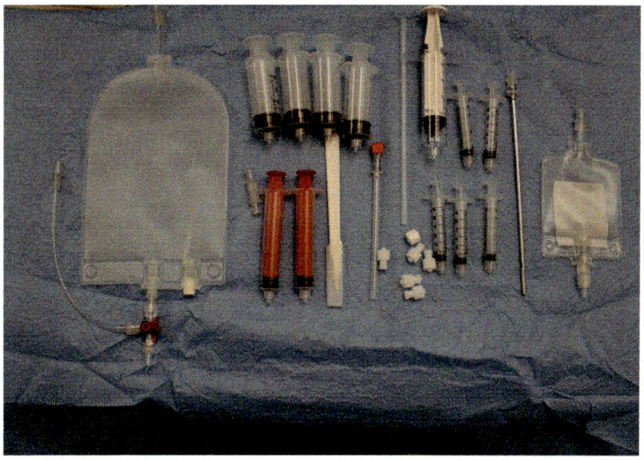

Fig. 10.25 The Fastkit system. (Published by kind permission of ©Mario Goisis 2018. All Rights Reserved)

pluripotency and able to differentiate in different adult cells. panel A showed the sub population in a patient of 35 years old, while pane B showed the sub population of a patient of 28 years old. In younger one the expression of two markers, so the pluripotent population is higher than in older patient. 23dAdipogenic induction of pluripotent mesenchymal stem-cells. these cells are capable to differentiate in different types of mature and adult cells, but they have the capability to differentiate into mature adipocytes in shorter time in comparison with multipotent stem-cells.

10.3.4 The PRL® Platelet-Rich Lipotransfer

The PRL® (Platelet-Rich Lipotransfer) method is the result of a multi-year experience in the use of fat tissue enriched with platelet-rich plasma (PRP) and stromal vascular fraction (SVF) in different surgical procedures.

The PRL system comprises three devices:

- The Fastkit SVF separation system for isolation of SVF
- The C.Punt system for preparation of PRP
- The Mixing system

The Fastkit is a method based on selective filtration of SVF and separation by centrifugation (Figs. 10.25, 10.26a, b, 10.27a, b, 10.28, 10.29a, b, and 10.30)

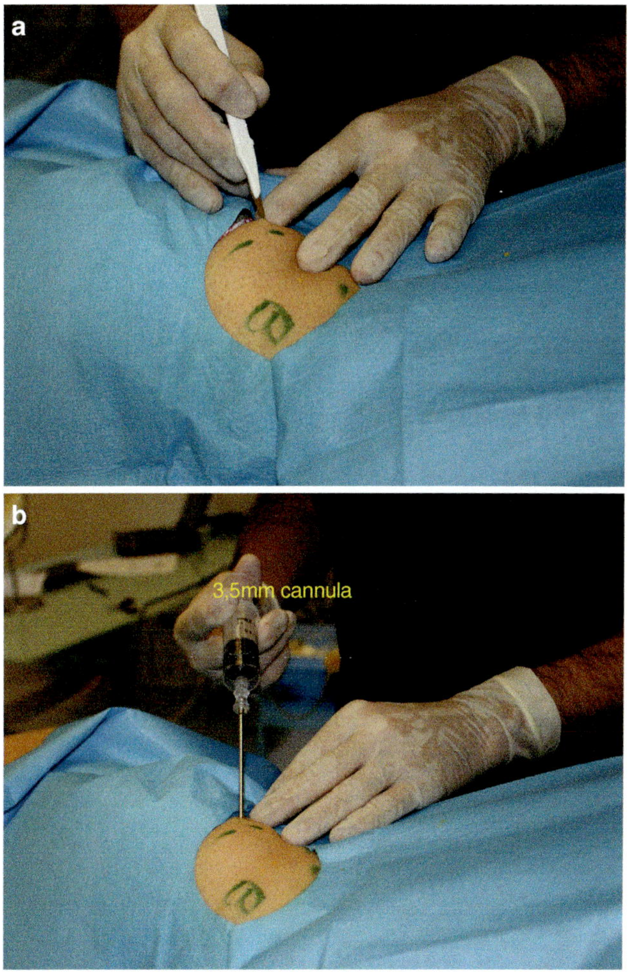

Fig. 10.26 (a, b) Liposuction is performed using a 3.5 mm cannula. (Published by kind permission of ©Mario Goisis 2018. All Rights Reserved)

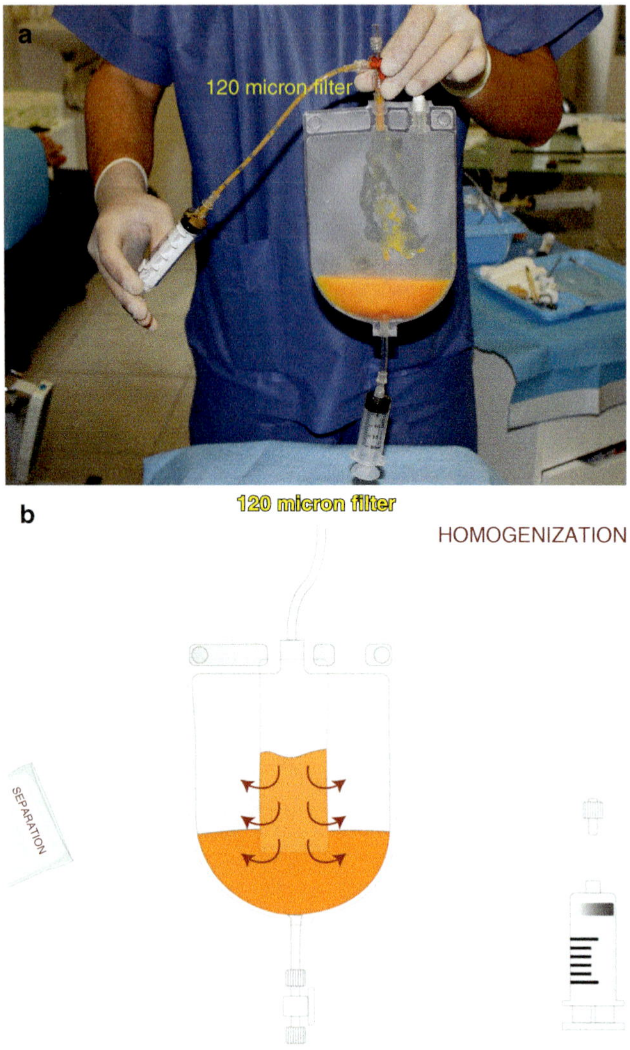

Fig. 10.27 (**a**, **b**) A first filtration is performed using a 120 μ filtre. (Published by kind permission of ©Mario Goisis 2018. All Rights Reserved)

10.3.5 Lipogems

The Lipogems system (Lipogems International S.R.L., Milan, Italy) is a nonenzymatic device used to obtain a fat tissue derivative highly enriched in pericyte-like elements.

It is based on a disposable device that gradually reduces the size of clusters of adipose tissue (from clusters with a diameter of 1–3.5 mm to clusters of 0.2–0.8 mm), while eliminating oil and red cells. The entire process occurs availing itself a full-immersion system. The standard 225 mL Lipogems device allows to process about 100–130 mL of lipoaspirate to obtain approximately 60–100 mL of final tissue product. This product is a fat tissue derivative with the appearances of a minimally manipulated product that can be injected. It does not require stem-cell expansion or manipulation, and therefore, it is not subjected to the regulatory restrictions of cGMP Guidelines. Histology of lipogem-derived product showed microfragmentated and damaged adipose tissue (Fig. 10.31).

Tremolada et al. reported a significantly higher percentage of mature pericytes and hMSCs, and lower amount of hematopoietic elements in Lipogems, compared with unprocessed lipoaspirate.

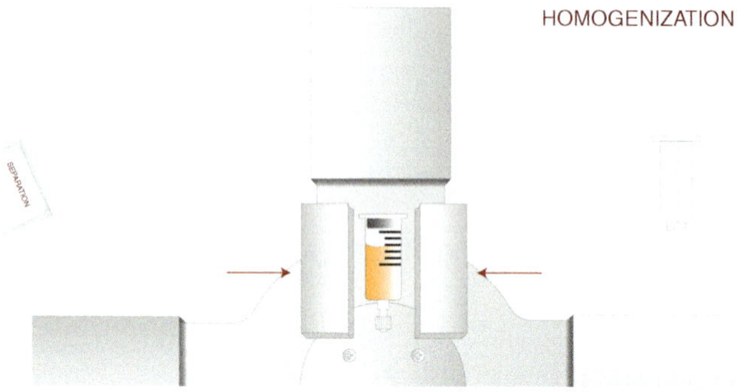

Fig. 10.28 Centrifugation is applied for 10 min. (Published by kind permission of ©Mario Goisis 2018. All Rights Reserved)

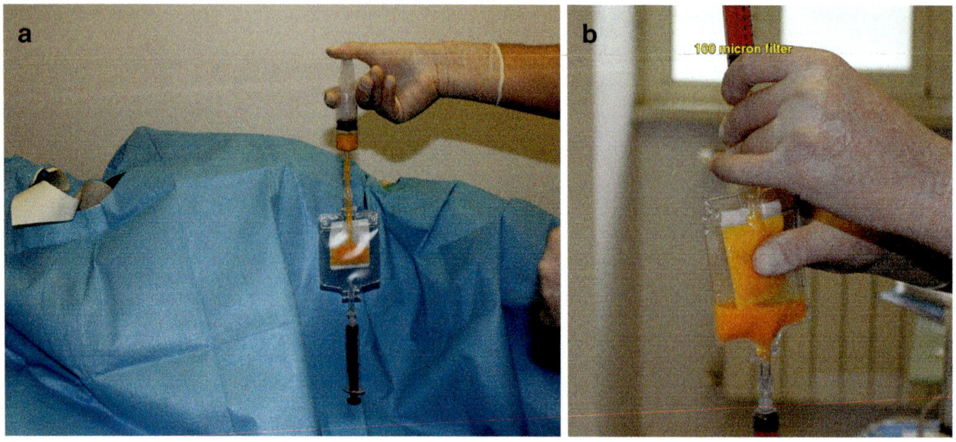

Fig. 10.29 (**a**, **b**) A second filtration, by means of mechanical separation of SVF, is applied. (Published by kind permission of ©Mario Goisis 2018. All Rights Reserved)

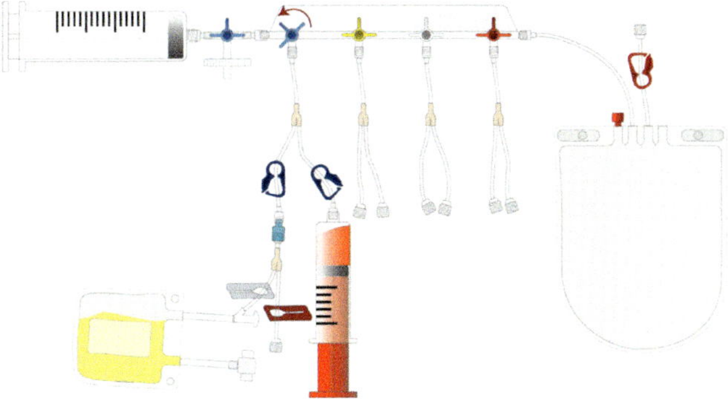

Fig. 10.30 The SVF, the fat, and the PRP are mixed in a closed system. (Published by kind permission of ©Mario Goisis 2018. All Rights Reserved)

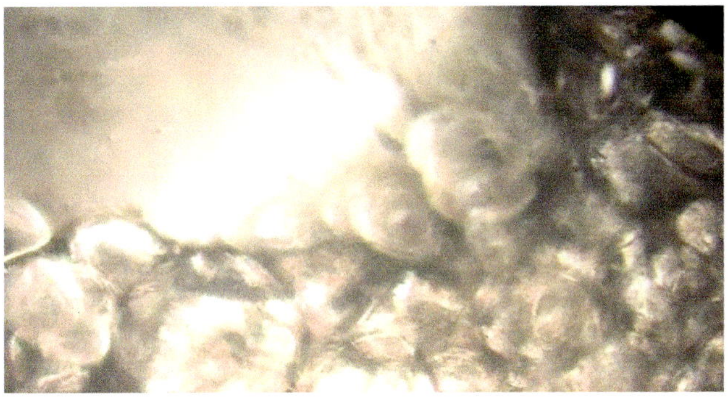

Fig. 10.31 Histological image of fat obtained using the Lipogems system. (Published by kind permission of ©Mario Goisis 2018. All Rights Reserved)

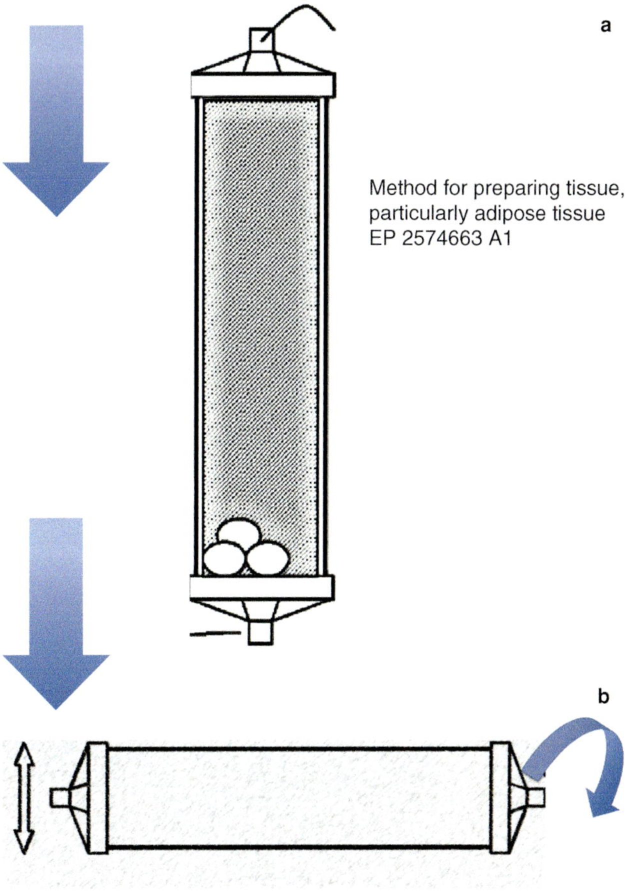

Fig. 10.32 (a, b) Illustration of the Lipogems system (public patent). (Published by kind permission of ©Mario Goisis 2018. All Rights Reserved)

Despite this, Lipogems needs to be classified as a system for harvesting, processing, and reinjecting human fat. In actual fact, Lipogems cannot isolate stem-cells. The final product (Lipogems) contains adult adipocytes mixed with stem-cells [1] (Fig. 10.32a–c).

10.3.6 Nanofat: Tonnard Technique

In 2013 Tonnard et al. published an innovative technique. The harvested fat was mechanically emulsified and filtered until a liquid suspension was obtained. Tonnard called this "nanofat" [25].

In particular, emulsification of the fat was achieved by moving the fat between two 10-cc syringes, coupled by a female-to-female Luer-Lok connector. After 30 passes, the fat became liquid and took on a whitish appearance (Fig. 10.33a, b). In fact, the fat was fragmented and changed into an emulsion. After emulsification, the fatty liquid was filtered through a sterile nylon cloth with a pore-size of 0.5 mm (Fig. 10.34a–c). The filtration was performed to remove the remnants of connective tissue that would block the fine needles during injection (Figs. 10.35a, b and 10.36).

The histology and viability evaluation shows that the nanofat has lost the normal structure of fatty tissue. In particular, adipocytes are destroyed and replaced by an oily emulsion. However, isolation and culture demonstrated that a large number of good-quality mesenchymal stem-cells are still present in the nanofat samples.

Tonnard considers nanofat as an in vivo tissue-engineering process. In fact, the major effect of nanofat is stem-cell activity.

In nanofat the stromal vascular fraction is not purified, but is mixed with oil and dead adipocyte fraction. However, in the opinion of Tonnard, isolating the stromal vascular fraction from the nanofat before injection would be complicated, time consuming, and expensive. Moreover, it is known that apoptotic cells attract macrophages that induce growth

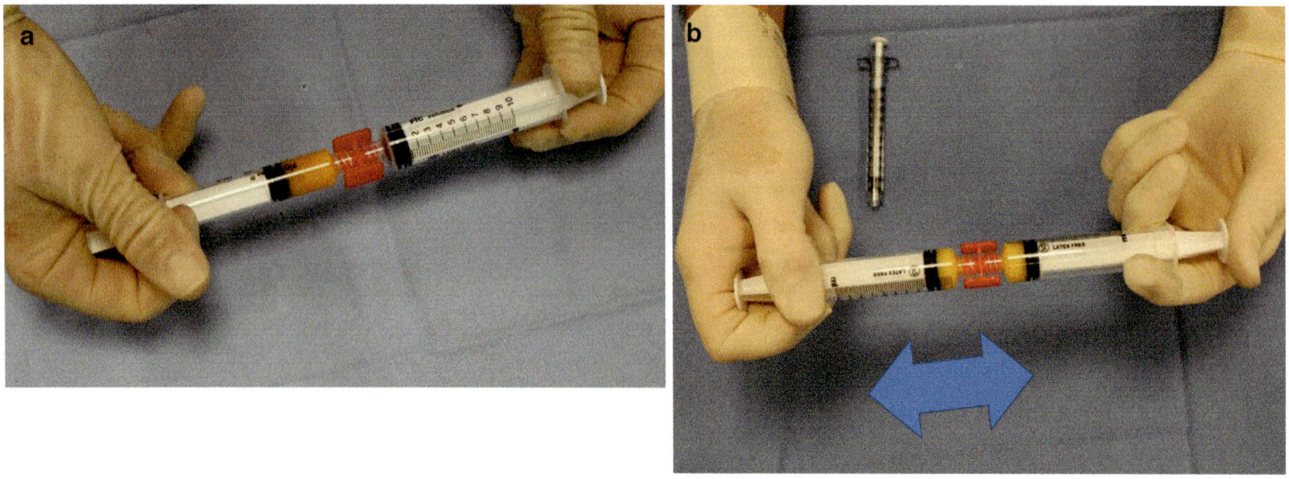

Fig. 10.33 (**a**, **b**) Emulsification of the fat is achieved by moving the fat between two 10-cc syringes. (Published by kind permission of ©Mario Goisis 2018. All Rights Reserved)

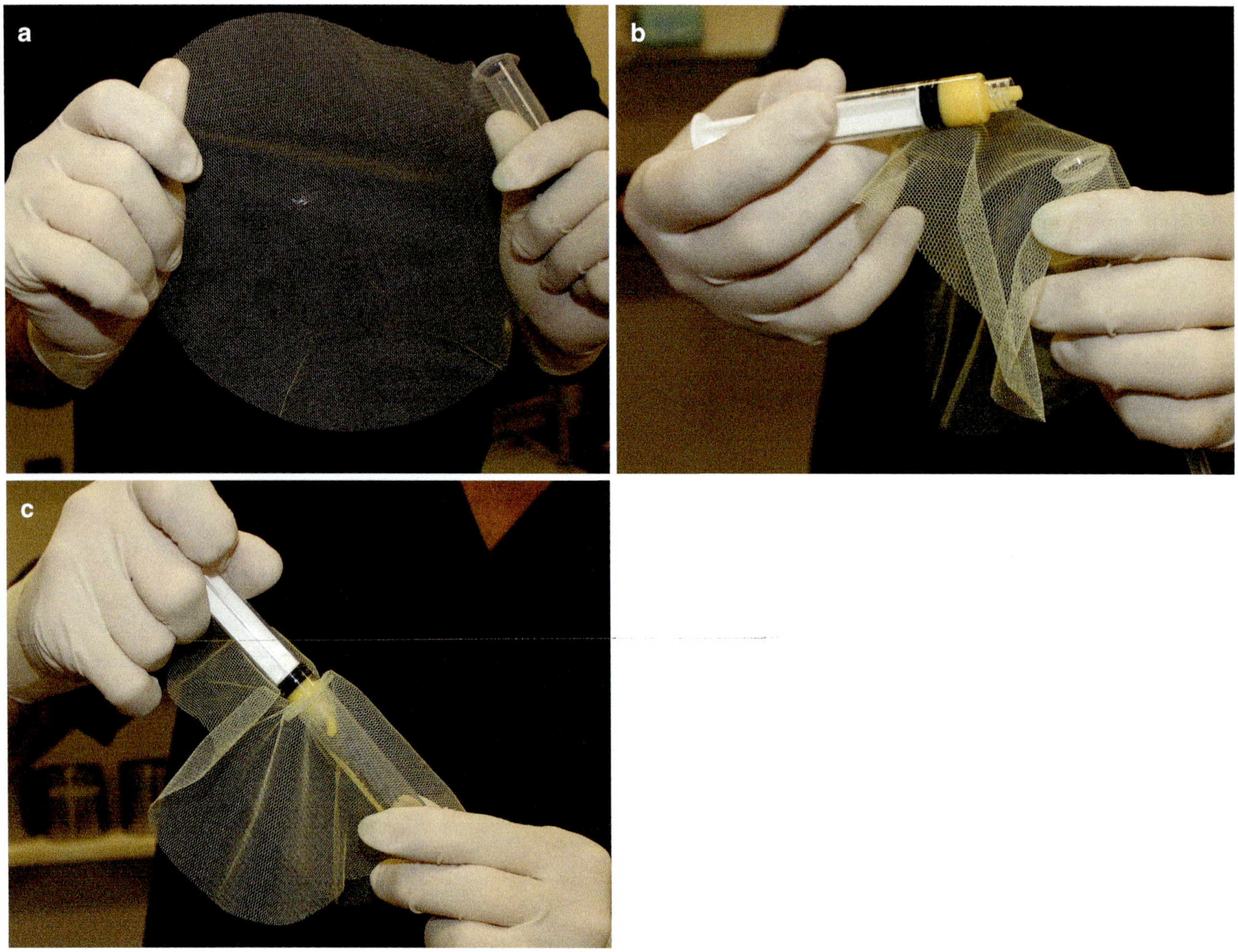

Fig. 10.34 (**a**–**c**) After emulsification, the fatty liquid is filtered through a sterile nylon cloth having a pore-size of 0.5 mm. (Published by kind permission of ©Mario Goisis 2018. All Rights Reserved)

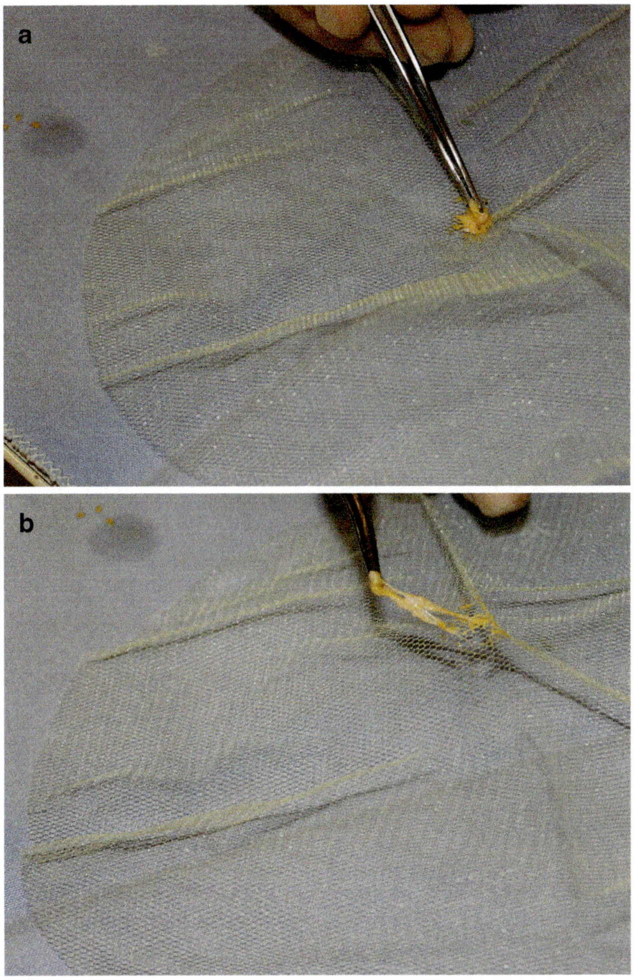

Fig. 10.35 (**a**, **b**) The filtration is performed to remove the connective tissue remnants that would block the fine needles during injection. These remnants are demonstrated here. (Published by kind permission of ©Mario Goisis 2018. All Rights Reserved)

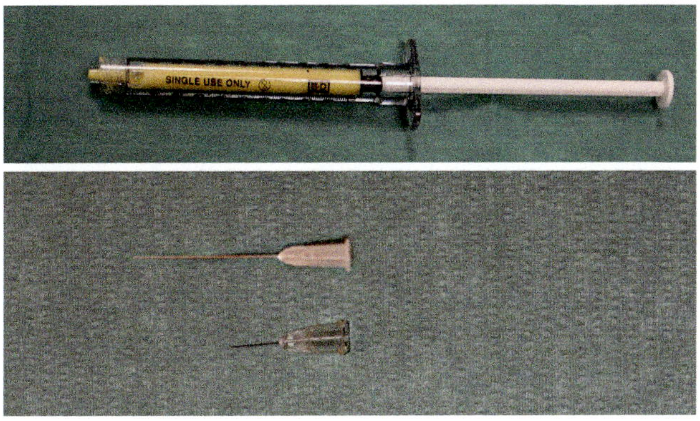

Fig. 10.36 Nanofat is injected using a 27-gauge cannula. (Published by kind permission of ©Mario Goisis 2018. All Rights Reserved)

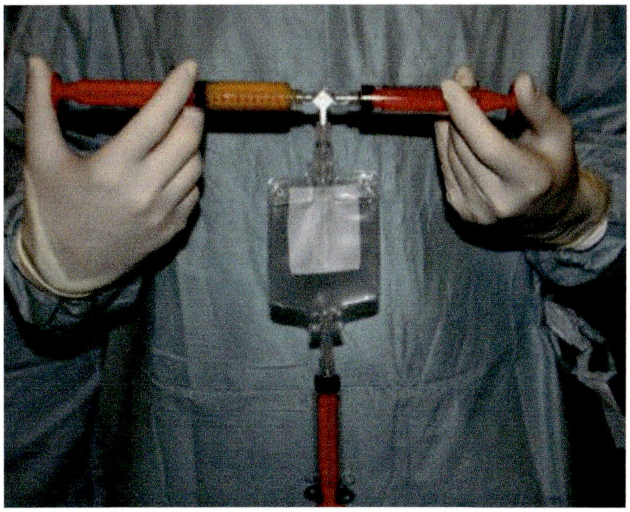

Fig. 10.37 With this device we can carry out the fat emulsification process, shifting fat 30 times from one syringe to another

factors and play an important role in regeneration of the damaged tissue. For this reason, injection of fragmented adipocytes may play a role in stem-cell differentiation and tissue regeneration (Fig. 10.37).

10.3.7 Nanograft: Planas Technique

The main aim of the Planas nanofat technique is to avoid exposure to the air.

For this reason, in his experience Planas did not resort to filtering the fat through nylon cloth as originally described by Tonnard et al., in an attempt to maintain the entire the procedure within a closed loop system, in order to reduce infection and oxidation of the tissue.

Because nylon cloth was not used, injection was initially performed using a sharp 25-GA sharp needle, slightly wider than the one used by Tonnard et al. The 25GA needle was used as a mechanical filter for those unemulsified particles, especially in connective tissue. Sometimes it was necessary to change the needle several times during the procedure because it gets clogged with this connective tissue.

Of course, the use of needles with a larger diameter increased the presence of ecchymosis after treatment.

An innovation was the introduction of the Nanofat Kit (Nanofat Planas Kit), which allows one to carry out the fat emulsification and filtration by means of a completely closed system.

This device consists of two syringes of 10 mL each connected to a three-way device, a 10-mL collecting bag with a 120 μ filtre inside, and another 10-ml collecting syringe for nanofat (Fig. 10.38).

A nylon mesh filtre with mesh openings of 120 μ was chosen as optimal with a view both to prevent the product from clumping or clogging and keep the stem-cells intact because small openings can damage the cell product to be collected.

With this device the fat emulsification is carried out, by shifting fat 30 times between two syringes, through the 3-way connector. Once this action has been accomplished, the connector is turned and sends the syringe contents into the collecting bag, where the residual particles are filtered; this content is aspirated directly through the 10 cc collecting syringe afterward (Figs. 10.38, 10.39, 10.40, and 10.41).

Through a Luer-Lok female-to-female connector the nanofat is transferred to Luer-Lok syringes of 1 mL, and later infiltrated using 27–30-GA needles (Figs. 10.42 and 10.43).

10.3.8 Stem-Cell Analysis of Nanofat

Emulsified fat samples were sent for tissue evaluation to the Stem-Cells and Cancer Laboratory, at the Vall d´Hebron Research Institute (Barcelona, Spain). Using flow cytometry, the presence of viable CD34+ cells was analysed. In addition, phase-contrast microscopy examination was used to show disrupted adipose tissue and apoptotic cells (Figs. 10.44 and 10.45, respectively).

Using fluorescence microscopy, Tonnard et al. demonstrated that nonviable adipocytes and non-normal adipose tissue-structures were detected when emulsified fat samples were analysed [25]. However, when this emulsion was passed through a magnetic-activated cell sorter for CD34+ cell selection, they obtained products containing up to

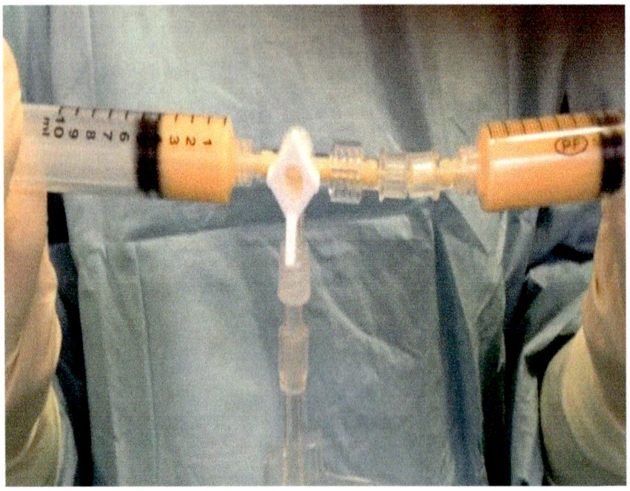

Fig. 10.38 With this device we can carry out the fat emulsification, shifting fat 30 times from one syringe to another

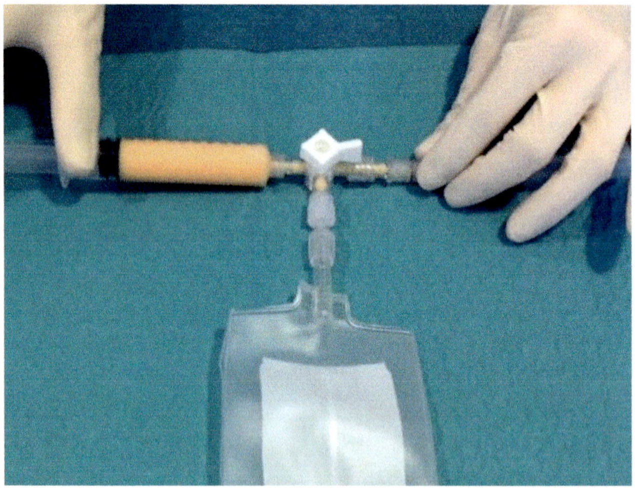

Fig. 10.39 Turn the connector on and send the syringe contents into the collecting bag, where the residual particles are filtered

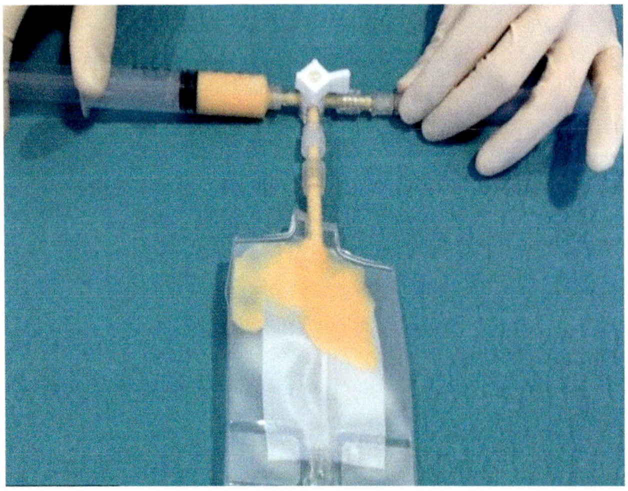

Fig. 10.40 Turn the connector on and send the syringe contents into the collecting bag, where the residual particles are filtered

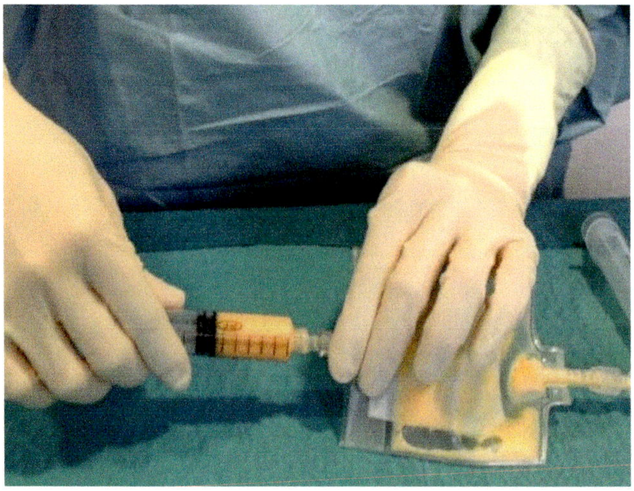

Fig. 10.41 Afterward, the content is aspirated directly through the 10-cc collecting syringe

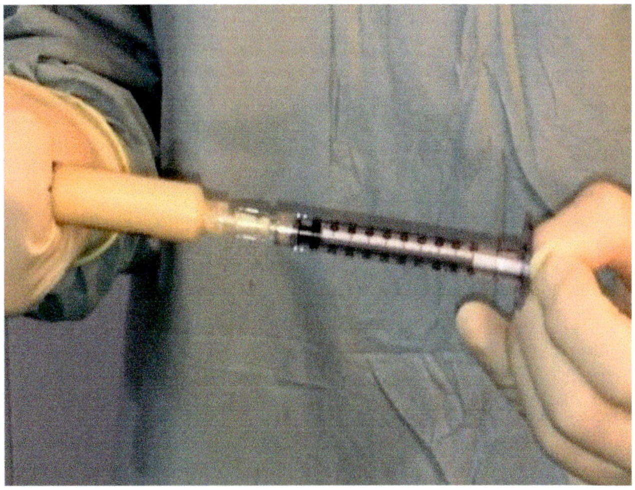

Fig. 10.42 Through a Luer-Lok female-to-female connector the nanofat is transferred to Luer-Lok syringes of 1 mL, and later infiltrated with needles of using 27–30-GA needles

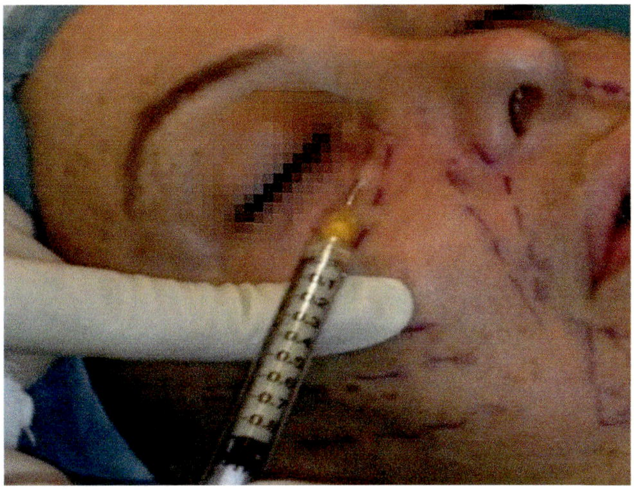

Fig. 10.43 Intradermal infiltration of nanofat, observing small yellowish wheal at dermis level

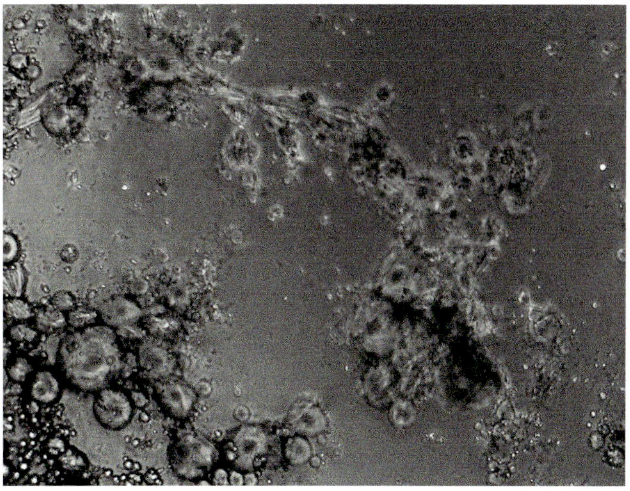

Fig. 10.44 Phase-contrast microscopy digital image showing disrupted adipose tissue and the presence of bright cells after tissue emulsification. Phase-contrast microscopy was used to view unstained specimens by using the light phase amplitude differences within microscopic biological materials

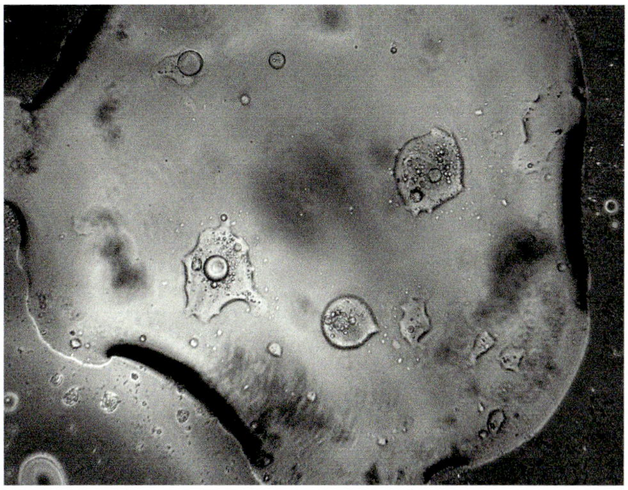

Fig. 10.45 Apoptosis detection using phase-contrast microscopy, showing nanofat containing cells with fragmented nuclear morphology as well as other specific hallmarks of programmed cell death. (Published by kind permission of ©Mario Goisis 2018. All Rights Reserved)

100,000 CD34+ cells per 100 mL of lipoaspirate. Magnetic cell-sorting enables fast separation of the desired cells with excellent yields and purities, and preserves cell functionality. Nevertheless, purity of sorted cells alone is not a sufficient performance parameter, and recovery of almost all of the stem-cells contained in the initial fat product is highly desirable.

In order to overcome the limitations associated with yield and/or recovery of stem-cell count after magnetic cell separation, we have performed direct immunofluorescence measurements for CD34+ absolute cell-counts using acoustic focusing flow cytometry. In our study, the remaining cells from emulsified fat were simultaneously stained with PE-CD34 and FITC-CD45 antibodies, and Vybrant(R) DyeCycle™ Violet (DCV), a cell-permeant nucleic acid stains that can penetrate the nucleus without cell fixation, and it is compatible with many live cell applications. Briefly, emulsified fat was filtered through a 52 μm nylon mesh, and the effluent was collected for flow cytometric assays. Nanofat aliquots (100 μL) were stained with PE-CD34, FITC-CD45, and DCV for 20 min at RT, protected from light.

10.3.9 Flow Cytometry Measurements

All cell measurements were carried out using the Attune® Acoustic Focusing Cytometer (Life Technologies, Carlsbad, CA). Nanofat samples were simultaneously stained with PE-CD34, PE-CD133, and FITC-CD45, and DCV. Filtre combination used consisted of 555 DLP, BP 530/30 (FITC), and 620 DLP, 574/26 (PE). Acquisition was stopped when a minimum of 10,000 live-gated DCV+ events were collected. FITC, PE, and DCV fluorescence were collected according to a logarithmic scale.

10.4 Results

10.4.1 Stem-Cell Analysis

CD34+ cells were detected in emulsified fat (>50% of total DCV cells; Fig. 10.46a), and near one-half of CD34+ cells co-expressed CD45 (43.22%; Fig. 10.46b), indicating their hematopoietic origin. These results showed an enrichment of CD34+ cells from nanofat specimens, suggesting that adipose tissue might constitute a hypoxic reservoir for CD34+ hematopoietic stem-cells. The enrichment in CD34 cells could be explained because adipose tissue may compose a trap to sequester peripheral blood circulating CD34+ cells. Adipose tissue is especially hypoxic (40–50 mmHg), and this could be an explanation for the appearance of CD34+ stem-cells, giving support to a growing body of evidence suggesting that various types of stem-cells exist in a hypoxic microenvironment.

10.4.2 Nanofat: Goisis Nanofat Kit

The Goisis kit (www.microfat.com) is a system for washing fat and the production of nanofat. All the procedure is carried out using a closed system. This way the risk of infection is reduced, and there is no contact between fat and air.

In particular, microfat is harvested using a microfat box (www.microfat.com).

The syringe filled with microfat is then connected to the DE nanofat kit. The production of nanofat is based on a closed system, without exposure to air.

The procedure is very fast and efficient. In particular, only 1.5 cc of fat are lost into the DE nanofat kit (Figs. 10.47, 10.48, 10.49a–c, 10.50, 10.51a, b, 10.52, and 10.53).

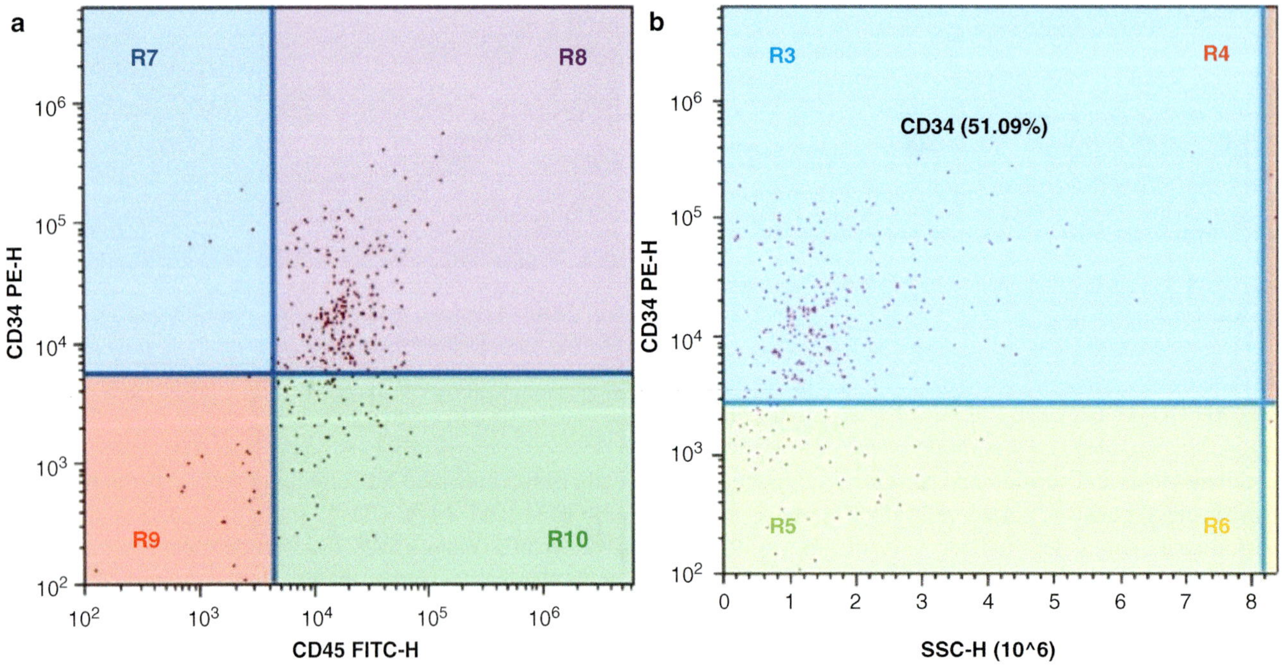

Fig. 10.46 (**a**) Representative CD34+/CD45+ measurements in nanofat. Flow cytometric dotplot displaying CD34+/CD45+ cells on an Attune Acoustic Focusing Cytometer (Life Technologies) equipped with a 50 mW violet laser emitting at 405 nm. (Published by kind permission of ©Mario Goisis 2018. All Rights Reserved). (**b**) Representative CD34+ measurements in nanofat. Flow cytometric dotplot displaying Side Scatter vs. CD34+ cells on an Attune Acoustic Focusing Cytometer (Life Technologies) equipped with a 50 mW violet laser emitting at 405 nm. (Published by kind permission of ©Mario Goisis 2018. All Rights Reserved)

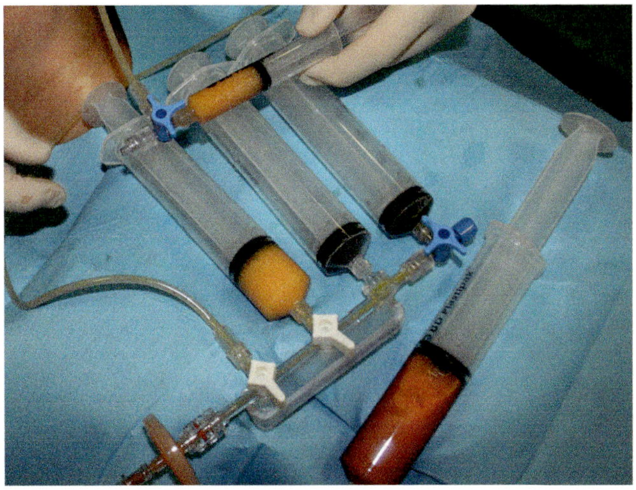

Fig. 10.47 5 cc of microfat are produced using the microfat box (www.microfat.com). (Published by kind permission of ©Mario Goisis 2018. All Rights Reserved)

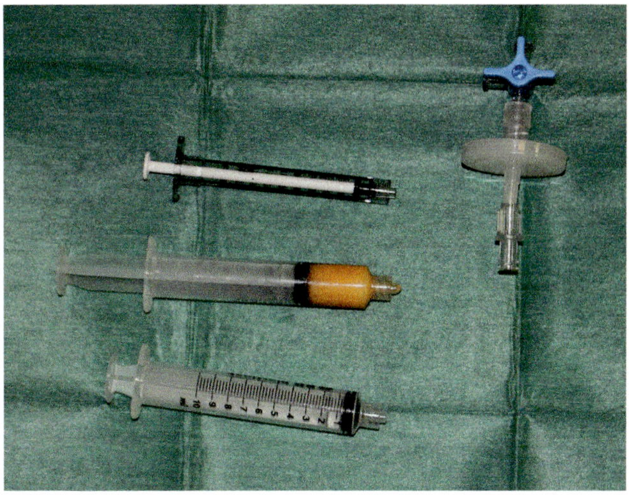

Fig. 10.48 The Goisis nanofat kit. (Published by kind permission of ©Mario Goisis 2018. All Rights Reserved)

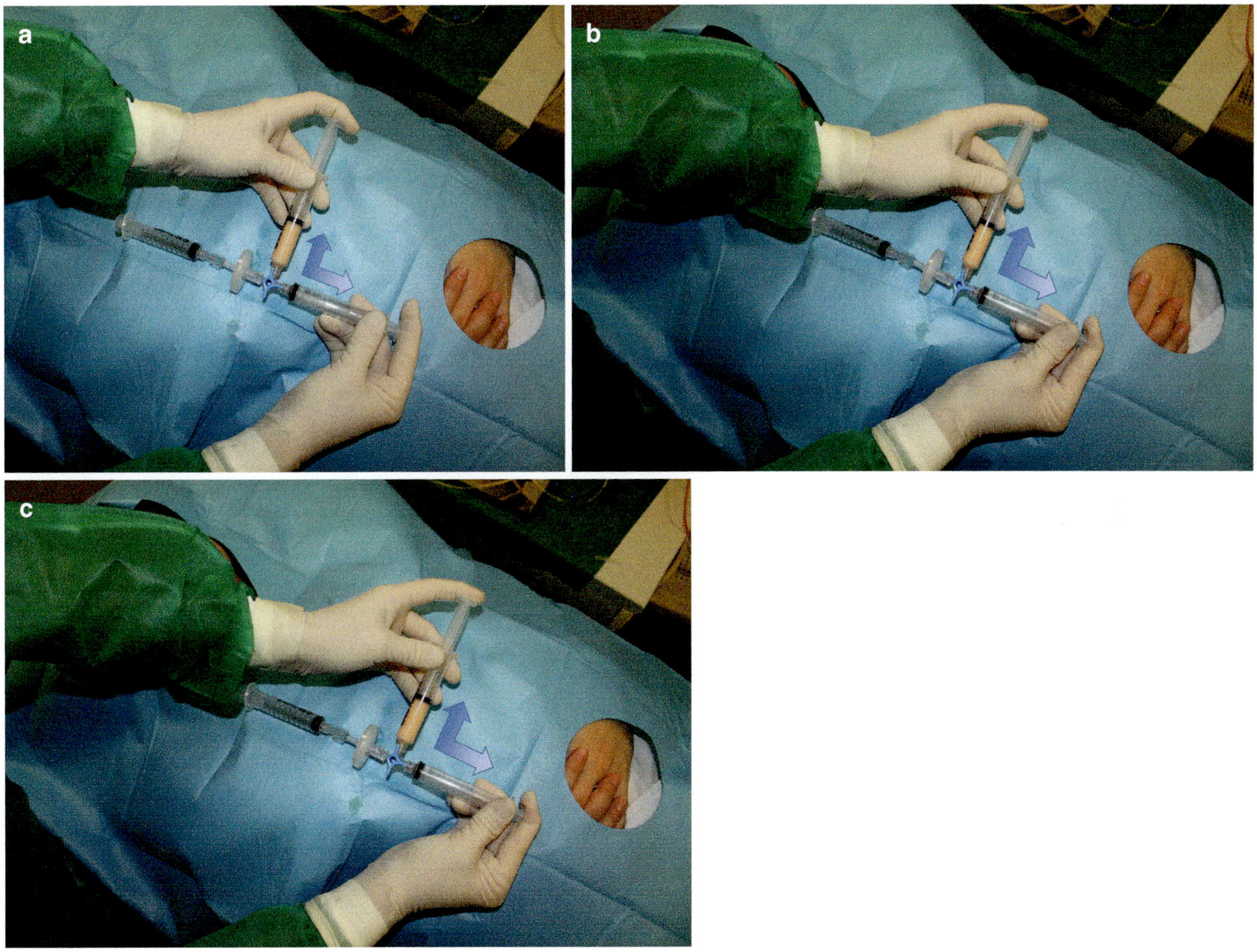

Fig. 10.49 (**a**) Three 10 cc syringes are connected to the kit. The fat is moved between the 2 syringes 30 times. (Published by kind permission of ©Mario Goisis 2018. All Rights Reserved). (**b**) Three 10 cc syringes are connected to the kit. The fat is moved rapidly between the 2 syringes 30 times. (Published by kind permission of ©Mario Goisis 2018. All Rights Reserved). (**c**) Three 10 cc syringes are connected to the kit. The fat is moved quickly between the 2 syringes 30 times. (Published by kind permission of ©Mario Goisis 2018. All Rights Reserved)

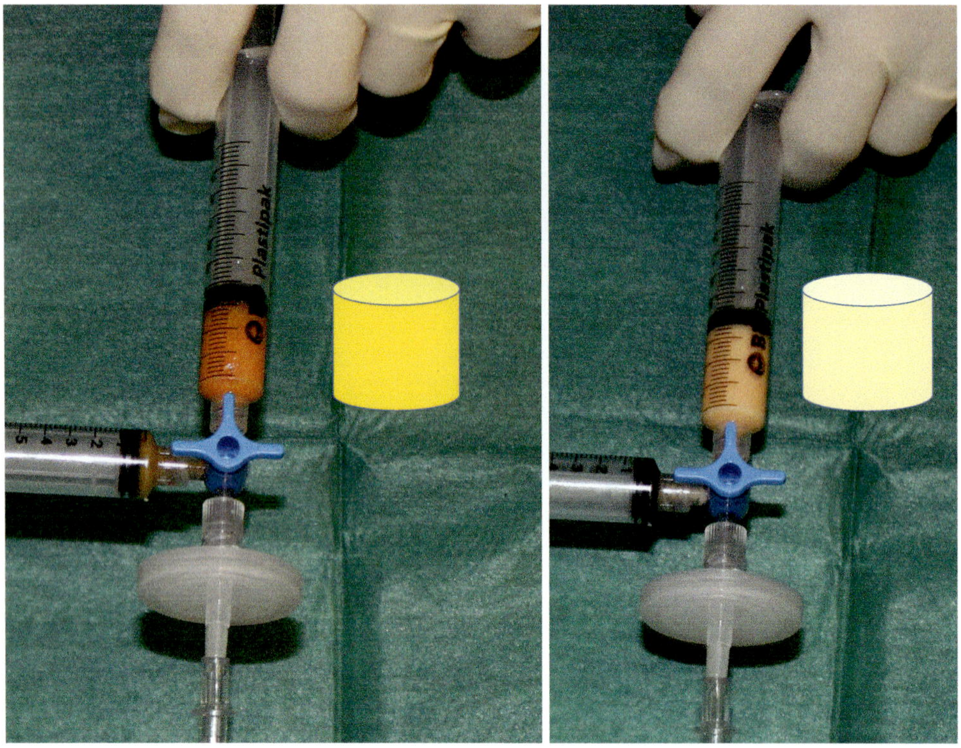

Fig. 10.50 The microfat has a yellow colour. After 30 passages, it is transformed in nanofat, which is whitish. (Published by kind permission of ©Mario Goisis 2018. All Rights Reserved)

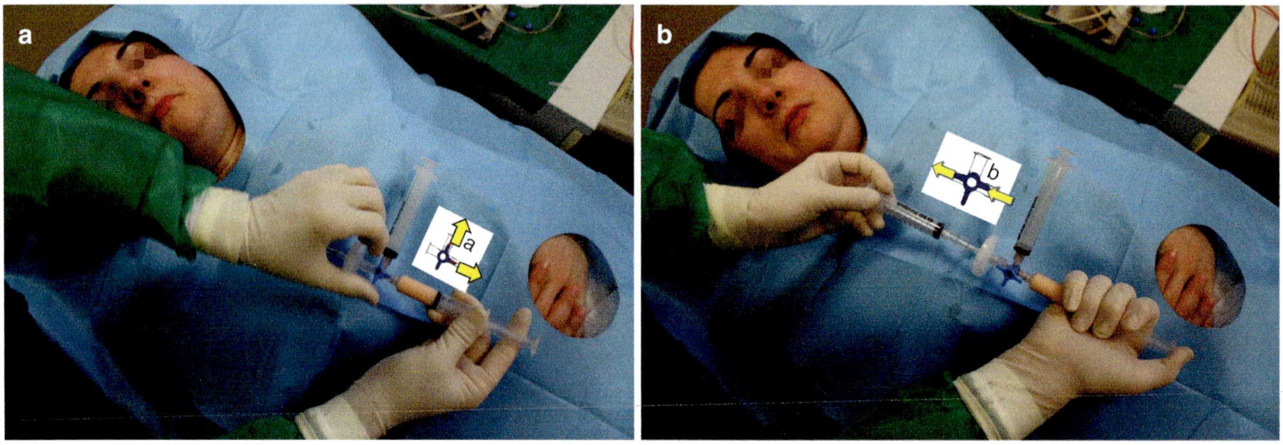

Fig. 10.51 (**a**, **b**) The stopcock is moved form position "a" to position "b". (Published by kind permission of ©Mario Goisis 2018. All Rights Reserved)

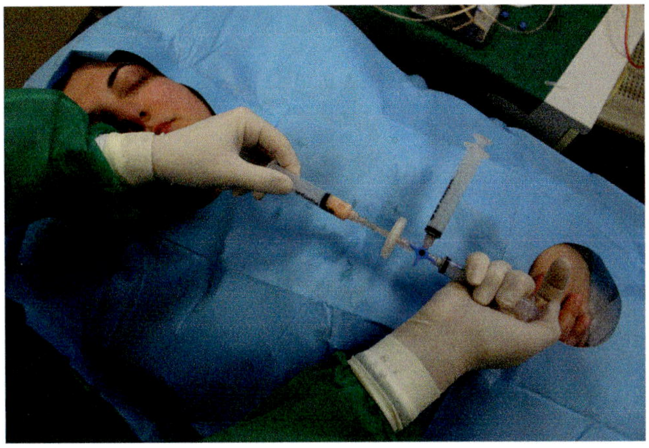

Fig. 10.52 This way, the fat is filtered and directly transferred into the third syringe. (Published by kind permission of ©Mario Goisis 2018. All Rights Reserved)

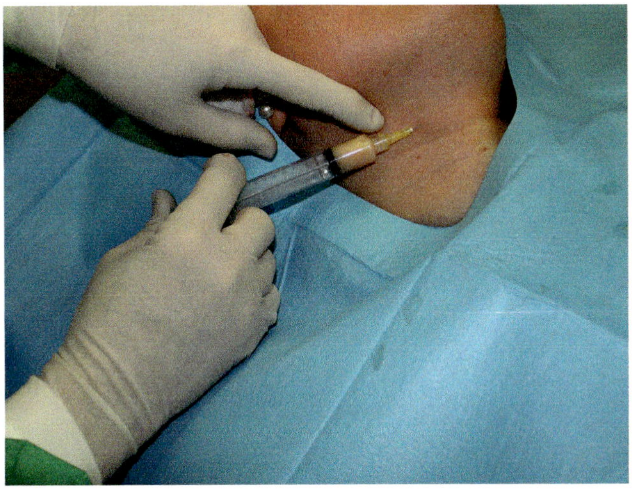

Fig. 10.53 Because of filtration, the fat can be injected directly using a 30-GA needle. (Published by kind permission of ©Mario Goisis 2018. All Rights Reserved)

References

1. Bianchi F, Maioli M, Leonardi E, Olivi E, Pasquinelli G, Valente S, Mendez AJ, Ricordi C, Raffaini M, Tremolada C, Ventura C. A new nonenzymatic method and device to obtain a fat tissue derivative highly enriched in pericyte-like elements by mild mechanical forces from human lipoaspirates. Cell Transplant. 2013;22(11):2063–77.
2. Ventura C, Cantoni S, Bianchi F, Lionetti V, Cavallini C, Scarlata I, Foroni L, Maioli M, Bonsi L, Alviano F, Fossati V, Bagnara GP, Pasquinelli G, Recchia FA, Perbellini A. Hyaluronan mixed esters of butyric and retinoic acid drive cardiac and endothelial fate in term placenta human mesenchymal stem cells and enhance cardiac repair in infarcted rat hearts. J Biol Chem. 2007;282(19):14243–52.
3. Cavallari G, Olivi E, Bianchi F, Neri F, Foroni L, Valente S, Manna GL, Nardo B, Stefoni S, Ventura C. Mesenchymal stem cells and islet cotransplantation in diabetic rats: improved islet graft revascularization and function by preconditioned with natural molecules. Cell Transplant. 2012;21(12):2771–81.
4. Stavely R, Robinson AM, Miller S, Boyd R, Sakkal S, Nurgali K. Human adult stem cells derived from adipose tissue and bone marrow attenuate enteric neuropathy in the guinea-pig model of acute colitis. Stem Cell Res Ther. 2015;6(1):244.
5. Wang W, He N, Feng C, Liu V, et al. Human adipose-derived mesenchymal progenitor cells engraft into rabbit articular cartilage. Int J Mol Sci. 2015;16:12076–91.
6. Chang YH, Liu HW, Wu KC, Ding DC. Mesenchymal stem cells and their clinical applications in osteoarthritis. Cell Transplant. 2016;25:937.
7. Sato M, Uchida K, Nakajima H, Miyazaki T, Guerrero AR, Watanabe S, Roberts S, Baba H. Direct transplantation of mesenchymal stem cells into the knee joints of Hartley strain guinea pigs with spontaneous osteoarthritis. Arthritis Res Ther. 2012;14(1):R31.
8. Jo CH, Lee YG, Shin WH, Kim H, Chai JW, Jeong EC, Kim JE, Shim H, Shin JS, Shin IS, Ra JC, Oh S, Yoon KS. Intra-articular injection of mesenchymal stem cells for the treatment of osteoarthritis of the knee: a proof-of-concept clinical trial. Stem Cells. 2014;32(5):1254–66.
9. Kølle SF, Fischer-Nielsen A, Mathiasen AB, Elberg JJ, Oliveri RS, Glovinski PV, Kastrup J, Kirchhoff M, Rasmussen BS, Talman ML, Thomsen C, Dickmeiss E, Drzewiecki KT. Enrichment of autologous fat grafts with ex-vivo expanded adipose tissue-derived stem cells for graft survival: a randomised placebo-controlled trial. Lancet. 2013;382(9898):1113–20.
10. Trojahn Kolle SF, Oliveri RS, Glovinski PV, et al. Pooled human platelet lysate versus fetal bovine serum—investigating the proliferation rate, chromosome stability and angiogenic potential of human adipose tissue-derived stem cells intended for clinical use. Cytotherapy. 2013;15:1086.
11. Chang H, Park JH, Min KH, Lee RS, Kim EK. Whitening effects of adipose-derived stem cells: a preliminary in vivo study. Aesthet Plast Surg. 2014;38(1):230–3.
12. Kim WS, Park SH, Ahn SJ, Kim HK, Park JS, Lee GY, Kim KJ, Whang KK, Kang SH, Park BS, Sung JH. Whitening effect of adipose-derived stem cells: a critical role of TGF-beta 1. Biol Pharm Bull. 2008;31(4):606–10.
13. Solano F, Briganti S, Picardo M, Ghanem G. Pigment Cell Res. 2006;19:550–71.
14. Won C. Hair growth promoting effects of adipose tissue-derived stem cells. J Dermatol Sci. 2010;57:132–46.
15. Shin H, Ryu HH, Kwon O, Park BS, Jo SJ. Clinical use of conditioned media of adipose tissue-derived stem cells in female pattern hair loss: a retrospective case series study. Int J Dermatol. 2015;54(6):730–5.
16. Fukuoka H, Suga H. Hair regeneration treatment using adipose-derived stem cell conditioned medium: follow-up with trichograms. Eplasty. 2015;15:e10.
17. Strioga M, Viswanathan S, Darinskas A, Slaby O, Michalek J. Same or not the same? Comparison of adipose tissue-derived versus bone marrow-derived mesenchymal stem and stromal cells. Stem Cells Dev. 2012;21:2724–52.
18. Tremolada C, Palmieri G, Ricordi C. Adipocyte transplantation and stem cells: plastic surgery meets regenerative medicine. Cell Transplant. 2010;19(10):1217–23.
19. Wang W, Fang XH, Williams SJ, et al. Lidocaine-induced ASC apoptosis (tumescent v. local anesthesia). Aesthet Plast Surg. 2014;38:1017–23.
20. Goldman JJ, Wang WZ, Fang XH, Williams SJ, Baynosa RC. Tumescent liposuction without lidocaine. Plast Reconstr Surg Glob Open. 2016;4(8):e829.
21. Bowen JE. Technical issues in harvesting and concentrating stem cells (bone marrow and adipose). PM R. 2015;7:S8–S18.
22. Vincent L, Chen W, Hong L. Inhibition of endothelial cell migration by cerivastatin, an HMG-CoA reductase inhibitor: contribution to its anti-angiogenic effect. FEBS Lett. 2001;495:159–66.

23. Raposio E, Caruana G, Bonomini S, Libondi G. A novel and effective strategy for the isolation of adipose-derived stem cells: minimally manipulated adipose-derived stem cells for more rapid and safe stem cell therapy. Plast Reconstr Surg. 2014;133(6):1406–9.
24. Trivisonno A, Di Rocco G, Cannistra C, Finocchi V, Torres Farr S, Monti M, Toietta G. Harvest of superficial layers of fat with a microcannula and isolation of adipose tissue-derived stromal and vascular cells. Aesthet Surg J. 2014;34(4):601–13.
25. Tonnard P, Verpaele A, Peeters G, Hamdi M, Cornelissen M, Declercq H. Nanofat grafting: basic research and clinical applications. Plast Reconstr Surg. 2013;132(4):1017–26. https://doi.org/10.1097/PRS.0b013e31829fe1b0.
26. Danilenko DM, Ring BD, Pierce GF. Growth factors and cytokines in hair follicle development and cycling: recent insights from animal models and the potentials for clinical therapy. Mol Med Today. 1996;2:460–7.
27. De Ugarte DA, Alfonso Z, Zuk PA, Elbarbary A, Zhu M, Ashjian P, Benhaim P, Hedrick MH, Fraser JK. Differential expression of stem cell mobilization-associated molecules on multilineage cells from adipose tissue and bone marrow. Immunol Lett. 2003;89(2-3):267–70.
28. De Ugarte DA, Morizono K, Elbarbary A, Alfonso Z, Zuk PA, Zhu M, Dragoo JL, Ashjian P, Thomas B, Benhaim P, Chen I, Fraser J, Hedrick MH. Comparison of multilineage cells from human adipose tissue and bone marrow. Cells Tissues Organs. 2003;174(3):101–9.
29. Lipworth BJ. Systemic adverse effects of inhaled corticosteroid therapy: a systematic review and meta-analysis. Arch Intern Med. 1999;159:941–55.
30. Zuk PA, Zhu M, Mizuno H, et al. Multilineage cells from human adipose tissue: implications for cell-based therapies. Tissue Eng. 2001;7:211–28.
31. Goisis M. A novel closed system for isolating stem cells. Face congress, London, 2017.
32. Mahdavian Delavary B, van der Veer WM, van Egmond M, Niessen FB, Beelen RH. Macrophages in skin injury and repair. Immunobiology. 2011;216:753–62.

Part II

Aesthetic Medicine Step by Step

Temporal Fossa

11

Mario Goisis, Sara Izzo, and Rand S. Al Yahya

Depression of the temporal area has a tendency to become much more visible with age. This is due in part to atrophy of the fat and in part to atrophy of the temporal muscle. In some subjects, the depression is visible already at an early age. Excavation in this area is often associated with a skull-like appearance. Temporal excavation is considered one of the worst anti-aesthetic signs of ageing regarding the upper-face approach.

11.1 Anatomy

The temporal fossa is a depression on each side of the skull bounded above by the insertion of the temporal muscle and terminating below at the level of the zygomatic arch. The anterior boundary is constituted by the posterior surface of the frontal process of the zygomatic bone and the posterior surface of the zygomatic process of the frontal bone. Superiorly, the fossa is delimited by a line that arches across the skull from the zygomatic process of the frontal bone to the supramastoid crest of the temporal bone. The inferior boundary is represented, laterally, by the zygomatic arch and, medially, by the infratemporal crest of the greater wing of the sphenoid (Fig. 11.1). Noble structures that are contained in the fossa temporalis which need to be preserved during treatment are the following:

- The superficial temporal artery which is a major artery of the head. It arises from the external carotid artery when it bifurcates into the superficial temporal and maxillary arteries. It begins in the parotid gland, behind the neck of the mandible, and passes superficially over the posterior root of the zygomatic process of the temporal bone; about 5 cm above this process, it divides into two branches, a frontal and a parietal. Its pulse is palpable above the zygomatic arch, around 1 cm in front of and above the tragus (Fig. 11.2, blue arrow).
- The uppermost branches of the seventh cranial nerve, also known as the frontal branch of the facial nerve, which cross the zygomatic arch to the temporal region, supplying the upper and anterior auricular muscles. The branches placed closest to the front supply the frontalis, the orbicularis oculi, and corrugator supercilii. The branch crosses the

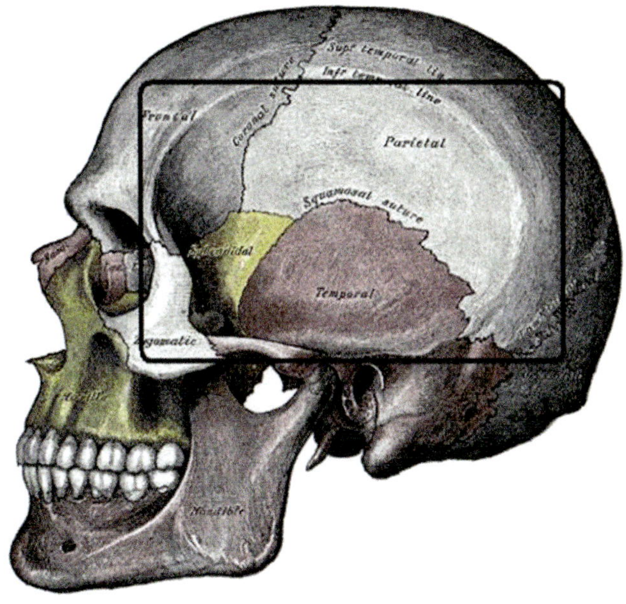

Fig. 11.1 Bone anatomy of temporal fossa. Reproduction of a lithograph plate from Gray's anatomy (Henry Gray, Anatomy: Descriptive and Surgical). (Published by kind permission of ©Mario Goisis 2018. All Rights Reserved)

M. Goisis (✉)
Maxillo-Facial and Aesthetic Surgeon, Go Easy Clinic, Milan, Italy

S. Izzo
Department of Plastic Surgery, University of Campania "Luigi Vanvitelli", Naples, Italy

R. S. Al Yahya
Prince Sattam Bin Abdulaziz University, Al Kharj, Saudi Arabia

M. Goisis (ed.), *Outpatient Regenerative Medicine*, https://doi.org/10.1007/978-3-319-44894-7_11

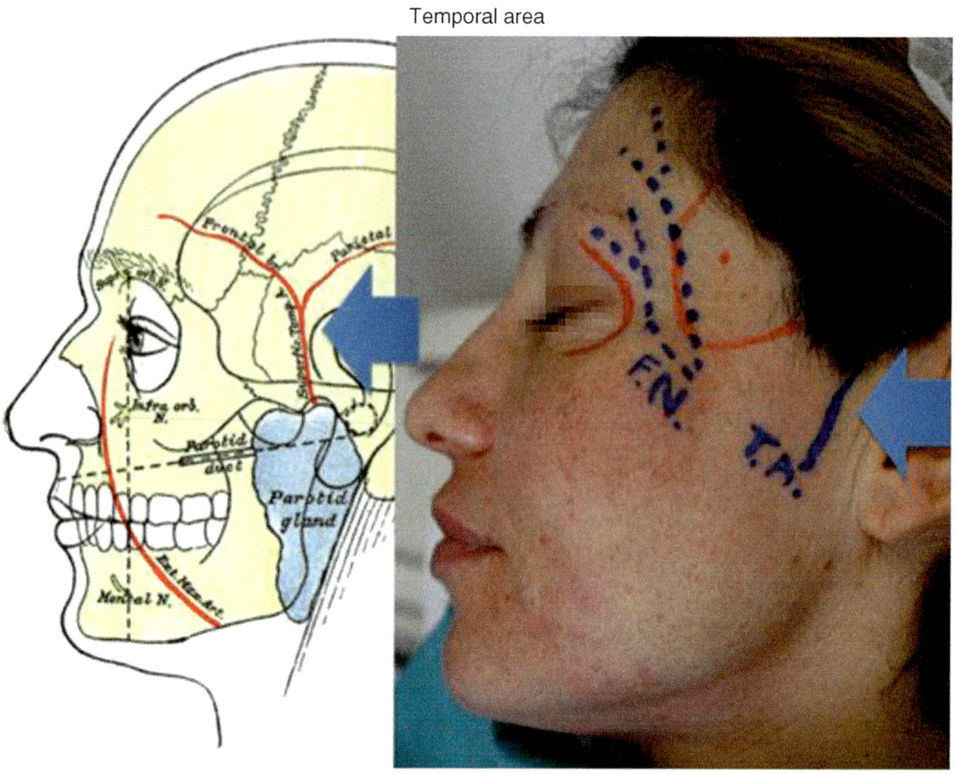

Fig. 11.2 The superficial temporal artery arises from the external carotid artery. It originates in the parotid gland, behind the neck of the mandible. Its pulse is palpable above the zygomatic arch, around 1 cm in front of and above the tragus (blue arrow). (Published by kind permission of ©Mario Goisis 2018. All Rights Reserved)

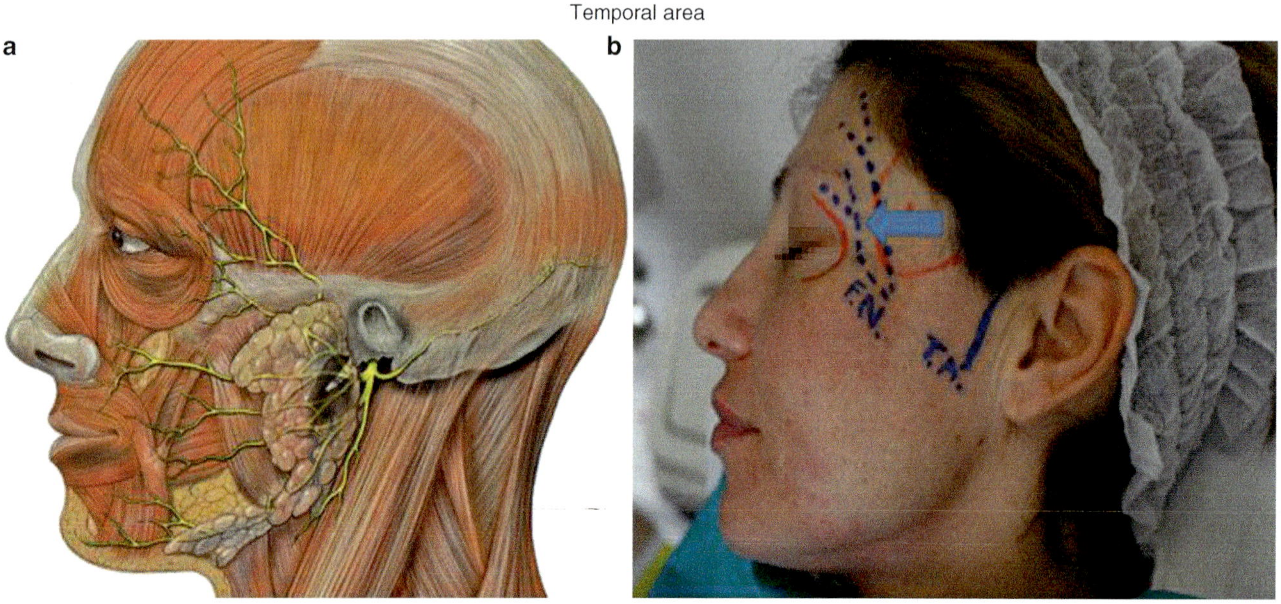

Fig. 11.3 (**a**, **b**) The frontal (**a**) (**b**) branch of the facial nerve crosses the zygomatic arch as far as the temporal region, supplying the superior and anterior auricular muscles. Most of the anterior branches (blue arrows) cross the zygomatic arch 3–4 cm anterior to the tragus and enters the temporal fossa spreading out just below the auriculotemporal fascia. (Published by kind permission of ©Mario Goisis 2018. All Rights Reserved)

zygomatic arch 3–4 cm anteriorly to the tragus and enters the temporal fossa decurring just below the auriculotemporal fascia. Accidental lesion of the temporal branch leads to facial asymmetry due to monolateral insufficient functioning of the frontalis muscle and corrugator supercilii (Fig. 11.3).

11.2 Pitfalls

The noble structures, such as the temporal artery and nerve, can be preserved by using the correct injection point (safe point). The safe point is located 2.5 cm to the side of the lateral margin of the orbital cavity (Fig. 11.4a, c) and 2.5 cm

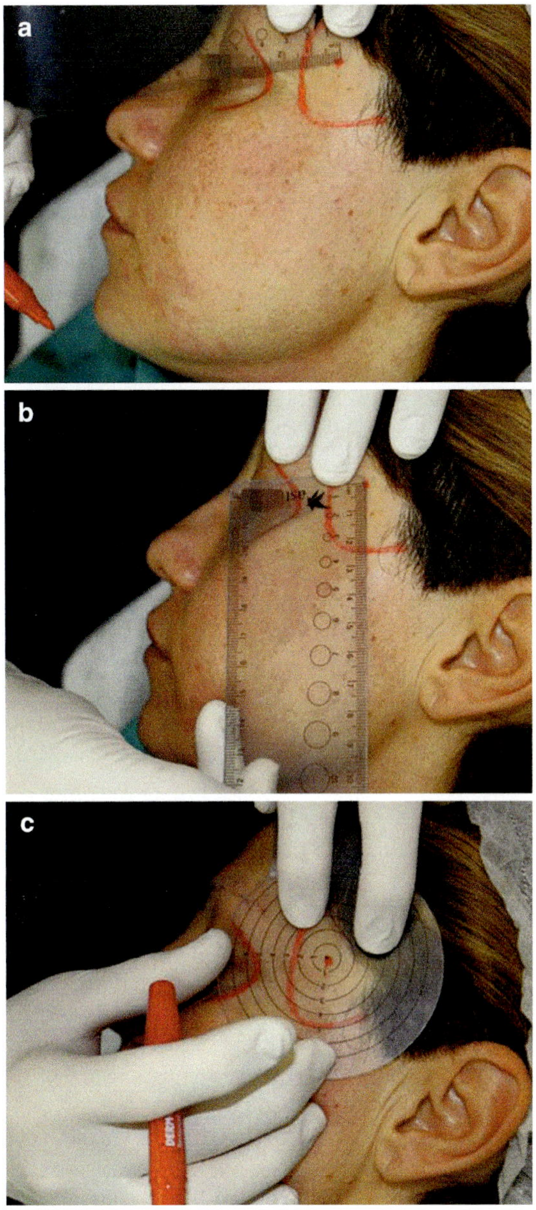

Fig. 11.4 (**a**, **b**, **c**) Anesthesia is performed in the safe point with 0.2 cc of Klein solution. The safe injection point is located 2 cm to the side of the lateral margin of the orbital cavity and 2 cm above the superior border of the zygomatic arch. (Published by kind permission of ©Mario Goisis 2018. All Rights Reserved)

above the superior border of zygomatic arch (Fig. 11.4b.). The temporal artery is palpalble to the finger. The pulse can be retrieved anteriorly to the tragus as far as the temporal area. The safe point is usually at least 2 cm to the front of this vessel (Fig. 11.4a, c). The facial nerve is usually located at least 2 cm below the safe point (Fig. 11.4a, c).

11.3 Augmentation of the Temporal Fossa

Correction of temporal excavation can lead to substantial improvement in the appearance of the face, bestowing a younger look on the patient. Augmentation of the temporal area is a simple procedure, performable in the medical surgery under local anesthesia. Only a few noble structures need to be preserved, but this can be accomplished simply.

11.4 Filling the Temporal Fossa with Microfat: Deep Technique

11.4.1 Indications

Marked excavation of the temporal area.

11.4.2 Contraindications

- Anatomical alterations due to previous trauma or surgical intervention (neurosurgery). Scarring often induces a displacement of the noble structures and can lead to perforation of the temporal artery or nerve section. It can also induce retracting scars that can cause asymmetry and unequal filling of the part treated.
- The fat should not be injected in areas that lack sufficient blood supply or affected by infection or inflammation.
- No injection should be carried out if the head has been previously treated with liquid silicone or other permanent fillers because a new injection might lead to inflammation or infection of the implants.

11.4.3 Operating Time

Once the fat is harvested, the procedure usually takes from 10 to 15 min.

11.4.4 Materials

- 2–4 cc of microfat on each side for injection of the microfat:
  - 21-gauge needle.
  - 22-gauge 4 cm blunt cannula.

  For microfat harvesting and processing:
  A standard system for microfat is used, in particular:

  - Microfat box (www.microfat.com), composed of a ramp with a closed system for washing and filtration.
  - 4 60-cc syringes.
  - 2 10-cc syringes.
  - One 1-cc syringe.
  - 30-gauge needle.

- 16-gauge needle.
- A 2-mm-diameter, 10-cm-long Goisis cannula for fat harvesting.
- A chlorhexidine-alcohol solution (2% chlorhexidine gluconate and 70% isopropyl alcohol), sterile drapes, or towels.
- Ice packs.
- Sterile 2 cm x 2 cm gauze squares.
- Occlusive dressing cover.

Medications include:

100 cc of cold saline solution.
120 cc of cold Klein solution.
1 litre of Klein solution is composed of 800 mg of lidocaine, 1 mg of epinephrine, 40 MEq of sodium bicarbonate, 1000 cc of saline solution.

Location: The microfat harvesting can be carried out in a small operating theatre/medical surgery. Oxygen, pulse oximetry, and a crash cart/box should be present.

Assistants: An assistant is useful for the transfer of items to the procedure field in a sterile manner during the first part of the procedure. Despite this, a single doctor may carry out the entire procedure alone.

Plane of injection: deep, intramuscular.

11.4.5 Methods

Procedure is shown in Figs. 11.4–11.8a. Ultrasound images of the procedure are shown in Fig. 11.8b, c. Cadaver dissection of deep injection technique in the temporal area (courtesy by doctor's equipe) is shown in Figs. 11.9–11.12.

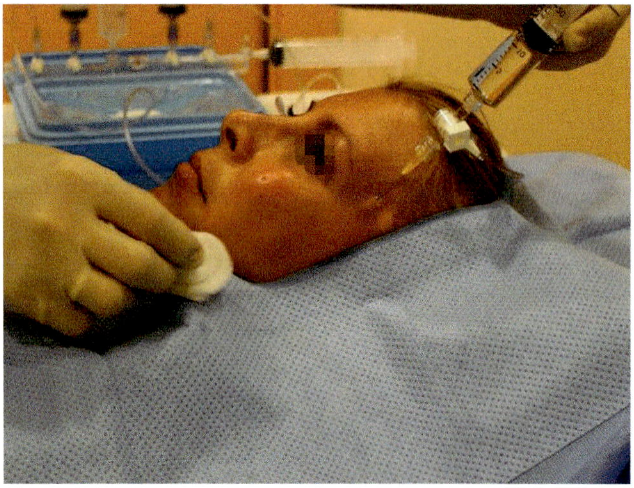

Fig. 11.5 A perforating 21G needle is inserted into the safe point (see text) at a 90° angle. When the periosteum is touched the needle is retracted by 1 mm. One cc of fat is injected in a retrograde way. (Published by kind permission of ©Mario Goisis 2018. All Rights Reserved)

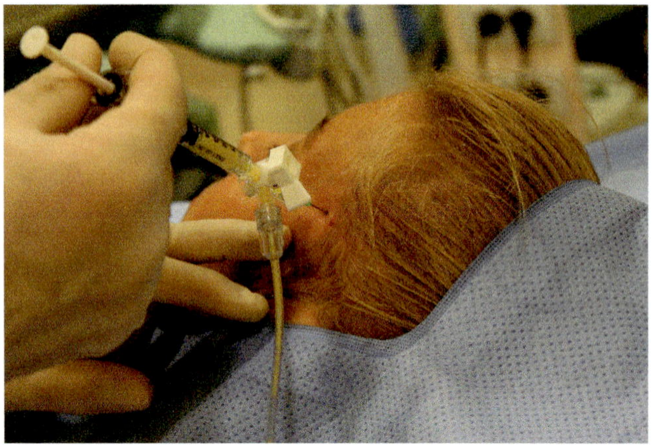

Fig. 11.6 A perforating 21G needle is inserted in the safe point (see text) at an angle of 90 degrees. The periostium is touched, then the needle is retracted by 1 mm. One cc of fat is injected in a retrograde way. (Published by kind permission of ©Mario Goisis 2018. All Rights Reserved)

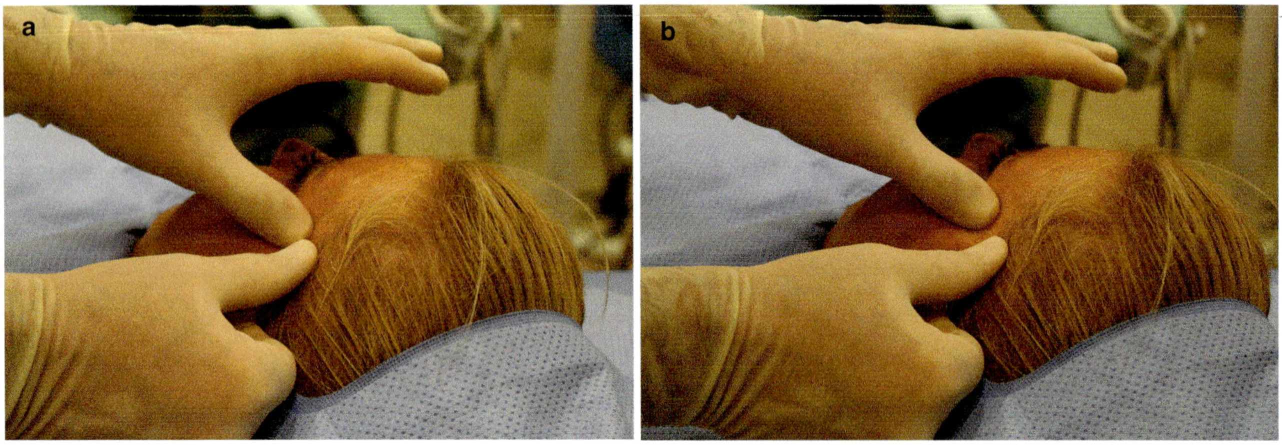

Fig. 11.7 (**a**, **b**) A strong massage is applied to the injected area. (Published by kind permission of ©Mario Goisis 2018. All Rights Reserved)

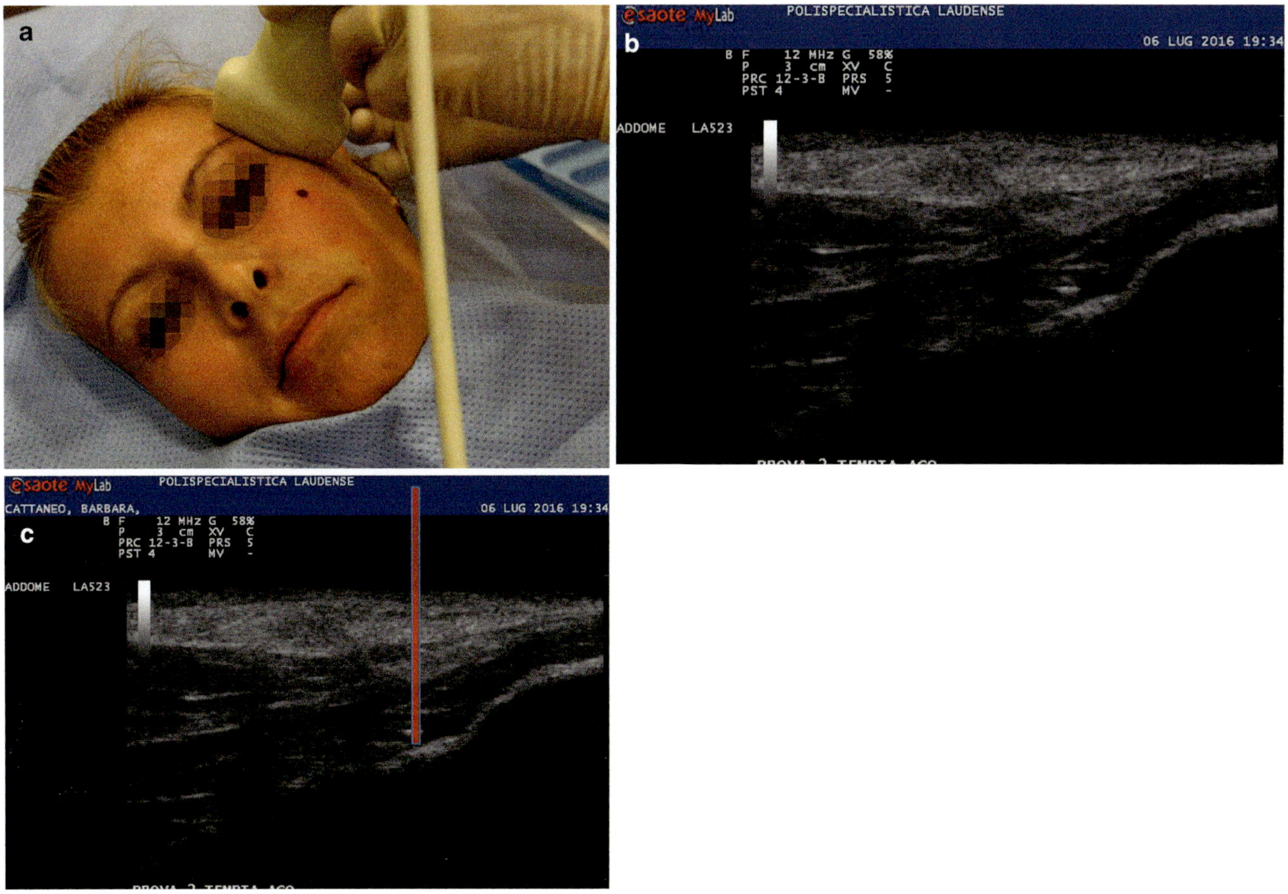

Fig. 11.8 (**a**, **b**, **c**) Ultrasound images of the procedure. The position of the sharp needle is demonstrated (Courtesy of the Doctor's Equipe). (Published by kind permission of ©Mario Goisis 2018. All Rights Reserved)

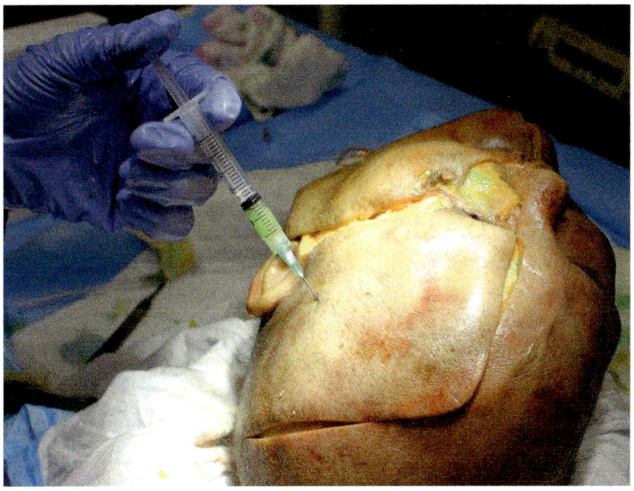

Fig. 11.9 The temporal area is filled using a single entry point. (Published kind permission of ©Mario Goisis 2018. All Rights Reserved)

11.4.6 Complications and Management

Early complications (within 72 hours after the injection) are transient erythema, oedema, induration, pruritus and ecchymosis. Possible perforation of the superficial temporal artery leads to sudden bleeding. If perforation occurrs treatment should be stopped immediately and bleeding controlled by bringing intense pressure of the finger to bear for about 5 mins. If the bleeding does not stop, a large-volume injection of diluted adrenaline in proximity of the arterial wall can be effective.

Delayed complications (days to weeks after the injection) include hypercorrection, local infection, necrosis of the skin, reactivation of herpes, discoloration and persistent local symptoms (erythema, oedema, induration, pruritus and hyperpigmentation).

Delayed complications include high rates of fat resorption and cysts.

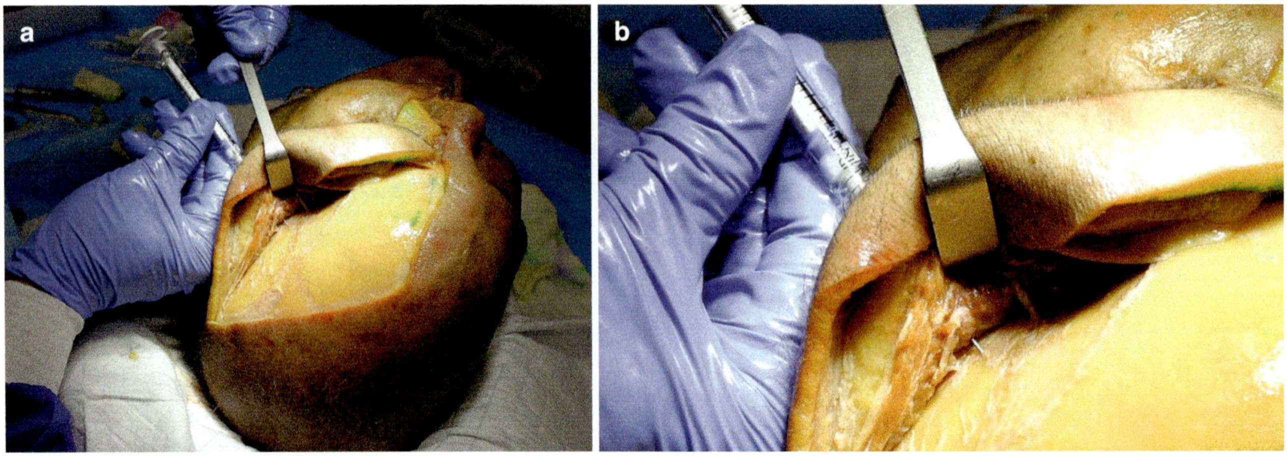

Fig. 11.10 (**a**, **b**) Demonstration of the position of the tip of the sharp needle. (Published by kind permission of ©Mario Goisis 2018. All Rights Reserved)

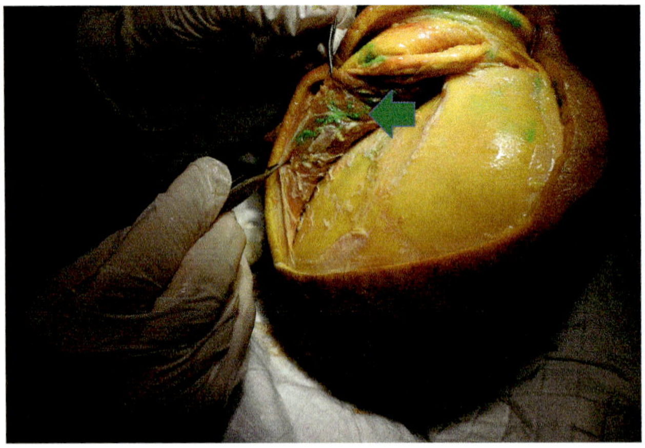

Fig. 11.11 After the injection of the fat, dissection is executed. The bone and muscular planes are exposed. Evidence of fat is shown in the temporal muscle plane (green arrow). (Published by kind permission of ©Mario Goisis 2018. All Rights Reserved)

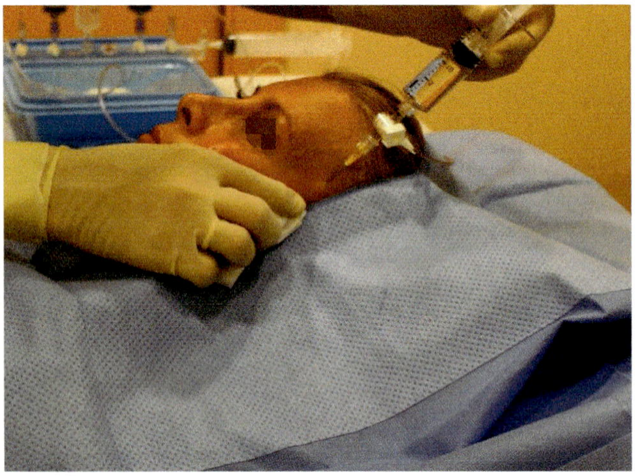

Fig. 11.12 Anesthesia is performed in the safe point using 0.2 cc of Klein solution. The safe injection point is located 2 cm to the side of the lateral margin of the orbital cavity and 2 cm above the superior border of malar arch. (Published by kind permission of ©Mario Goisis 2018. All Rights Reserved)

11.5 Filling of the Temporal Fossa with Microfat: Superficial Technique

11.5.1 Indications

Excavation of the temporal area.

11.5.2 Contraindications

- Anatomical alterations due to previous trauma or surgical intervention (neurosurgery). Scarring often induces a displacement of the noble structures and can lead to temporal artery perforation or nerve section. It can also induce retracting scars that can cause asymmetry and unequal filling of the part treated.
- The fat should not be injected in areas that lack sufficient blood supply or that have an infection or inflammation.
- No injection should be done if the head has been previously treated with liquid silicone or other permanent fillers because new injection could lead to inflammation or infection of the implants.

11.5.3 Operating Time

Once the fat is harvested, the procedure usually takes from 10 to 15 min.

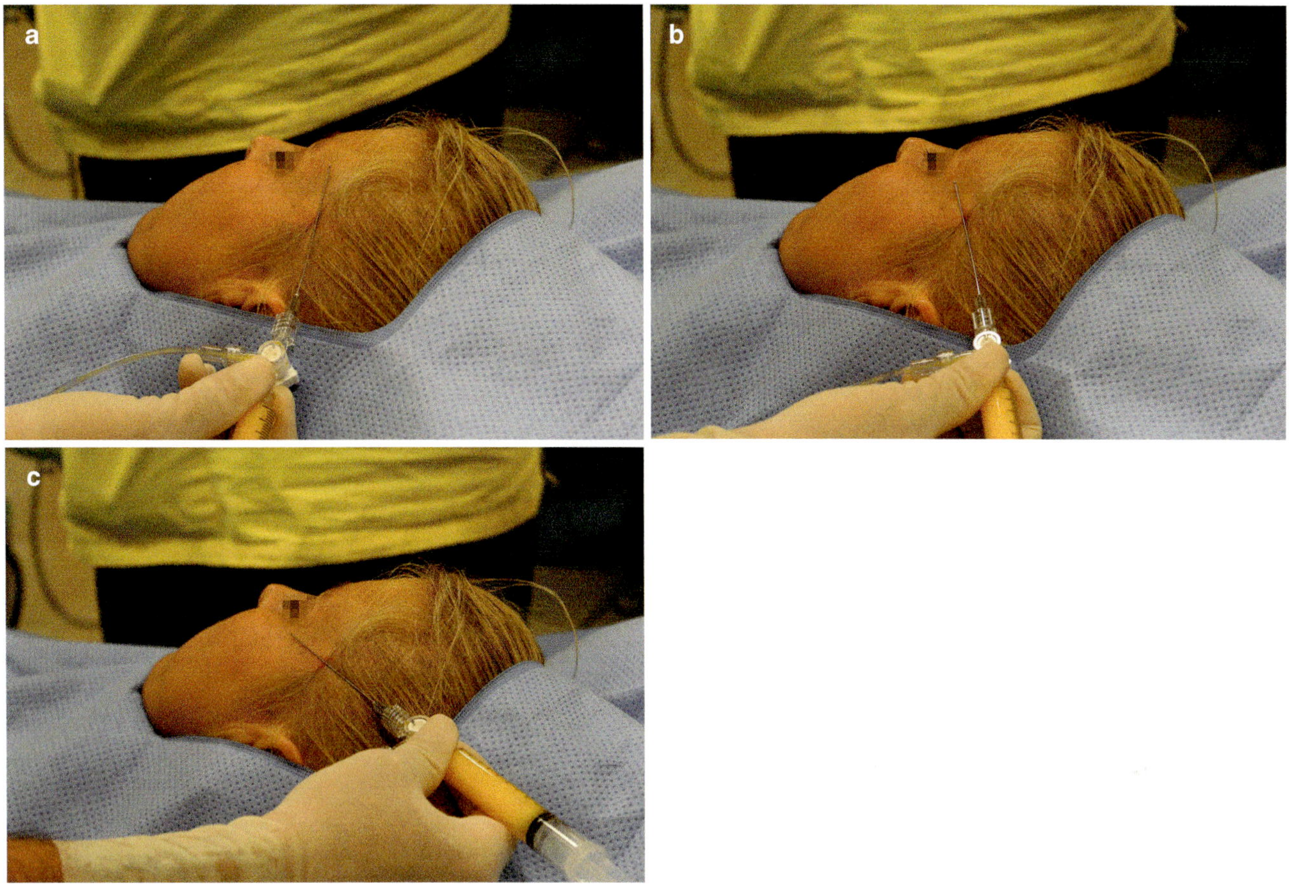

Fig. 11.13 (**a**, **b**, **c**) The route of the cannula is demonstrated here. (Published by kind permission of ©Mario Goisis 2018. All Rights Reserved)

11.5.4 Materials

- 1–2 cc of microfat on each side for injection of microfat:
  - 21-gauge needle.
  - 22-gauge 4-cm blunt cannula.

  For microfat harvesting and processing:
  A standard system for microfat is used, in particular:

  - Microfat box (www.microfat.com), composed of a ramp with a closed a system for washing and filtration.
  - 4 60-cc syringes.
  - 2 10-cc syringes.
  - One 1-cc syringe.
  - 30-gauge needle.
  - 16-gauge needle.
  - A 2-mm-diameter, 10-cm-long Goisis cannula for fat harvesting.
  - A chlorhexidine-alcohol solution (2% chlorhexidine gluconate and 70% isopropyl alcohol), sterile drapes, or towels.
  - Ice packs.
  - Sterile 2 cm x 2 cm gauze squares.
  - Occlusive dressing cover.

Medications include:

100 cc of cold saline solution.
120 cc of cold Klein solution.
1 litre of Klein solution is composed of 800 mg of lidocaine, 1 mg of epinephrine, 40 MEq of sodium bicarbonate, 1000 cc of saline solution.

Location: The microfat harvesting can be carried out in a small operating theatre/medical surgery. Oxygen, pulse oximetry, and a crash cart/box should be present.

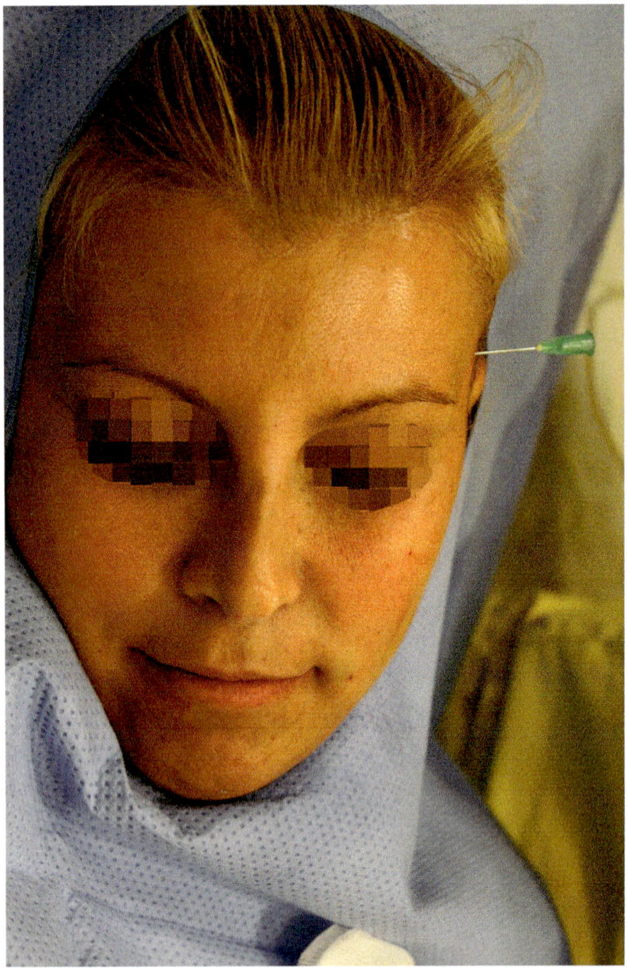

Fig. 11.14 An opening is created at the level of the safe point using a 21-G needle. (Published by kind permission of ©Mario Goisis 2018. All Rights Reserved)

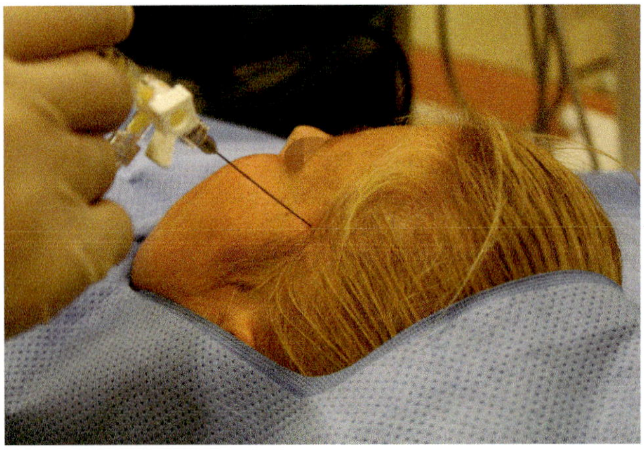

Fig. 11.15 A 22-G blunt-tip cannula is inserted perpendicularly to the skin's surface, and the cannula is then pivoted parallel to the plane of the skin. (Published by kind permission of ©Mario Goisis 2018. All Rights Reserved)

Assistants: An assistant is useful for the transfer items to the procedure field in a sterile manner during the first part of the procedure. Despite this, a single doctor may carry out the entire procedure alone.

Plane of injection: superficial, subcutaneous (Figs. 11.16, 11.17, 11.18, 11.19, 11.20, 11.21, 11.22, 11.23, 11.24, 11.25, 11.26, 11.27, 11.28, and 11.29).

11.5.5 Methods

- Procedure is shown in (Fig. 11.17a).
- Ultrasound images of the procedure are shown in (Fig. 11.17b, c).
- Cadaver dissection of deep injection technique in the temporal area (courtesy by doctor's equipe) are shown in (Figs. 11.19–11.23).

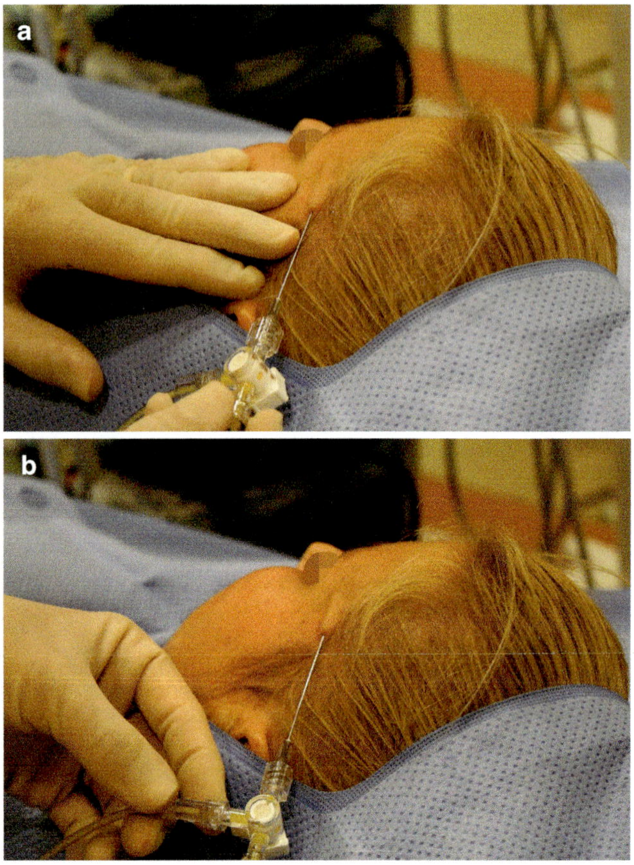

Fig. 11.16 (**a**, **b**) The fat is delivered slowly, while the cannula is withdrawn by retrograde injection. The fat is injected into the subcutaneous plane, on the surface of the superficial temporal fascia. (Published by kind permission of ©Mario Goisis 2018. All Rights Reserved)

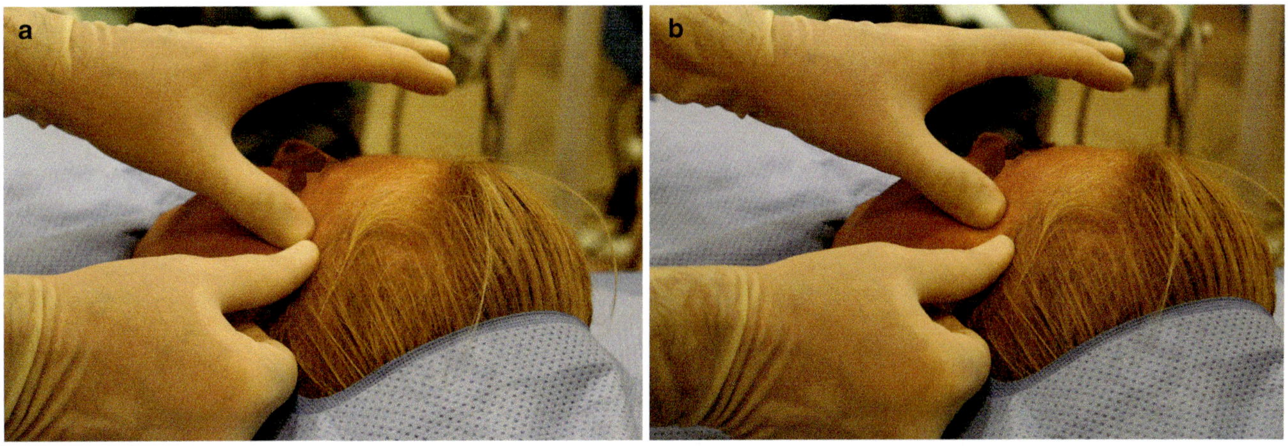

Fig. 11.17 (**a**, **b**) A strong massage is applied to the injected area. (Published by kind permission of ©Mario Goisis 2018. All Rights Reserved)

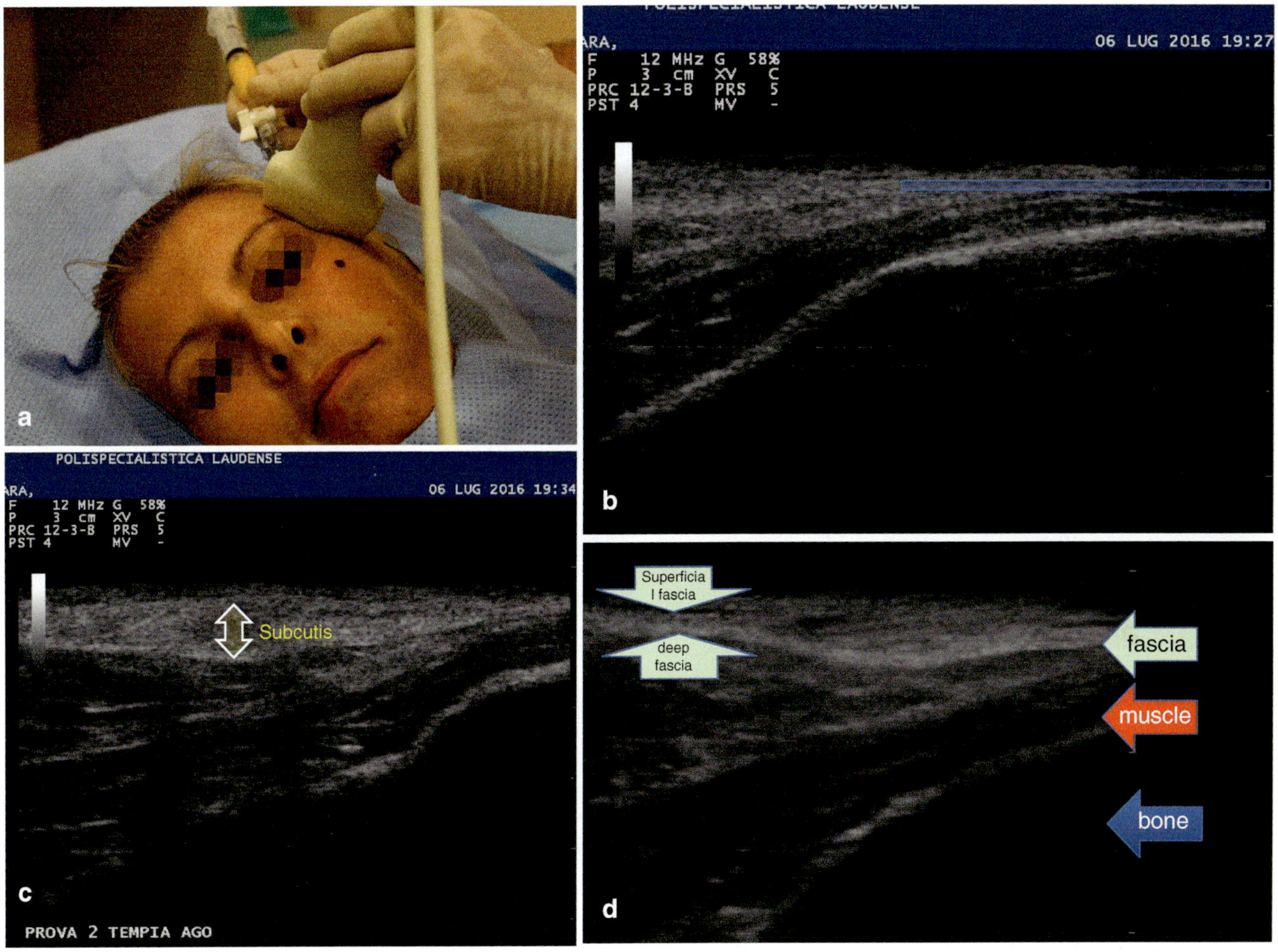

Fig. 11.18 (**a**, **b**, **c**, **d**) Ultrasound images of the procedure. The position of the blunt cannula is demonstrated here. In particular, the cannula is inserted into the subcutaneous-superficial plane of the fat. (Published by kind permission of ©Mario Goisis 2018. All Rights Reserved)

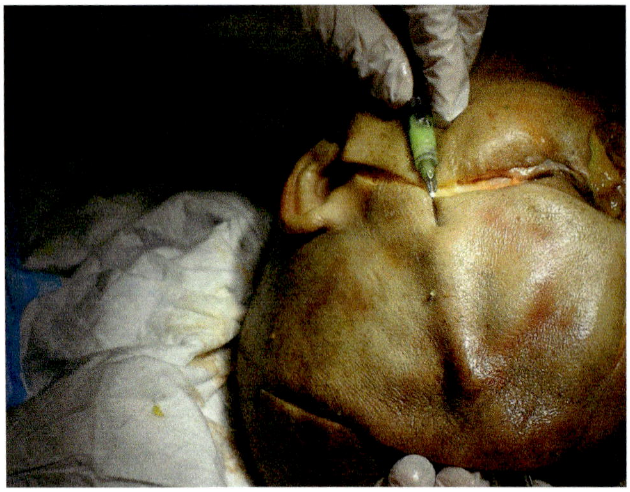

Fig. 11.19 The temporal area is filled using a single entry point with a fan technique. (Published by kind permission of ©Mario Goisis 2018. All Rights Reserved)

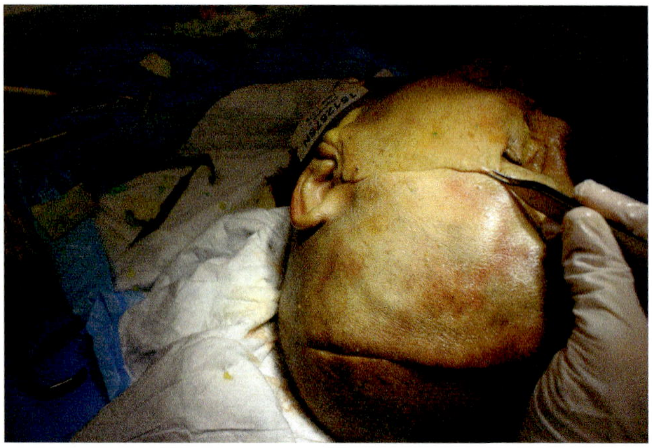

Fig. 11.21 The cutaneous plane. (Published by kind permission of ©Mario Goisis 2018. All Rights Reserved)

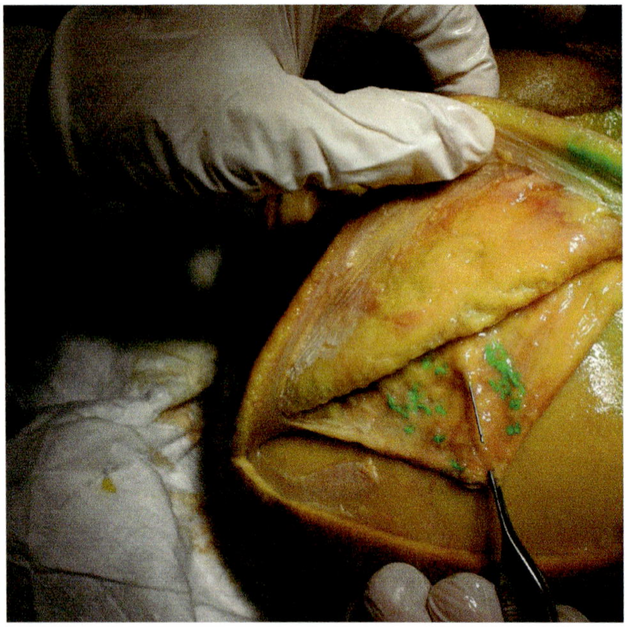

Fig. 11.20 Demonstration of the position of the blunt cannula. (Published by kind permission of ©Mario Goisis 2018. All Rights Reserved)

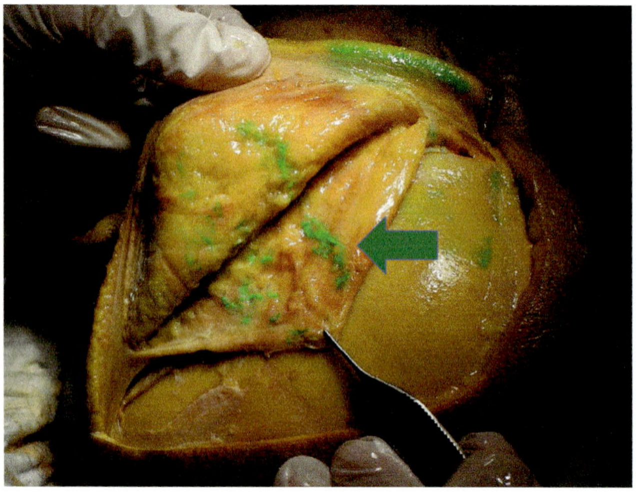

Fig. 11.22 The subcutaneous plane. The presence of fat is demonstrated (green arrow). (Published by kind permission of ©Mario Goisis 2018. All Rights Reserved)

11.6 Temporal Amelioration with Nanofat

11.6.1 Indications

Amelioration of acne scars in the temporal area. The use of the small blunt-tip cannula allows for an atraumatic dissection of the tissue and placing of nanofat into the subcutaneous plane, in order to obtain significantly less pain and bruising.

11.6.2 Contraindications

- The nanofat should not be injected into areas that lack sufficient blood supply or that have an infection or inflammation in course.
- No injection should be carried out if the head has been previously treated with liquid silicone or other permanent fillers because a new injection might lead to inflammation or infection of the nanofat.

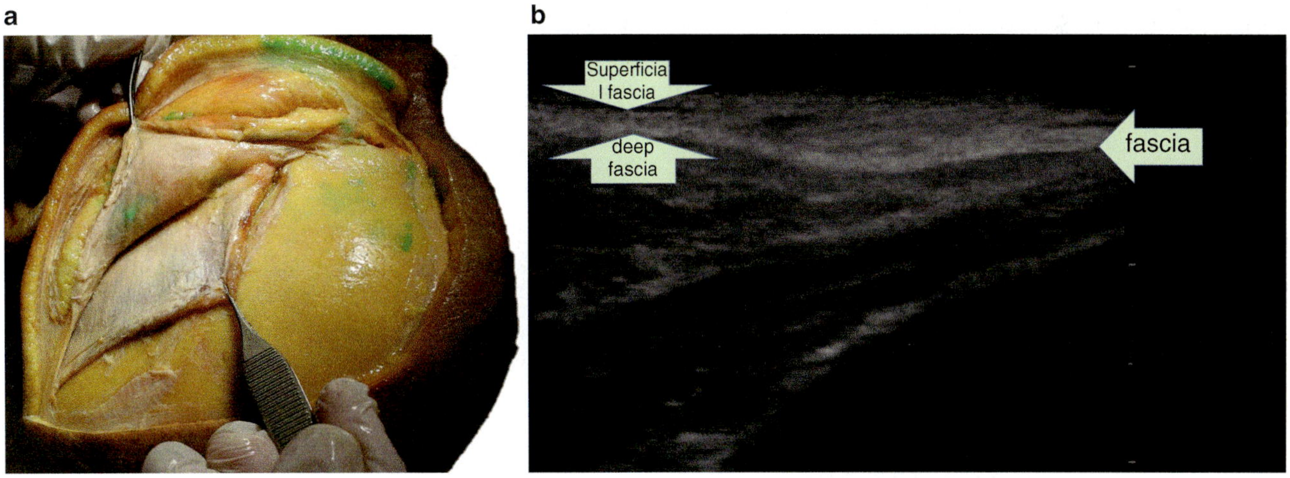

Fig. 11.23 (**a**, **b**) The plane between the split of the temporal fascia: no fat is shown. (Published kind permission of ©Mario Goisis 2018. All Rights Reserved)

11.6.3 Operating Time

The procedure usually takes from 10 to 15 min, once the nanofat has been produced.

Plane of injection: hypodermis-superficial fat compartment

11.6.4 Materials

- *1–2 cc of nanofat on each side for injection of nanofat:*
  - *26-gauge needle.*
  - *27-gauge 3, 7 cm blunt cannula.*

A standard system for producing nanofat is used, in particular:

- Nanofat system (www.microfat.com) composed of a connector with a closed system for emulsion of microfat and filtration.
- 2 10-cc syringes.

For microfat harvesting and processing:

A standard system for microfat is used, in particular:

- Microfat box (www.microfat.com), composed of a ramp with a closed system for washing and filtration.
- 4 60-cc syringes.
- 2 10-cc syringes.
- One 1-cc syringe.
- 30-gauge needle.
- 16-gauge needle.
- A 2-mm-diameter, 10-cm-long Goisis cannula for fat harvesting
- A chlorhexidine-alcohol solution (2% chlorhexidine gluconate and 70% isopropyl alcohol), sterile drapes, or towels.
- Ice packs.
- Sterile 2 cm x 2 cm gauze squares.
- Occlusive dressing cover.

Medications include:

100 cc of cold saline solution.
120 cc of cold Klein solution.
1 litre of Klein solution is composed of 800 mg of lidocaine, 1 mg of epinephrine, 40 MEq of sodium bicarbonate, 1000 cc of saline solution.

Location: The microfat harvesting can be carried out in a small operating theatre. The oxygen, pulse oximetry, and a crash cart/box should be present.

Assistants: An assistant is useful to transfer items to the procedure field in a sterile manner in the first part of the procedure. Despite that, a single doctor can execute all the procedure.

Plane of injection: hypodermis-superficial fat compartment

11.6.5 Methods

The method is shown in (Figs. 11.24–11.27).

Cadaver dissection after Nanofat injection into the temporal area is shown in Fig. 11.28.

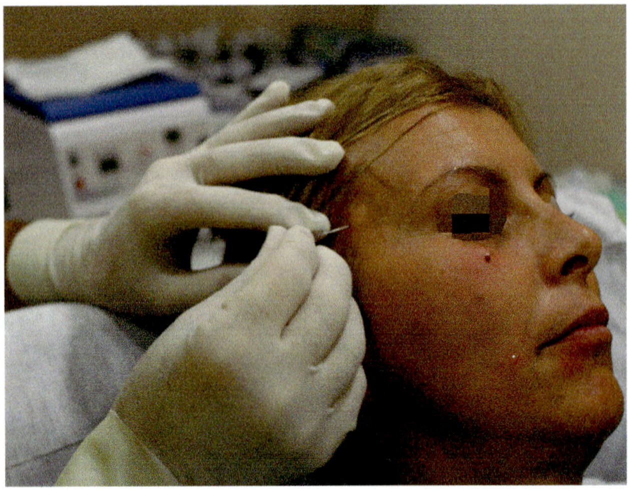

Fig. 11.24 Nanofat injection technieque. An opening is created with a 25-G needle at the level of the temporal safe point. (Published by kind permission of ©Mario Goisis 2018. All Rights Reserved)

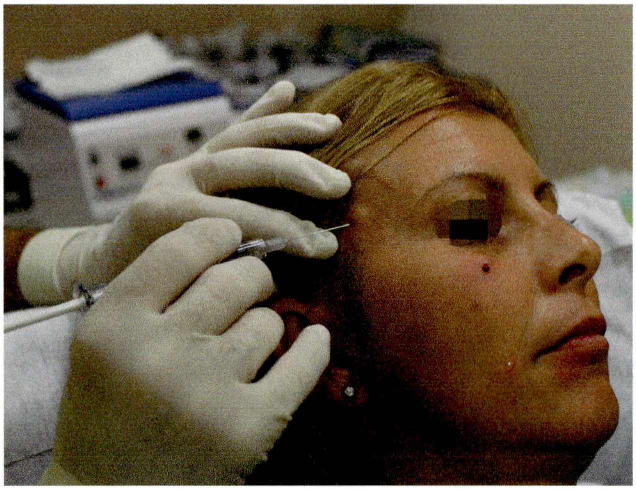

Fig. 11.25 A 27-G blunt-tip cannula is inserted perpendicularly to skin's surface. (Published by kind permission of ©Mario Goisis 2018. All Rights Reserved)

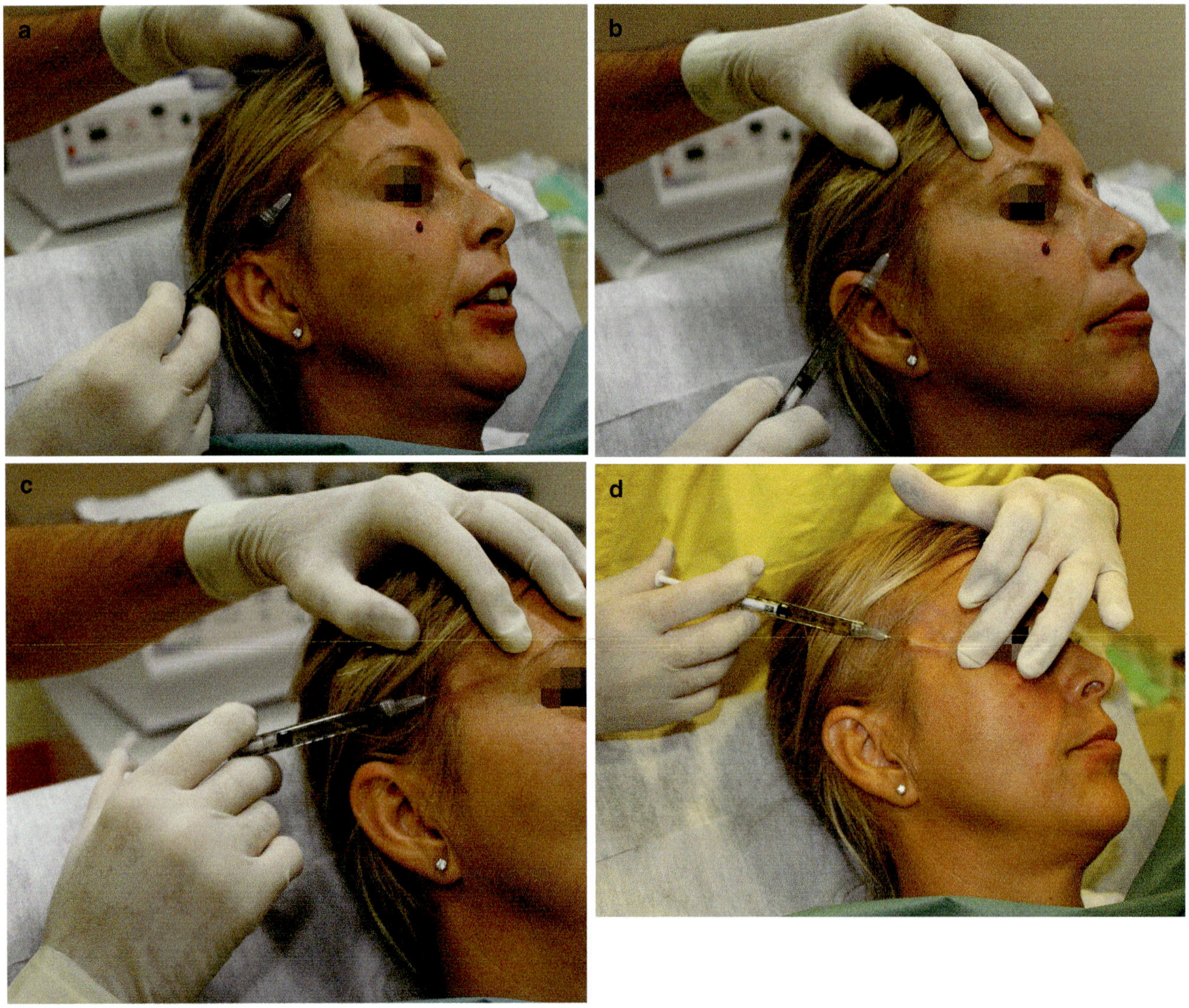

Fig. 11.26 (**a**, **b**, **c**, **d**, **e**) The cannula is then pivoted parallel to the plane of the skin and the nanofat is delivered slowly, while the cannula is withdrawn by retrograde injection. The injection is performed with a fan technique. (Published by kind permission of ©Mario Goisis 2018. All Rights Reserved)

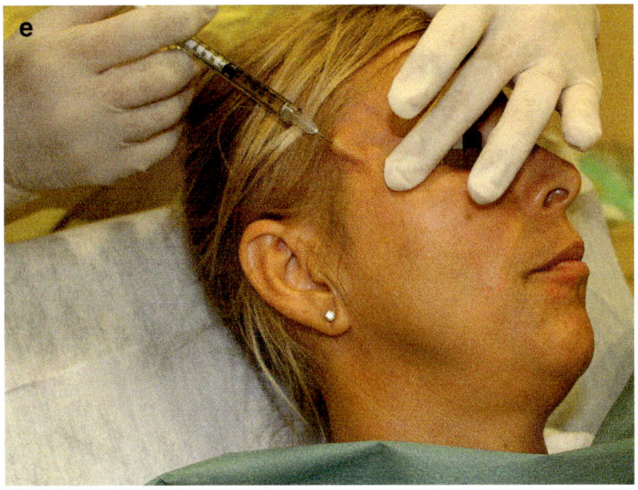

Fig. 11.26 (continued)

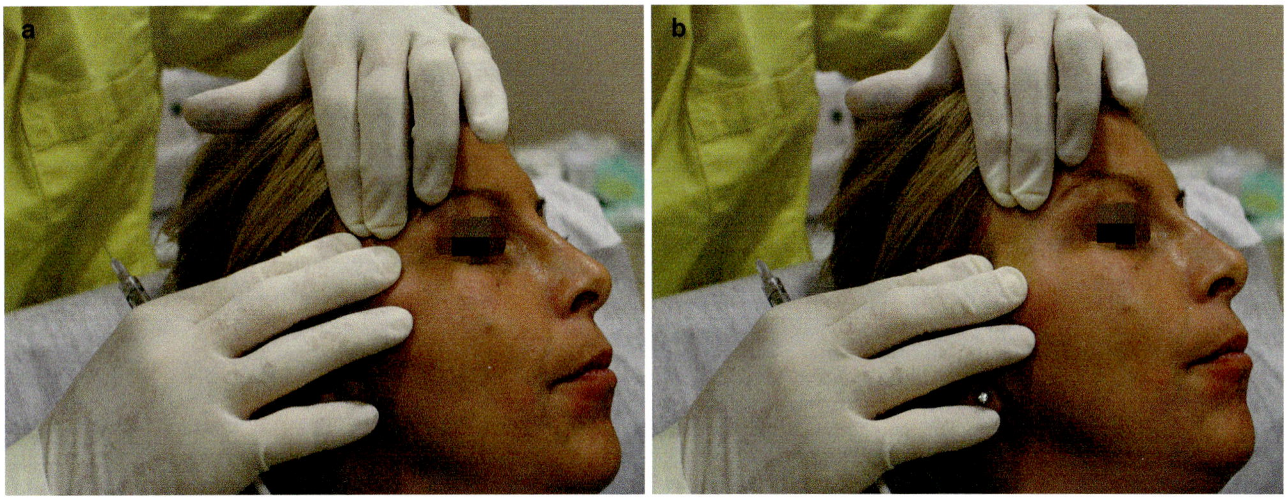

Fig. 11.27 (**a**, **b**) A strong massage is applied to the area of treatment. (Published by kind permission of ©Mario Goisis 2018. All Rights Reserved)

Fig. 11.28 After nanofat injection, temporal dissection is executed and the subcutaneous plane is exposed. The presence of the injected nanofat is shown in the subcutaneous plane. (Published by kind permission of ©Mario Goisis 2018. All Rights Reserved)

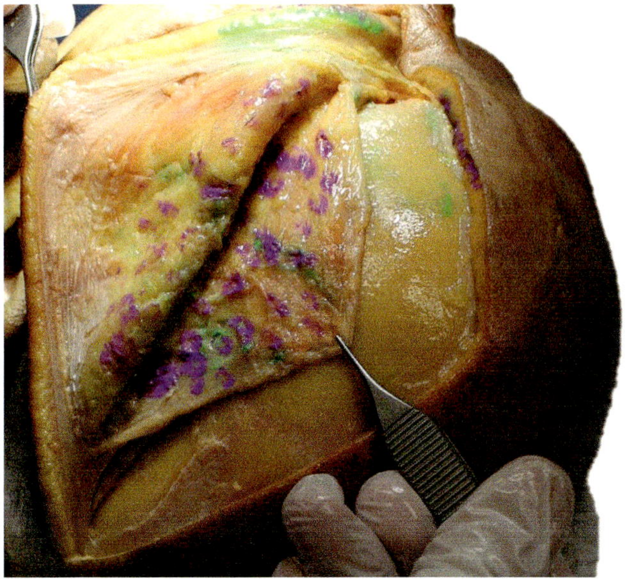

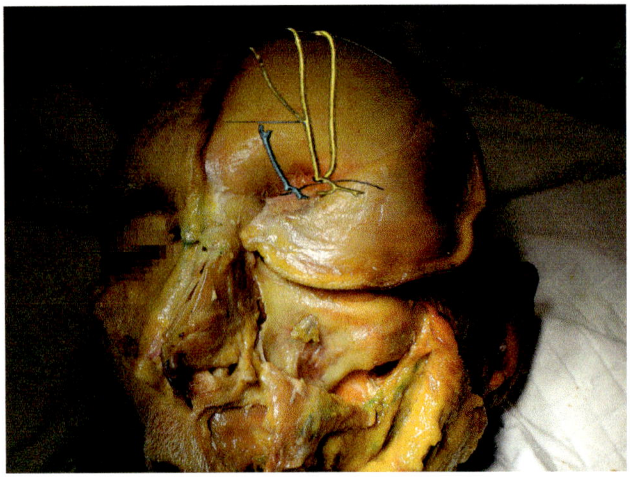

Fig. 12.2 The supratrochlear nerve (blue). It is smaller than the supraorbital nerve. It exits the orbit between the pulley of the superior oblique and the supraorbital foramen, curves up onto the forehead close to the bone, and ascends beneath the frontalis muscles. It supplies the skin of the lower part of the forehead, close to the midline and the skin of the upper eyelid (courtesy of the Doctor's Equipe). (Published by kind permission of ©Mario Goisis 2018. All Rights Reserved)

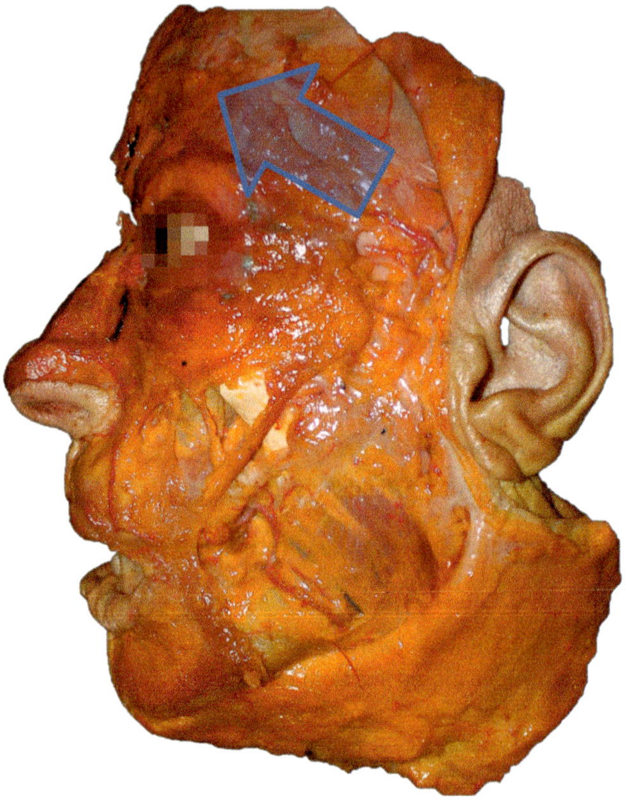

Fig. 12.3 The frontalis muscle is a thin quadrilateral muscle (courtesy of the Doctor's Equipe). (Published by kind permission of ©Mario Goisis 2018. All Rights Reserved)

- Ice packs.
- Sterile 2 cm x 2 cm gauze squares.
- Occlusive dressing cover.

Medications include:

- 100 cc of cold saline solution.
- 120 cc of cold Klein solution.
- 1 litre of Klein solution is composed of 800 mg of lidocaine, 1 mg of epinephrine, 40 MEq of sodium bicarbonate, 1000 cc of saline solution.

Location: The microfat harvesting can be carried out in a small opèerating theatre/the physician's own surgery. Oxygen, pulse oximetry, and a crash cart/box should be present.

Assistance: An assistant may prove useful for the transfer of items to the procedure field in a sterile manner during the first stage of the procedure. Nevertheless, a single doctor can perform the entire procedure alone.

Injection plane: SMAS

12.4 Operating Time

Once the fat is harvested, the procedure usually takes from 5 to 15 mins.

12.5 Complications and Management

Immediate complications (within 72 h after injection) are transient erythema, oedema, induration, pruritus, and ecchymosis.

Early complications (days to weeks after injection) include hypercorrection, local infection, necrosis of the skin, reactivation of herpes, discoloration, and persistent local symptoms (erythema, oedema, induration, pruritus, and hyperpigmentation).

Later or delayed complications include high rates of fat resorption, cysts.

12.6 Method

The procedure is illustrated.

Plane of injection: Frontalis muscle (Figs. 12.4, 12.5, 12.6, 12.7, 12.8, 12.9, 12.10, 12.11, 12.12, 12.13, 12.14, 12.15, 12.16, 12.17, and 12.18)

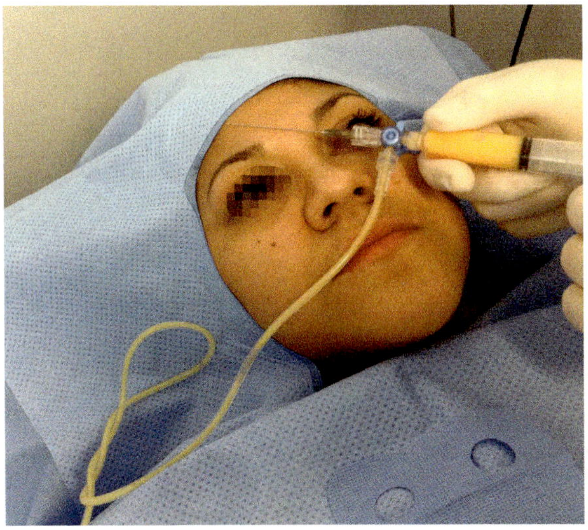

Fig. 12.4 The route of the cannula used for injection of the fat. (Published by kind permission of ©Mario Goisis 2018. All Rights Reserved)

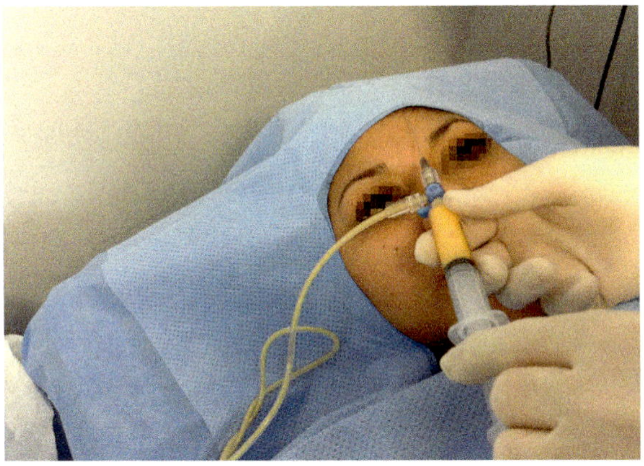

Fig. 12.5 The route of the cannula used to inject the fat. (Published by kind permission of ©Mario Goisis 2018. All Rights Reserved)

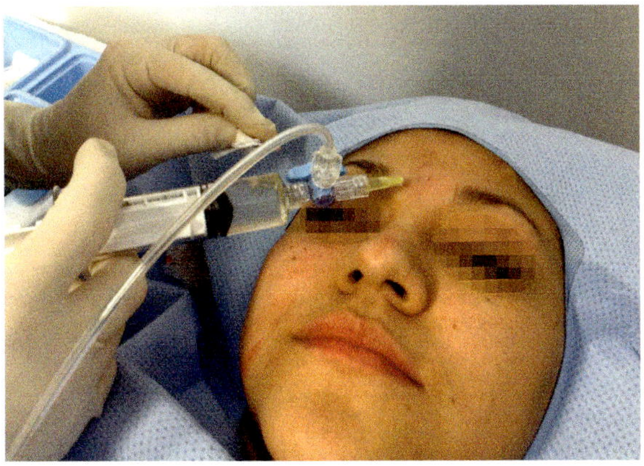

Fig. 12.6 The local anaesthesia is performed on the glabella. (Published by kind permission of ©Mario Goisis 2018. All Rights Reserved)

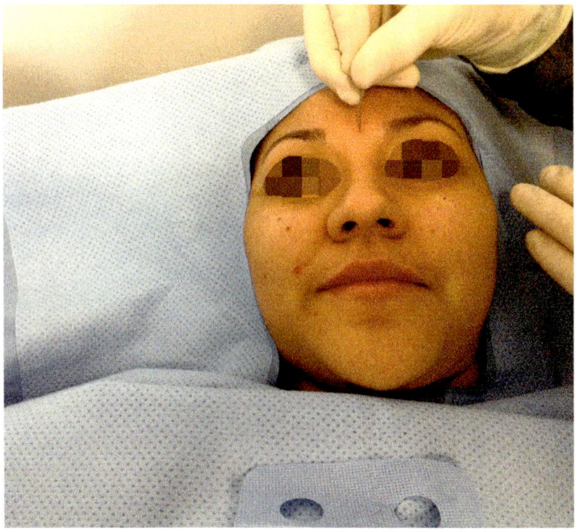

Fig. 12.7 Perforation of the plane of the skin using a 21-G needle. (Published by kind permission of ©Mario Goisis 2018. All Rights Reserved)

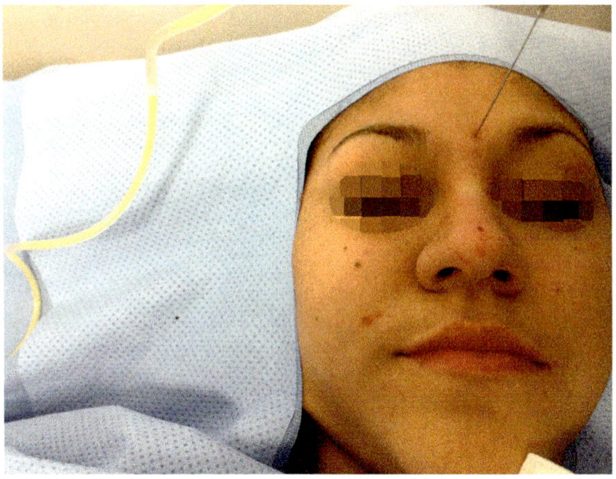

Fig. 12.8 A 22-G blunt-tip cannula is inserted perpendicularly into surface of the skin. (Published by kind permission of ©Mario Goisis 2018. All Rights Reserved)

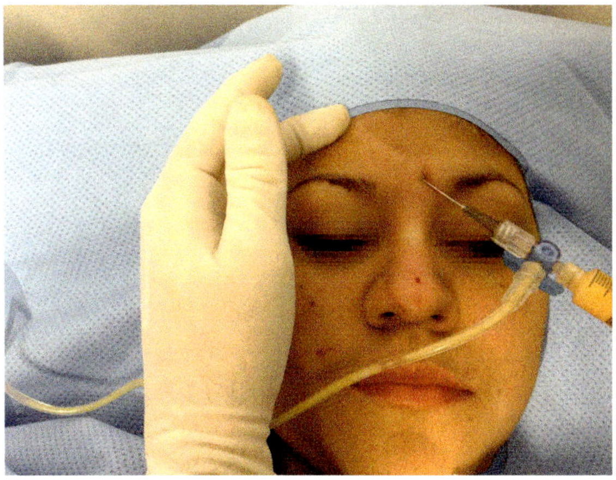

Fig. 12.9 The cannula is then pivoted parallel to the plane of the skin and slid in the direction of the frontal region with a 45° angle respect at the bipupillary line. (Published by kind permission of ©Mario Goisis 2018. All Rights Reserved)

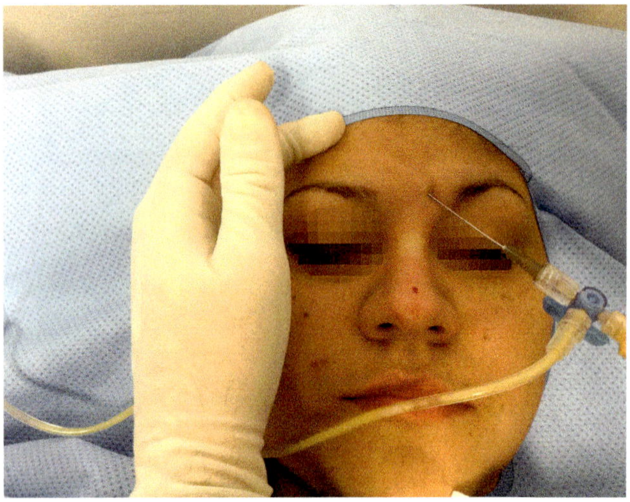

Fig. 12.10 The fat is delivered slowly, while the cannula is withdrawn by retrograde injection. (Published by kind permission of ©Mario Goisis 2018. All Rights Reserved)

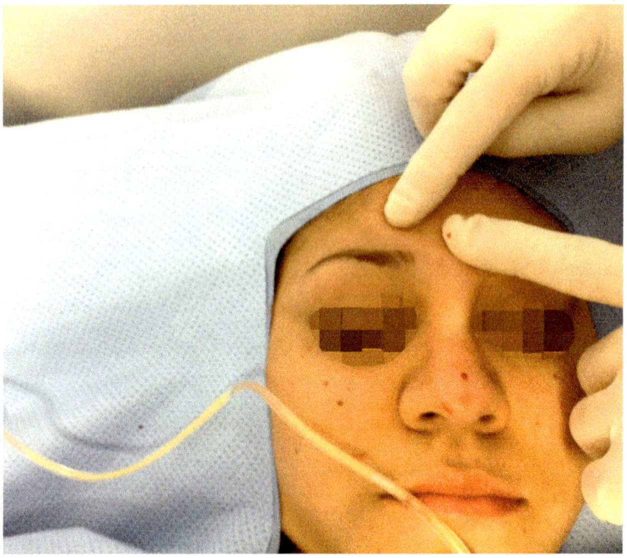

Fig. 12.11 At the end of the treatment, a massage is applied to the injected area. (Published by kind permission of ©Mario Goisis 2018. All Rights Reserved)

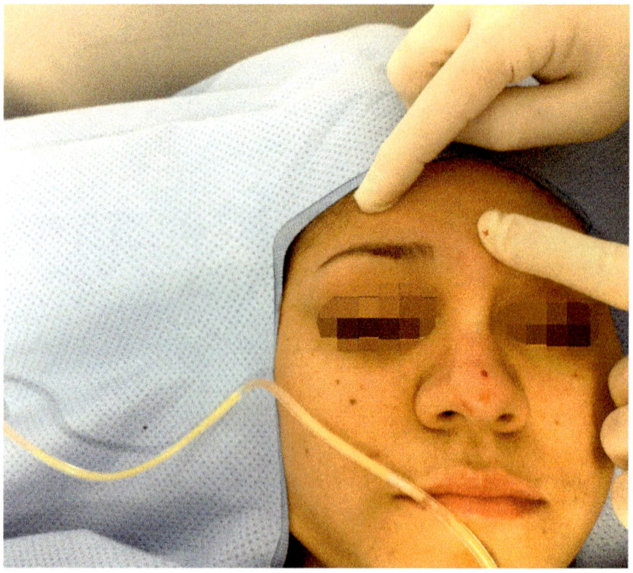

Fig. 12.12 At the end of the treatment, a massage is applied to the injected area. (Published by kind permission of ©Mario Goisis 2018. All Rights Reserved)

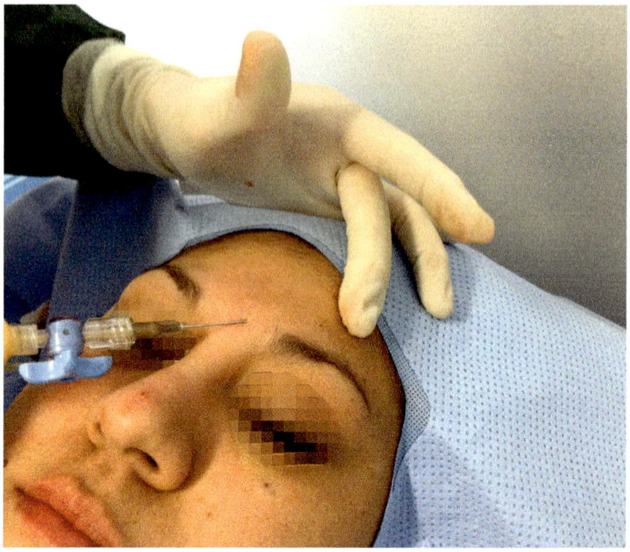

Fig. 12.13 On the opposite side too, the cannula is pivoted parallel to the plane of the skin and slid toward the frontal region at a 45° angle with respect to the bipupillary line. (Published by kind permission of ©Mario Goisis 2018. All Rights Reserved)

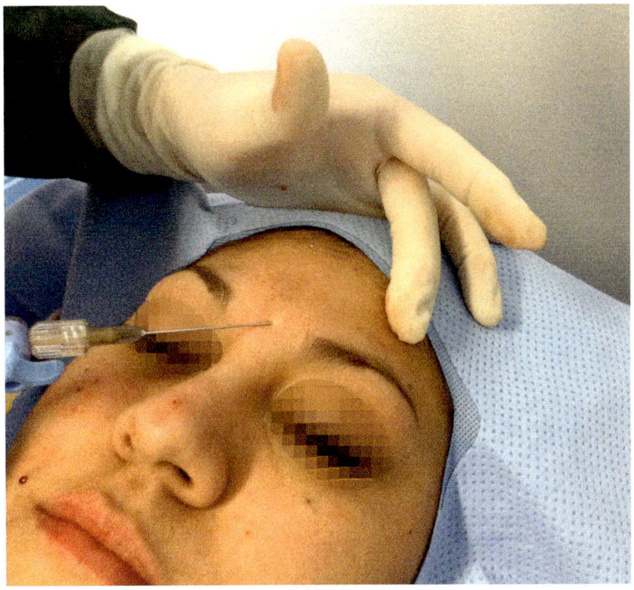

Fig. 12.14 The fat is delivered slowly, while the cannula is withdrawn by retrograde injection. (Published by kind permission of ©Mario Goisis 2018. All Rights Reserved)

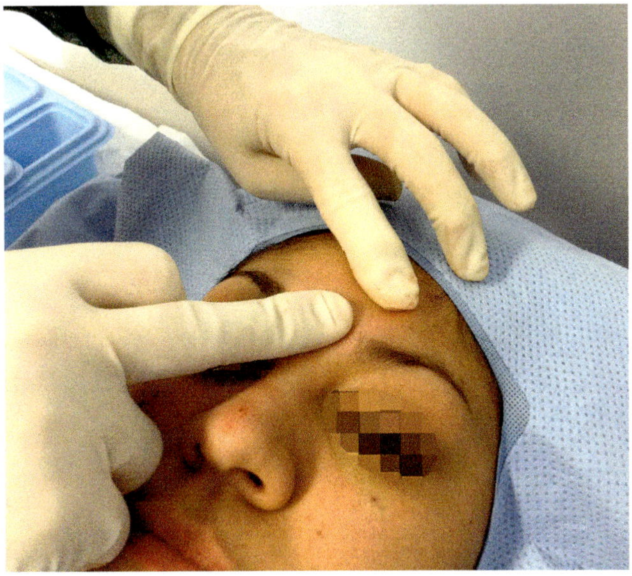

Fig. 12.15 At the end of the treatment, a massage is applied to the injected area. (Published by kind permission of ©Mario Goisis 2018. All Rights Reserved)

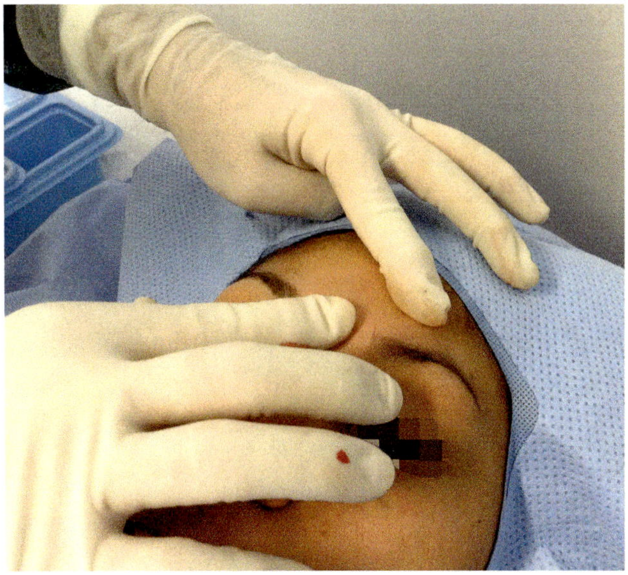

Fig. 12.16 At the end of the treatment, the injected area is massaged. (Published by kind permission of ©Mario Goisis 2018. All Rights Reserved)

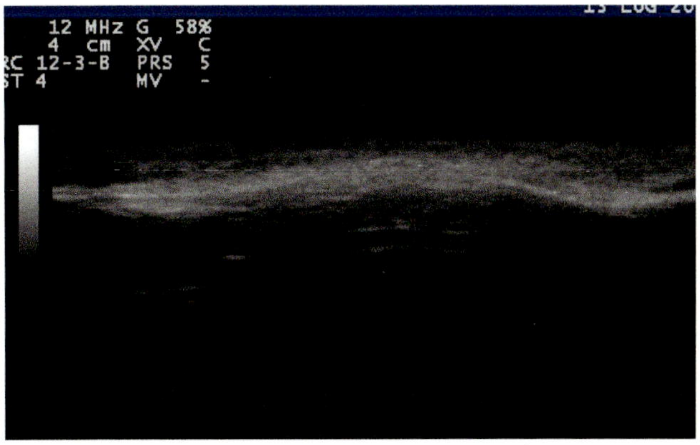

Fig. 12.17 Ultrasound images of the injection into the frontal area: the cannula is inserted into the frontalis muscle. Depth: 1 cm (courtesy of the Doctor's Equipe). (Published by kind permission of ©Mario Goisis 2018. All Rights Reserved)

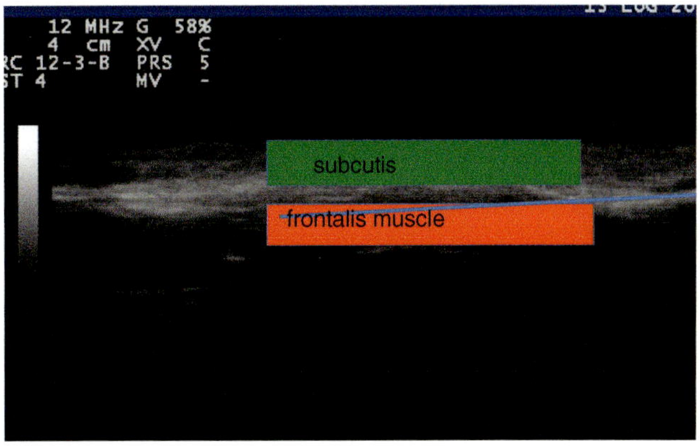

Fig. 12.18 Ultrasound images of the injection into the frontal area: the cannula is inserted into the frontalis muscle. Depth: 1 cm (courtesy of the Doctor's Equipe). (Published by kind permission of ©Mario Goisis 2018. All Rights Reserved)

12.7 Cadaveric Dissection of Fat Step by Step (Figs. 12.19, 12.20)

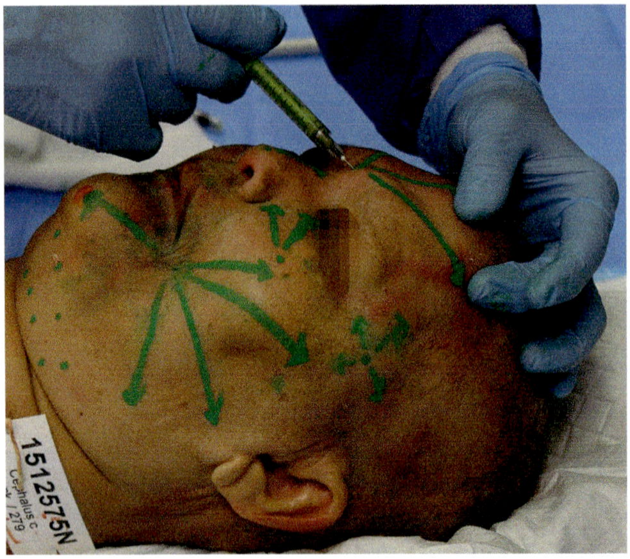

Fig. 12.19 The fat is delivered slowly into the muscle, while the cannula is withdrawn by retrograde injection (courtesy Doctor's Equipe). (Published with kind permission of ©Mario Goisis 2018. All Rights Reserved)

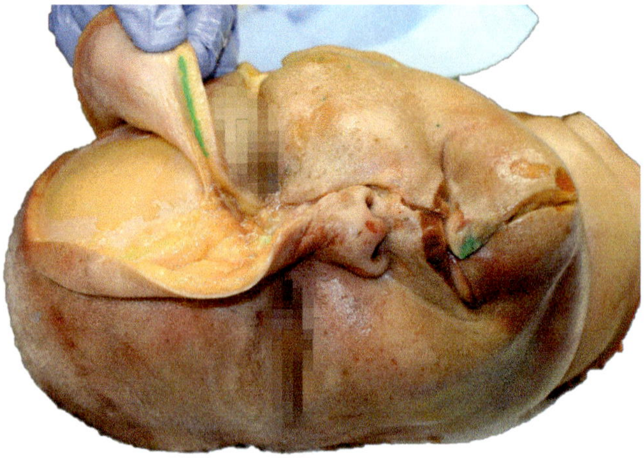

Fig. 12.20 Demonstration of the plane of injection: the injected fat (green) is transferred into the intramuscular plane (courtesy of the Doctor's Equipe). (Published by kind permission of ©Mario Goisis 2018. All Rights Reserved)

13 Malar Area

Mario Goisis, Giuseppe A. Ferraro, Sara Izzo, and Giovanni Francesco Nicoletti

Augmentation of the malar area is a simple procedure, than can be carried out in the physician's own surgery under local anaesthesia. Augmentation of the malar area is one of the best treatments for quality of results, as far as the midface approach is concerned.

13.1 Anatomy

The malar bone, or zygomatic bone, creates the prominence of the cheek and belongs to the lateral wall and floor of the orbit and to that of the temporal and infratemporal fossa.

Some important structures have to be preserved during this procedure:

- The infraorbital nerve exits the infraorbital foramen of the maxilla and is a branch of the maxillary nerve. This nerve innervates the lower eyelid, upper lip, and part of the nasal vestibule (Fig. 13.1, see the yellow arrow).
- The infraorbital foramen is an opening in the skull located below the infraorbital margin of the orbit. It permits the passage of the infraorbital artery, vein, and nerve. The distance of the infraorbital foramen from the lower margin of the orbit varies between 6.10 and 10.9 mm. It is often palpable 1 cm below the lower margin of the orbit, along the axis of the pupil (see Figs. 13.2, 13.3, 13.4, and 13.5).

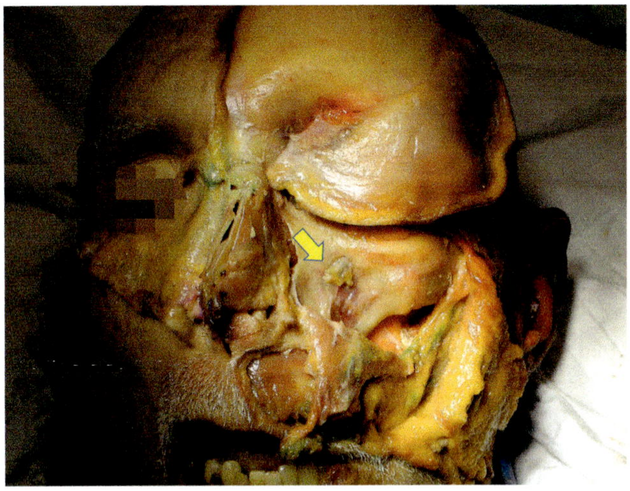

Fig. 13.1 The yellow arrow shows the infraorbital nerve emerging from the infraorbital foramen. The infraorbital foramen is an opening in the skull located below the infraorbital margin of the orbit. It creates a passage for the infraorbital artery, vein, and nerve. The distance of the infraorbital foramen from the lower margin of the orbit varies between 6.10 and 10.9 mm. It is often palpable 1 cm below the lower margin of the orbit, along the axis of the pupil (courtesy of the Doctor's Equipe). (Published by kind permission of ©Mario Goisis 2018. All Rights Reserved)

13.2 Pitfalls

It is essential to plan the treatment correctly: traditionally, a set of easy lines defined the areas where there was no risk of damaging the infraorbital nerve. These lines are called Hinderer's lines or the Hinderer lines. The practitioner should draw one line joining the external cantus of the eye to the lateral rim of the mouth and a second line going from the nasal wing to the tragus, on the patient's face. By intersecting, the two lines delineate four quadrants. The superomedial quadrant represents the high-risk area.

M. Goisis (✉)
Maxillo-Facial and Aesthetic Surgeon, Go Easy Clinic, Milan, Italy

G. A. Ferraro · S. Izzo · G. F. Nicoletti
Department of Plastic Surgery, University of Campania "Luigi Vanvitelli", Naples, Italy
e-mail: giuseppe.ferraro@unicampania.it; giovannifrancesco.nicoletti@unicampania.it

M. Goisis (ed.), *Outpatient Regenerative Medicine*, https://doi.org/10.1007/978-3-319-44894-7_13

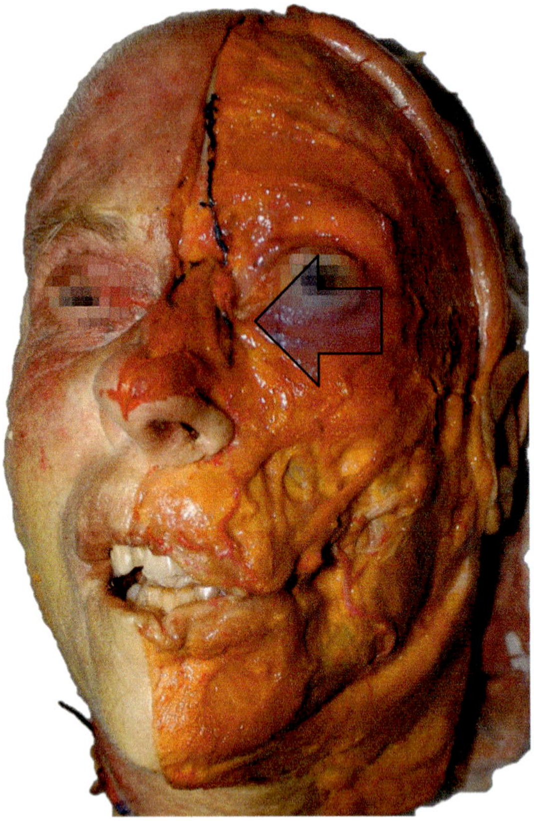

Fig. 13.2 The angular artery is the terminal part of the facial artery; it ascends to the medial angle of the eye's orbit, imbedded in the fibres of the angular head of the quadratus labii superioris and accompanied by the angular vein (see the blue arrows) (courtesy of the Doctor's Equipe). (Published by kind permission of ©Mario Goisis 2018. All Rights Reserved)

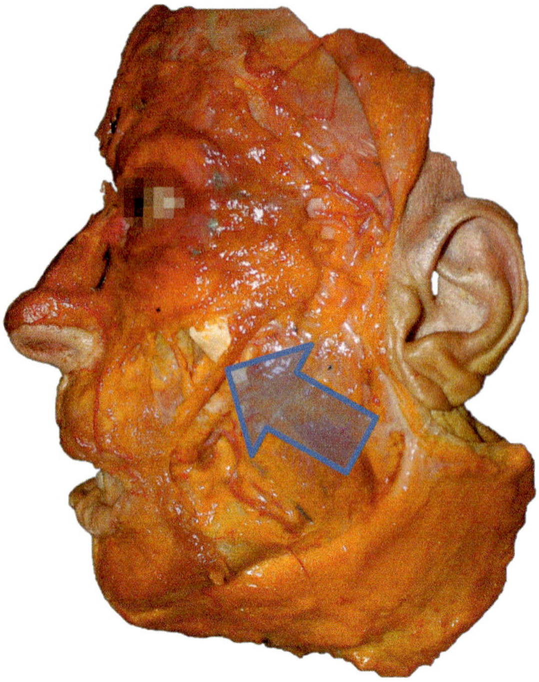

Fig. 13.4 Anatomical dissections of the ztygomaticus major muscle (see the blue arrow) (courtesy of the Doctor's Equipe). (Published by kind permission of ©Mario Goisis 2018. All Rights Reserved)

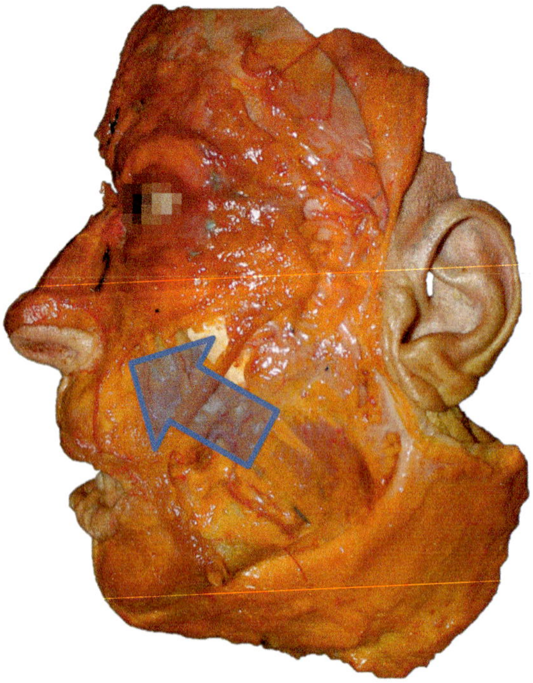

Fig. 13.3 Anatomical dissections of the levator labii muscle (blue arrow) (courtesy of the Doctor's Equipe). (Published by kind permission of ©Mario Goisis 2018. All Rights Reserved)

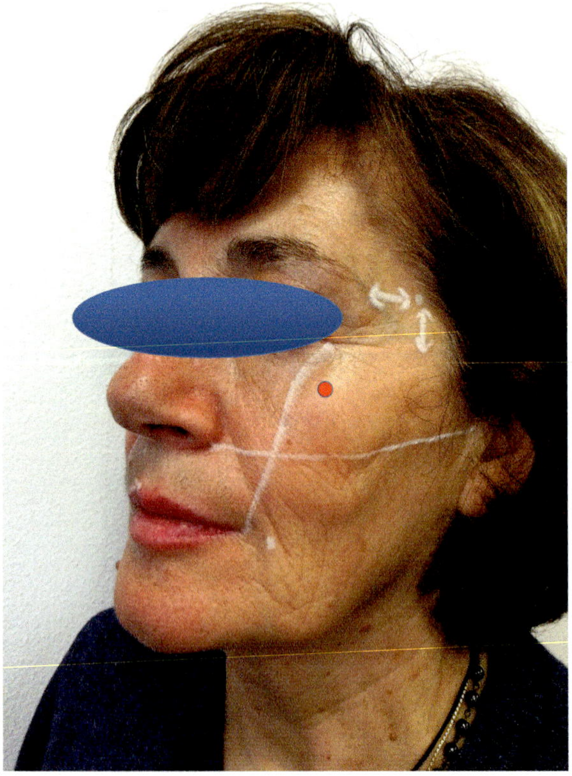

Fig. 13.5 The Hinderer lines are represented here. The safe injection points are indicated by the red circles. (Published by kind permission of ©Mario Goisis 2018. All Rights Reserved)

Safe point: The deep-injection point is situated in the superolateral quadrant determined using Hinderer's lines.

13.3 Indications

Malar atrophy is often congenital but can be also age-related. It has been calculated that the malar area loses approximately 3 mm of lateral thickness due to bone reabsorption between the ages of 25 and 60. This causes soft tissues of the middle part of the face to collapse, due to gravity. Comparing patient's older pictures with more recent ones, this phenomenon can often be emphasised. Collapse of midface tissues is responsible for the formation of nasolabial folds, marionette lines, and prejowl sulcus (Figs. 13.6, 13.7, 13.8, 13.9, and 13.10). Correction of age-related malar atrophy is often the best treatment to perform on patients with collapse of midface tissue, and this often represents the sole treatment capable of resolving this important problem in a sole session, with very little pain, excellent results, and great satisfaction for the patient and the surgeon. The conditions that this treatment is best suited for are reduced trophism, reduced lateral projection of the malar area, correction of the prejowl sulcus, correction of the marionette lines, and correction of the nasolabial folds. Malar augmentation can also be useful for correction of asymmetry.

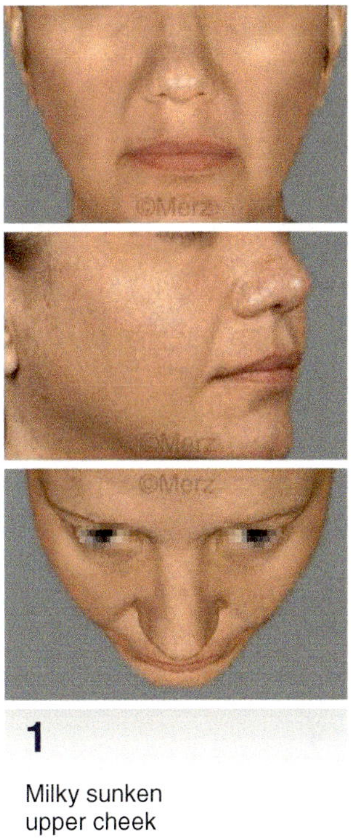

Fig. 13.7 Age-related atrophy of the malar area (by courtesy of the Merz company). (Published by kind permission of ©Mario Goisis 2018. All Rights Reserved)

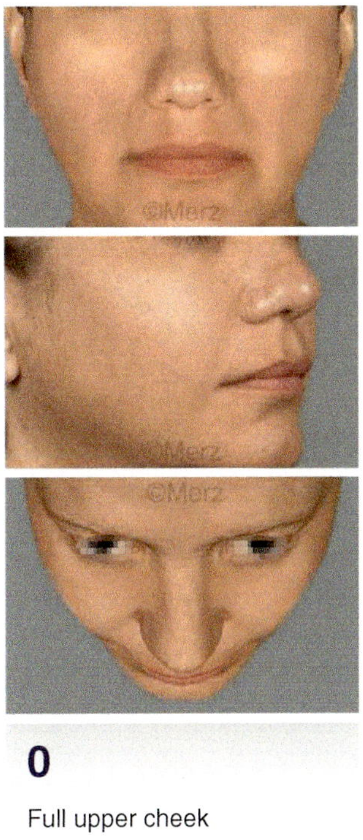

Fig. 13.6 Age-related atrophy of the malar area (by courtesy of the Merz company). (Published by kind permission of ©Mario Goisis 2018. All Rights Reserved)

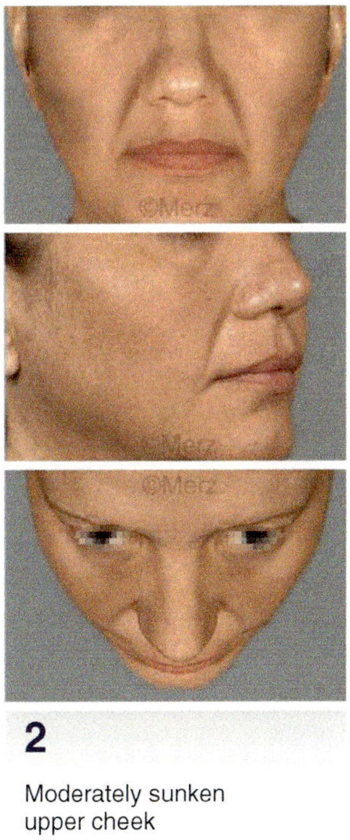

Fig. 13.8 Age-related atrophy of the malar area (by courtesy of the Merz company). (Published by kind permission of ©Mario Goisis 2018. All Rights Reserved)

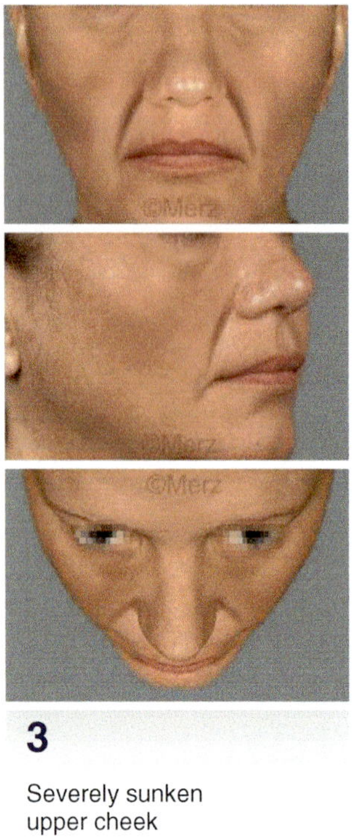

Fig. 13.9 Age-related atrophy of the malar area (by courtesy of the Merz company). (Published by kind permission of ©Mario Goisis 2018. All Rights Reserved)

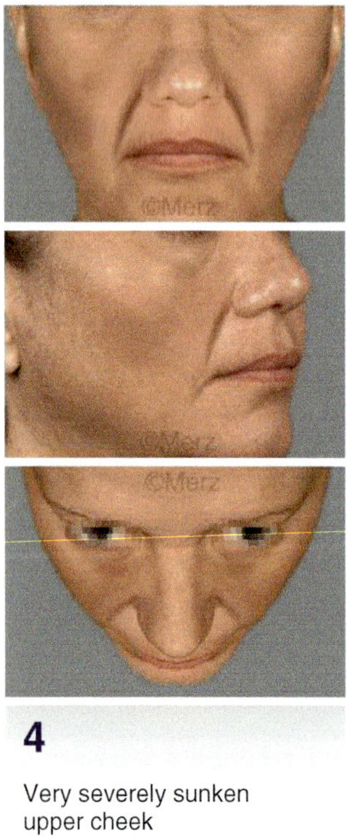

Fig. 13.10 Age-related atrophy of the malar area (by courtesy of the Merz company). (Published by kind permission of ©Mario Goisis 2018. All Rights Reserved)

13.4 Augmentation of the Malar Area Using Microfat Grafting Plus PRP

13.4.1 Indications

Correction of the age-related malar atrophy.

13.4.2 Contraindications

- Relative contraindications are anatomical alterations due to previous trauma or surgical intervention (maxillofacial surgery). Scarring often induces a displacement of the noble structures and can lead to perforation of the artery or resection of the nerve. It can also induce retracting scars that can cause asymmetry and unequal filling of the part treated.
- The fat should not be injected in areas that lack sufficient blood supply or affected by infection or inflammation.
- No injection should be carried out if the area has been previously treated with liquid silicone or other permanent fillers because new injections might lead to inflammation or infection of the implants.

13.4.3 Operating Time

Once the fat harvesting has been done, the procedure usually takes 5 min.

13.4.4 Materials

- 2–4 cc of microfat for injection into either side
  - *21-gauge needle*
  - *22-gauge 4 cm blunt cannula*

  For microfat harvesting and processing:
  A standard system for microfat is used, in particular:

- A Microfat box (www.microfat.com), composed of a ramp with a closed system for washing and filtration
- Four 60-cc syringes
- Two 10-cc syringes
- One 1-cc syringe
- One 30-gauge needle
- One 16-gauge needle

- A 2-mm-diameter, 10-cm-long Goisis cannula for fat harvesting
- A chlorhexidine-alcohol solution (2% chlorhexidine gluconate and 70% isopropyl alcohol), sterile drapes or towels
- Ice packs
- Sterile 2 cm by 2-cm gauze squares
- Occlusive dressing cover

Medications include:

- 100 cc of cold saline solution.
- 120 cc of cold Klein solution.
- One litre of Klein solution is composed of 800 mg of lidocaine, 1 mg of epinephrine, 40 MEq of sodium bicarbonate, and 1000 cc of saline solution.

Location: The microfat harvesting may be carried out in a small operating theatre /the physician's own surgery. Oxygen, pulse oximetry, and a crash cart/box should be present.

Assistance: An assistant can prove useful for the transfer of items to the procedure field in a sterile manner during the first stage of the procedure. Despite this, a single doctor may perform the procedure alone and unassisted.

13.4.5 Complications and Management

Immediate complications (within 72 h after injection) include transient erythema, oedema, induration, pruritus, and ecchymosis.

Early complications (days to weeks after injection) include hypercorrection, local infection, necrosis of the skin, reactivation of herpes, discoloration, and persistent local symptoms (erythema, oedema, induration, pruritus, and hyperpigmentation).

Later complications include high rates of fat resorption and cysts.

13.4.6 Method

The procedure is shown in Figs. 13.9, 13.10, 13.11, 13.12, 13.13, 13.14, 13.15, 13.16, and 13.17.

Injection plane: Smas

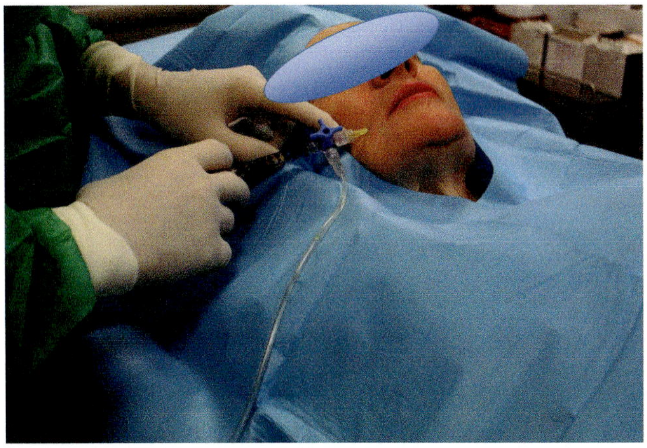

Fig. 13.11 An injection of 0.5 cc of local anaesthesia is carried out at the level of the modiolus. (Published by kind permission of ©Mario Goisis 2018. All Rights Reserved)

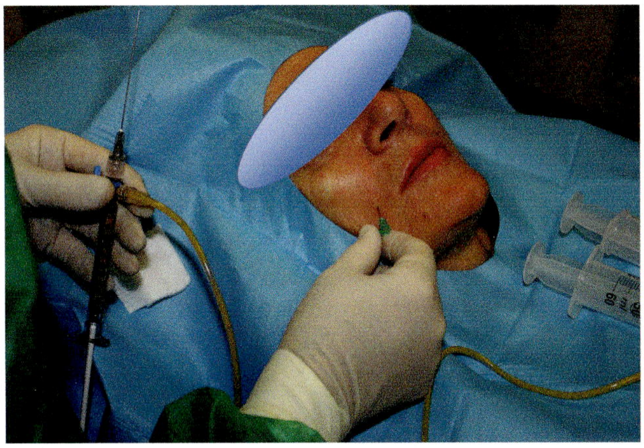

Fig. 13.12 After the local anaesthesia hastaken effect, an initial opening is made using a 21-G needle. (Published by kind permission of ©Mario Goisis 2018. All Rights Reserved)

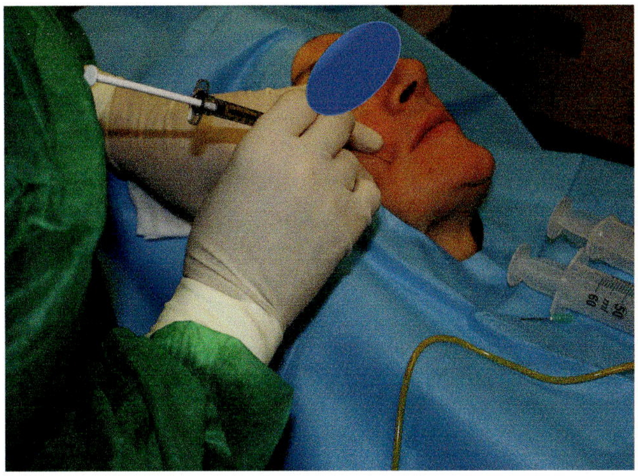

Fig. 13.13 A 22-G, blunt-tip cannula is inserted perpendicularly into the skin surface through the ad-hoc hole created. (Published by kind permission of ©Mario Goisis 2018. All Rights Reserved)

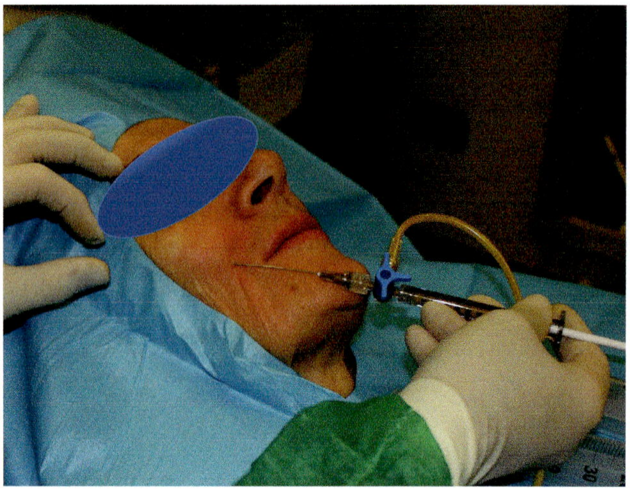

Fig. 13.14 The tip of the cannula is pushed forward along and inside the zygomaticus major muscle. (Published by kind permission of ©Mario Goisis 2018. All Rights Reserved)

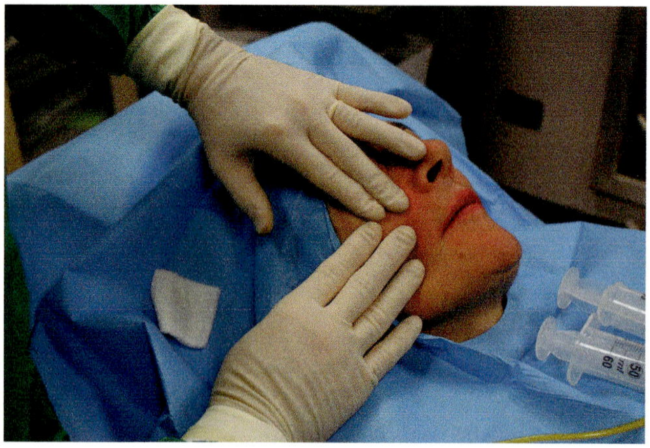

Fig. 13.16 After the injection of the fat the malar region is massaged. (Published by kind permission of ©Mario Goisis 2018. All Rights Reserved)

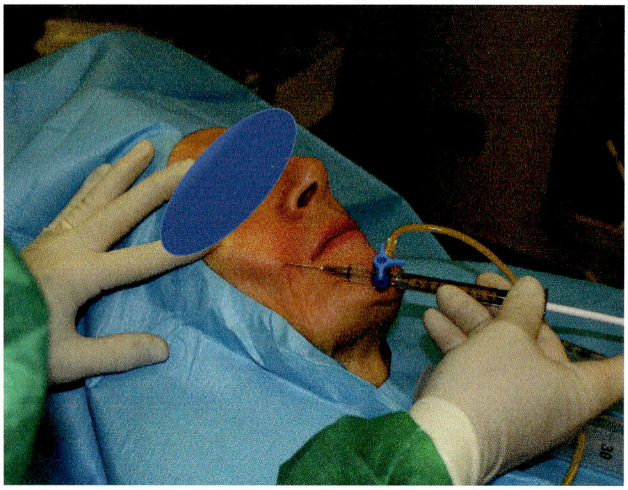

Fig. 13.15 The fat is delivered slowly while the cannula is withdrawn by retrograde injection. (Published by kind permission of ©Mario Goisis 2018. All Rights Reserved)

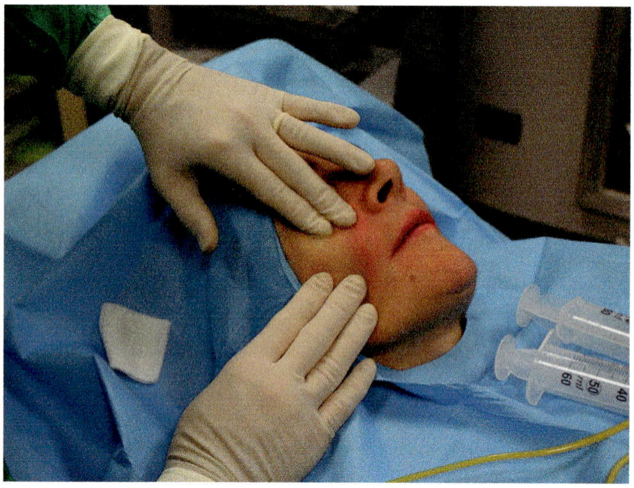

Fig. 13.17 After injection of the fat the malar region is massaged. (Published by kind permission of ©Mario Goisis 2018. All Rights Reserved)

13.4.7 Cadaver Dissection After Injection of Fat into the Malar (Figs. 13.18, 13.19, 13.20, 13.21, 13.22, and 13.23) (Courtesy by Doctor's Equipe)

13.5 Amelioration of the Malar Area Using PRP

13.5.1 Indications

Correction of small age-related wrinkles.

13.5.2 Operating Time

The procedure usually takes 15 min, due mostly to the time required for PRP harvesting.

Injection plane: dermis, subcutis

13.5.3 Materials

Tubes for PRP preparation, empty and with anticoagulant (www.microfat.com)

Bandages and antiseptic solutions (Figs. 13.23, 13.24, 13.25, and 13.26)

2 cc of local anaesthetic (2% lidocaine or 2% mepivacaine) with epinephrine 1:100000

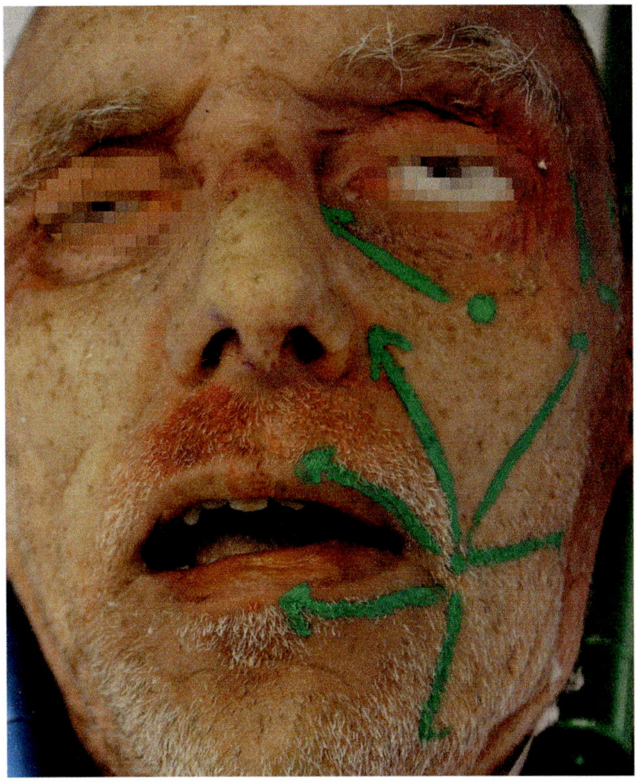

Fig. 13.18 The malar region is augmented using a single entry-point located 1.5–2 cm laterally to the oral rim. (Published by kind permission of ©Mario Goisis 2018. All Rights Reserved)

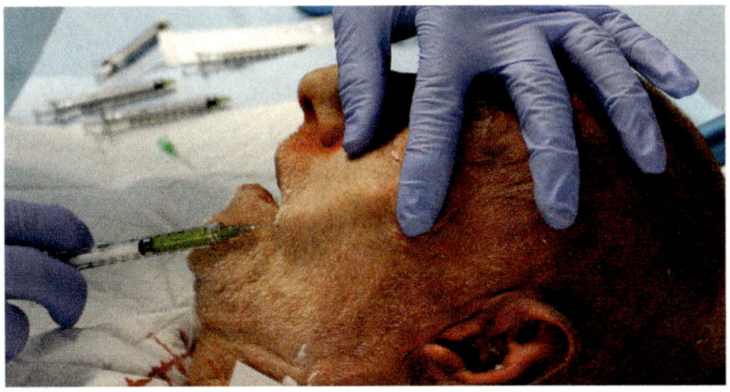

Fig. 13.19 The fat is delivered slowly while the cannula is withdrawnby retrograde injection. (Published by kind permission of ©Mario Goisis 2018. All Rights Reserved)

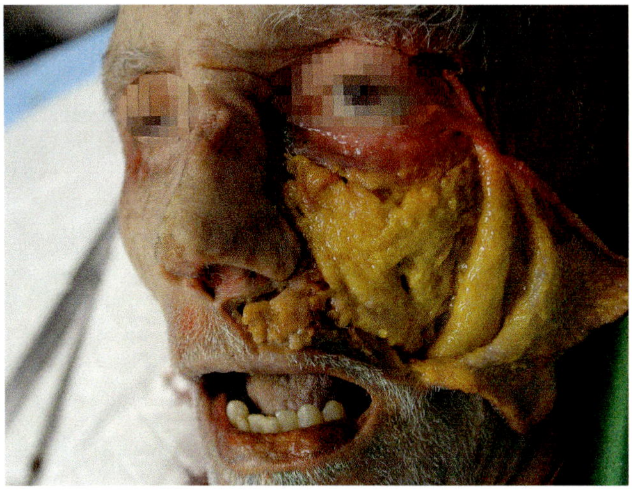

Fig. 13.20 After finjection of the fat, midfacial dissection is executed starting from a subciliary incision of the lower lid which continues downwards to the internal cantus following a paranasal route to the labial filter as far as the vermilion border and all along it. The subcutaneous plane is thus exposed. No evidence of fat is shown in the subcutaneous plane. (Published by kind permission of ©Mario Goisis 2018. All Rights Reserved)

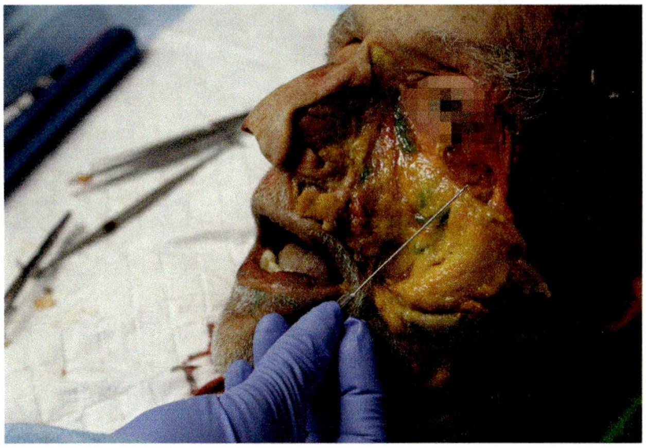

Fig. 13.21 The image shows the relationships of the 22-G cannula with the surrounding anatomical structures once the subcutaneous plane has been removed. The coloured fat can be retrieved on the muscular plane. (Published by kind permission of ©Mario Goisis 2018. All Rights Reserved)

One 1 -cc Luer lock syringe
One 30-G needle
One 26-G needle
One 27-G blunt cannula
1–2 cc of activated PRP (thrombin serum)

13.5.4 Method

The Method is illustrated in Figs. 13.27, 13.28, 13.29, 13.30, 13.31, 13.32, 13.33, 13.34, 13.35, 13.36, 13.37, 13.38, and 13.39 below.

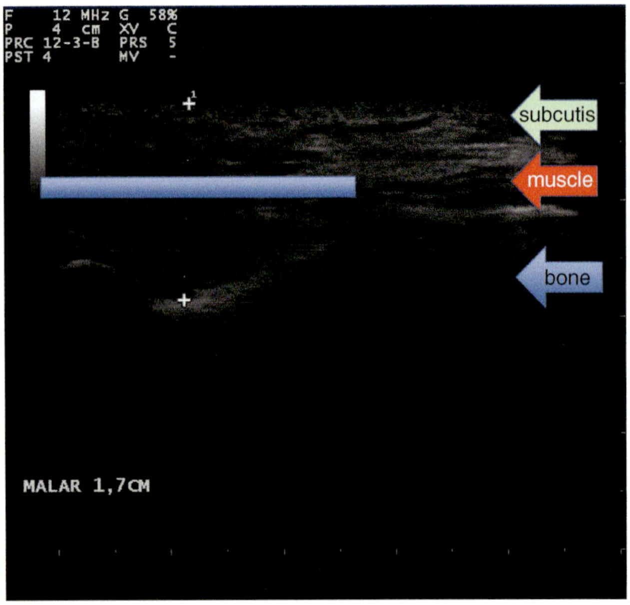

Fig. 13.22 An ultrasound image of the injection plane of microfat: the cannula is inserted into the muscle. (Published by kind permission of ©Mario Goisis 2018. All Rights Reserved)

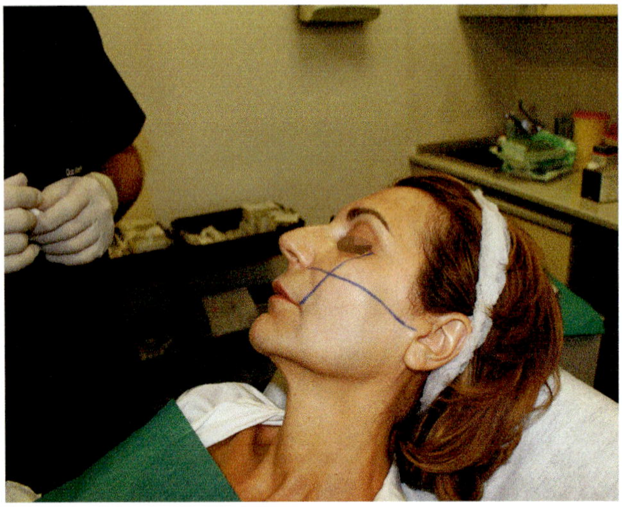

Fig. 13.23 Tecnique of injection of PRP: The Hinderer lines are drawn on the face of the patient. (Published by kind permission of ©Mario Goisis 2018. All Rights Reserved)

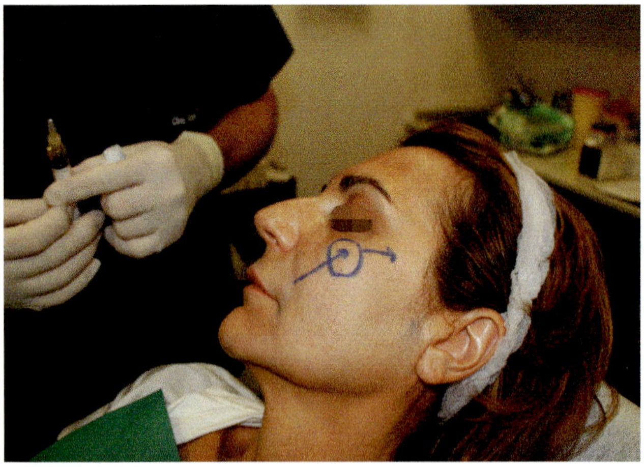

Fig. 13.24 The point of injection and movement of the cannula are represented here. (Published by kind permission of ©Mario Goisis 2018. All Rights Reserved)

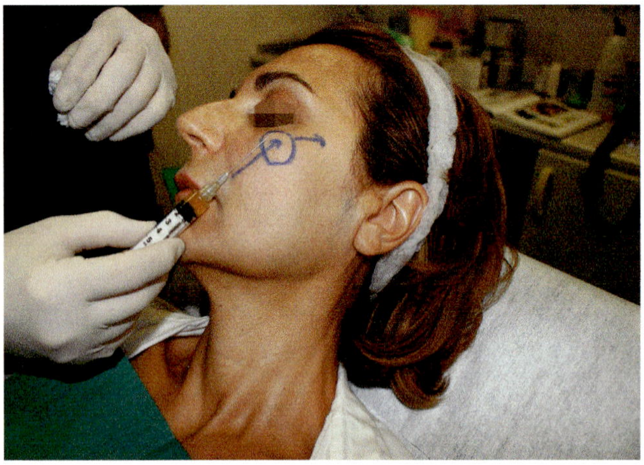

Fig. 13.25 The point of injection and movement of the cannula are represented here. (Published by kind permission of ©Mario Goisis 2018. All Rights Reserved)

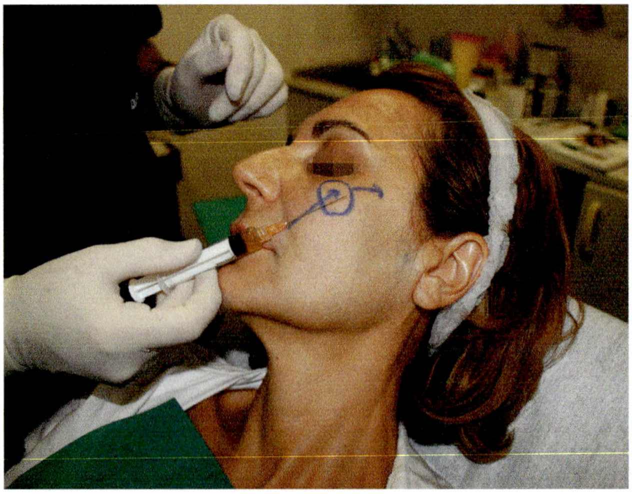

Fig. 13.26 The point of injection and movement of the cannula are represented here. (Published by kind permission of ©Mario Goisis 2018. All Rights Reserved)

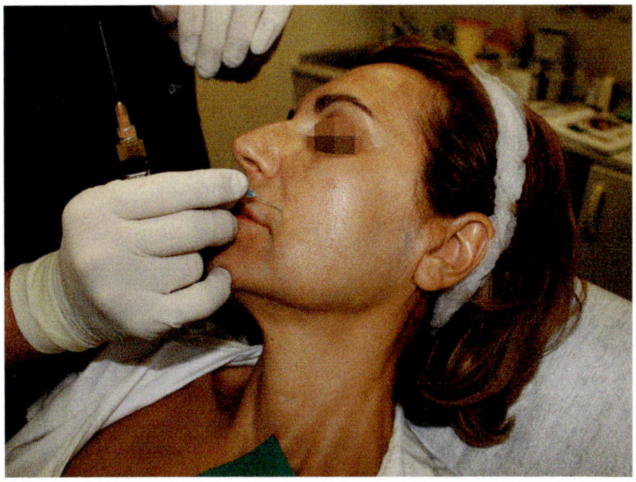

Fig. 13.27 After the local anaesthesia takes effect, an opening is created with a 23-G needle at the base of the nasolabial fold. (Published by kind permission of ©Mario Goisis 2018. All Rights Reserved)

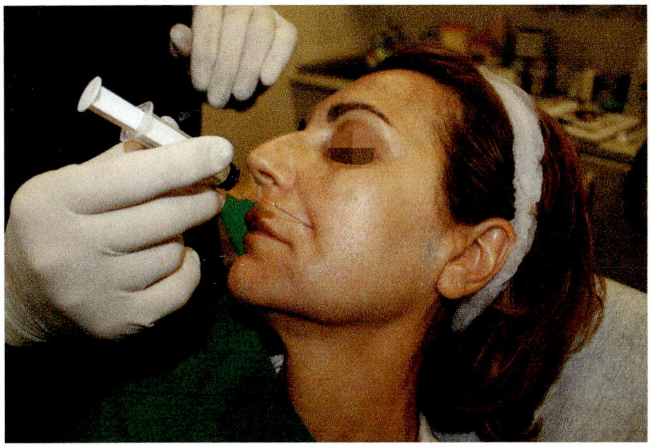

Fig. 13.28 A 25-G blunt-tip cannula is inserted perpendicularly into the skin's surface. (Published by kind permission of ©Mario Goisis 2018. All Rights Reserved)

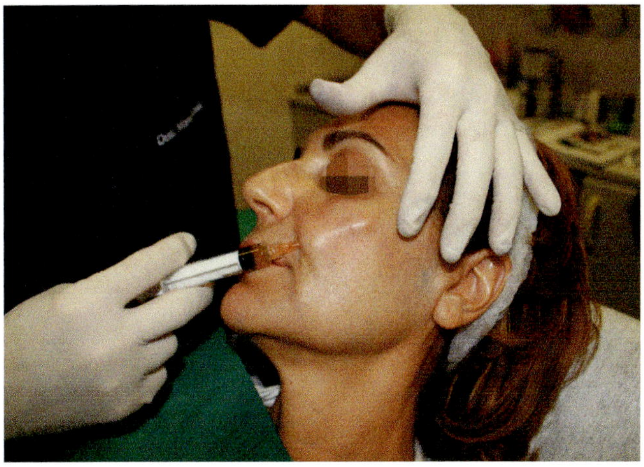

Fig. 13.29 The cannula is then pivoted parallel to the plane of the skin and slid forward in the direction of the body of the malar bone. (Published by kind permission of ©Mario Goisis 2018. All Rights Reserved)

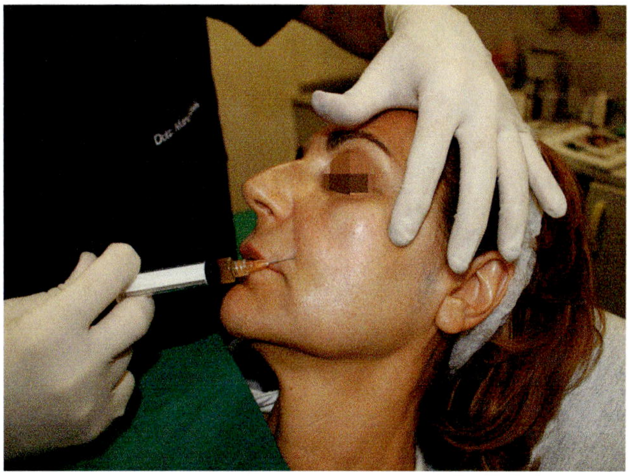

Fig. 13.30 The activated PRP is delivered slowly, while the cannula is withdrawn by retrograde injection along the entire length of malar bone from the arch to the medial section.. (Published by kind permission of ©Mario Goisis 2018. All Rights Reserved)

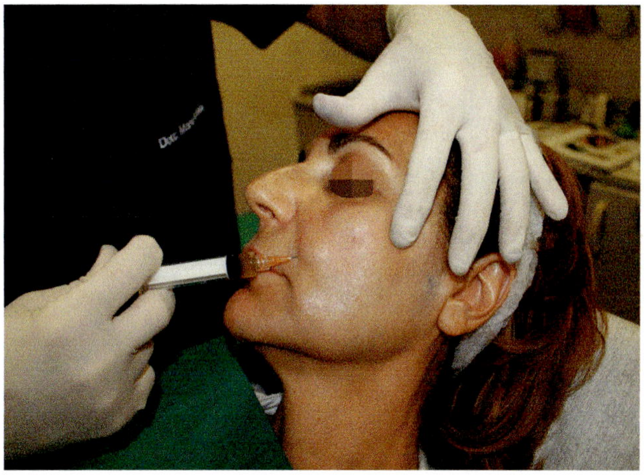

Fig. 13.31 The activated PRP is delivered slowly. (Published by kind permission of ©Mario Goisis 2018. All Rights Reserved)

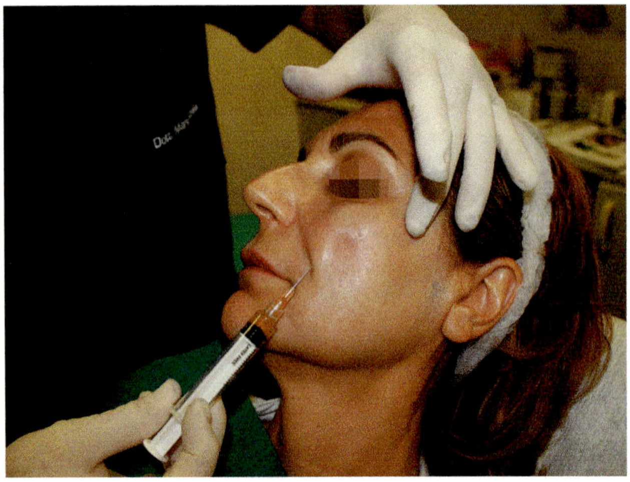

Fig. 13.32 The cannula is withdrawn by retrograde injection along the entire length of the malar bone from the arch to the medial section. (Published by kind permission of ©Mario Goisis 2018. All Rights Reserved)

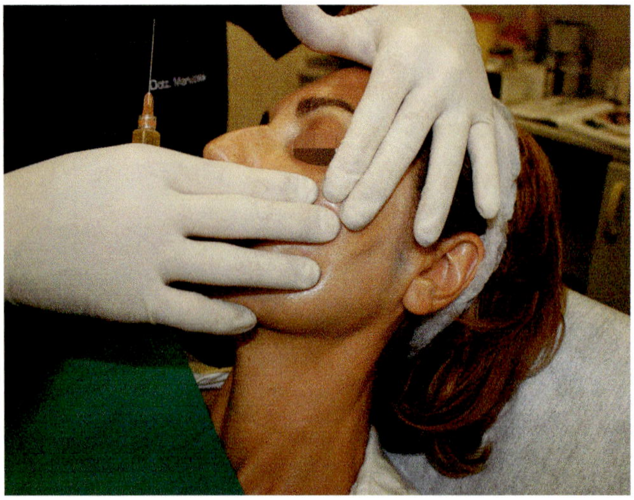

Fig. 13.34 When the treatment has been completed, the area is massaged. (Published by kind permission of ©Mario Goisis 2018. All Rights Reserved)

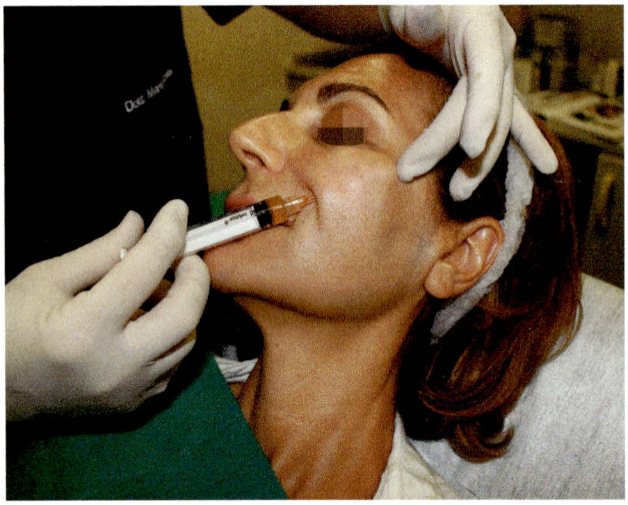

Fig. 13.33 The cannula is withdrawn. (Published by kind permission of ©Mario Goisis 2018. All Rights Reserved)

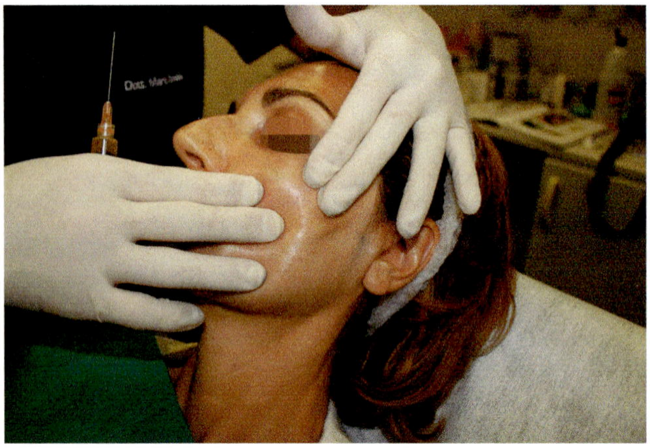

Fig. 13.35 When the treatment has been completed, the area is massaged. (Published by kind permission of ©Mario Goisis 2018. All Rights Reserved)

13.6 Amelioration of the Malar Area Using Nanofat

13.6.1 Indications

Correction of small age-related wrinkles and correction of acne scars.

13.6.2 Operating Time

The procedure usually takes 10 min, due mostly to the time required for PRP harvesting.

13.6.3 Contraindications

- Platelet dysfunction syndrome
- Critical thrombocytopenia
- Local infection at the site of the procedure
- Consistent use of NSAIDs within the 48 hours prior to procedure
- Corticosteroid injection at treatment site during the month prior to procedure
- Systemic use of corticosteroids during the 2 weeks prior to procedure
- Cancer – especially if haematopoietic or of bone
- HIV, HCV

13.6.4 Materials

- 1–2 cc of nanofat for injection into each side
  - *a 26-gauge needle*
  - *a 27-gauge 3.7 cm blunt cannula*

A standard system for producing nanofat is used, in particular:

- The Nanofat system (www.microfat.com), composed of a connector with a closed system for emulsion of microfat and filtration
- Two 10-cc syringes

For microfat harvesting and processing:
A standard system for microfat is used, in particular:

- A Microfat box (www.microfat.com), composed of a ramp with a closed system for washing and filtration
- Four 60-cc syringes
- Two 10-cc syringes
- One 1-cc syringe
- One 30-gauge needle
- One 16-gauge needle
- One 2-mm-diameter, 10-cm-long Goisis cannula for fat harvesting
- A chlorhexidine-alcohol solution (2% chlorhexidine gluconate and 70% isopropyl alcohol), sterile drapes or towels
- Ice packs
- Sterile 2 cm by 2-cm gauze squares
- Occlusive dressing cover

Medications include:

- 100 cc of cold saline solution.
- 120 cc of cold Klein solution.

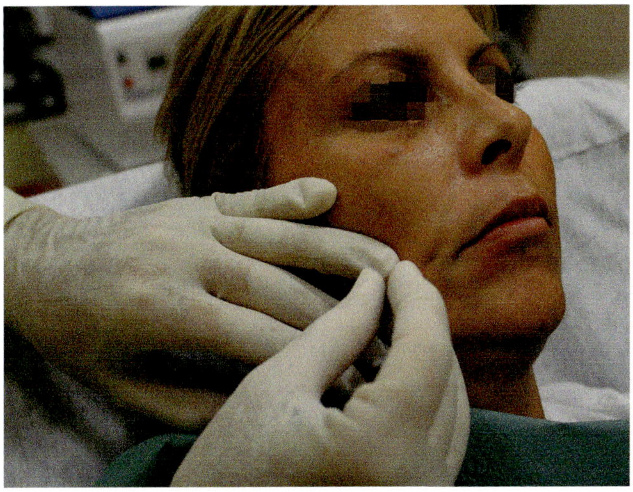

Fig. 13.36 An opening is created at the base of the nasolabial fold using a 26-G needle. (Published by kind permission of ©Mario Goisis 2018. All Rights Reserved)

- One litre of Klein solution is composed of 800 mg of lidocaine, 1 mg of epinephrine, 40 MEq of sodium bicarbonate, and 1000 cc of saline solution.

Location: The microfat harvesting can be in a small operating theatre/the physician's own surgery. Oxygen, pulse oximetry, and a crash cart/box should be present.

Assistance: An assistant can prove useful for the transfer items to the procedure field in a sterile manner during the first phase of the procedure. Despite this, a single doctor may perform the entire procedure unaided.

13.6.5 Method

The method is shown in Figs. 13.37, 13.38, and 13.39 below.

Injection plane: subcutis

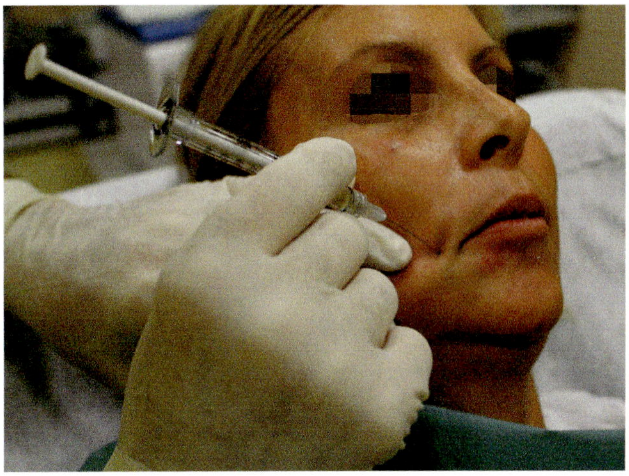

Fig. 13.37 The cannula is then pivoted parallel to the plane of the skin and slid in the direction of the malar bone. (Published by kind permission of ©Mario Goisis 2018. All Rights Reserved)

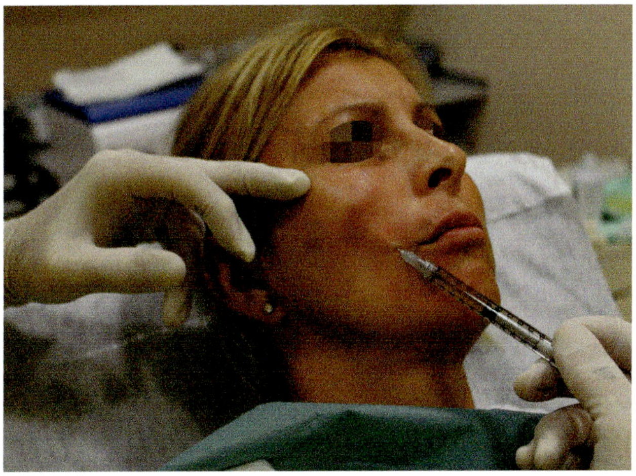

Fig. 13.38 The nanofat is delivered slowly, while the cannula is withdrawn by retrograde injection. (Published by kind permission of ©Mario Goisis 2018. All Rights Reserved)

13.6.6 Cadaver Dissection After Nanofat Injection (Figs. 13.40, 13.41, 13.42, 13.43, and 13.44) (Courtesy of the Doctor's Equipe)

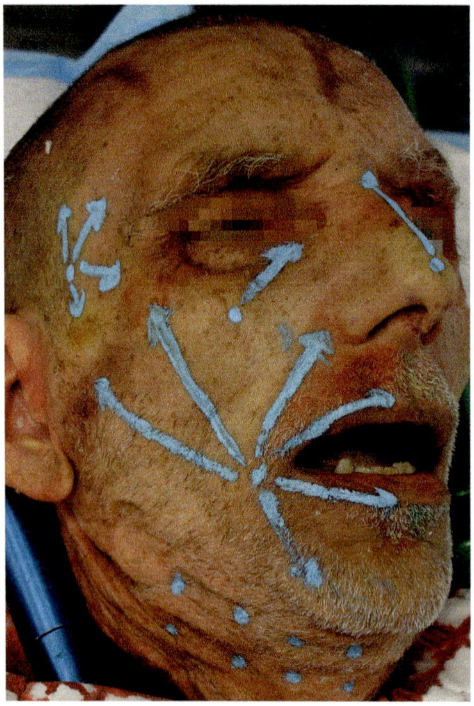

Fig. 13.39 Malar regions are treated using a single entry-point located 1.5–2 cm laterally to the oral rim. (Published by kind permission of ©Mario Goisis 2018. All Rights Reserved)

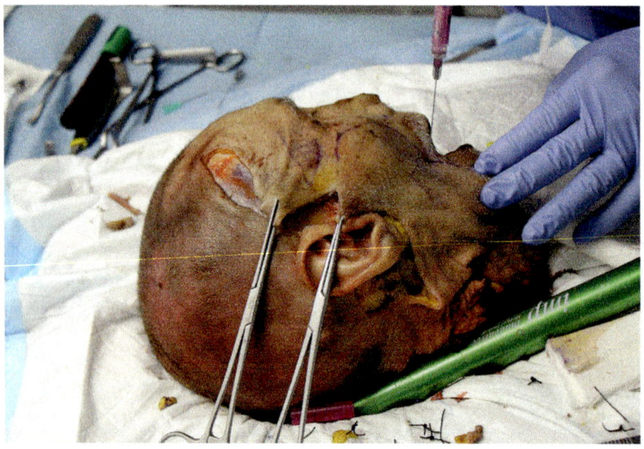

Fig. 13.40 An opening is created using a 25-G needle. A 27-G, blunt-tip cannula is inserted perpendicularly into the skin's surface through a hole created for that purpose. (Published by kind permission of ©Mario Goisis 2018. All Rights Reserved)

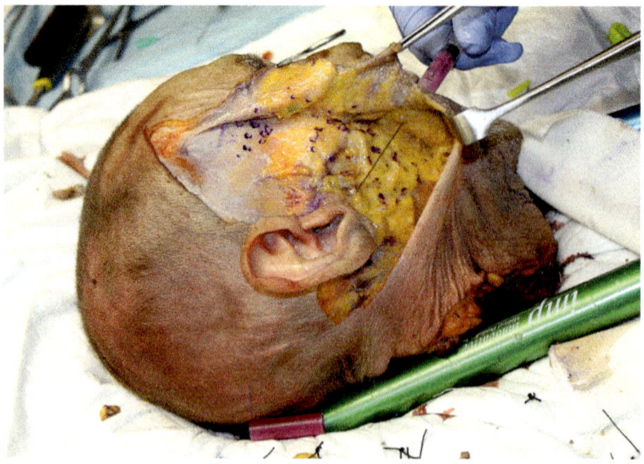

Fig. 13.41 After the nanofat injection, midfacial dissection is executed and the subcutaneous plane exposed. The presence of the injected nanofat is shown in this plane. (Published by kind permission of ©Mario Goisis 2018. All Rights Reserved)

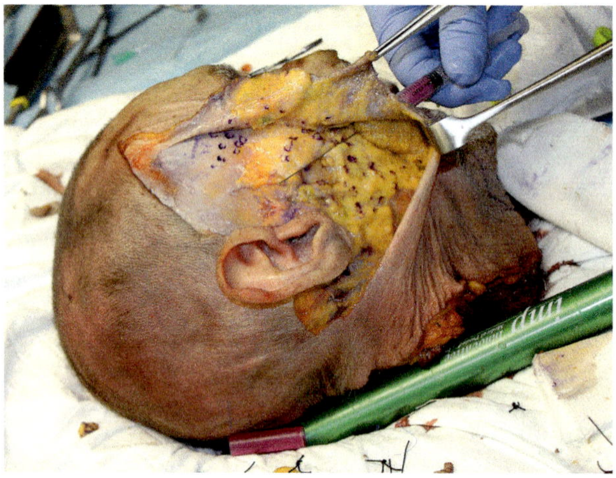

Fig. 13.42 After the nanofat injection, the midfacial dissection is executed and the subcutaneous plane exposed. The presence of the injected nanofat is shown in this plane. (Published by kind permission of ©Mario Goisis 2018. All Rights Reserved)

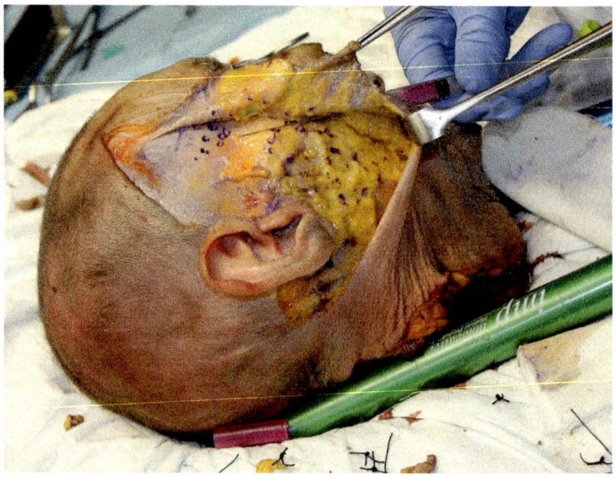

Fig. 13.43 After the nanofat injection, the midfacial dissection is executed and the subcutaneous plane exposed. The presence of the injected nanofat is shown in this plane. (Published by kind permission of ©Mario Goisis 2018. All Rights Reserved)

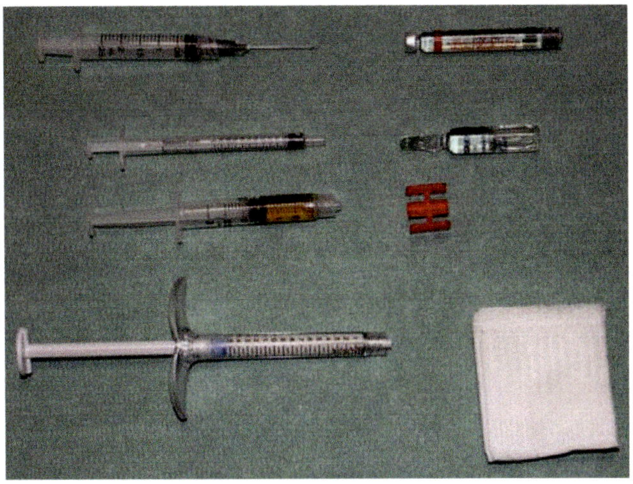

Fig. 13.44 Materials. (Published by kind permission of ©Mario Goisis 2018. All Rights Reserved)

13.7 Augmentation of the Malar Area Using Calcium Hydroxylapatite and PRP

13.7.1 Indications

Correction of age-related malar atrophy.

13.7.2 Pitfalls

- The product has to be injected deeply into a sovra-periosteal space. The product needs to be injected slowly. The fingers of the free hand need to be positioned in such a way as to be able to feel the product under the tips of the fingers while it is being injected.
- If a sudden pain is felt in the area of the skin innerved by the infraorbital nerve during insertion of the needle or injection of the product, treatment should be immediately stopped, and no further product injected so as to avoid possible compression of the infraorbital nerve.
- The product may be diffused during injection or after treatment by massage the length of the lateral margin of the orbit. This is not a serious side effect but can turn out to be anti-aesthetic. If the product tends to migrate upwards, the surgeon should block the migration of the product with his/her finger, compressing the lateral margin of the orbit.

13.7.3 Contraindications

- Platelet dysfunction syndrome
- Critical thrombocytopenia
- Local infection at the site of the procedure
- Consistent use of NSAIDs 48 h prior to the procedure
- Corticosteroid injection at the treatment site 1 month prior to the procedure
- Systemic use of corticosteroids 2 weeks prior to treatment
- Cancer – especially if haematopoietic or of the bone
- HIV, HCV

13.7.4 Operating Time

The procedure usually takes 15 min, though most of the time is employed to obtain the platelet-enriched plasma (PRP).

Injection plane: deep plane (sovra-periosteal plane)

13.7.5 Materials

REGEN BCT Kit

- 1.5 calcium hydroxylapatite
- A 28-G needle
- A 22-G needle
- 2 cc of local anaesthetic (2% lidocaine or 2% mepivacaine) with epinephrine 1:100000
- A 1-mL syringe
- A 3-mL Luer lock syringe
- A connector for the Luer lock syringes
- Bandages and alcohol

13.7.6 Choice of Material

Radiesse and kit for the production of PRP

13.7.7 Method

The procedure is shown in Figs. 13.45, 13.46, 13.47, 13.48, 13.49, 13.50, 13.51, 13.52, 13.53, 13.54, 13.55, 13.56, and 13.57. (courtesy of Springer, injection in aesthetic medicine).

13.7.8 Contraindications

- The mix of Radiesse and PRP should not be injected into areas that lack sufficient blood supply or suffering from infection or inflammation.
- No injection should be if the area has been previously treated with liquid silicone or other permanent fillers

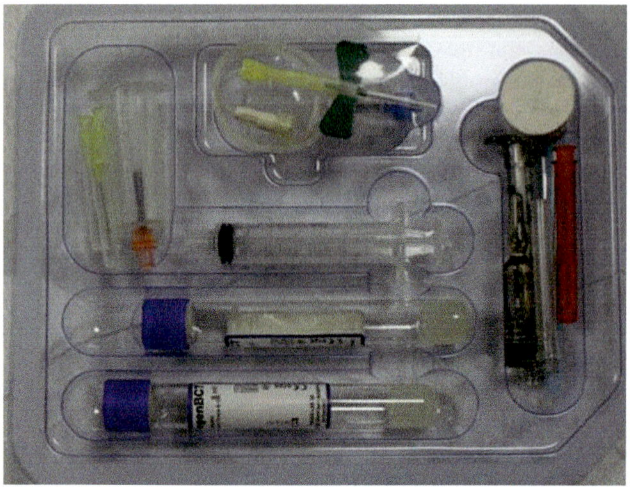

Fig. 13.45 The Regen kit is used by us to obtain the PRP. (Published by kind permission of ©Mario Goisis 2018. All Rights Reserved)

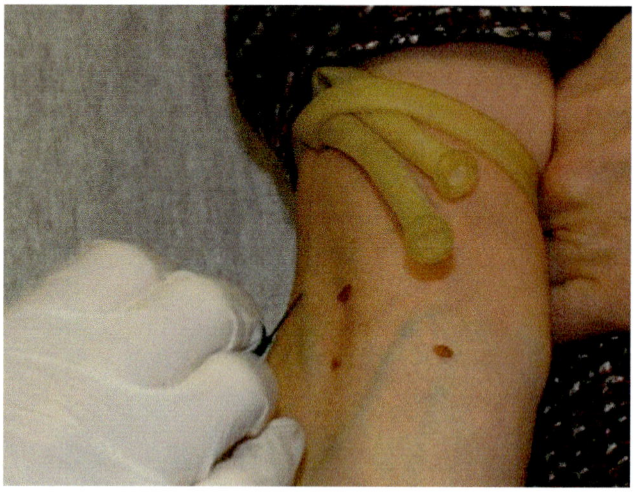

Fig. 13.47 A whole blood sample collected in an appropriate tube. (Published by kind permission of ©Mario Goisis 2018. All Rights Reserved)

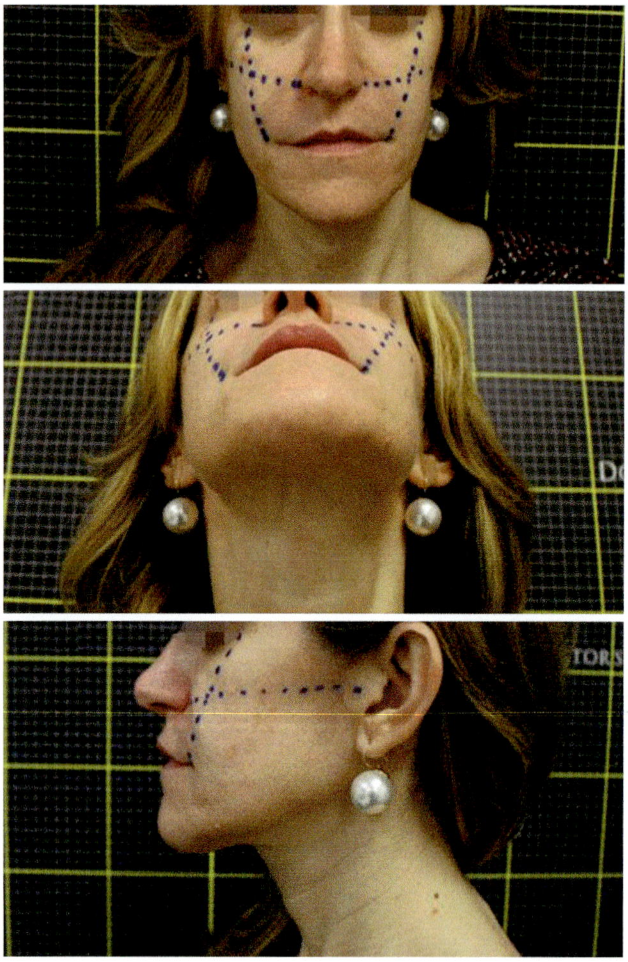

Fig. 13.46 The patient is evaluated from three different positions to show the hypoplasia of the maxillary bone to be corrected. (Published by kind permission of ©Mario Goisis 2018. All Rights Reserved)

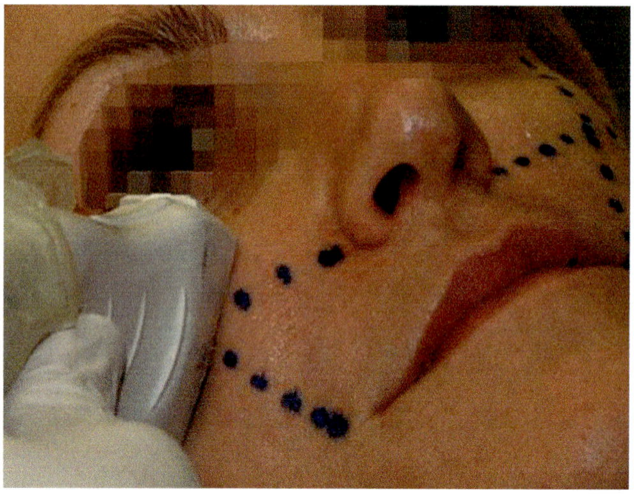

Fig. 13.48 An ultrasound evaluation test is performed, to compare the part before and after treatment. (Published with kind permission of ©Mario Goisis 2018. All Rights Reserved)

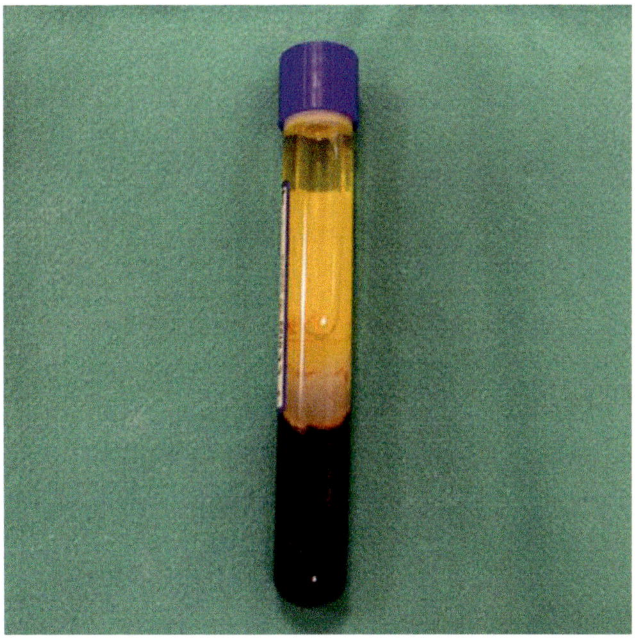

Fig. 13.49 Result of the separation of the PRP from the red blood-cells. (Published by kind permission of ©Mario Goisis 2018. All Rights Reserved)

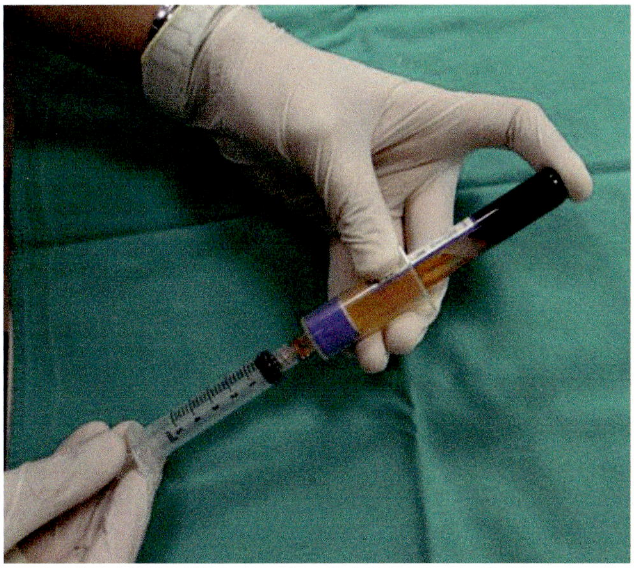

Fig. 13.50 The PRP is transferred into a 3-mL syringe leaving the red blood-cells in the test-tube, thanks to the specific gel that has favoured separation during centrifugation. (Published by kind permission of ©Mario Goisis 2018. All Rights Reserved)

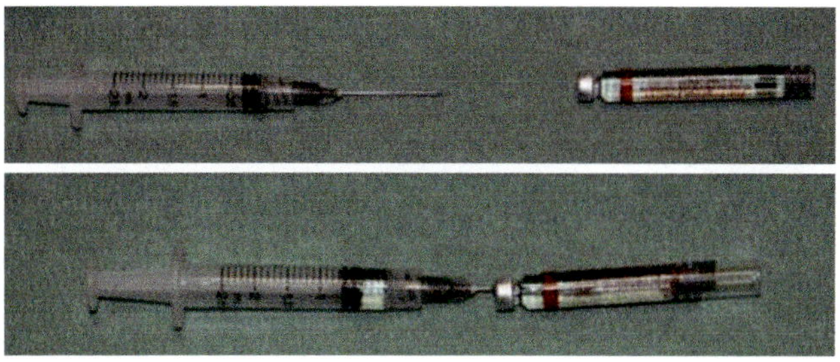

Fig. 13.51 0.5 mLs of local anaesthetic (lidocaine, mepivacaine) are aspired into a 3-mL syringe. (Published by kind permission of ©Mario Goisis 2018. All Rights Reserved)

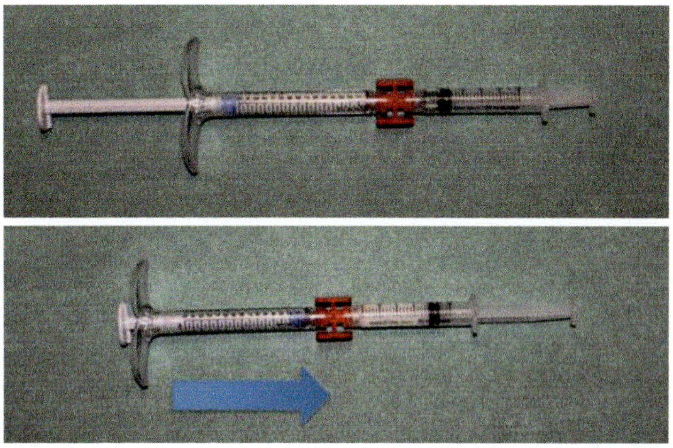

Fig. 13.52 1.5 cc of calcium hydroxylapatite is mixed with the 0.5 mL of local anaesthetic. (Published by kind permission of ©Mario Goisis 2018. All Rights Reserved)

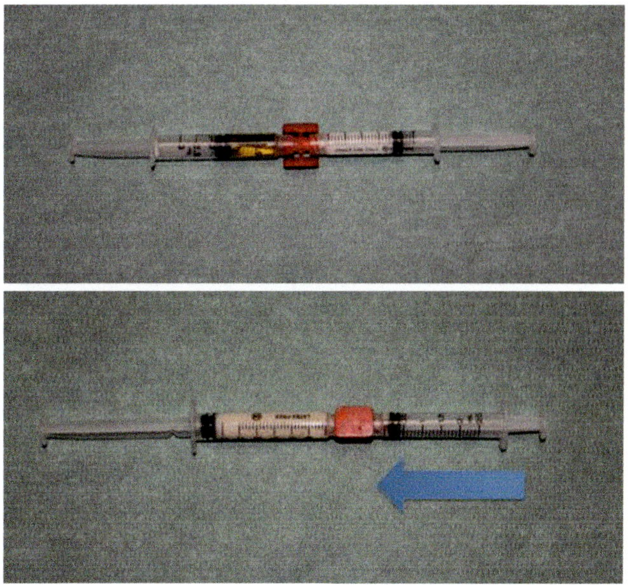

Fig. 13.53 The PRP is mixed with calcium hydroxylapatite plus anaesthesia. (Published by kind permission of ©Mario Goisis 2018. All Rights Reserved)

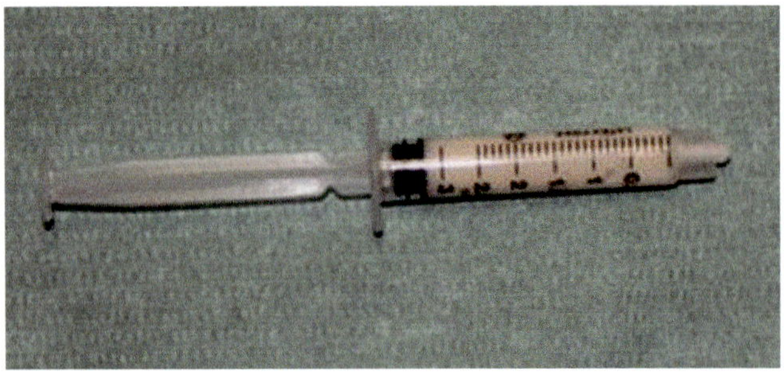

Fig. 13.54 The product is ready; it is composed of 1.5 mL of PRP, 0.5 cc of local anaesthesia, 1.5 cc of calcium hydroxylapatite. (Published by kind permission of ©Mario Goisis 2018. All Rights Reserved)

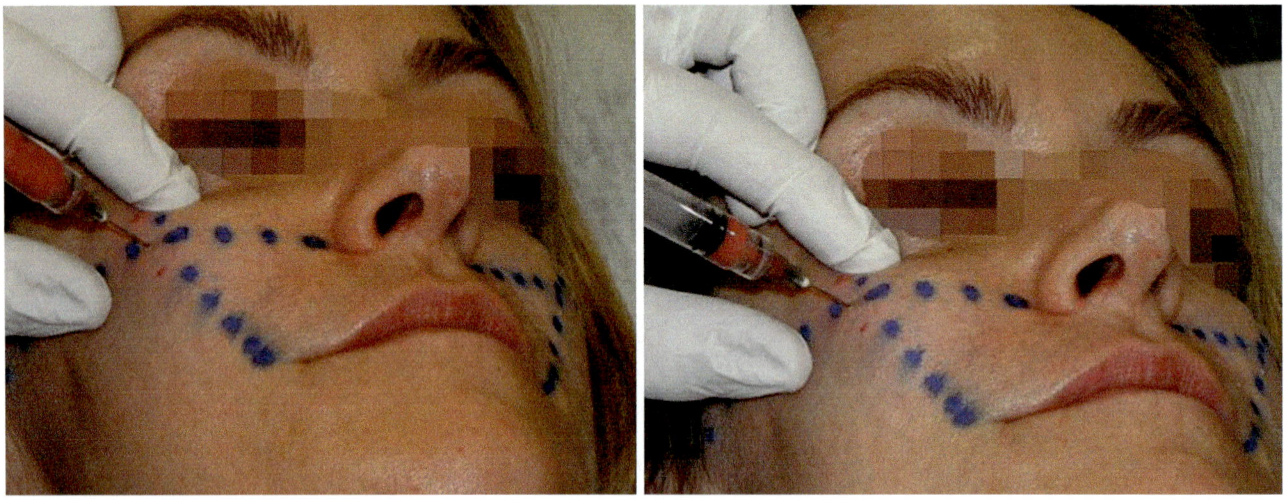

Fig. 13.55 After preparing the material, the needle has to be inserted deep into the malar area. The surgeon should touch the malar bone with the tip of the needle. Half of the syringe (1.5 cc of the 3 cc in the syringe) is slowly injected as a bolus into the risk-free area previously delimited (the safe point is right above the intersection of the Hinderer lines). (Published with kind permission of ©Mario Goisis 2018. All Rights Reserved)

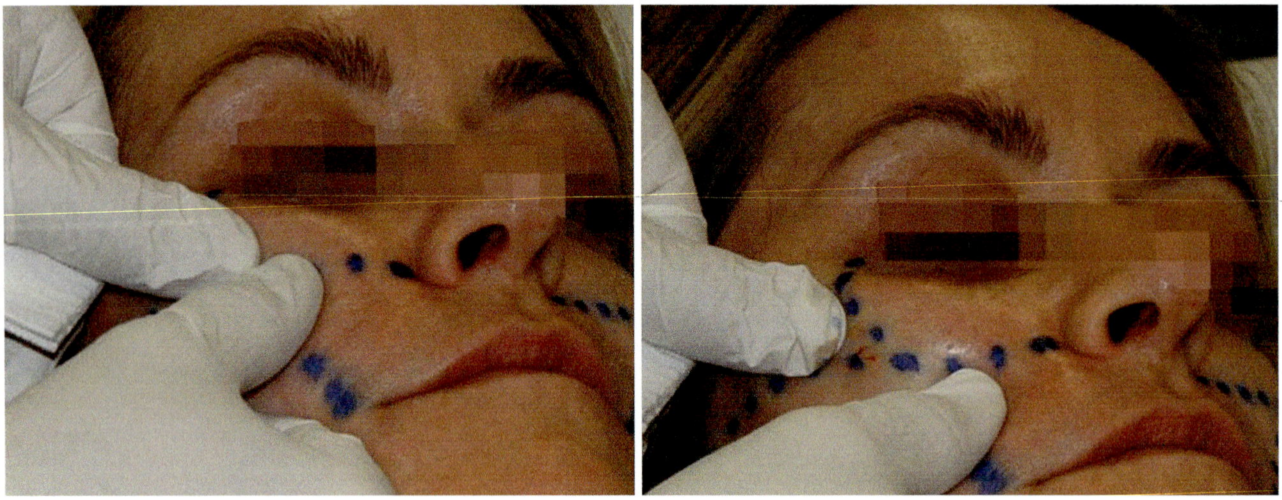

Fig. 13.56 After the injection, the surgeon should massage the area of injection firmly. The massage should be carried out from the medial to the lateral part of the malar bone. Attention needs to be paid to possible migration of the material along the lateral margin of the orbit during vigorous massage. This should be avoided by bringing firm pressure to bear on the lateral margin of the orbit with the finger. Mild tenderness and discrete swelling on the malar area are to be expected during the week following treatment and should not worry the patient or the surgeon. (Published by kind permission of ©Mario Goisis 2018. All Rights Reserved)

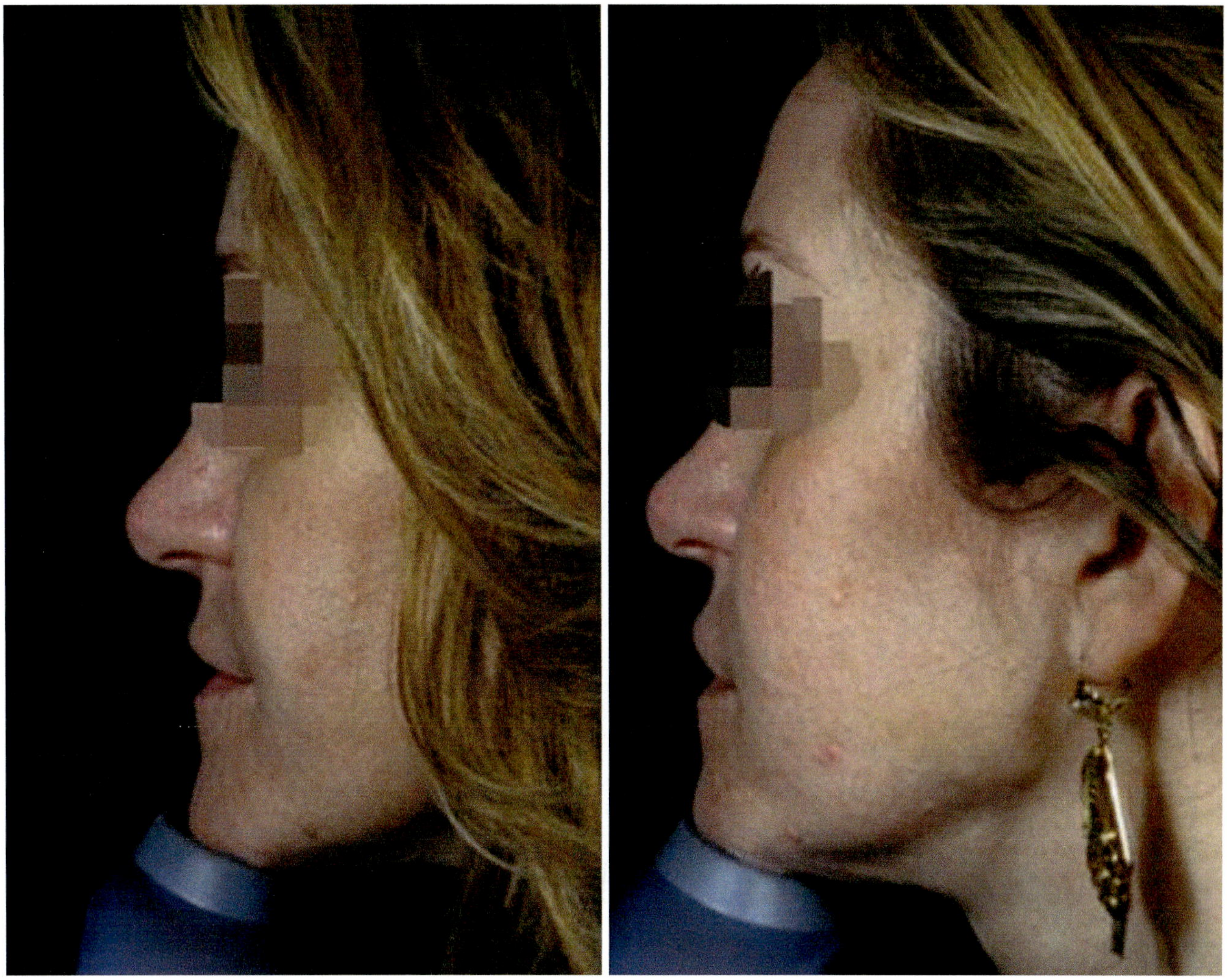

Fig. 13.57 Pictures of pretreatment (left) and of posttreatment (right). (Published by kind permission of ©Mario Goisis 2018. All Rights Reserved)

because new injections might lead to inflammation or infection of the implants.

13.7.9 Complications and Management

Immediate complications (within 72 h after injection) include transient erythema, oedema, induration, pruritus, and ecchymosis. Attention should be paid to possible migration of the material along the lateral margin of the orbit during vigorous massage. This should be avoided by applying firm pressure on the lateral margin of the orbit with the finger.

Early complications (days to weeks after injection) include hyper correction, local infection, necrosis of the skin, and reactivation of herpes.

Late complications include infection, filler migration, foreign-body granuloma, and scarring.

Tear Trough Amelioration

14

Mario Goisis, Claudio Rinna, and Rand S. Al Yahya

14.1 Anatomy

Tear trough or lacrimal groove lies on the nasal surface of the body of the maxilla, in front of the opening of the sinus. The lacrimal groove is converted into the nasolacrimal canal, by the lacrimal bone and inferior nasal concha; this canal opens into the inferior meatus of the nose and transmits the nasolacrimal duct. The lateral margin of the lacrimal fossa is named the anterior lacrimal crest and continues below with the inferior orbital rim (Fig. 14.1).

The eyelid is made up of several layers, from superficial to deep, which are the skin, subcutaneous tissue, orbicularis oculi, orbital septum and tarsal plates, and palpebral conjunctiva. The skin is similar to areas elsewhere but is relatively thin and has more pigment cells. It contains sweat glands and hairs, the latter becoming eyelashes as they meet the border of the eyelid. The orbital septum is a membranous sheet that acts as the anterior boundary of the orbit. It extends from the orbital rims to the eyelids. It forms the fibrous portion of the eyelids.

The angular artery is the terminal part of the facial artery; it ascends to the medial angle of the eye's orbit, imbedded in the fibers of the angular head of the quadratus labii superioris, and accompanied by the angular vein (Fig. 14.2).

Orbicularis oculi muscle: The orbicularis oculi is a muscle in the face that closes the eyelids. It arises from the nasal part of the frontal bone, from the frontal process of the maxilla in front of the lacrimal groove, and from the anterior surface and borders of a short fibrous band, the medial palpebral ligament. From this origin, the fibers are directed lateralward, forming a broad and thin layer, which occupies the eyelids or palpebrae, surrounds the circumference of the orbit, and spreads over the temple, and downward on the cheek. This muscle is thin and pale, forms a series of concentric curves, and is inserted into the lateral palpebral. The lacrimal part (tensor tarsi) is a small, thin muscle, about 6 mm in breadth and 12 mm in length, situated behind the medial palpebral ligament and lacrimal sac. It arises from the posterior crest and adjacent part of the orbital surface of the lacrimal bone and, passing behind the lacrimal sac, divides into two slips, upper and lower, which are inserted into the superior and inferior tarsi medial to the puncta lacrimalia. The muscle acts to close the eye and is the only muscle capable of doing so (Fig. 14.3).

The infraorbital nerve exits the infraorbital foramen of the maxilla and is a branch of the maxillary nerve. This nerve innervates the lower eyelid, upper lip, and part of the nasal vestibule. The infraorbital foramen is an opening in the skull located below the infraorbital margin of the orbit. It allows the passage for the infraorbital artery, vein, and nerve. The infraorbital foramen distance varies between 6.10 and 10.9 mm from the infraorbital margin. It is often palpable 1 cm below the lower orbit margin, on the pupil axis (Fig. 14.4).

14.2 Pitfalls

Caution should be paid around the infraorbital foramen (Fig. 14.5): It is useful to locate it with the finger before performing the pinch. The periorbital area is prone to bruising, and in the main structures, we have to pay attention to the angular vein and arteries. The safer technique is to use a blunt-tipped cannula, to minimize the chance of injuring the vessels.

M. Goisis (✉)
Maxillo-Facial and Aesthetic Surgeon, Go Easy Clinic, Milan, Italy

C. Rinna
Doctor's Equipe, Milan, Italy

R. S. Al Yahya
Prince Sattam Bin Abdulaziz University, Al Kharj, Saudi Arabia

M. Goisis (ed.), *Outpatient Regenerative Medicine*, https://doi.org/10.1007/978-3-319-44894-7_14

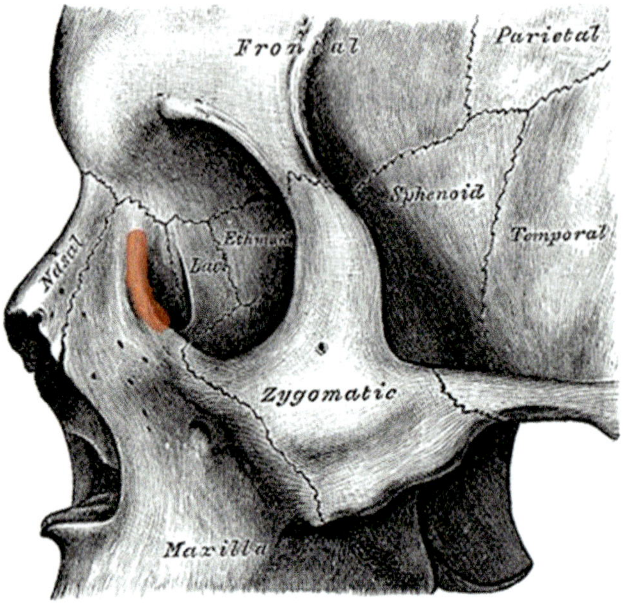

Fig. 14.1 Lacrimal crest in red. Reproduction of a lithograph plate from Gray's anatomy (Henry Gray, Anatomy: 1918). (Published with kind permission of ©Mario Goisis 2018. All Rights Reserved)

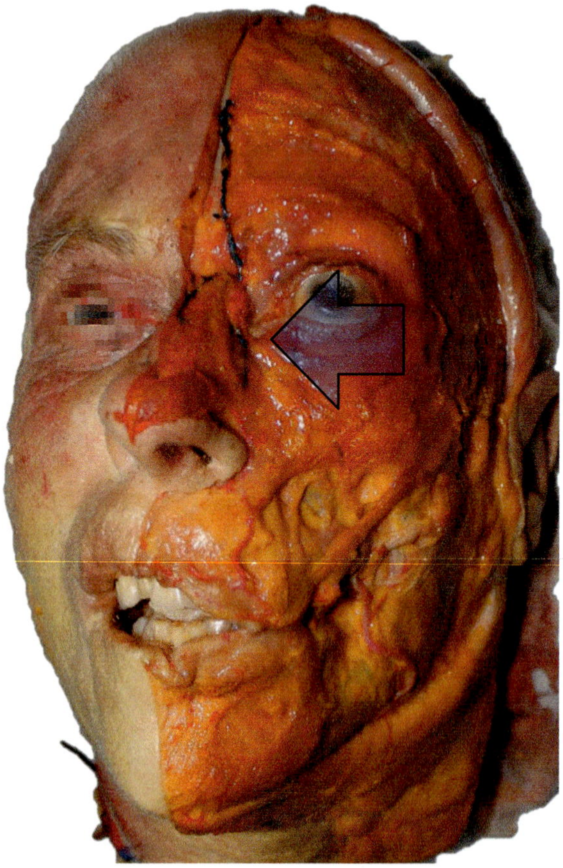

Fig. 14.2 Angular aretery and vien (blue arrows) (courtesy by DE). (Published with kind permission of ©Mario Goisis 2018. All Rights Reserved)

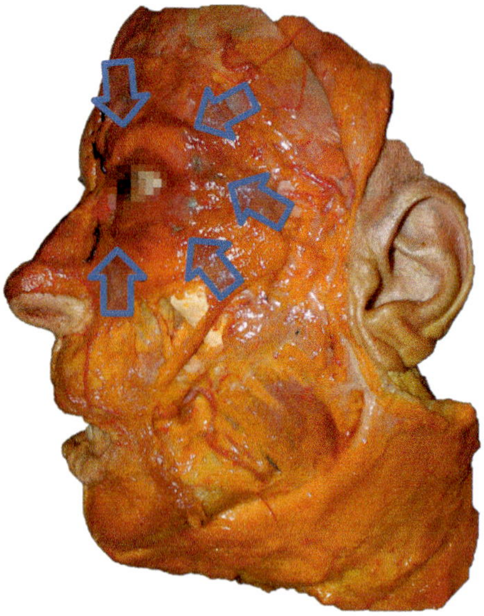

Fig. 14.3 Orbicularis oculi muscle anatomy. (courtesy by DE). (Published with kind permission of ©Mario Goisis 2018. All Rights Reserved)

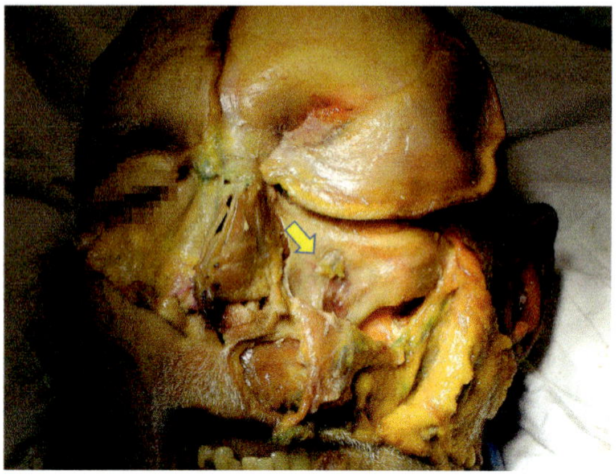

Fig. 14.4 Infraorbital nerve anatomy. (courtesy by DE). (Published with kind permission of ©Mario Goisis 2018. All Rights Reserved)

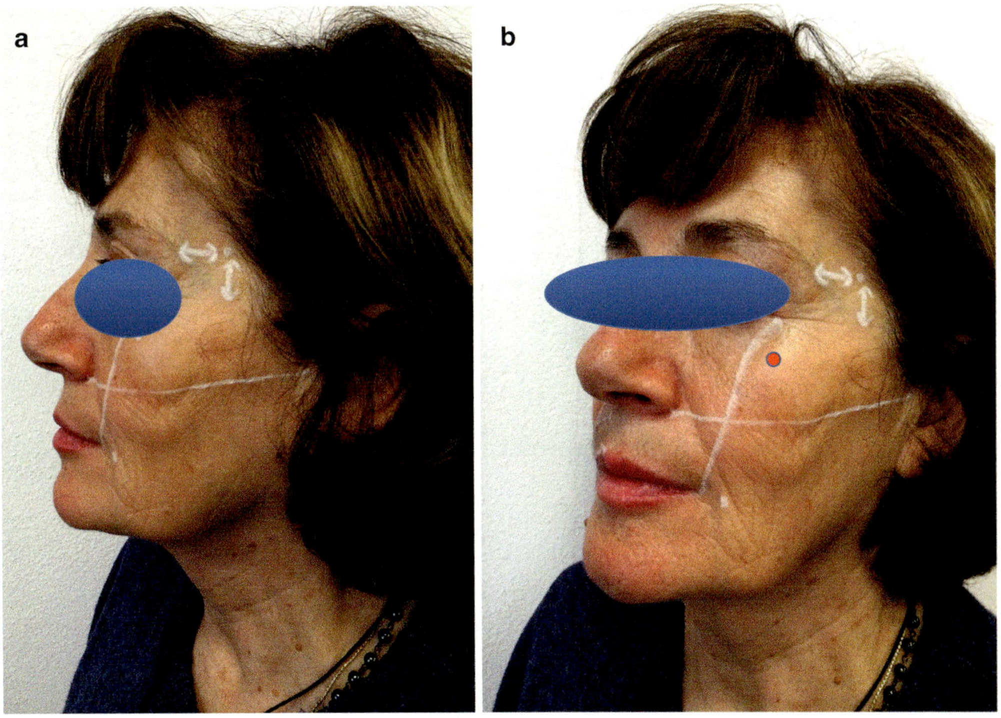

Fig. 14.5 The Hinderer's lines. A first line joining the external cantus of the eye to the lateral rim of the mouth and a second line going from the nasal wing to the tragus. The safe entry point (red circle) is located in the upper later quadrant of the area. (Published with kind permission of ©Mario Goisis 2018. All Rights Reserved)

14.3 Correction of Tear Trough Deformity with Microfat

14.3.1 Indications

The correction of the tear trough deformity is addressed to those people having a dip under the eye that casts a shadow and gives them a tired look. This condition can be part of the normal aging process, or following lower eyelid surgery when too much fat has been removed.

14.3.2 Contraindications

- Anatomical malformations of lacrimal ducts.
- Presence of severe skin laxity or atrophy and large bulgy fat pads will lead to unsatisfactory results.
- Anatomical alterations due to previous trauma or surgical intervention (maxillofacial surgery, titanium plates). Scarring often induces a displacement of the noble structures. It can also induce retracting scars that can cause asymmetry and unequal filling of the part treated.
- No injection should be done if the area has been previously treated with liquid silicone or other permanent fillers because new injection could lead to inflammation or infection of the implants.

14.3.3 Materials

- *0.5–1 cc of microfat on each side for injection:*
  - *21-gauge needle*
  - *22-gauge 4 cm blunt cannula*

For microfat harvesting and processing, a standard system for microfat is used, in particular:

- Microfat box (www.microfat.com), composed by a ramp with a closed a system for washing and filtration
- 4 60-cc syringes
- 2 10-cc syringes
- one 1-cc syringe
- 30-gauge needle
- 16-gauge needle
- A 2-mm-diameter, 10-cm-long Goisis cannula for fat harvesting
- A chlorhexidine-alcohol solution (2% chlorhexidine gluconate and 70% isopropyl alcohol), sterile drapes, or towels
- Ice packs
- Sterile 2 cm for 2 cm gauze squares
- Occlusive dressing cover

Medications include:

- 100 cc of cold saline solution

- 120 cc of cold Klein solution
- One liter of Klein solution is composed by 800 mg of lidocaine, 1 mg of epinephrine, 40 MEq of sodium bicarbonate, and 1000 cc of saline solution

Location: The microfat harvesting can be done in a small/office operating room. The oxygen, pulse oximetry, and a crash cart/box should be present.

Assistants: An assistant is useful to transfer items to the procedure field in a sterile manner in the first part of the procedure. Despite of that, a single doctor can execute all the procedure.

14.3.4 Complications and Management

Immediate complications (within 72 h after injection) include transient erythema, edema, induration, pruritus, and ecchymosis.

Early complications (days to weeks after injection) include overcorrection, local infection, skin necrosis, herpes reactivation, discoloration, and persistent local symptoms (erythema, edema, induration, pruritus, and hyperpigmentation).

Late complications include high rate of fat resorption, cysts, and lumpiness.

14.3.5 Operating Time

Once the fat has been harvested, the procedure usually takes from 2 to 5 min.

Plane of injection: intramuscular and submuscular

14.3.6 Method

Procedure is shown in Figs. 14.6, 14.7, 14.8, 14.9, 14.10, 14.11, and 14.12.

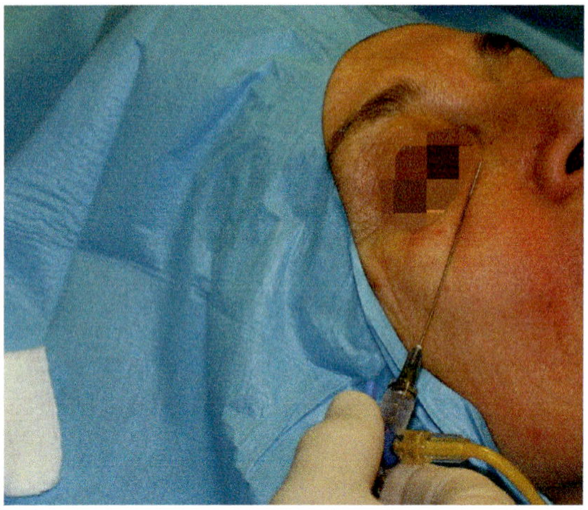

Fig. 14.6 Route of the cannula on the area of injection. (Published with kind permission of ©Mario Goisis 2018. All Rights Reserved)

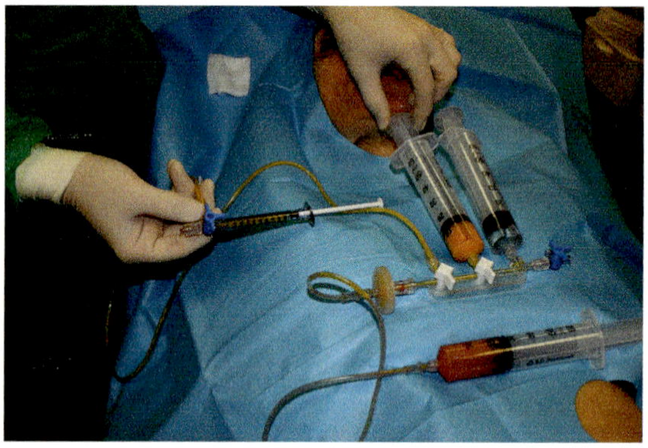

Fig. 14.8 The 1 cc syringe is filled by microfat. (Published with kind permission of ©Mario Goisis 2018. All Rights Reserved)

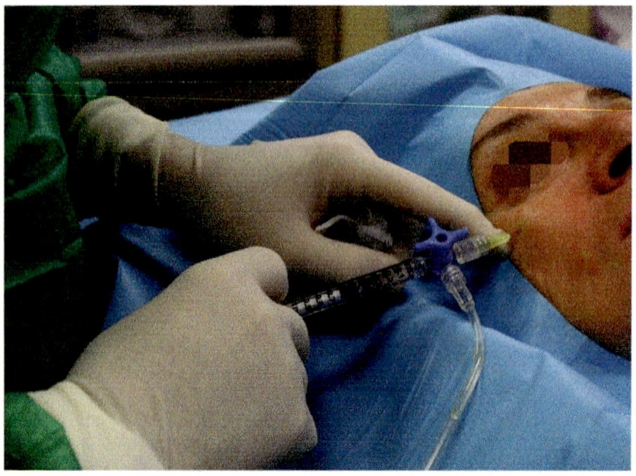

Fig. 14.7 To see better tear trough deformity, the patient should be kept in an semi-seated position rather than laid down. 1 cc of Klein solution can be used to anasthetize the area in the safe entry point. Taking this precaution, the treatment with the blunt-tip cannula will not give any pain to the patient. (Published with kind permission of ©Mario Goisis 2018. All Rights Reserved)

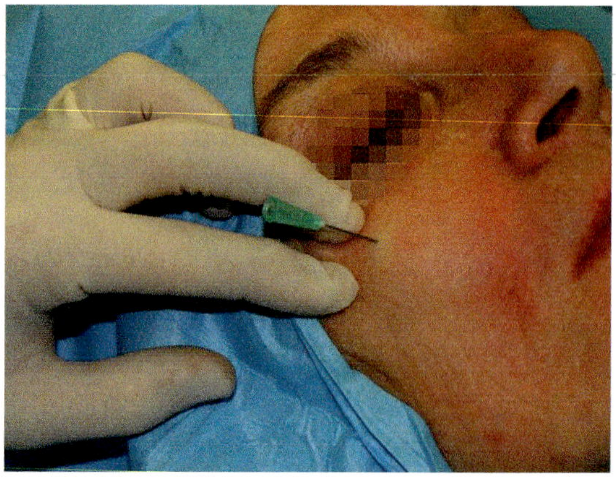

Fig. 14.9 A little hole is created in the safe point. A 21-G needle is used for this purpose. (Published with kind permission of ©Mario Goisis 2018. All Rights Reserved)

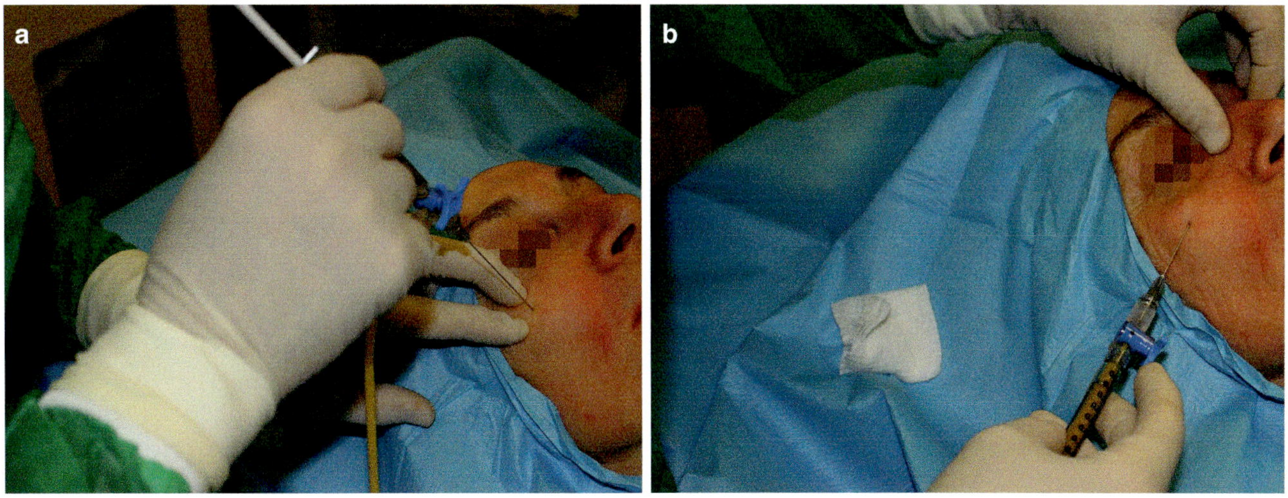

Fig. 14.10 Perpendicular insertion of a 22-G blunt-tip cannula. The cannula is plunged deep into the skin under the orbicular muscle, advancing to the periosteum. The cannula is then directed diagonally up toward the medial cantus of the eye and made it slide forward to the top of the tear trough. The tip of the cannula is showed through the skin to be just above the lacrimal crest. In fact, the tip of the cannula should be positioned over the lacrimal crest, touching the bone. (Published with kind permission of ©Mario Goisis 2018. All Rights Reserved)

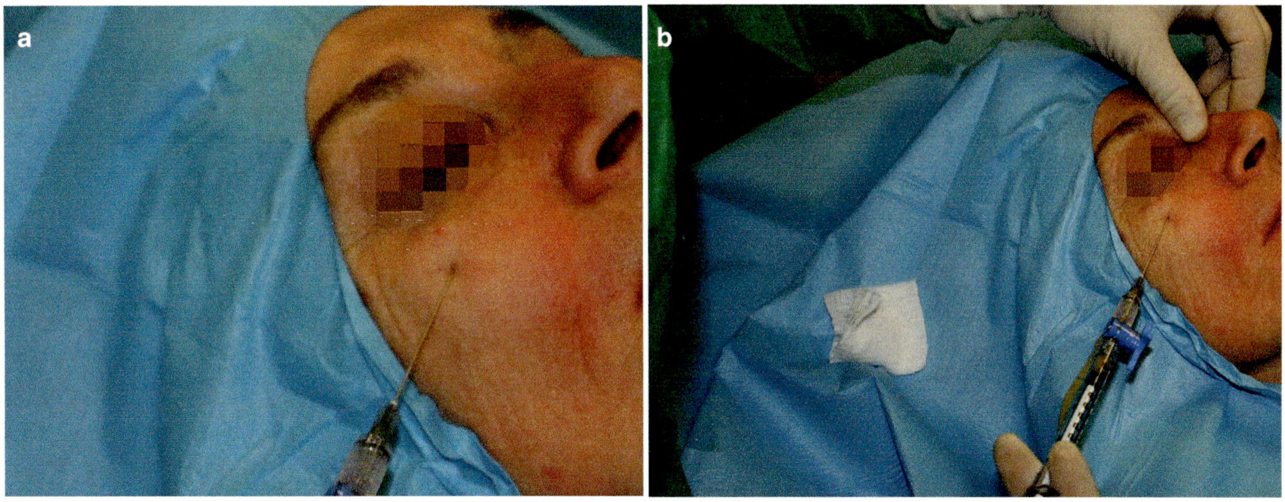

Fig. 14.11 0.5–1 cc of fat is injected with a retrograde technique. (Published with kind permission of ©Mario Goisis 2018. All Rights Reserved)

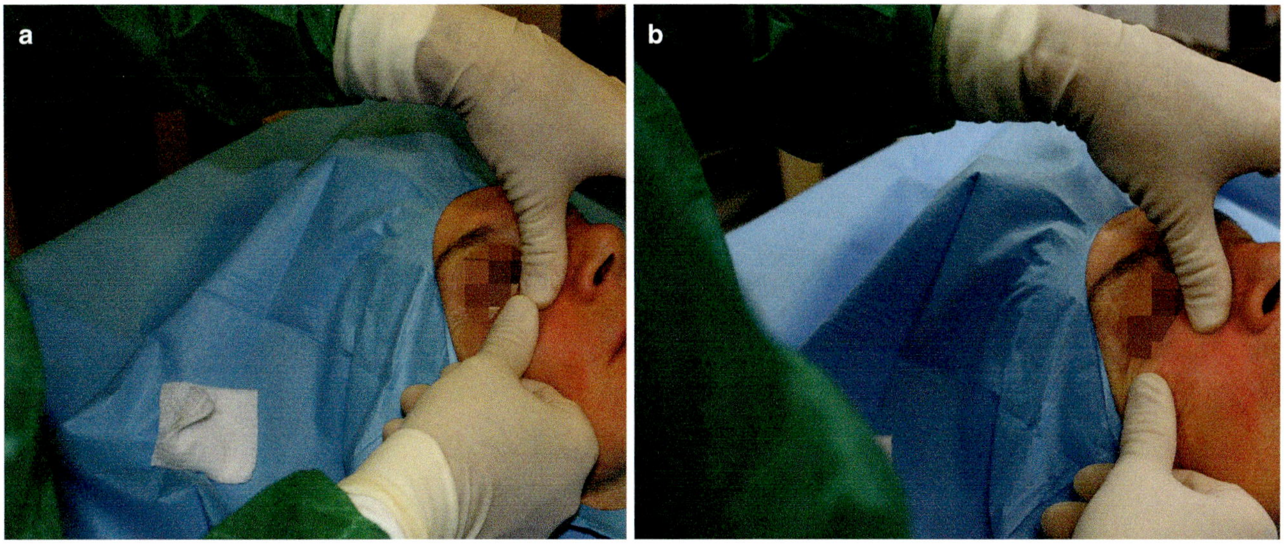

Fig. 14.12 The trough is gently massaged to smooth down lumps and irregularities of the fat graft. (Published with kind permission of ©Mario Goisis 2018. All Rights Reserved)

14.3.7 Cadaver Dissection After Tear Drop Correction with Colored Fat (Courtesy by DE) (Fig. 14.13)

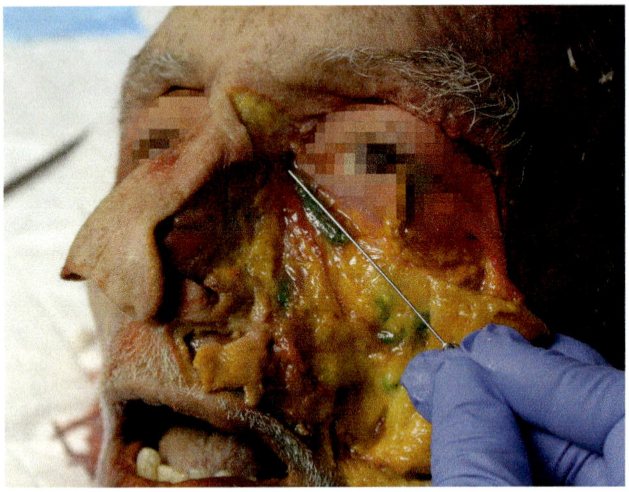

Fig. 14.13 After subcutaneous facial dissection, the colored fat is covered by the subcutaneous layer and by the orbicularis oculi on the inferior eyelid. Turning the orbicularis oculi upward, the cannula shows the colored fat that can be seen under the orbicularis oculi muscle on the periosteal plane (courtesy Doctor's Equipe). (Published with kind permission of ©Mario Goisis 2018. All Rights Reserved)

14.4 Amelioration of Tear Trough Aging and Pigmentation Deformity with Nanofat

14.4.1 Indications

The correction of the tear trough pigmentation

In fact, nanograft and ASCs have a whitening effect via a paracrine mechanism. In particular, tyrosinase activity, which plays a key role in melanin synthesis, was inhibited by ASCs in a dose-dependent manner.

14.4.2 Contraindications

- Anatomical malformations of lacrimal ducts.
- Presence of severe skin laxity or atrophy and large bulgy fat pads will lead to unsatisfactory results.
- Anatomical alterations due to previous trauma or surgical intervention (maxillofacial surgery, titanium plates). Scarring often induces a displacement of the noble structures. It can also induce retracting scars that can cause asymmetry and unequal filling of the part treated.
- No injection should be done if the area has been previously treated with liquid silicone or other permanent fillers because new injection could lead to inflammation or infection of the implants.

14.4.3 Materials

- *0.5–1 cc of nanofat on each side for injection:*
  - *26-gauge needle*
  - *27-gauge 3.7 cm blunt cannula*

A standard system for producing nanofat is used, in particular:

- Nanofat system (www.microfat.com), composed by a connector with a closed system for emulsion of microfat and filtration
- 2 10-cc syringes

For microfat harvesting and processing, a standard system for microfat is used, in particular:

- Microfat box (www.microfat.com), composed by a ramp with a closed a system for washing and filtration
- 4 60-cc syringes
- 2 10-cc syringes
- One 1-cc syringe
- 30-gauge needle
- 16-gauge needle
- A 2-mm-diameter, 10-cm-long Goisis cannula for fat harvesting
- A chlorhexidine-alcohol solution (2% chlorhexidine gluconate and 70% isopropyl alcohol), sterile drapes, or towels
- Ice packs
- Sterile 2 cm for 2 cm gauze squares
- Occlusive dressing cover

Medications include:

- 100 cc of cold saline solution
- 120 cc of cold Klein solution
- One liter of Klein solution is composed by 800 mg of lidocaine, 1 mg of epinephrine, 40 MEq of sodium bicarbonate, and 1000 cc of saline solution

Location: The microfat harvesting can be done in a small/office operating room. The oxygen, pulse oximetry, and a crash cart/box should be present.

Assistants: An assistant is useful to transfer items to the procedure field in a sterile manner in the first part of the procedure. Despite of that, a single doctor can execute all the procedure

14.4.4 Operating Time

Once the microfat has been harvested, the procedure usually takes from 2 to 5 min.

Plane of injection: subcutaneous

14.4.5 Method

Procedure is shown in Figs. 14.14, 14.15, 14.16, 14.17, and 14.18

Plane of injection: Hypodermis

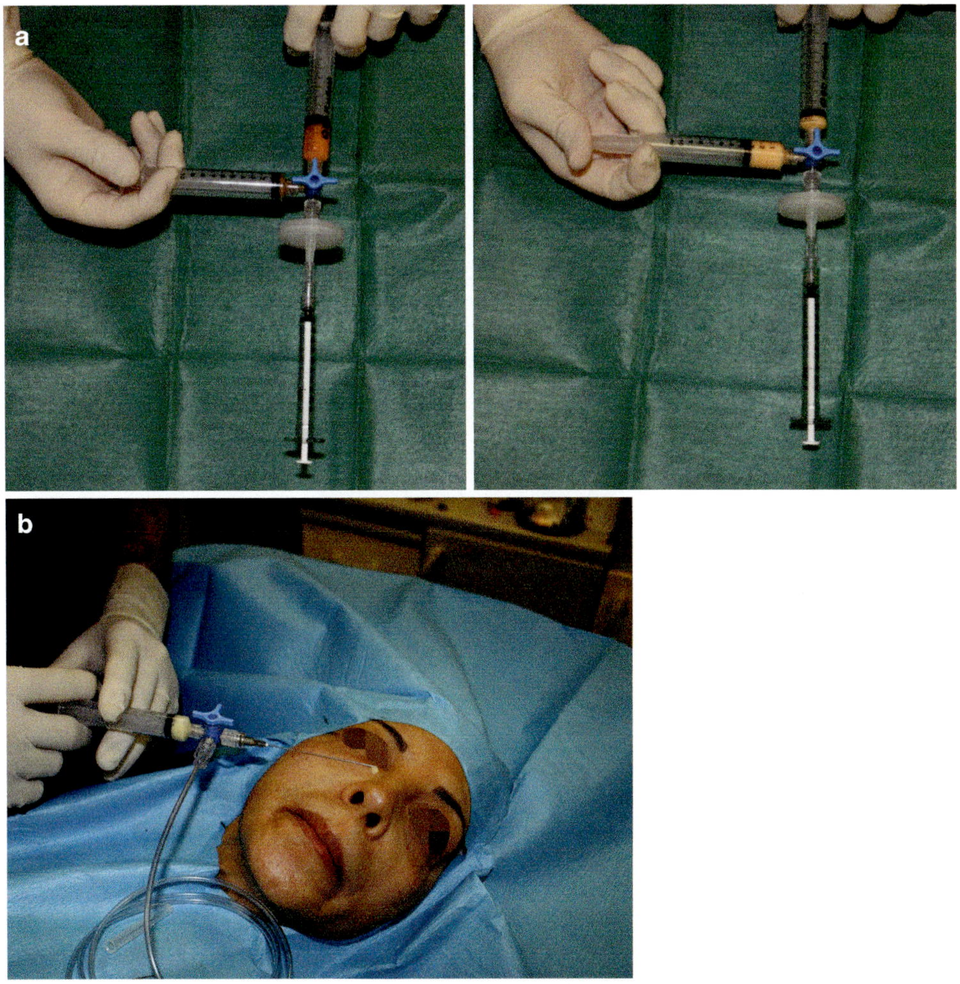

Fig. 14.14 The microfat is transformed in nanofat with nanofat system (www.microfat.com). (Published with kind permission of ©Mario Goisis 2018. All Rights Reserved)

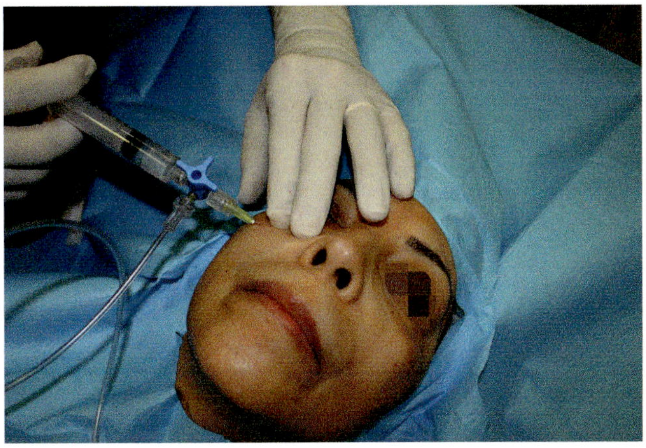

Fig. 14.15 0.2 cc of local anesthetic (Klein solution) can be used. Taking this precaution, the treatment with the blunt-tip cannula will not give any pain to the patient. (Published with kind permission of ©Mario Goisis 2018. All Rights Reserved)

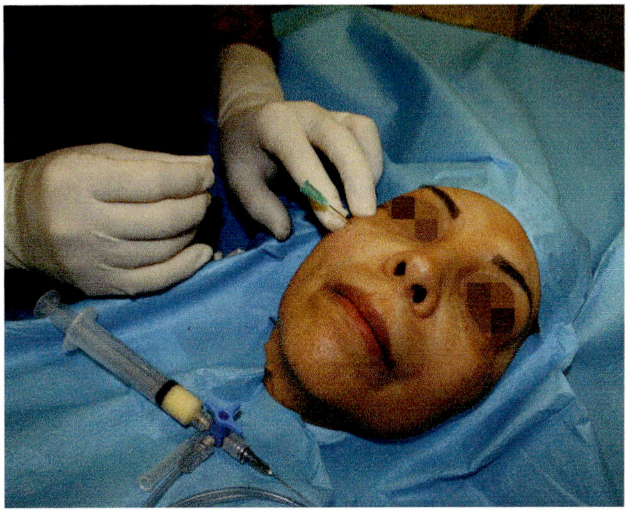

Fig. 14.16 A little hole is created with 26-G needle in the safe entry point. (Published with kind permission of ©Mario Goisis 2018. All Rights Reserved)

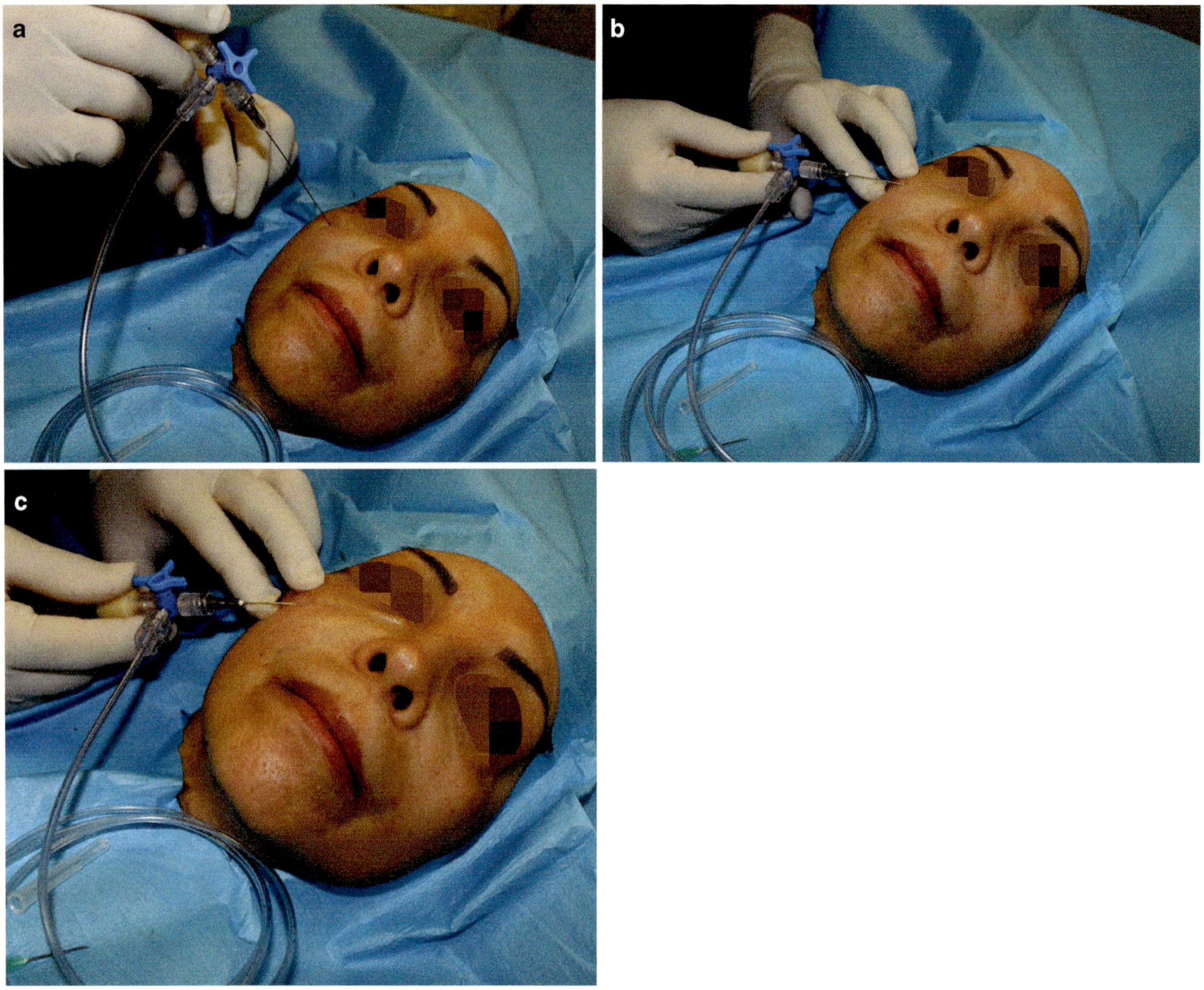

Fig. 14.17 Perpendicular insertion of a 22-G blunt-tip cannula. The cannula is plunged deep into the skin through the orbicular muscle, advancing to the periosteum. (Published with kind permission of ©Mario Goisis 2018. All Rights Reserved)

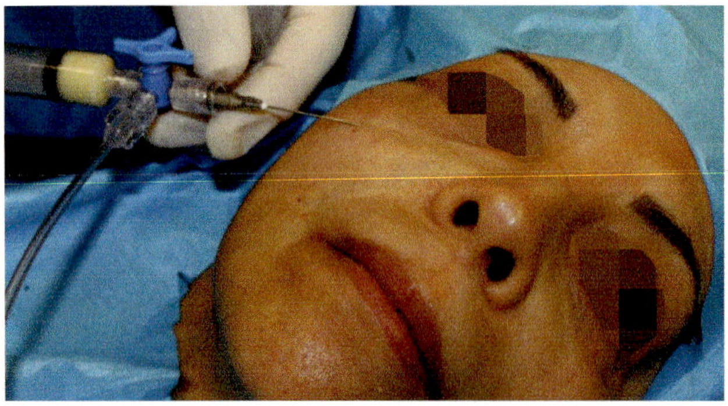

Fig. 14.18 The cannula is then directed diagonally up toward the medial cantus of the eye and made it slide forward to the top of the tear trough. The tip of the cannula is showed through the skin to be just above the lacrimal crest. In fact, the tip of the cannula should be positioned over the lacrimal crest, touching the bone. (Published with kind permission of ©Mario Goisis 2018. All Rights Reserved)

14.4.6 Cadaver Dissection After Tear Drop Correction with Nanofat (Courtesy by DE) (Fig. 14.19)

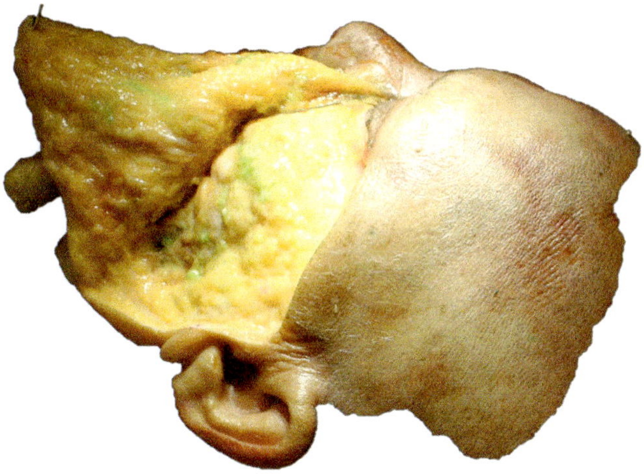

Fig. 14.19 After subcutaneous facial dissection, the colored nanofat is contained into the subcutaneous layer (courtesy Doctor's Equipe). (Published with kind permission of ©Mario Goisis 2018. All Rights Reserved)

14.5 Injection of PRP

14.5.1 Materials

Tubes for PRP preparation, empty and with anticoagulant (www.microfat.com)

- 1–2 cc of PRP on each side
- 1 cc Luer lock syringe
- 27G Blunt-tip cannula
- 25G Entrance needle
- Local anesthetic (lidocaine, mepivacaine) with adrenaline 1:200,000 (equal to 1 mg/40 mL of solution)
- Bandages and antiseptic solution

Plane of injection: Hypodermis

14.5.2 Operating Time

Once the PRP is harvested, the procedure usually takes from 5 to 15 min.

14.5.3 Method (Figs. 14.20, 14.21, 14.22, 14.23, 14.24, 14.25 and 14.26)

Pre- and post-treatment with nanofat is shown in (Figs. 14.27 and 14.28)

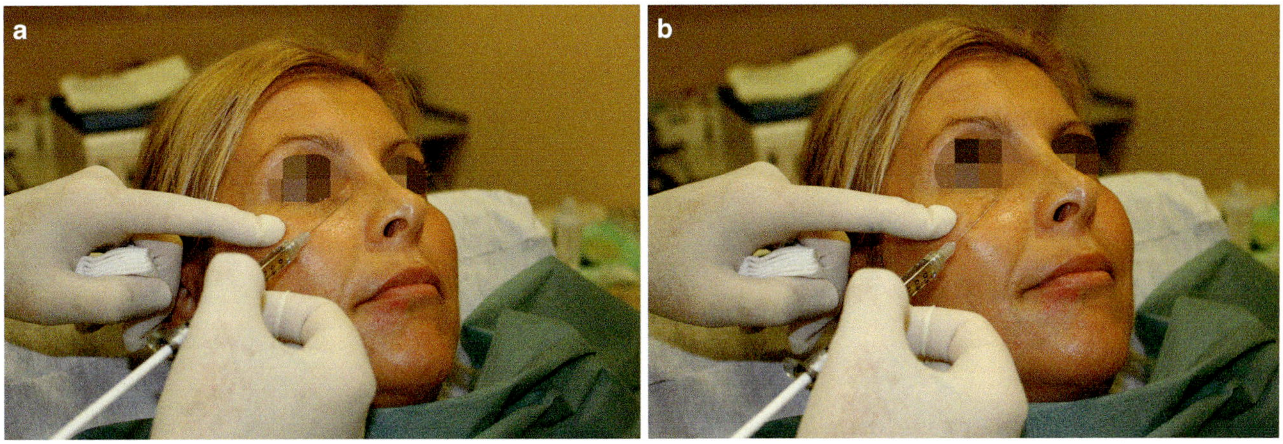

Fig. 14.20 Route of the cannula. (Published with kind permission of ©Mario Goisis 2018. All Rights Reserved)

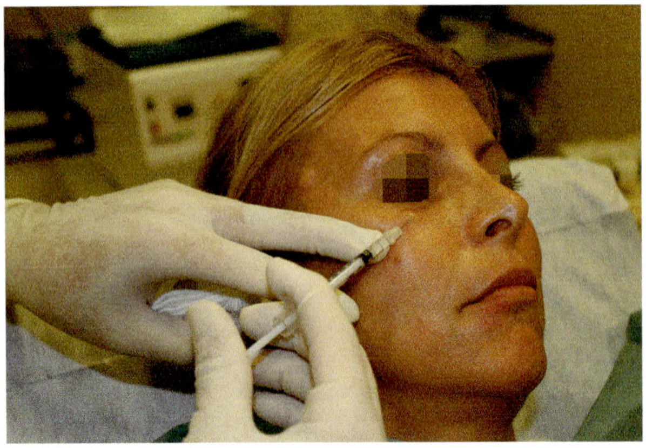

Fig. 14.21 Local anesthetic (lidocaine, mepivacaine) with adrenaline 1:200,000 (equal to 1 mg/40 mL of solution) can be used. Taking this precaution, the treatment with the blunt-tip cannula will not give any pain to the patient. (Published with kind permission of ©Mario Goisis 2018. All Rights Reserved)

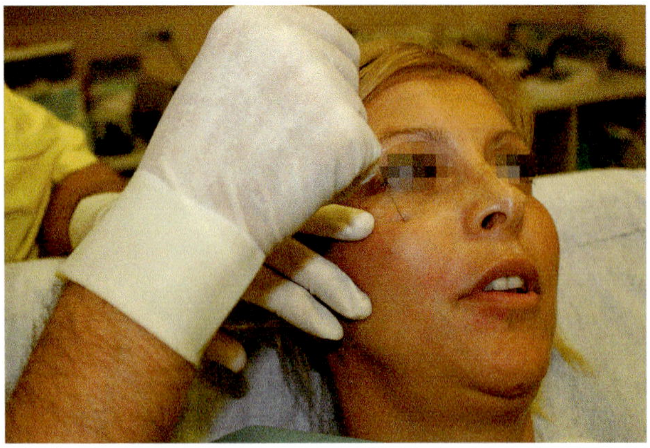

Fig. 14.23 Perpendicular insertion of a 27-G blunt-tip cannula. The cannula is advanced in subcutaneous plane superficial to the orbicularis muscle. (Published with kind permission of ©Mario Goisis 2018. All Rights Reserved)

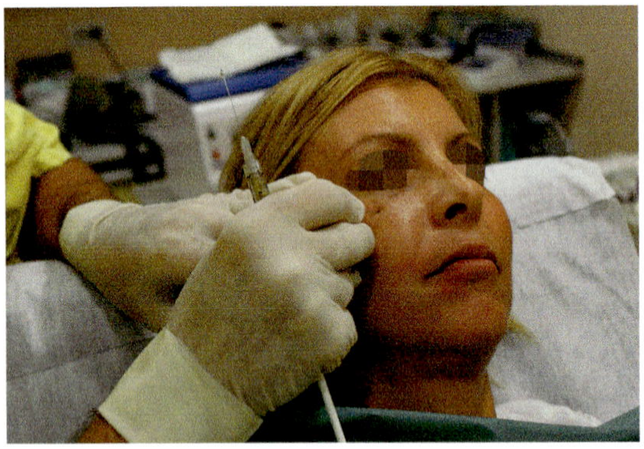

Fig. 14.22 A little hole is created with 25-G needle in the safe entry point. (Published with kind permission of ©Mario Goisis 2018. All Rights Reserved)

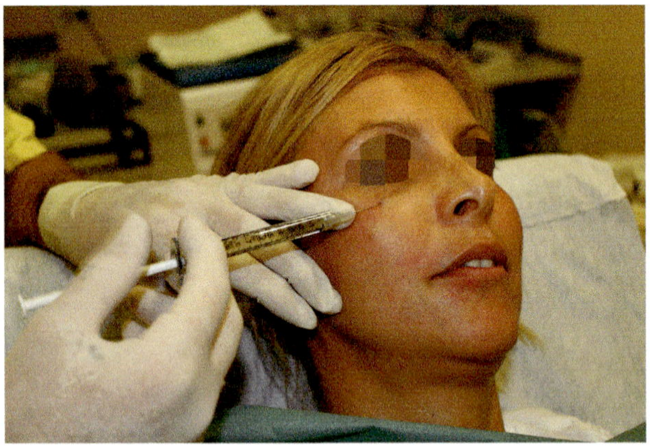

Fig. 14.24 The cannula is then directed diagonally up toward the medial cantus of the eye and made it slide forward to the top of the tear trough. The tip of the cannula is showed through the skin to be just above the lacrimal crest. In fact, the tip of the cannula should be positioned over the lacrimal crest, touching the bone. (Published with kind permission of ©Mario Goisis 2018. All Rights Reserved)

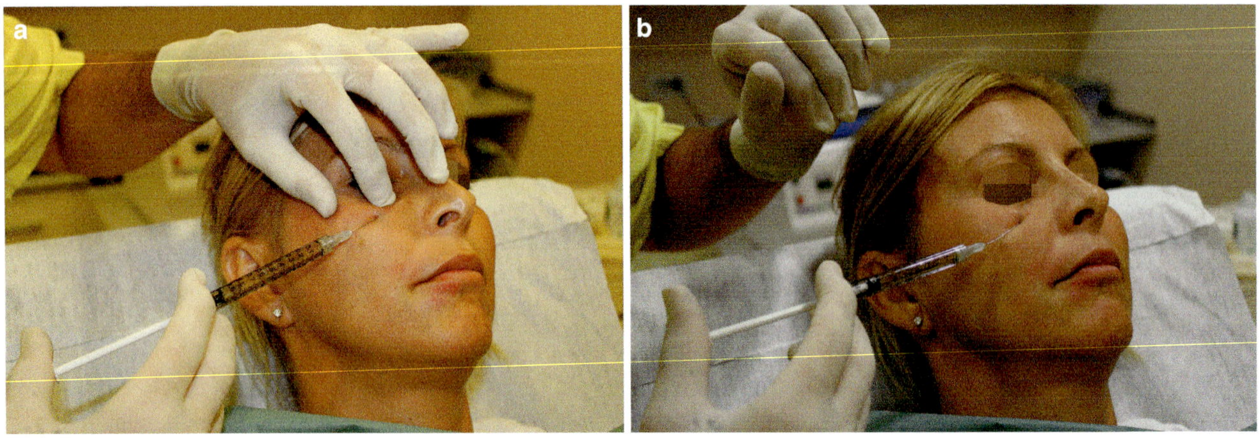

Fig. 14.25 0.1–0.5 cc of PRP is injected with a retrograde technique along the dip. (Published with kind permission of ©Mario Goisis 2018. All Rights Reserved)

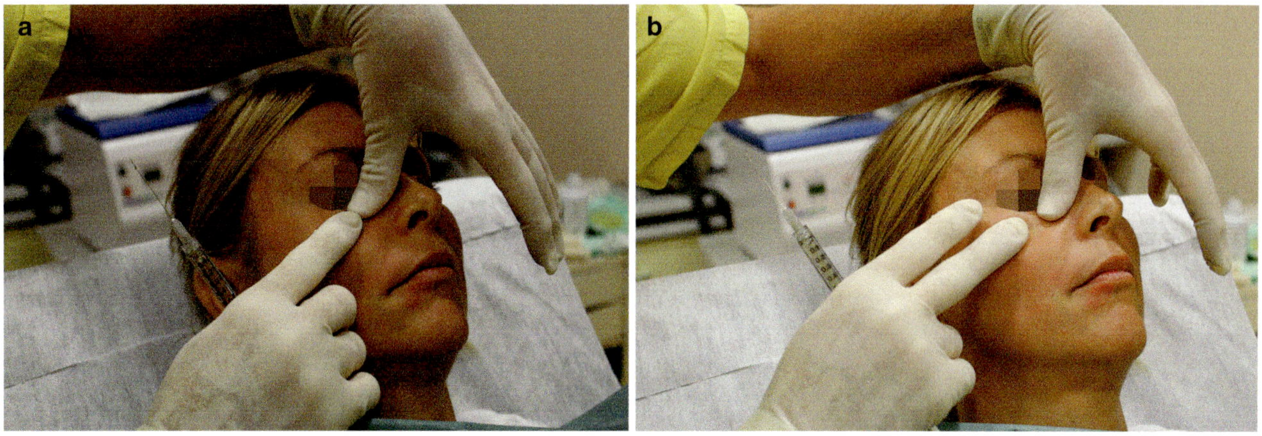

Fig. 14.26 The trough is gently massaged (Published with kind permission of ©Mario Goisis 2018. All Rights Reserved)

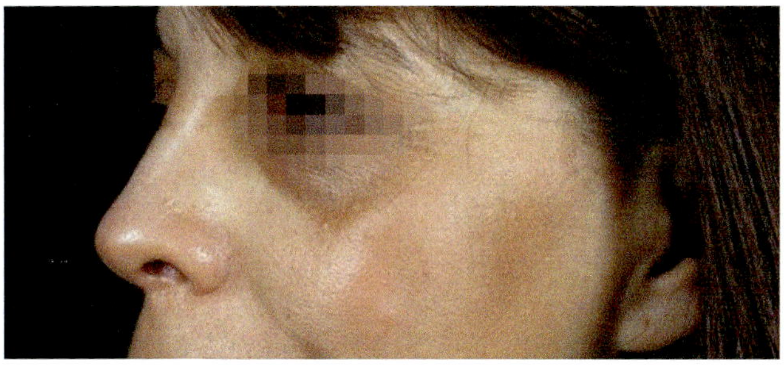

Fig. 14.27 Pretreatment with nanofat (courtesy by DE). (Published with kind permission of ©Mario Goisis 2018. All Rights Reserved)

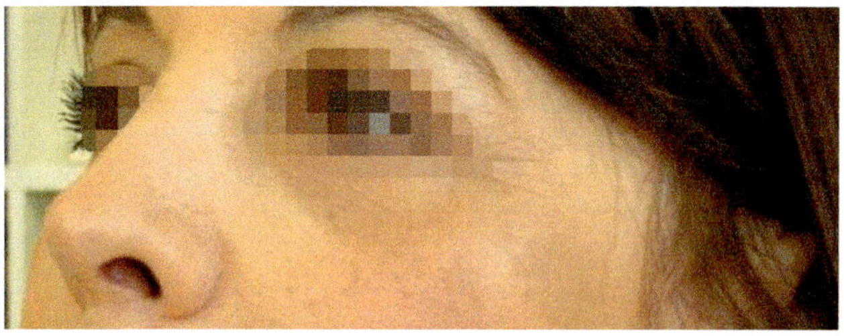

Fig. 14.28 Post-treatment with nanofat (courtesy by DE). (Published with kind permission of ©Mario Goisis 2018. All Rights Reserved)

Nasolabial Folds

15

Rand S. Al Yahya and Mario Goisis

Nasolabial folds give the face tired and sagging appearance (Fig. 15.1).

15.1 Anatomy

Nasolabial folds are creases that separate the upper lip from the cheeks and extend from the sides of the nose to the corners of the mouth. Figures 15.2 and 15.3 are anatomical images to show the muscular plane of the nasolabial folds. The facial artery, together with the anterior facial vein, crosses the inferior mandibular border just anteriorly to the masseter muscle. The vessels continue in superiorly and anteriorly lying just superficially to the buccinator muscle (Fig. 15.4).

15.2 Correction of Nasolabial Folds with Micrograft

15.2.1 Indications

Moderate, severe, and very severe nasolabial folds.

15.2.2 Contraindications

Attention should be paid if the area had been previously treated with permanent fillers. The filler should not be injected in areas that lack sufficient blood supply or affected by infection or inflammation.

R. S. Al Yahya
Prince Sattam Bin Abdulaziz University, Al Kharj, Saudi Arabia

M. Goisis (✉)
Maxillo-Facial and Aesthetic Surgeon, Go Easy Clinic, Milan, Italy

15.2.3 Materials

- *2–4 cc of microfat on each side for injection of the microfat:*
  - *21-gauge needle*
  - *22-gauge 4 cm blunt cannula*

For microfat harvesting and processing:
A standard system for microfat is used, in particular:

- Microfat box (www.microfat.com), composed of a ramp with a closed system for washing and filtration
- Four 60 cc syringes
- Two 10 cc syringes
- One 1 cc syringe
- 30-gauge needle
- -16-gauge needle
- A 2-mm-diameter, 10-cm-long Goisis cannula for fat harvesting
- A chlorhexidine-alcohol solution (2% chlorhexidine gluconate and 70% isopropyl alcohol), sterile drapes or towels
- Ice packs
- Sterile 2 × 2-cm gauze squares
- Occlusive dressing cover

Medications include:

100 cc of cold saline solution.
120 cc of cold Klein solution.
One liter of Klein solution is composed of 800 mg of lidocaine, 1 mg of epinephrine, 40 MEq of sodium bicarbonate, and 1000 cc of saline solution.

Location: The microfat harvesting can be done in a small/office operating room. The oxygen, pulse oximetry, and a crash cart/box should be present.

M. Goisis (ed.), *Outpatient Regenerative Medicine*, https://doi.org/10.1007/978-3-319-44894-7_15

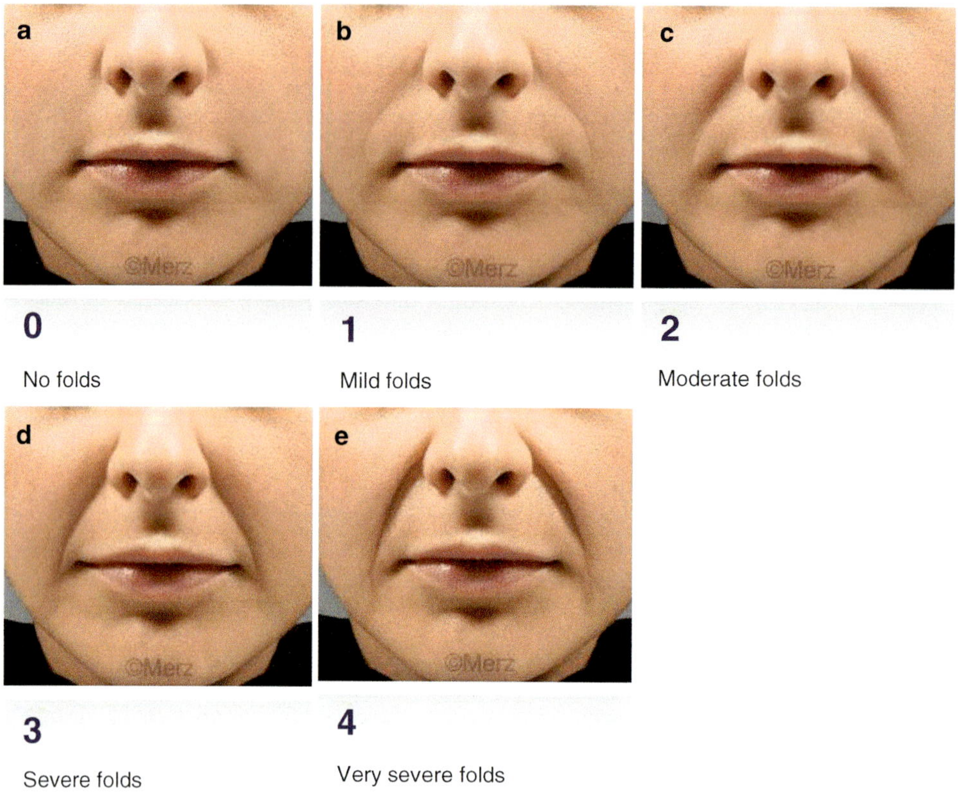

Fig. 15.1 Graduation of nasolabial folds from absent to very severe. (Published by kind permission of ©Mario Goisis 2018. All Rights Reserved)

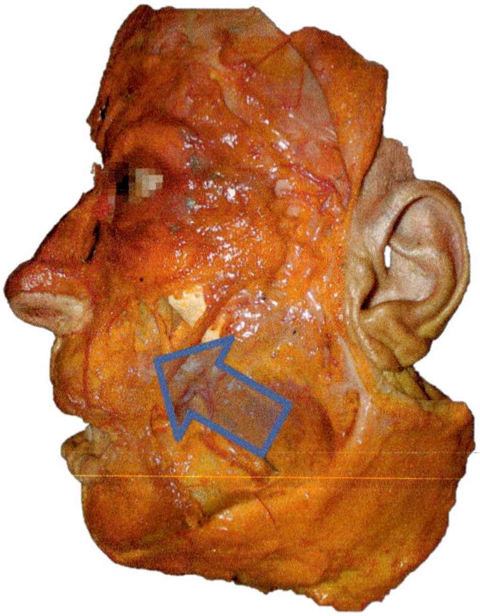

Fig. 15.2 Anatomical dissections of the levator anguli oris (caninus) muscle (blue arrow). It arises from the canine fossa, immediately below the infraorbital foramen, and inserts into the angle of the mouth, intermingling with the zygomaticus major and orbicularis oris muscle(Published with kind permission of ©Mario Goisis 2018. All Rights Reserved)

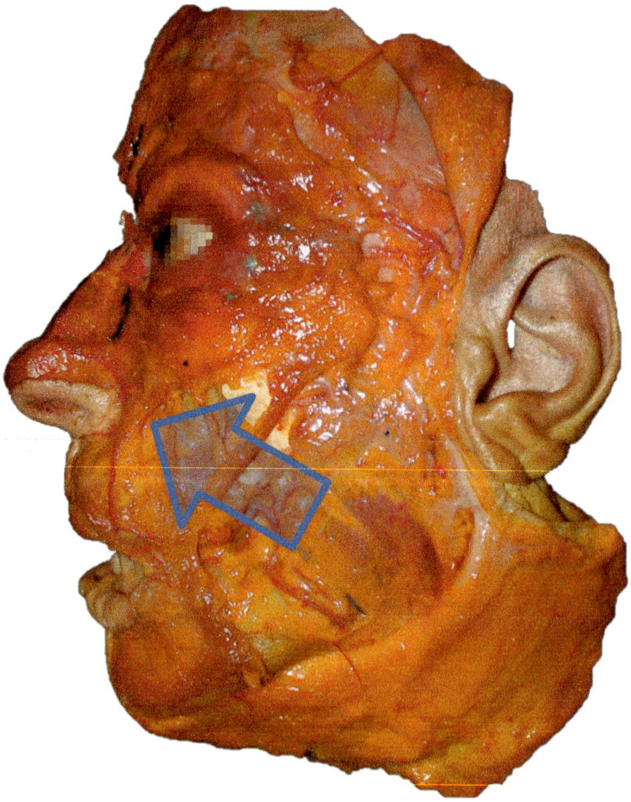

Fig. 15.3 Anatomical dissections of the *levator labii superioris (also described as the* intermediate portion of the *levator labii superioris* or *quadratus labii superioris). It* arises from the lower margin of the orbit immediately in correspondence of the maxilla and zygomatic bone (blue arrow). (Published with kind permission of ©Mario Goisis 2018. All Rights Reserved)

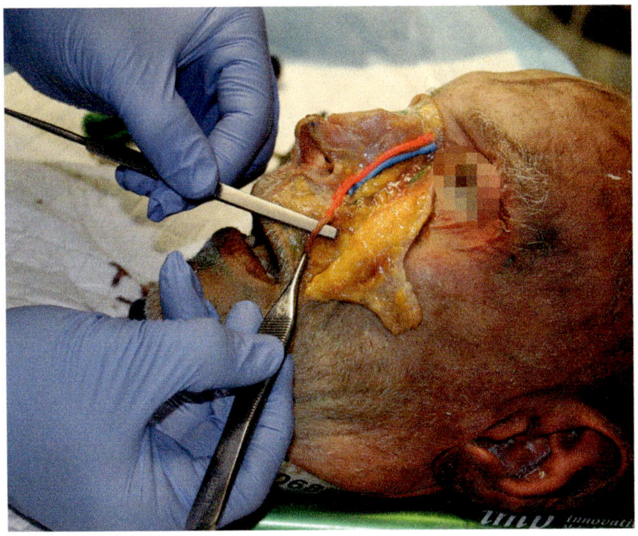

Fig. 15.4 The facial artery and vien. (courtesy by Doctor's Equipe). (Published with kind permission of ©Mario Goisis 2018. All Rights Reserved)

Assistants: An assistant is useful to transfer items to the procedure field in a sterile manner in the first part of the procedure. Despite that, a single doctor can execute all the procedure.

15.2.4 Complications and Management

Immediate complications (within 72 h after injection) include transient erythema, edema, induration, pruritus, and ecchymosis.

Early complications (days to weeks after injection) include overcorrection, local infection, skin necrosis, herpes reactivation, discoloration, and persistent local symptoms (erythema, edema, induration, pruritus, and hyperpigmentation).

Late complications include high rate of fat resorption and cyst.

Plane of injection: SMAS

15.2.5 Operating Time

Once the fat is harvested, the procedure usually takes from 5 to 15 min.

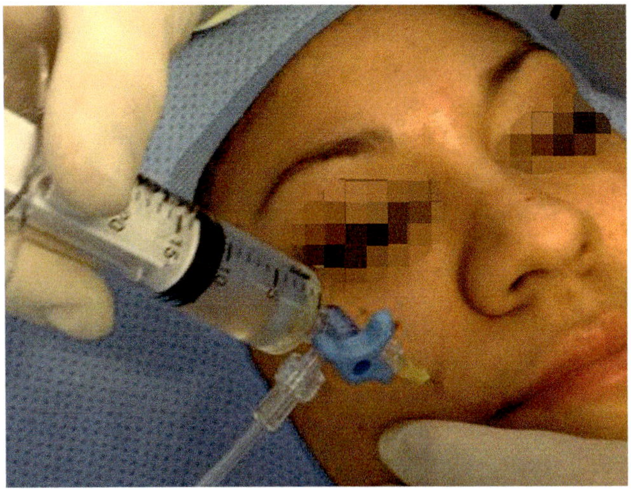

Fig. 15.5 Anesthesia is performed in the entrance point at the base of the nasolabial fold with 0.2 cc of local Klein solution. (Published with kind permission of ©Mario Goisis 2018. All Rights Reserved)

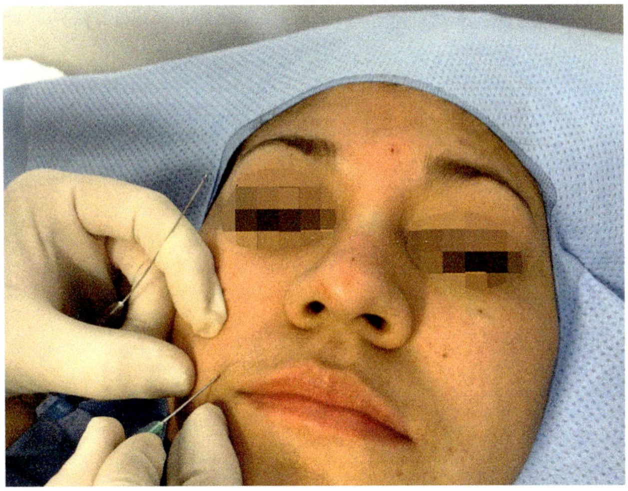

Fig. 15.6 An opening is created with a 21-G needle at the base of the nasolabial fold. (Published with kind permission of ©Mario Goisis 2018. All Rights Reserved)

15.2.6 Method

Procedure is shown in Fig. 15.5, 15.6, 15.7, 15.8, 15.9, and 15.10.

The fat is delivered slowly, while the cannula is withdrawn with retrograde injection (Figs. 15.9, 15.10, 15.11, 15.12, 15.13, 15.14, 15.15, 15.16, 15.17, 15.18, and 15.19).

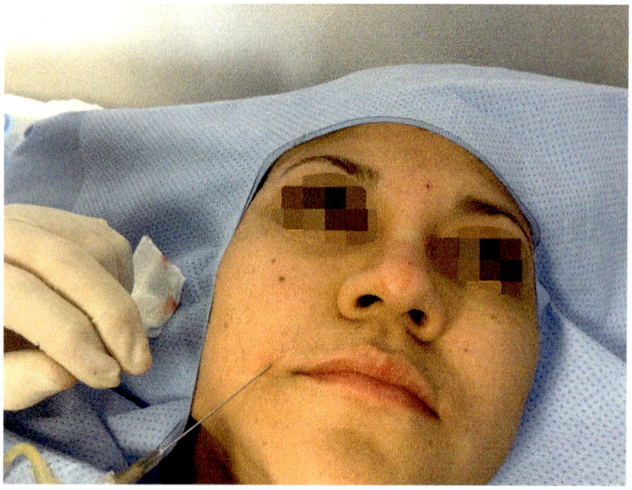

Fig. 15.7 A 22-G blunt-tip cannula is inserted perpendicularly to skin surface, and the cannula is then pivoted parallel to the skin plane into the muscular plane and slid toward the top of the nasolabial fold. (Published with kind permission of ©Mario Goisis 2018. All Rights Reserved)

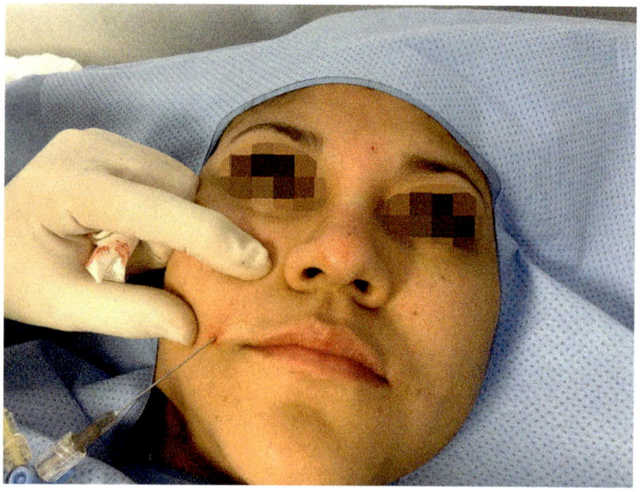

Fig. 15.8 The cannula crosses the lip levators under the nasolabial fold and thus helps with correction of nasolabial contours. In particular, the fat is injected into the levator labii superioris and levator anguli oris (caninus). The fat is delivered slowly, while the cannula is withdrawn with retrograde injection. (Published with kind permission of ©Mario Goisis 2018. All Rights Reserved)

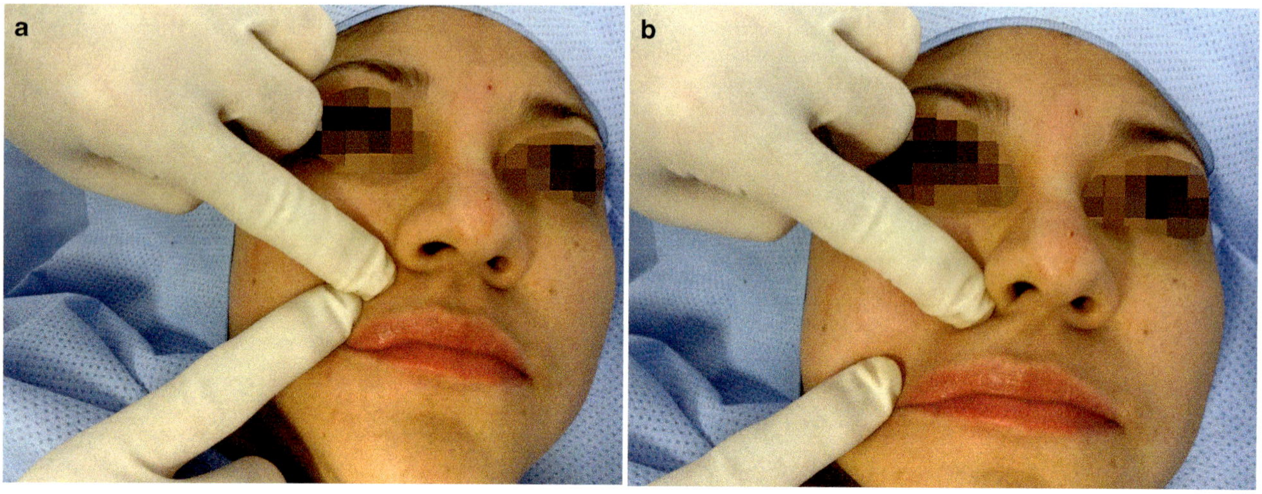

Fig. 15.9 (**a**, **b**) At the end of the treatment, a massage is applied over the area injected. (Published with kind permission of ©Mario Goisis 2018. All Rights Reserved)

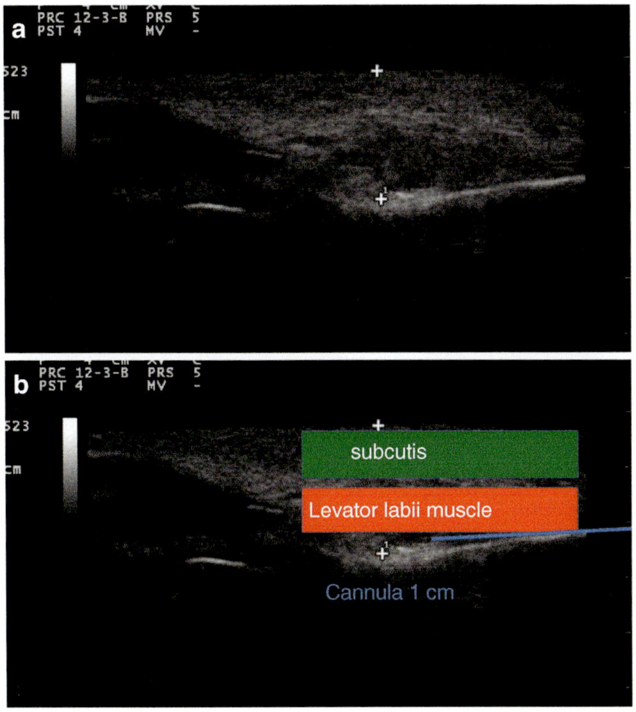

Fig. 15.10 (**a**, **b**) Ultrasound demonstration of the procedure: the cannula is inserted into the muscular plane. The deep of the cannula is 10 mm. In particular, the fat is injected into the levator labii superioris and levator anguli oris (caninus). (Published with kind permission of ©Mario Goisis 2018. All Rights Reserved)

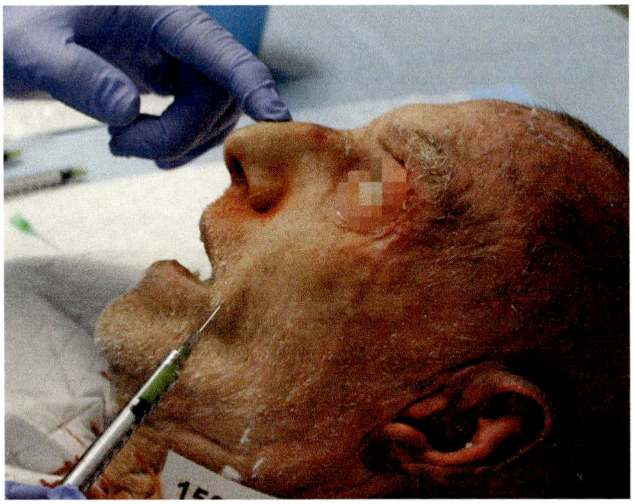

Fig. 15.11 The cannula crosses the lip levators under the nasolabial fold and thus helps with correction of nasolabial contours. In particular, the fat is injected into the levator labii superioris and levator anguli oris (caninus). The fat is delivered slowly, while the cannula is withdrawn with retrograde injection (courtesy by Doctor's Equipe). (Published with kind permission of ©Mario Goisis 2018. All Rights Reserved)

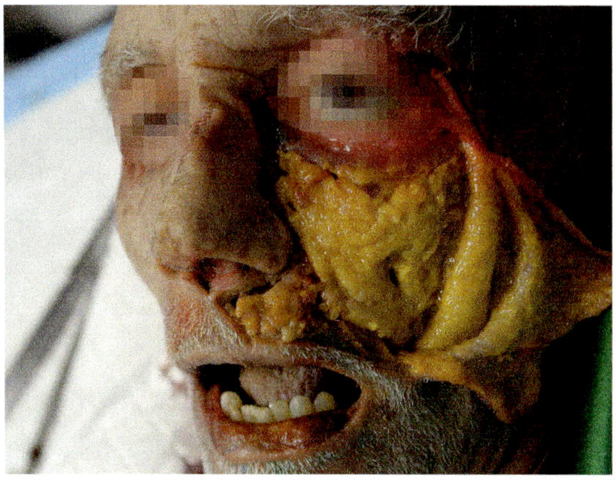

Fig. 15.12 After fat injection, midfacial dissection is executed starting from a subciliary incision of the lower lid which continues at the internal cantus inferiorly in a paranasal route to the labial filter until the vermilion border and all along it. Subcutaneous plane is exposed. No evidence of fat is shown in the subcutaneous plane (courtesy by Doctor's Equipe). (Published with kind permission of ©Mario Goisis 2018. All Rights Reserved)

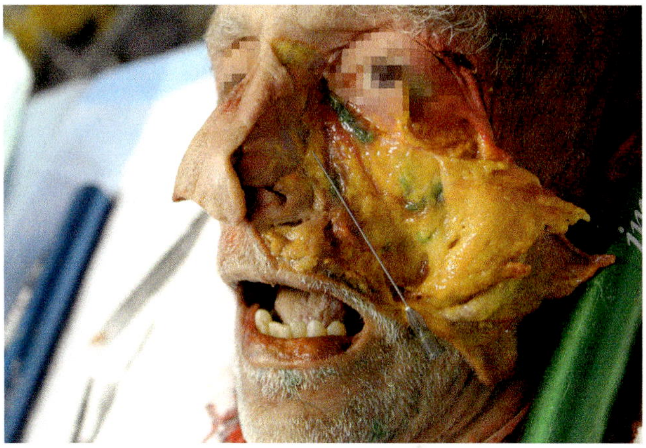

Fig. 15.13 Anatomical demonstration of the muscular plane of injection: the levator labii superioris and levator anguli oris (caninus) (courtesy by Doctor's Equipe). (Published with kind permission of ©Mario Goisis 2018. All Rights Reserved)

15.2.7 Cadaver Dissection After Microfat Injection of Nasolabial Folds (Figs. 15.11, 15.12, and 15.13)

15.3 Amelioration of Nasolabial Folds with Nanofat

15.3.1 Indications

Mild nasolabial folds.

15.3.2 Contraindications

Attention should be paid if the area had been previously treated with permanent fillers. The filler should not be injected in areas that lack sufficient blood supply or affected by infection or inflammation.

15.3.3 Materials

- *1–2 cc of nanofat on each side for injection of nanofat:*
  - *26-gauge needle*
  - *27-gauge 3.7 cm blunt cannula*

A standard system for producing nanofat is used, in particular:

- Nanofat system (www.microfat.com), composed of a connector with a closed system for emulsion of microfat and filtration
- Two 10 cc syringes

For microfat harvesting and processing:

A standard system for microfat is used, in particular:

- Microfat box (www.microfat.com), composed of a ramp with a closed system for washing and filtration
- Four 60 cc syringes
- Two 10 cc syringes
- One 1 cc syringe
- 30-gauge needle
- 16-gauge needle
- A 2-mm-diameter, 10-cm-long Goisis cannula for fat harvesting
- A chlorhexidine-alcohol solution (2% chlorhexidine gluconate and 70% isopropyl alcohol), sterile drapes or towels
- Ice packs
- Sterile 2 cm for 2-cm gauze squares
- Occlusive dressing cover

Medications include:

100 cc of cold saline solution.
120 cc of cold Klein Solution.
One liter of Klein solution is composed of 800 mg of lidocaine, 1 mg of epinephrine, 40 MEq of sodium bicarbonate, and 1000 cc of saline solution.

Location: The microfat harvesting can be done in a small/office operating room. The oxygen, pulse oximetry, and a crash cart/box should be present.

Assistants: An assistant is useful to transfer items to the procedure field in a sterile manner in the first part of the procedure. Despite that, a single doctor can execute all the procedure

Plane of injection: Hypodermis and dermis

15.3.4 Operating Time

Once the microfat is harvested, the procedure usually takes from 5 to 15 min.

15.3.5 Method

Procedure is shown in Figs. 15.14, 15.15, 15.16, 15.17, 15.18, 15.19, and 15.20.

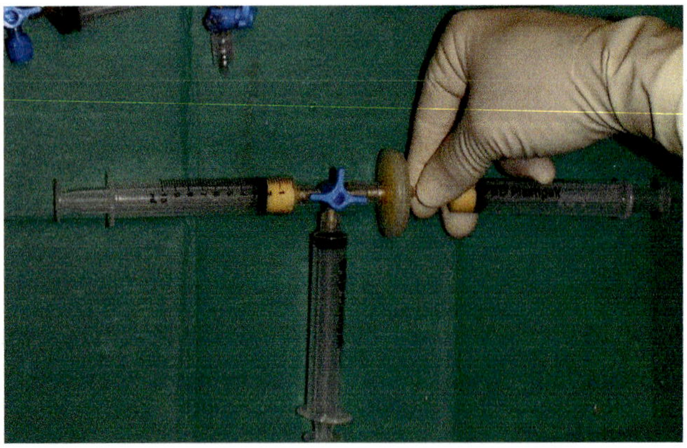

Fig. 15.14 The nanofat is produced with the nanofat kit (www.nanofat.com). (Published with kind permission of ©Mario Goisis 2018. All Rights Reserved)

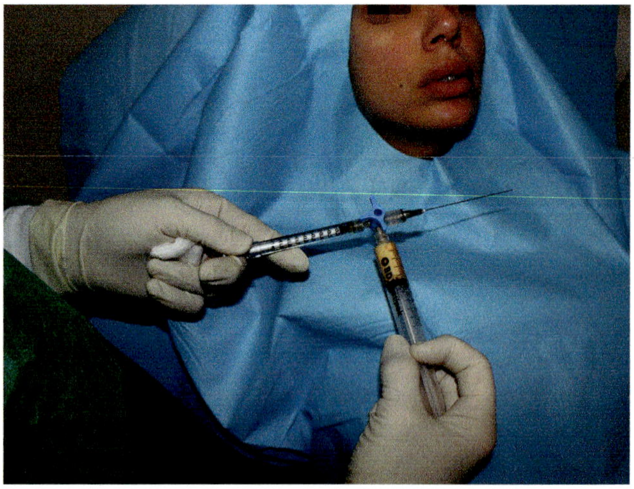

Fig. 15.15 A 10-cc syringe is filled with nanofat and is connected with a 1-cc syringe. (Published with kind permission of ©Mario Goisis 2018. All Rights Reserved)

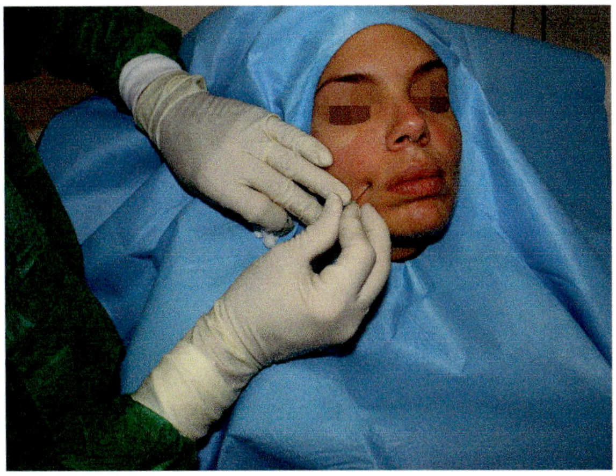

Fig. 15.16 An opening is created with 26-G needle at the base of the nasolabial fold. (Published with kind permission of ©Mario Goisis 2018. All Rights Reserved)

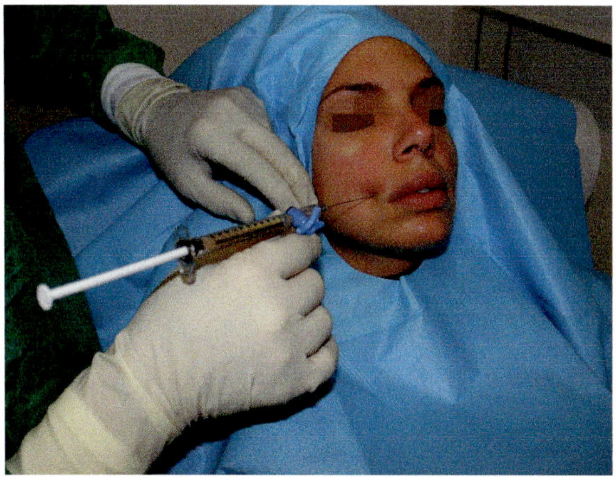

Fig. 15.17 A 27-G blunt-tip cannula is inserted perpendicularly to skin surface. (Published with kind permission of ©Mario Goisis 2018. All Rights Reserved)

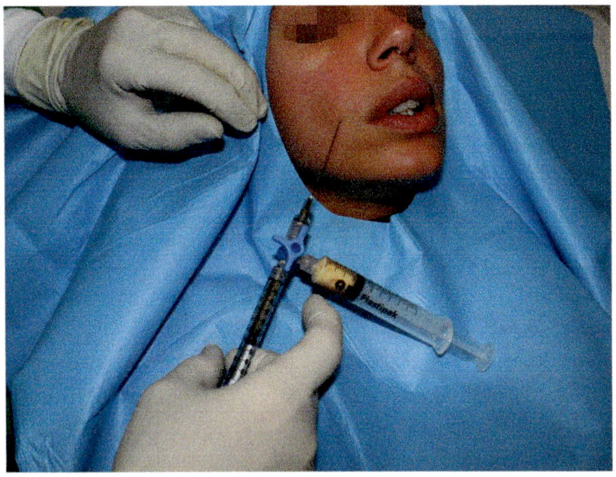

Fig. 15.18 The cannula is then pivoted parallel to the skin plane and slid toward the top of the nasolabial fold. (Published with kind permission of ©Mario Goisis 2018. All Rights Reserved)

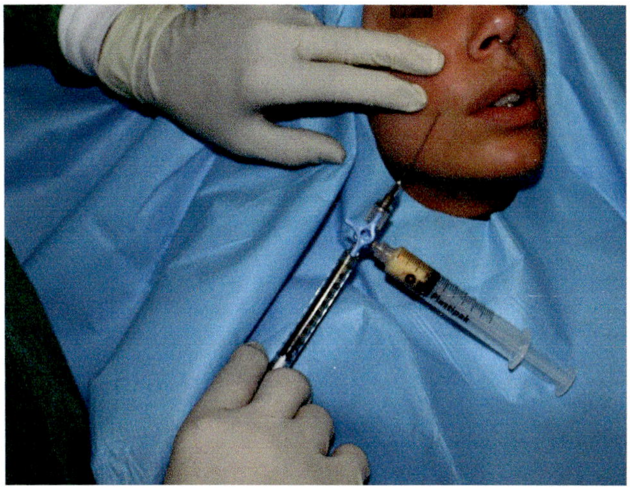

Fig. 15.19 The nanofat is delivered slowly, while the cannula is withdrawn with retrograde injection. (Published with kind permission of ©Mario Goisis 2018. All Rights Reserved)

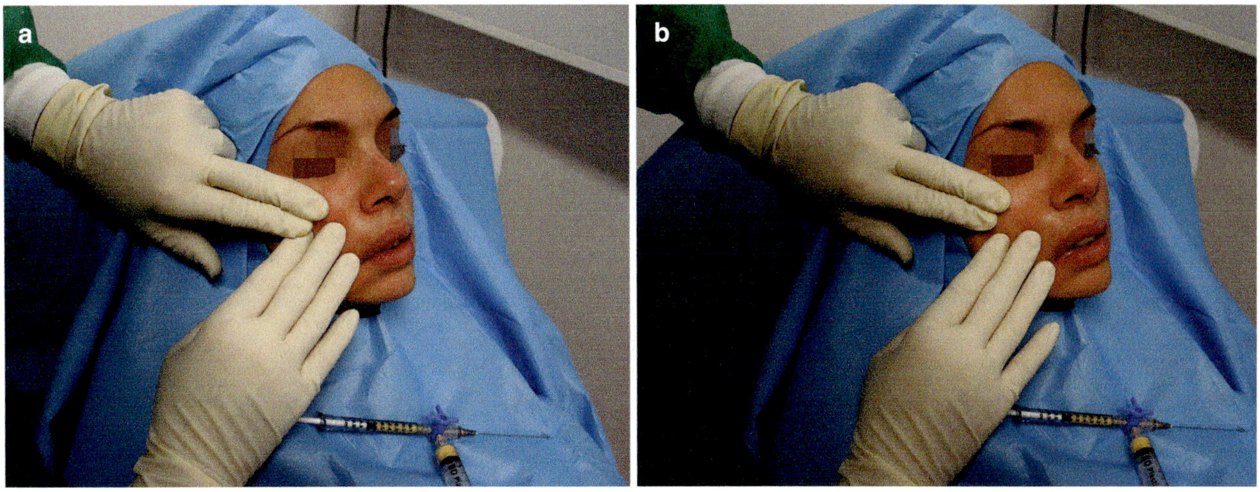

Fig. 15.20 (a, b) At the end of the treatment, massage is applied over the area. (Published with kind permission of ©Mario Goisis 2018. All Rights Reserved)

15.4 Amelioration of Nasolabial Folds with PRP

15.4.1 Indications

Mild nasolabial folds.

15.4.2 Contraindications

Attention should be paid if the area had been previously treated with permanent fillers. The filler should not be injected in areas that lack sufficient blood supply or affected by infection or inflammation.

15.4.3 Materials

Bandages and antiseptic solution

0.2 cc of local anesthetic (2% lidocaine or 2% mepivacaine) with epinephrine 1:100000

1 cc Luer lock syringe

26-G needle

27-G blunt cannula

Tubes for PRP preparation, empty and with anticoagulant (www.microfat.com)

1–2 cc of PRP

Plane of injection: Hypodermis

15.4.4 Operating Time

Once the PRP is produced, the procedure usually takes from 5 to 15 min.

15.4.5 Method

Procedure is shown in Figs. 15.21, 15.22, 15.23, 15.24, 15.25, and 15.26

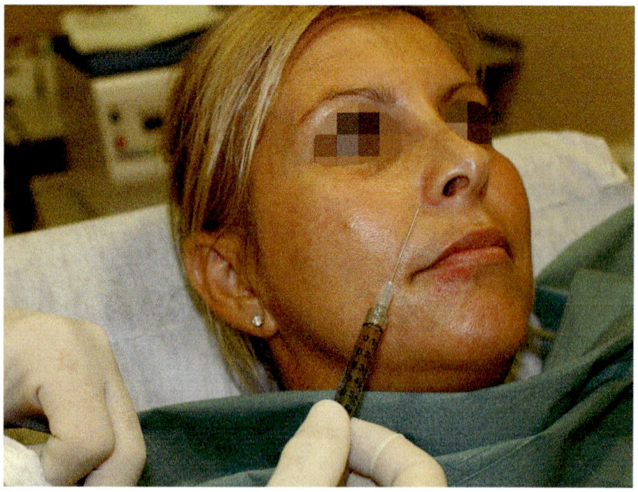

Fig. 15.21 Nasolabial folds are treated using a single entry point located 1.5–2 cm laterally to the oral rim. (Published with kind permission of ©Mario Goisis 2018. All Rights Reserved)

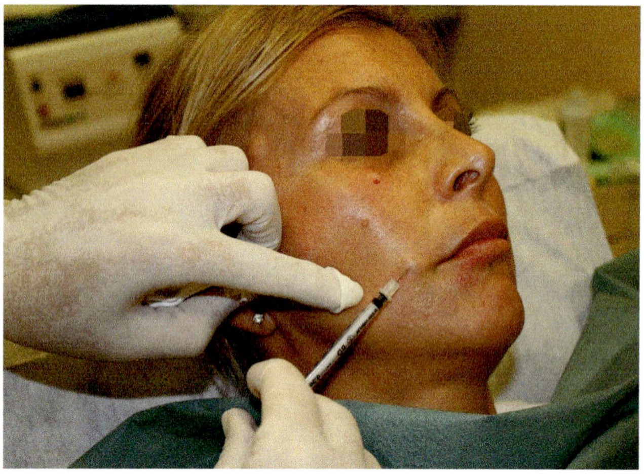

Fig. 15.22 Anesthesia is performed in the entrance point at the base of the nasolabial fold with 0.2 cc of local anesthetic (lidocaine, mepivacaine) with adrenaline. (Published with kind permission of ©Mario Goisis 2018. All Rights Reserved)

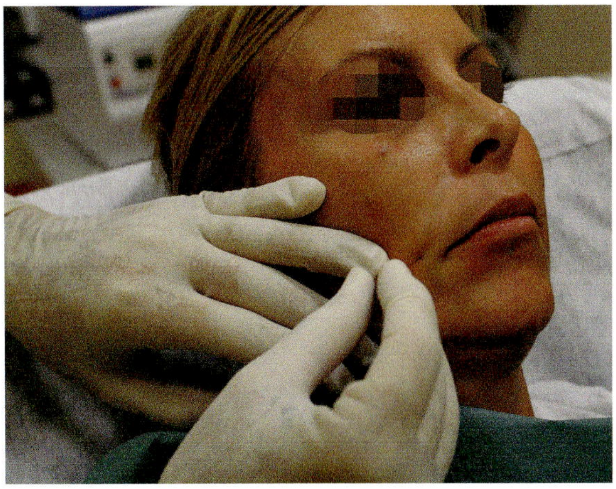

Fig. 15.23 An opening is created with a 25-G needle. A 27-G, blunt-tip cannula is inserted perpendicularly to the skin surface through the hole created. (Published with kind permission of ©Mario Goisis 2018. All Rights Reserved)

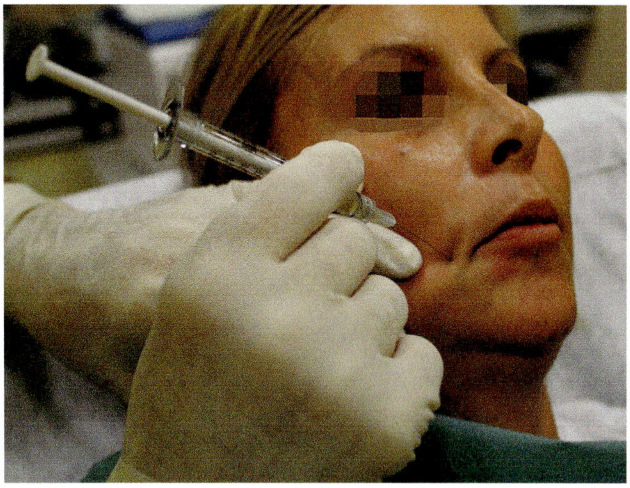

Fig. 15.24 The cannula is then pivoted parallel to the skin plane and slid toward the top of the nasolabial fold. (Published with kind permission of ©Mario Goisis 2018. All Rights Reserved)

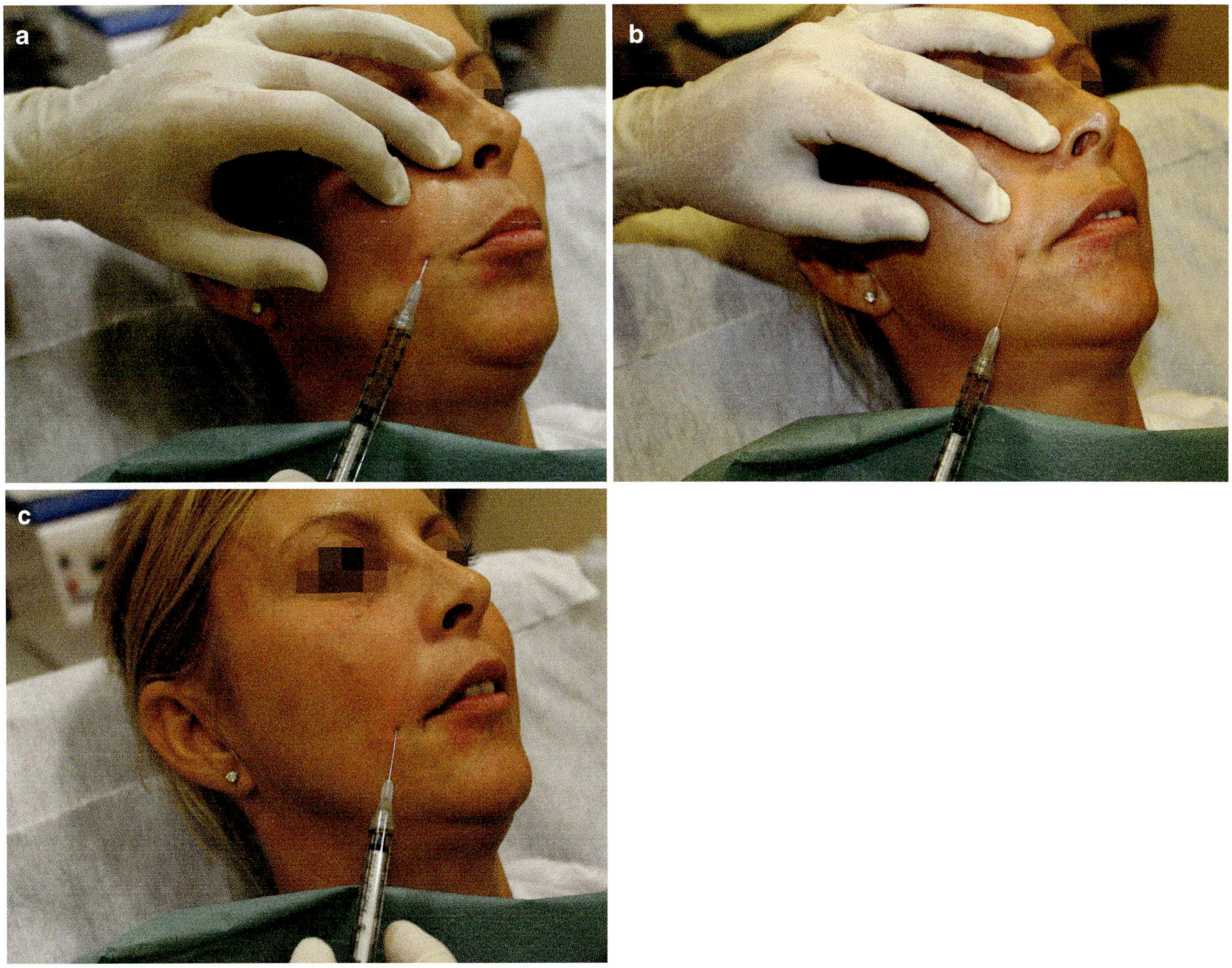

Fig. 15.25 (**a**–**c**) The PRP is delivered slowly, while the cannula is withdrawn with retrograde injection. (Published with kind permission of ©Mario Goisis 2018. All Rights Reserved)

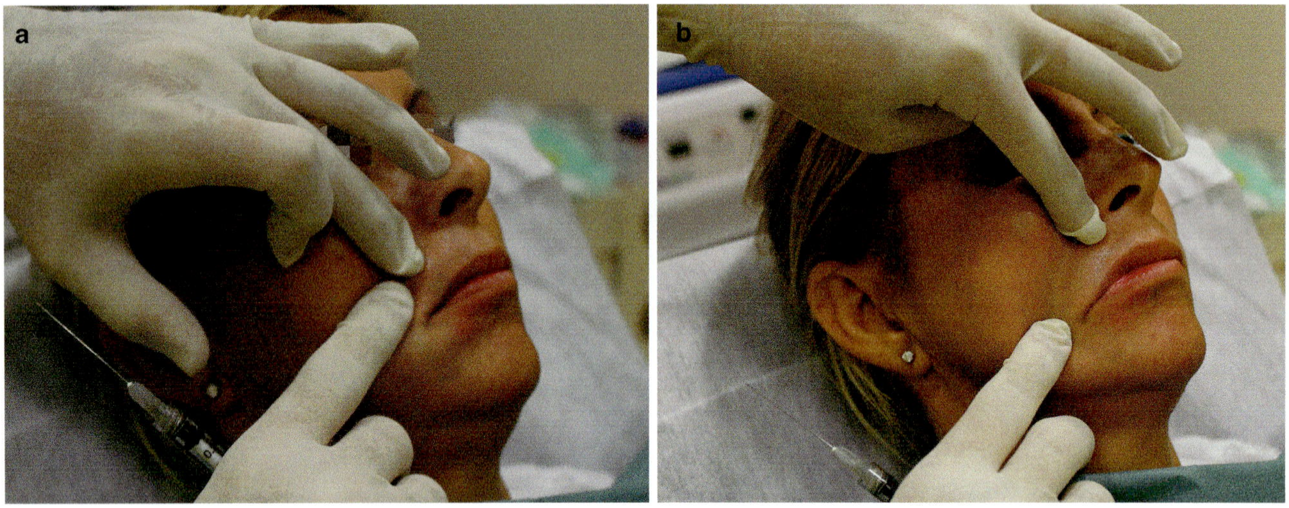

Fig. 15.26 (**a**, **b**) At the end of the treatment, a massage is applied over the area. (Published with kind permission of ©Mario Goisis 2018. All Rights Reserved)

Medical Microfat Rhinoplasty

16

Sara Izzo, Mario Goisis, Lorenzo Rosset, Giuseppe A. Ferraro, and Giovanni Francesco Nicoletti

16.1 Anatomy

The nose dominates the middle third of the face. In the upper region of the nose, the nasal bones are attached to the frontal bone. Above and to the side (superolaterally), the paired nasal bones are connected to the lacrimal bones, and below and to the side (inferolaterally), they attach they join to the ascending processes of the maxilla bones (Figs. 16.1, 16.2, 16.3, 16.4, 16.5, 16.6, 16.7, 16.8, 16.9, 16.10, 16.11, 16.12, and 16.13).

16.2 Pitfalls

By filling it with fat, the nasal dorsum permits modification of the nasofrontal angle and models the dorsum itself slightly. This procedure is performed by injecting the fat very slowly in order to prevent arteries compression and ischemic injury.

Before injecting, the profile of the patient's nose is carefully evaluated, paying attention to the nasofrontal and nasolabial angles; the right dimensions should be the following:

- The nasofrontal angle: between 115 and 135 degrees
- The dorsal angle, normally straight
- The nasolabial angle, between 90 and 110 degrees

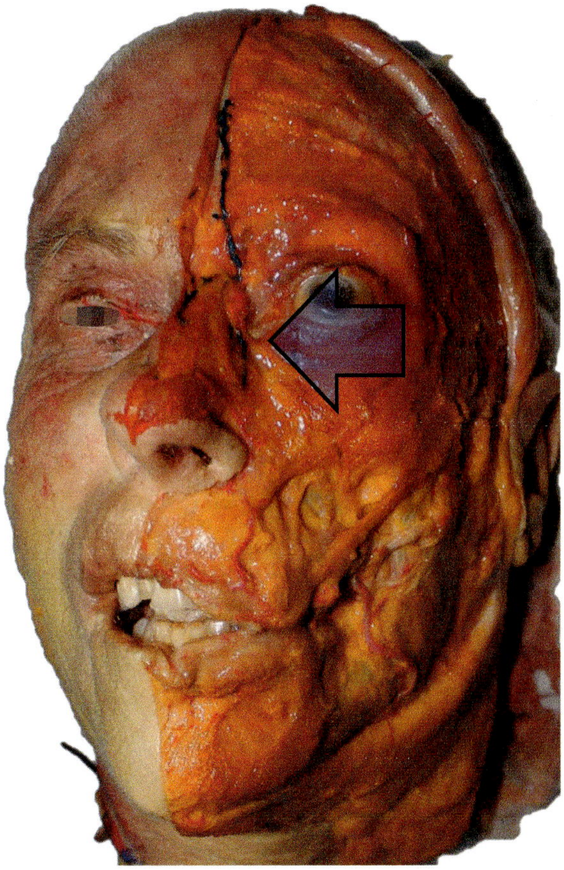

Fig. 16.1 The blue arrow indicates the relationship existing between the nose and the facial vessels after cadaver dissection along the muscular plane. The facial vessels meet the root of the nose in proximity of the internal cantus (courtesy of the Doctor's Equipe). (Published by kind permission of ©Mario Goisis 2018. All Rights Reserved)

16.3 Indications

Medical rhinoplasty can be the solution in cases where patients are reluctant to undergo surgery for the correction of minor imperfections of the nose.

S. Izzo (✉) · G. A. Ferraro · G. F. Nicoletti
Department of Plastic Surgery, University of Campania "Luigi Vanvitelli", Naples, Italy
e-mail: giuseppe.ferraro@unicampania.it; giovannifrancesco.nicoletti@unicampania.it

M. Goisis
Maxillo-Facial and Aesthetic Surgeon, Go Easy Clinic, Milan, Italy

L. Rosset
Doctor's Equipe, Milan, Italy

M. Goisis (ed.), *Outpatient Regenerative Medicine*, https://doi.org/10.1007/978-3-319-44894-7_16

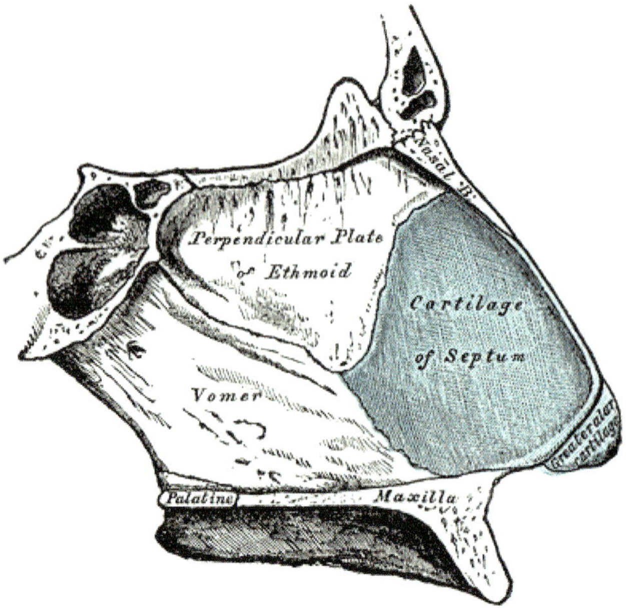

Fig. 16.2 The bony part of the nose is formed by the nasal septum, the nasal bones, and medial parts of the maxillae, palatine, and frontal bones; the cartilaginous part is formed by two lateral cartilages, two alar cartilages, and a septal cartilage. Reproduction of a lithographic plate from *Gray's Anatomy* (Henry Gray, Anatomy: Descriptive and Surgical). (Published by kind permission of ©Mario Goisis 2018. All Rights Reserved)

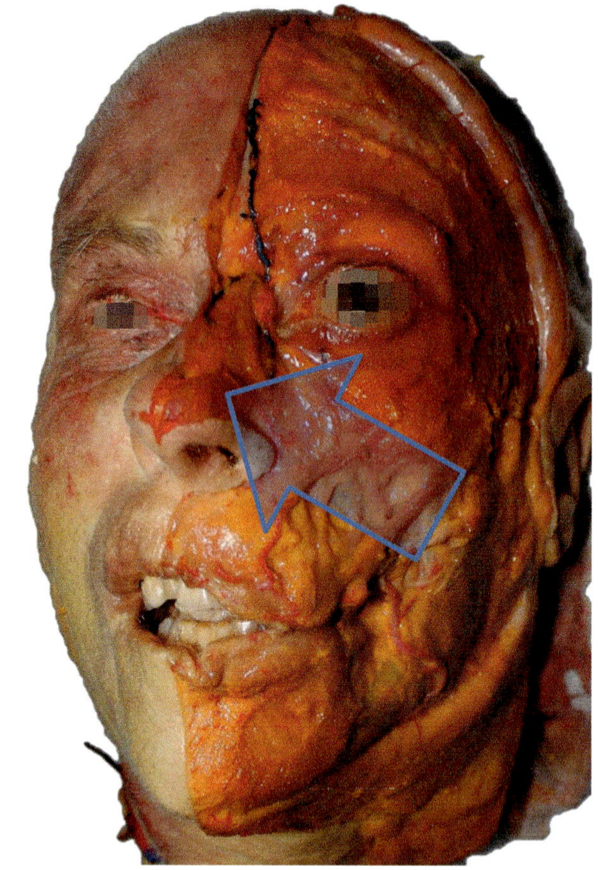

Fig. 16.4 The nasalis is a sphincter-like muscle of the nose whose function it is to compress the nasal cartilages. It is the muscle responsible for the "flaring" of the nostrils. The blue arrows (Figs. 16.5 and 16.6) show the relationship existing between the nasal pyramid and the nasalis muscle. (Published by kind permission of ©Mario Goisis 2018. All Rights Reserved)

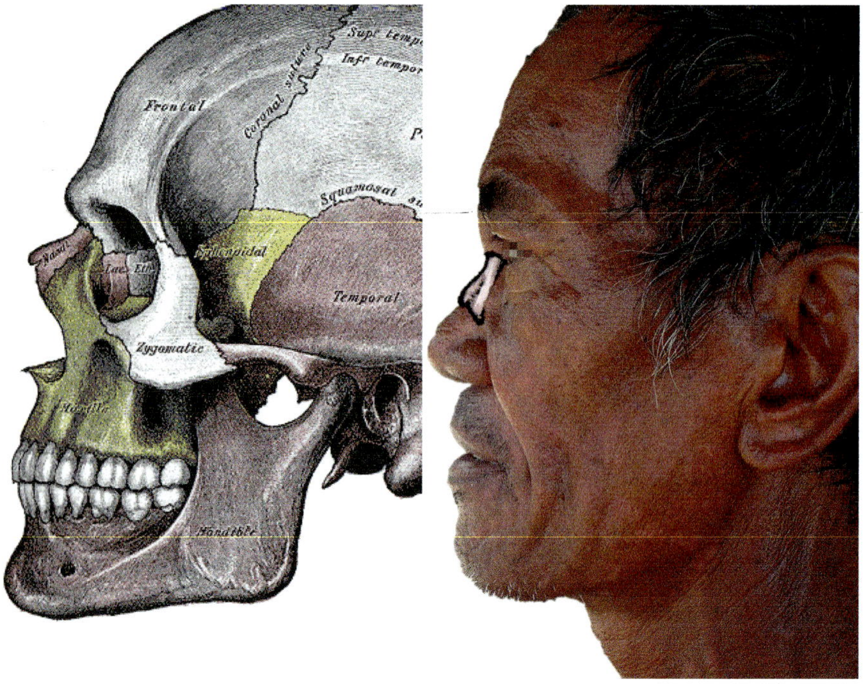

Fig. 16.3 The relationship between the skull and the nasal bones. On the left the reproduction of a lithograph plate from *Gray's Anatomy* (Henry Gray, Anatomy: Descriptive and Surgical) (courtesy of the Doctor's Equipe). (Published by kind permission of ©Mario Goisis 2018. All Rights Reserved)

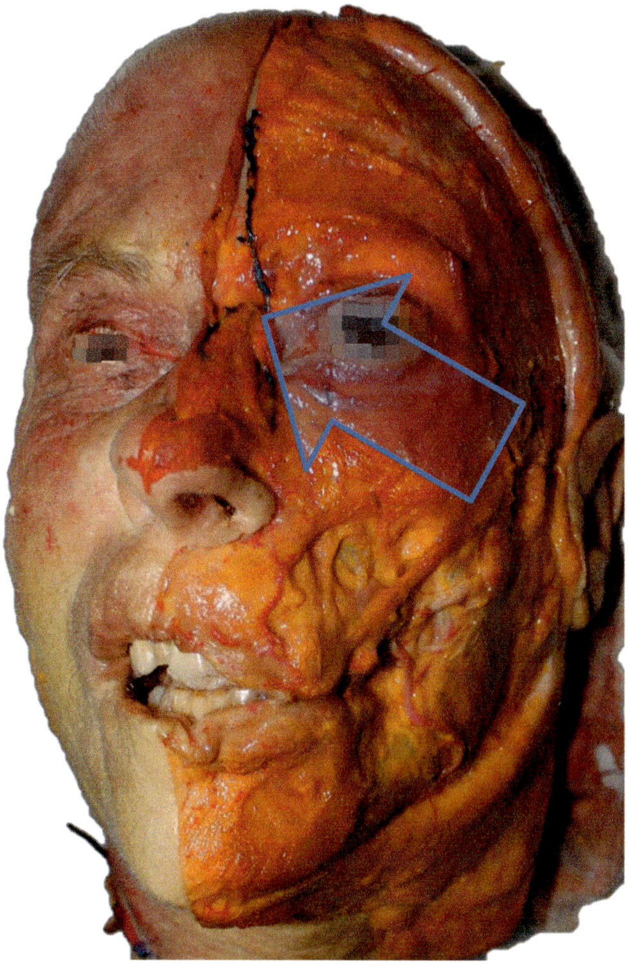

Fig. 16.5 The procerus stems by means of tendinous fibres from the fascia covering the lower part of the nasal bone and upper part of the lateral nasal cartilage. It is inserted into the skin over the lower part of the forehead between the two eyebrows on either side of the midline, its fibres merge with those of the frontalis. The blue arrows (Fig. 16.8) show the relationship between the nasal pyramid and the procerus muscle (courtesy Doctor's Equipe). (Published by kind permission of ©Mario Goisis 2018. All Rights Reserved)

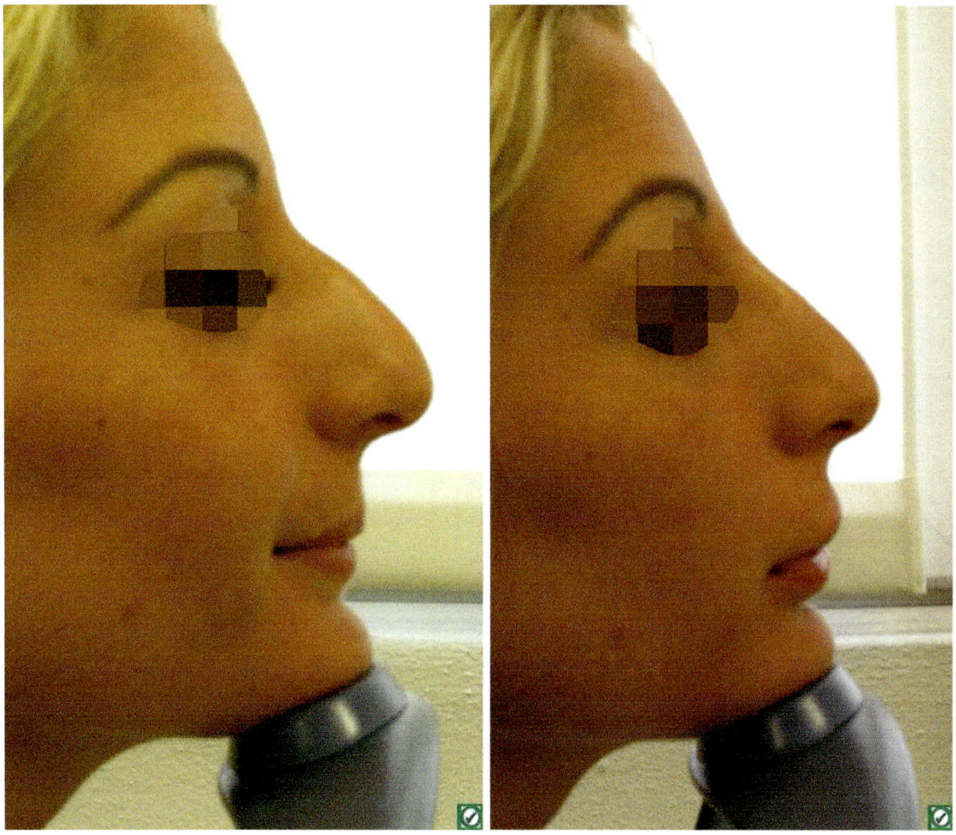

Fig. 16.6 Preoperative photos on the left and, on the right, postoperative photos taken 11 months after correction of the fronto-nasal and nasolabial angles using microfat. (Published by kind permission of ©Mario Goisis 2018. All Rights Reserved)

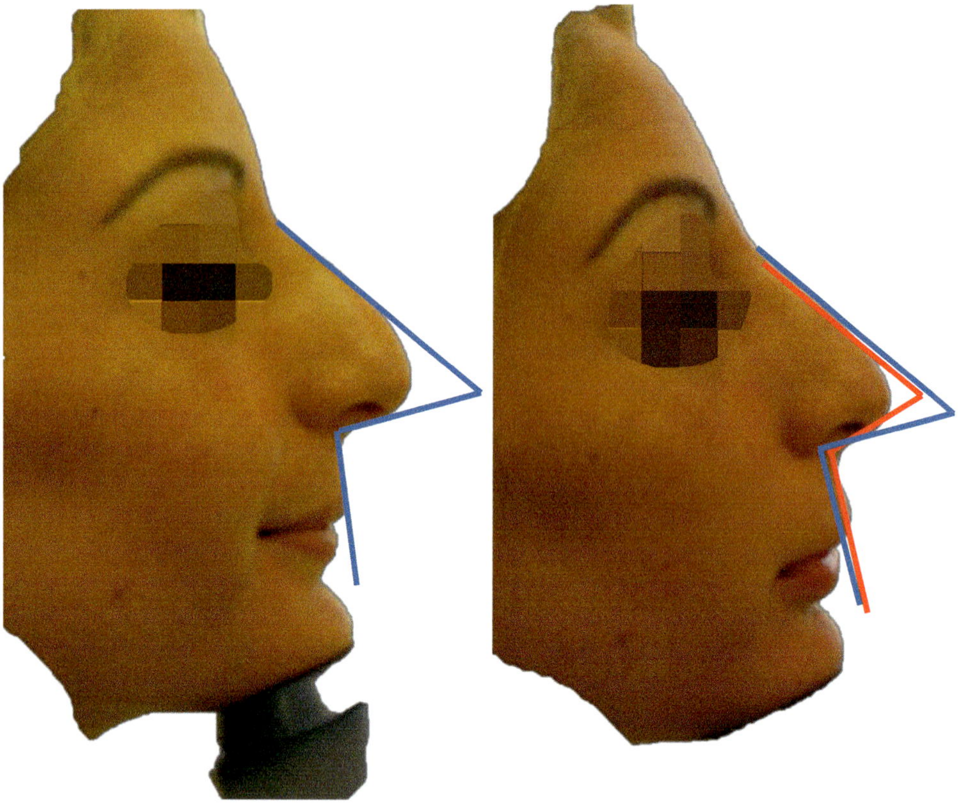

Fig. 16.7 Preoperative photos left composed to postoperative photos, right, the latter taken 11 months after correction of the fronto-nasal and nasolabial angles using microfat. (Published by kind permission of ©Mario Goisis 2018. All Rights Reserved)

16.4 Contraindications

Severe malformations requiring surgery.

Patients who have undergone surgical rhinoplasty or who have a previous history of trauma should be evaluated carefully before receiving similar medical treatment.

16.5 Correction of the Nasal Dorsum Using Microfat

16.5.1 Materials

- *1–2 cc of microfat on each side for injection of microfat:* 1–2 cc of microfat to the injected on each side
  - *A 21-gauge needle*
  - *A 22-gauge, 4 cm blunt cannula*

Harvesting and processing microfat:

A standard system for harvesting and processing microfat is used, in particular:

- A microfat box (www.microfat.com), composed of a ramp with a closed system for washing and filtration
- 4 60-cc syringes
- 2 10-cc syringes
- One 1-cc syringe
- A 30-gauge needle
- A 16-gauge needle
- A 2-mm-diameter, 10-cm-long Goisis cannula for fat harvesting
- A chlorhexidine-alcohol solution (2% chlorhexidine gluconate and 70% isopropyl alcohol), sterile drapes or towels
- Ice packs
- Sterile 2 cm × 2 cm gauze squares
- Occlusive dressing cover

Medications include:

100 cc of cold saline solution.

120 cc of cold Klein solution.

One litre of Klein solution is composed of 800 mg of lidocaine, 1 mg of epinephrine, 40 MEq of sodium bicarbonate, and 1000 cc of saline solution.

Location: The microfat harvesting can be carried out in a small operating theatre/medical surgery. Oxygen, pulse oximetry, and a crash cart/box should be present.

Assistants: An assistant is useful for the transfer of items to the procedure field in a sterile manner during the first part of the procedure. Despite this, a single doctor may carry out the entire procedure alone.

16.5.2 Complications and Management

Immediate complications (within 72 h after injection) include transient erythema, oedema, induration, pruritus, and ecchymosis.

Early complications (days to weeks after injection) include hypercorrection, local infection, necrosis of the skin, reactivation of herpes, discoloration, and persistent local symptoms (erythema, oedema, induration, pruritus, and hyperpigmentation).

Late or delayed complications include high rates of fat resorption and cysts.

16.5.3 Operating Time

Once the microfat is ready, the procedure usually takes from 5 to 15 min.

Plane of injection: intramuscular

16.5.4 Method

The procedure is illustrated in Figs. 16.8, 16.9, 16.10, 16.11, 16.12, 16.13, 16.14, 16.15, and 16.16.

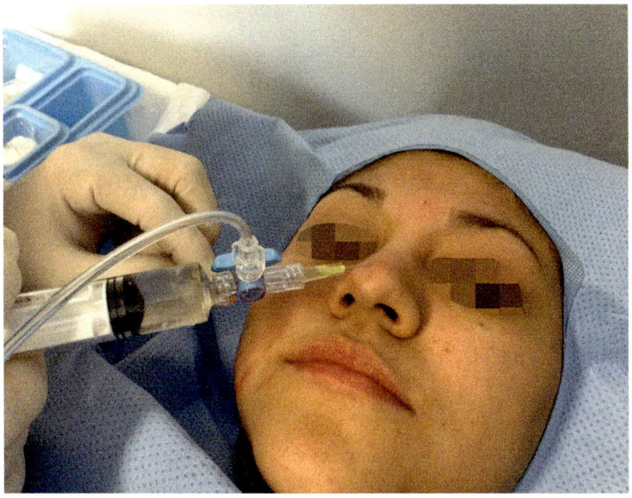

Fig. 16.8 Local anaesthesia is performed on the tip of the nose. (Published by kind permission of ©Mario Goisis 2018. All Rights Reserved)

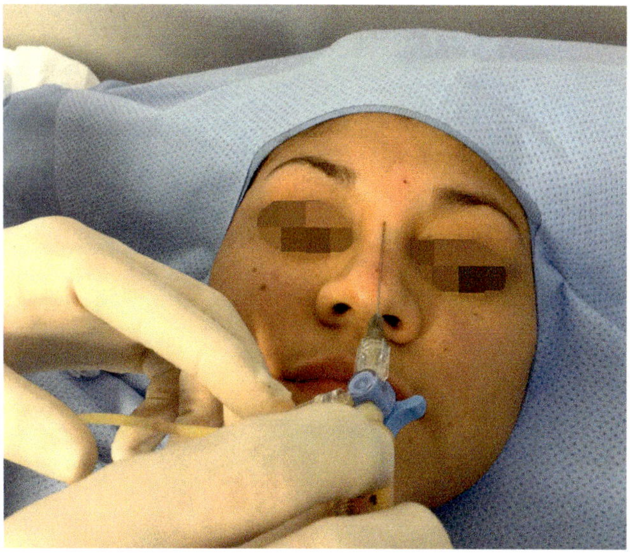

Fig. 16.9 The route of the cannula in the nasal dorsum. (Published by kind permission of ©Mario Goisis 2018. All Rights Reserved)

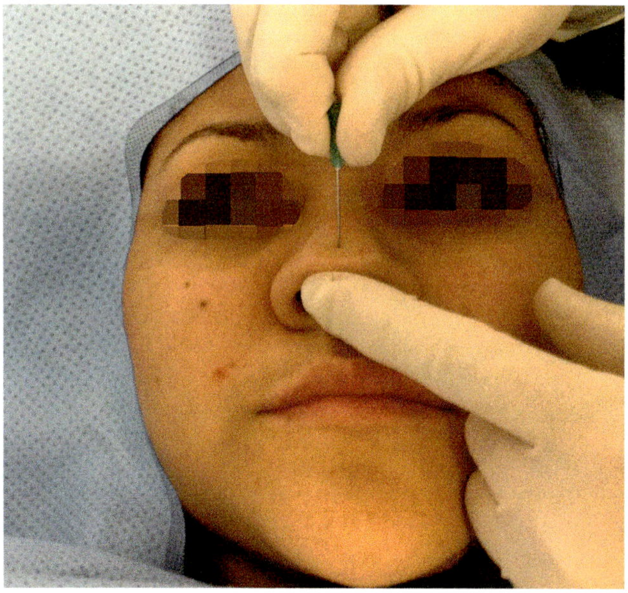

Fig. 16.10 Perforation of the plane of the skin using a 21-G needle. (Published by kind permission of ©Mario Goisis 2018. All Rights Reserved)

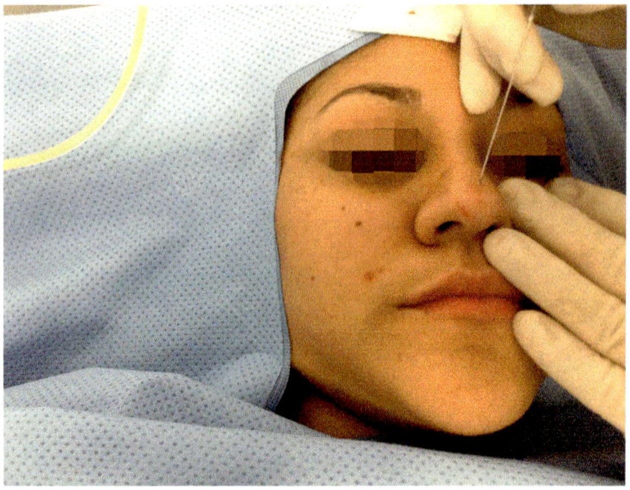

Fig. 16.11 A 22-G blunt-tip cannula is inserted perpendicularly into the surface of the skin. (Published by kind permission of ©Mario Goisis 2018. All Rights Reserved)

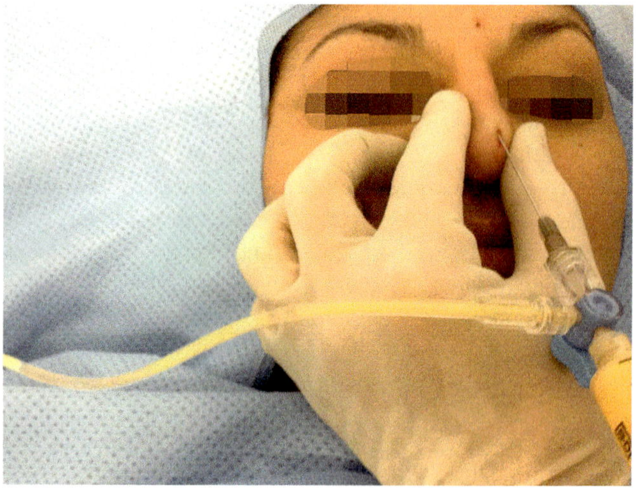

Fig. 16.13 The microfat is delivered slowly while the cannula is withdrawn by retrograde injection. (Published by kind permission of ©Mario Goisis 2018. All Rights Reserved)

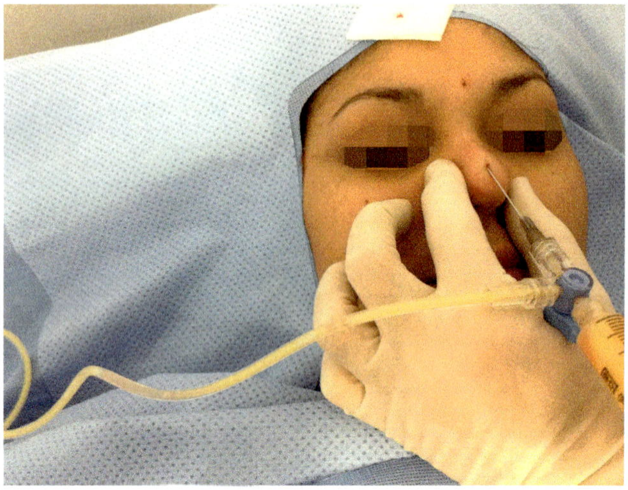

Fig. 16.12 The cannula is then pivoted parallel to the plane of the skin and slid toward the top of the nasal dorsum. (Published by kind permission of ©Mario Goisis 2018. All Rights Reserved)

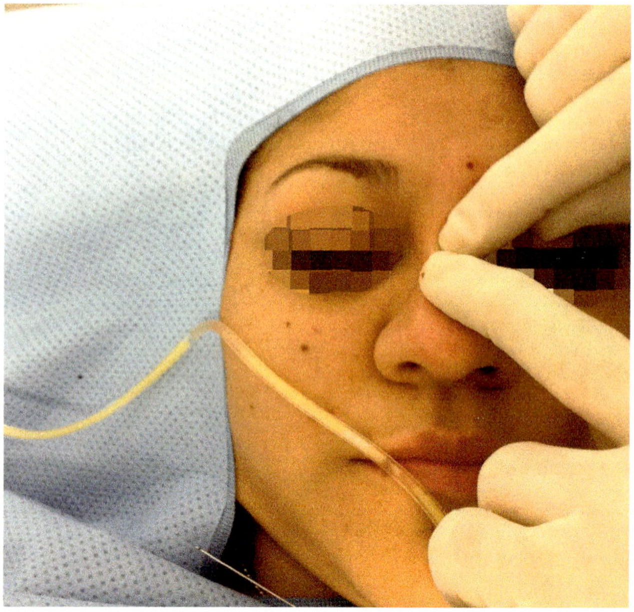

Fig. 16.14 At the end of the treatment, the injected area is massaged. (Published by kind permission of ©Mario Goisis 2018. All Rights Reserved)

16.5.5 Cadaver Dissection After Injection of Coloured Microfat into the Nasal Dorsum (Courtesy of the Doctor's Equipe) (Figs. 16.17, 16.18, 16.19, 16.20, 16.21, 16.22, and 16.23)

16.6 Augmentation of the Nasolabial Angle Using Microfat Mixed with PRP

16.6.1 Materials

- *2–4 cc of microfat on each side for injection of microfat: 2–4 cc of microfat for injection into both sides:*
  - *A 21-gauge needle*
  - *A 22-gauge, 4 -cm blunt cannula*

To harvest and process microfat:
A standard system is used, in particular:

- A microfat box (www.microfat.com), composed of a ramp with a closed system for washing and filtration
- 4 60-cc syringes
- 2 10-cc syringes
- One 1-cc syringe
- A 30-gauge needle

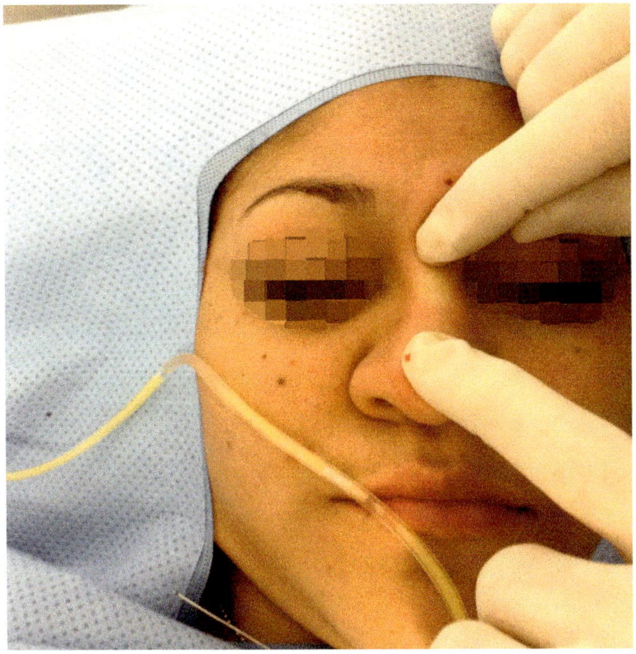

Fig. 16.15 At the end of the treatment, the injected area is massaged. (Published by kind permission of ©Mario Goisis 2018. All Rights Reserved)

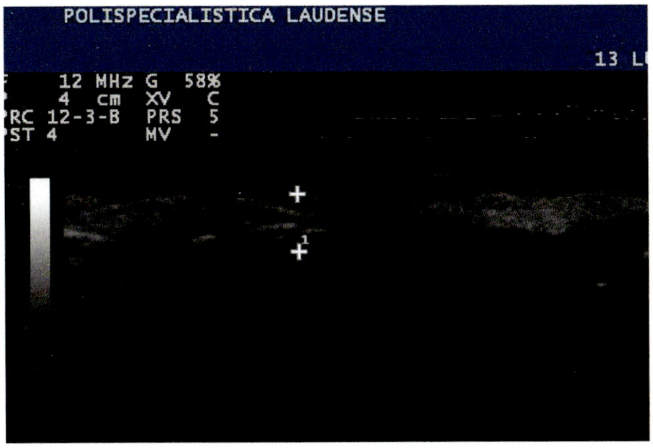

Fig. 16.16 Ultrasound evaluation of correction of the nasal dorsum: under the cutaneous and subcutaneous plane, there is a thin layer of muscle (Fig. 16.39). The fat needs to be injected deeply into this thin layer (Fig. 16.40) (courtesy of the Doctor's Equipe). (Published by kind permission of ©Mario Goisis 2018. All Rights Reserved)

- A 16-gauge needle
- A 2-mm-diameter, 10-cm-long Goisis cannula for fat harvesting
- A chlorhexidine-alcohol solution (2% chlorhexidine gluconate and 70% isopropyl alcohol), sterile drapes or towels
- Ice packs
- Sterile 2 cm × 2-cm gauze squares
- Occlusive dressing cover

Tubes for PRP preparation, empty and with anticoagulant (www.microfat.com)

Medications include:

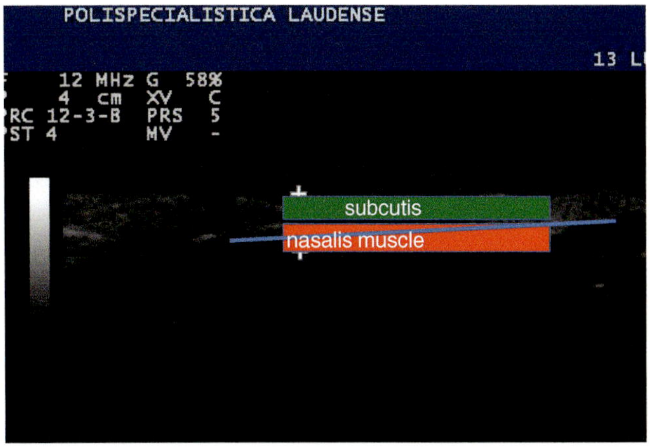

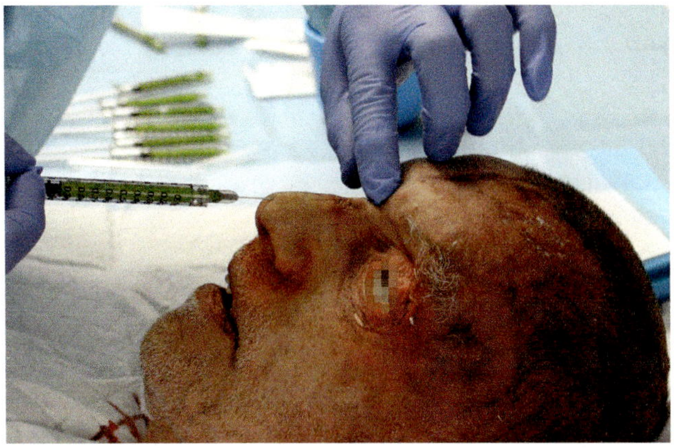

Fig. 16.17 The fat is injected onto the nasal dorsum starting from a single injection-point between the alar cartilages. The fat is delivered slowly, while the cannula is withdrawn retrograde fasion. (Published by kind permission of ©Mario Goisis 2018. All Rights Reserved)

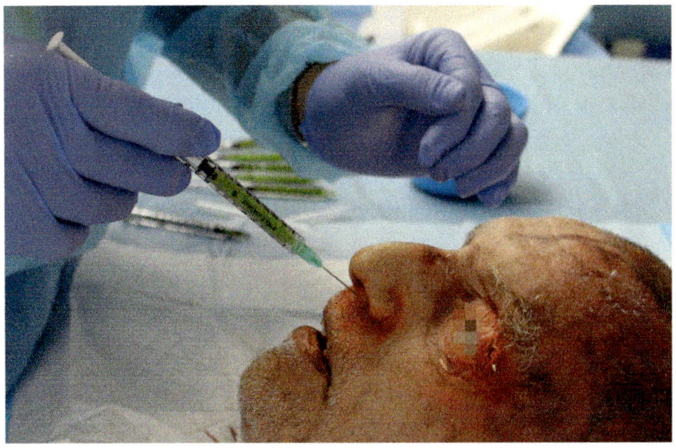

Fig. 16.18 The nasolabial angle can be augmented injecting the fat onto the anterior nasal spine. Fat is injected using a 21-G needle which enters at an angle of 45° between the columella and the upper lip. (Published by kind permission of ©Mario Goisis 2018. All Rights Reserved)

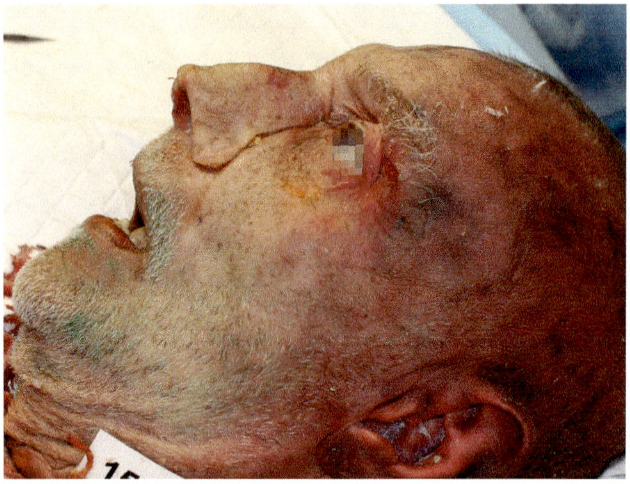

Fig. 16.19 After injecting the fat, a cadaver dissection of the supraperiosteal plane was carried out. (Published by kind permission of ©Mario Goisis 2018. All Rights Reserved)

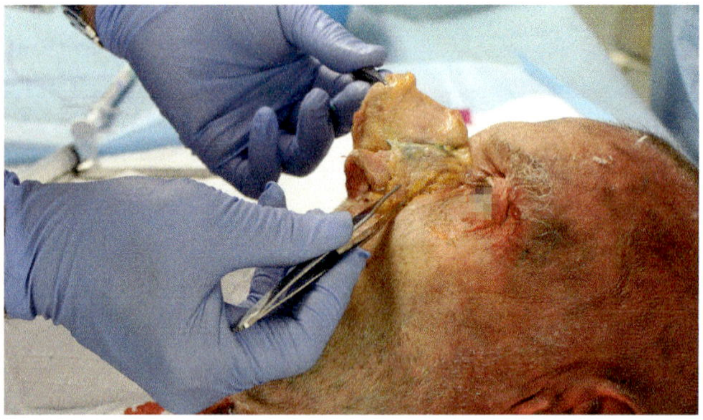

Fig. 16.20 The coloured fat can be retrieved from the subcutaneous plane, under the thick nasal dermis and over the periosteal plane. (Published by kind permission of ©Mario Goisis 2018. All Rights Reserved)

100 cc of cold saline solution.

120 cc of cold Klein solution.

One litre of Klein solution is composed of 800 mg of lidocaine, 1 mg of epinephrine, 40 MEq of sodium bicarbonate, and 1000 cc of saline solution.

Location: Microfat harvesting can be carried out in a small operating theatre/medical surgery. Oxygen, pulse oximetry, and a crash cart/box should be present.

Assistants: An assistant can prove useful when transferring items to the procedure field in a sterile manner during the first stage of the procedure. Nevertheless, a single doctor can perform the procedure single-handed.

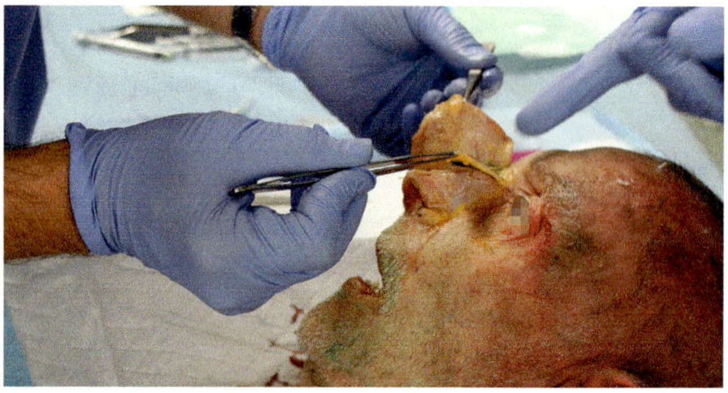

Fig. 16.21 The coloured fat can be retrieved from the subcutaneous plane, under the thick nasal dermis and over the periosteal plane. (Published by kind permission of ©Mario Goisis 2018. All Rights Reserved)

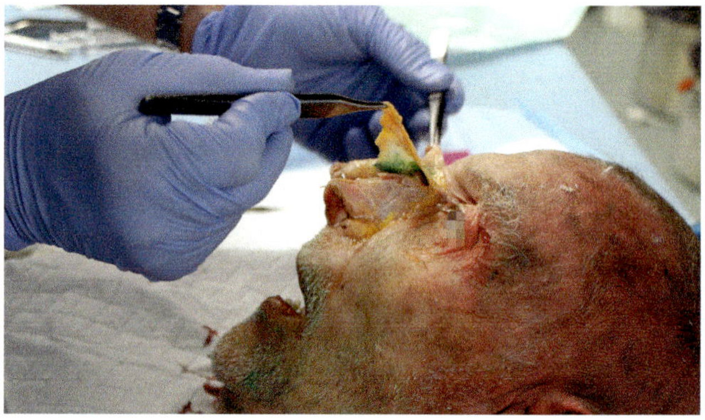

Fig. 16.22 The coloured fat can be retrieved from the subcutaneous plane, under the thick nasal dermis and over the periosteal plane. (Published by kind permission of ©Mario Goisis 2018. All Rights Reserved)

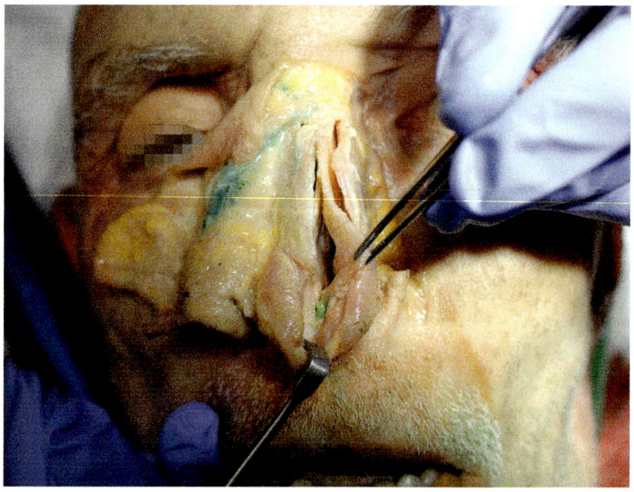

Fig. 16.23 Detail of the injection-point located under the orbital septum. (Published by kind permission of ©Mario Goisis 2018. All Rights Reserved)

16.6.2 Complications and Management

Immediate complications (within 72 h after injection) include transient erythema, oedema, induration, pruritus, and ecchymosis.

Early complications (days to weeks after injection) include hypercorrection, local infection, necrosis of the skin, reactivation of herpes, discoloration, and persistent local symptoms (erythema, oedema, induration, pruritus, and hyperpigmentation).

Later or delayed complications include high rates of fat resorption and cyst.

16.6.3 Operating Time

Once the microfat and PRP are ready, the procedure usually takes from 5 to 15 min.

16.6.4 Method

The procedure is illustrated in Figs. 16.24, 16.25, and 16.26.

16.7 Amelioration of Nasal Dorsum with PRP and a Blunt-Tip Cannula

16.7.1 Materials

Tubes for PRP preparation, empty and with anticoagulant (www.microfat.com)

Bandages and antiseptic solution

0.2 cc of local anaesthetic (2% lidocaine or 2% mepivacaine) with epinephrine 1:100000

1 cc Luer lock syringe

A 26-G needle

A 27-G blunt cannula

1–2 cc of PRP

16.7.2 Methods

The method is shown in Figs. 16.27, 16.28, 16.29, 16.30, 16.31, and 16.32.

16.7.3 Cadaver Dissection After PRP Injection in the Nasal Dorsum (Figs. 16.33 and 16.34)

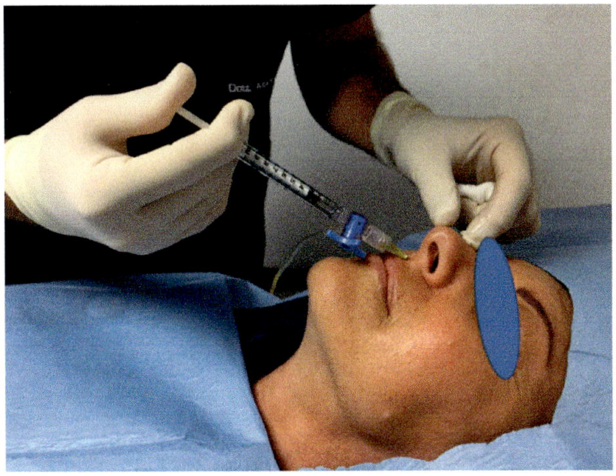

Fig. 16.24 Augmentation of the nasolabial anngle by injection of Microfat mixed with PRP. Local anaesthesia is injected by means of a 30-G needle into the anterior nasal spine. The needle enters the cutaneous plane between the labial filter and the columella and is then directed towards the anterior nasal spine. The local anaesthesia is then injected, retrograde fashion. (Published by kind permission of ©Mario Goisis 2018. All Rights Reserved)

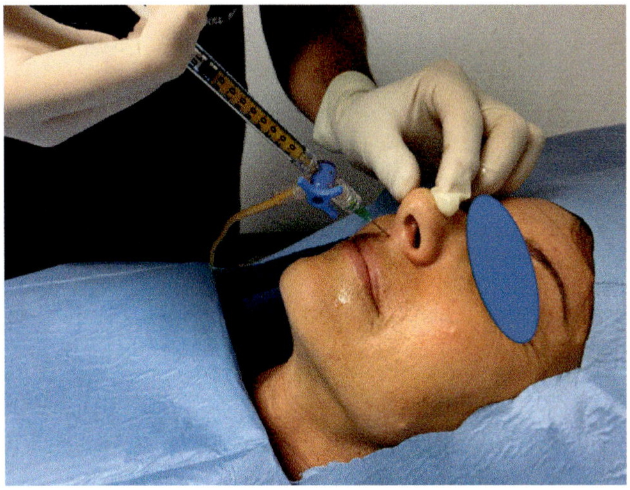

Fig. 16.25 The mix of PRP and micrograft is injected by means of a 21-gauge needle. The needle enters the cutaneous plane between the labial filter and the columella and is then directed towards the anterior nasal spine. (Published by kind permission of ©Mario Goisis 2018. All Rights Reserved)

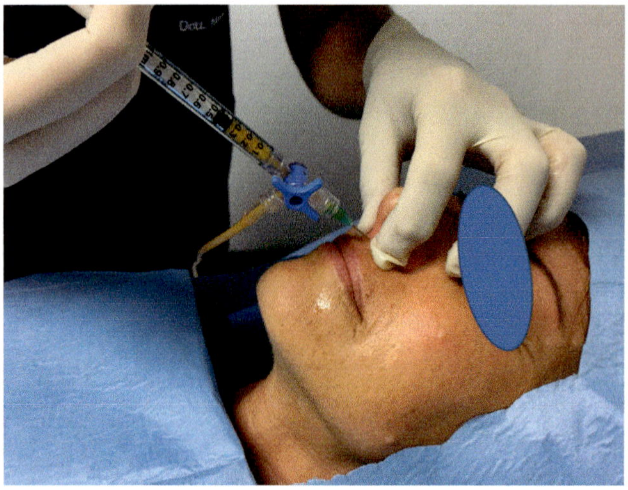

Fig. 16.26 Once the needle reaches the anterior nasal spine, the mix of micrograft and PRP is injected. It is useful to hold the labial filter tightly between the fingers in order to avoid loss of definition of the labial filter. (Published by kind permission of ©Mario Goisis 2018. All Rights Reserved)

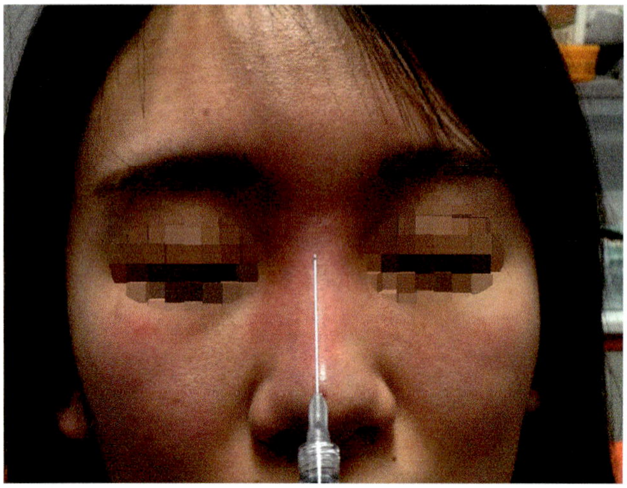

Fig. 16.27 The route of the cannula in the nasal dorsum. (Published by kind permission of ©Mario Goisis 2018. All Rights Reserved)

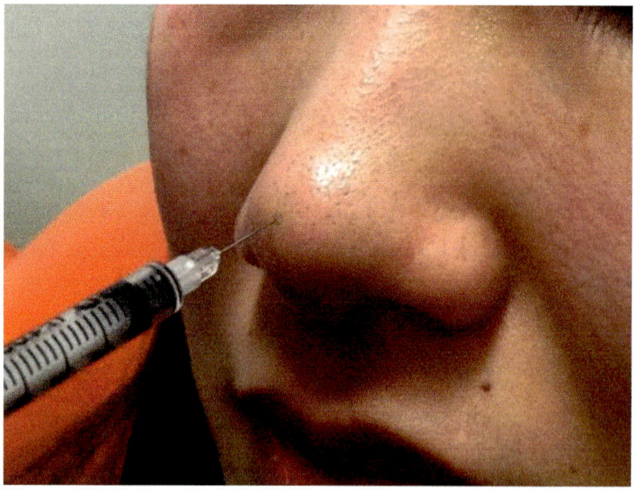

Fig. 16.28 Amelioration of Nasal Dorsum with PRP and a Blunt-Tip Cannula. Local anaesthesia is performed on the tip of the nose. (Published by kind permission of ©Mario Goisis 2018. All Rights Reserved)

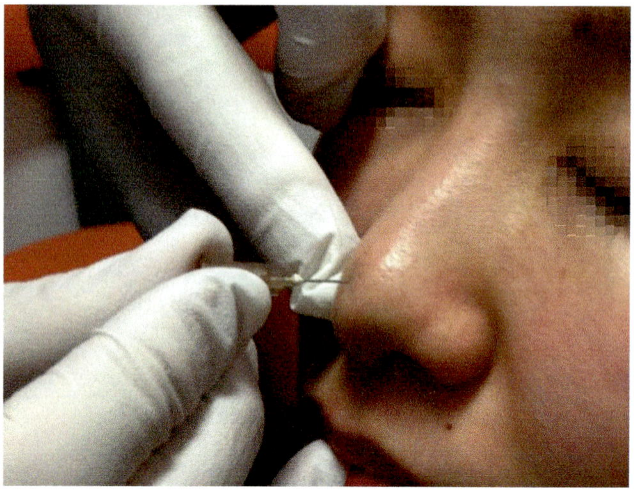

Fig. 16.29 Perforation of the skin plane using a 26-G needle. (Published by kind permission of ©Mario Goisis 2018. All Rights Reserved)

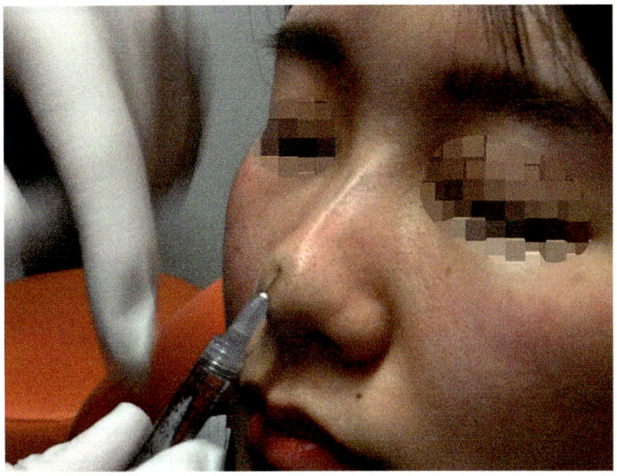

Fig. 16.30 A blunt-tip 27-G cannula is inserted perpendicularly into the skin's surface. The cannula is then pivoted parallel to the plane of the skin and slid toward the top of the nasal dorsum. The PRP and HA mix is delivered slowly, while the cannula is withdrawn by retrograde injection. (Published by kind permission of ©Mario Goisis 2018. All Rights Reserved)

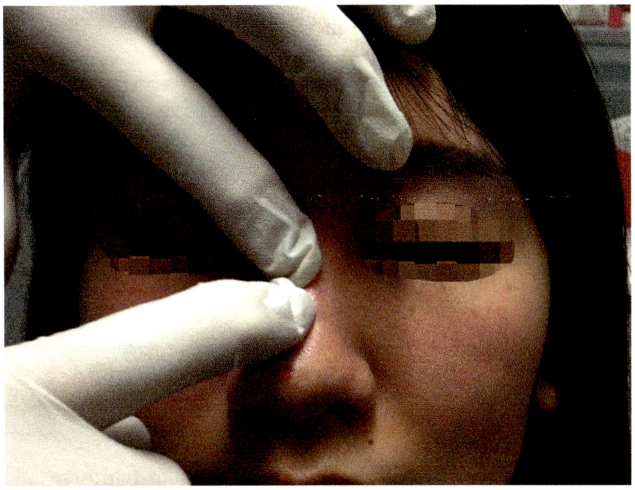

Fig. 16.31 At the end of the treatment, the injected area is massaged. (Published by kind permission of ©Mario Goisis 2018. All Rights Reserved)

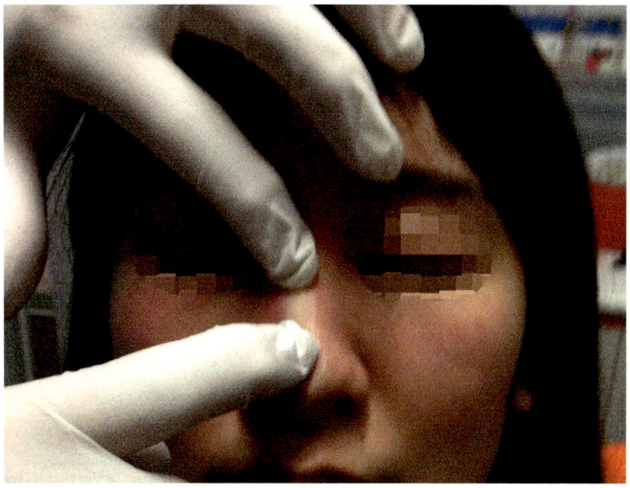

Fig. 16.32 At the end of the treatment, a massage is applied over the area injected the injected area is massaged. (Published by kind permission of ©Mario Goisis 2018. All Rights Reserved)

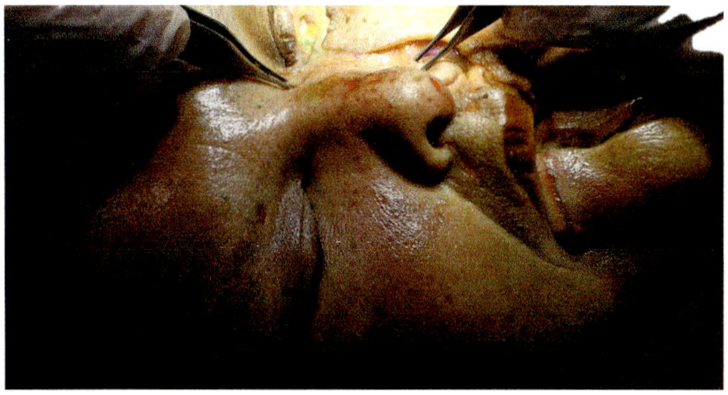

Fig. 16.33 Cadaver dissection shows the presence of coloured PRP in the subcutis of the perialar and nasal dorsum area (courtesy of the Doctor's Equipe). (Published by kind permission of ©Mario Goisis 2018. All Rights Reserved)

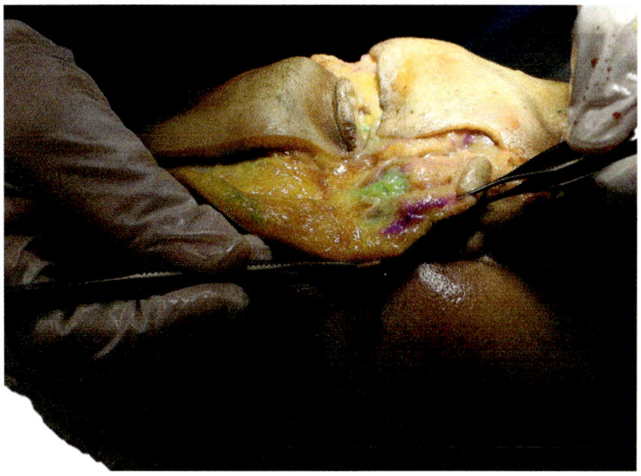

Fig. 16.34 This cadaver dissection shows the presence of coloured PRP in the subcutis of the perialar and nasal dorsum area (courtesy of the Doctor's Equipe). (Published by kind permission of ©Mario Goisis 2018. All Rights Reserved)

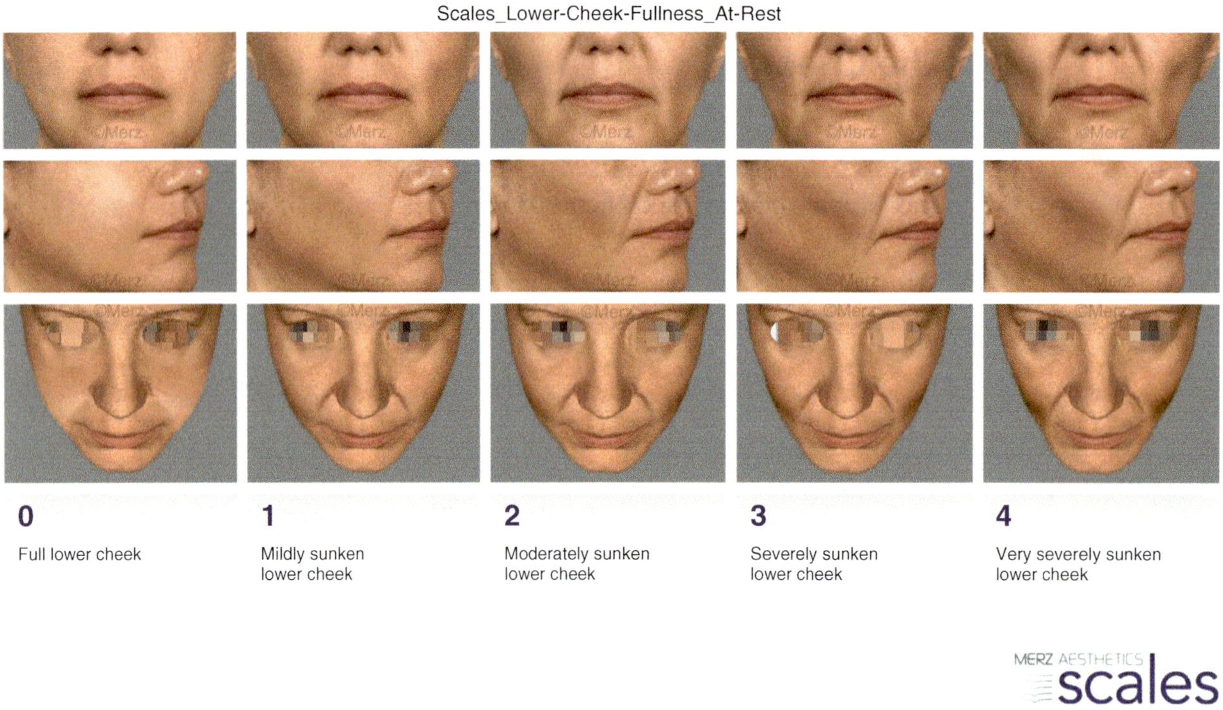

Fig. 17.1 Different degrees of sunken cheeks (courtesy of the Merz company). (Published by kind permission of ©Mario Goisis 2018. All Rights Reserved)

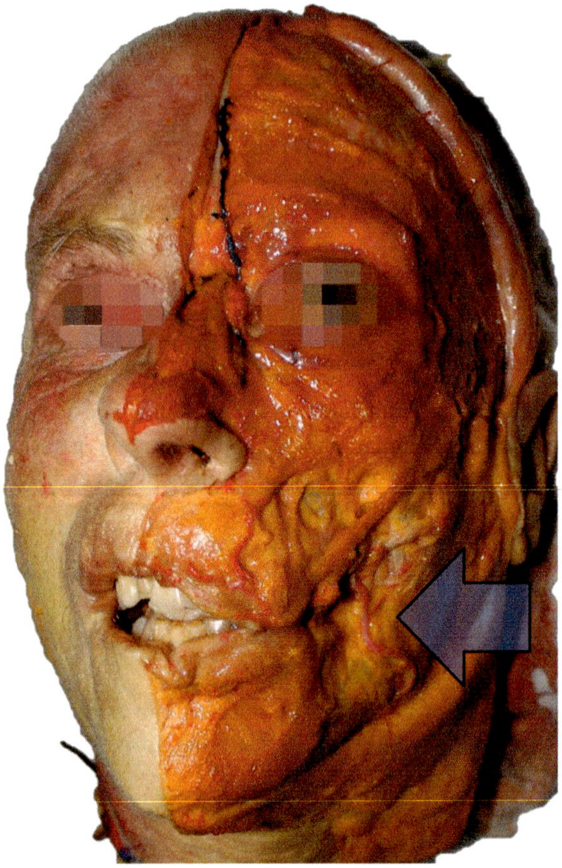

Fig. 17.2 In the anatomic dissection, the acial vein and artery are evident (courtesy of the Doctor's Equipe). (Published by kind permission of ©Mario Goisis 2018. All Rights Reserved)

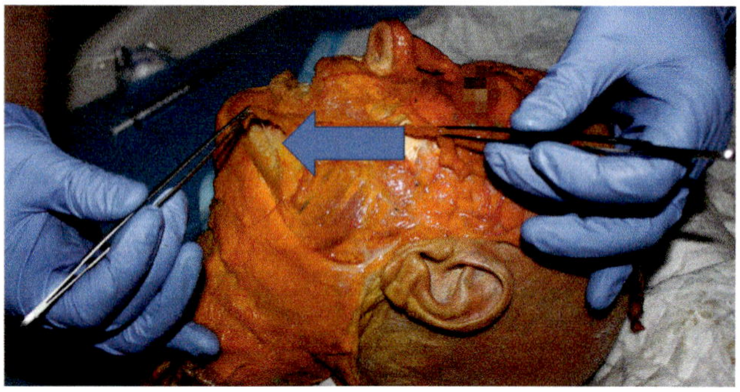

Fig. 17.3 The marginal mandibular branch of the facial nerve is indicated (see the blue arrow) (courtesy of the Doctor's Equipe). (Published by kind permission of ©Mario Goisis 2018. All Rights Reserved)

17.5.3 Complications and Management

Immediate complications (within 72 h after injection) include transient erythema, oedema, induration, pruritus, and ecchymosis.

Early complications (days to weeks after injection) include hypercorrection, local infection, necrosis of the skin, reactivation of herpes, discoloration, and persistent local symptoms (erythema, oedema, induration, pruritus, and hyperpigmentation).

Later or delayed complications include high rates of fat resorption and cysts.

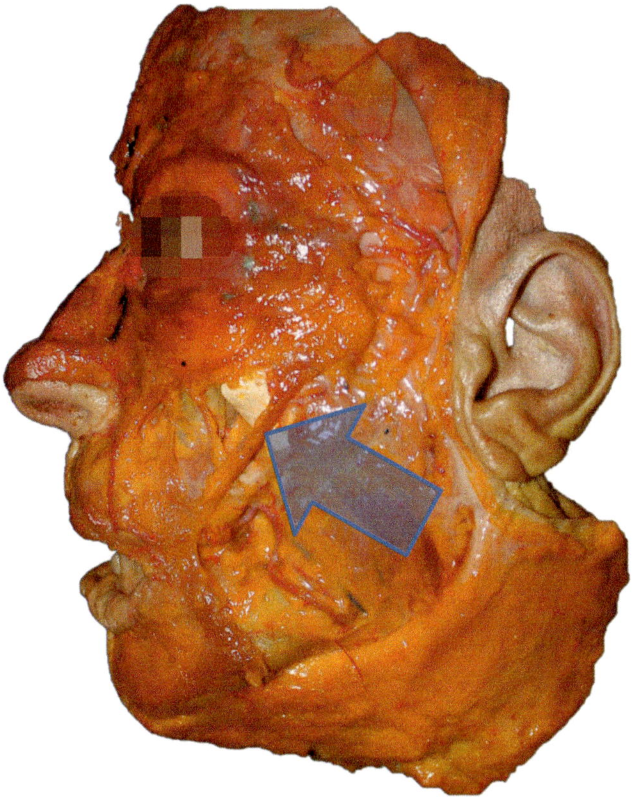

Fig. 17.4 The muscles which contribute to facial mimicry in the cheek area: see the blue arrow indicating the zygomaticus major muscle (courtesy of the Doctor's Equipe). (Published by kind permission of ©Mario Goisis 2018. All Rights Reserved)

17.5.4 Materials

- *1–2 cc of microfat on each side for injection of microfat: [1-2 cc of microfat for injection on either side]*
  - *A 21-gauge needle.*
  - *A 22-gauge 4-cm blunt cannula.*

To harvest and process microfat
A standard system is used, in particular:

- A Microfat box (www.microfat.com), composed of a ramp with a closed system for washing and filtration.
- 4 60-cc syringes.
- 2 10-cc syringes.
- One 1-cc syringe 1 cc.
- A 30-gauge needle.
- A 16-gauge needle.
- A 2-mm diameter, 10-cm long Goisis cannula for fat harvesting.
- A chlorhexidine-alcohol solution (2% chlorhexidine gluconate and 70% isopropyl alcohol), sterile drapes, or towels.
- Ice packs.
- Sterile 2 cm × 2-cm gauze squares.
- Occlusive dressing cover.

Medications include:

100 cc of cold saline solution.
120 cc of cold Klein solution.
1 litre of Klein solution is composed of 800 mg of lidocaine, 1 mg of epinephrine, 40 MEq of sodium bicarbonate, and 1000 cc of saline solution.

Location: Microfat harvesting can be carried out in a small operating theatre/physician's surgery. Oxygen, pulse oximetry, and a crash cart/box should be present.

Assistance: An assistant can prove useful when transferring items to the procedure field in a sterile manner during the first stage of the procedure. Nevertheless, a single doctor can easily perform the entire procedure alone.

Plane of injection: SMAS

17.5.5 Operating Time

Once the fat has been harvested the procedure usually takes from 5 to 15 min.

17.5.6 Methods

The procedure is described in Figs. 17.5, 17.6, 17.7, 17.8, 17.9, 17.10, and 17.11.

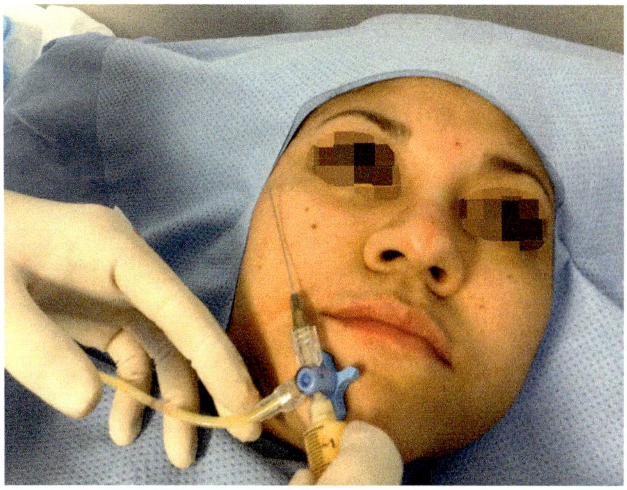

Fig. 17.5 The route of the cannula. (Published by kind permission of ©Mario Goisis 2018. All Rights Reserved)

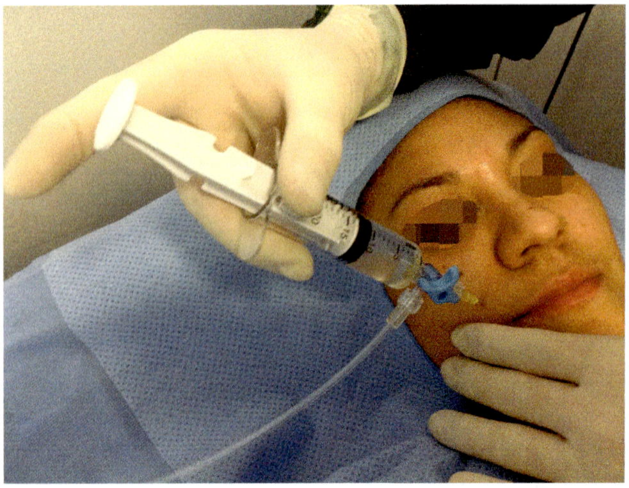

Fig. 17.6 Anaesthesia is performed at the entry-point at the level of the modiolus using 0.2 cc of Klein solution. (Published by kind permission of ©Mario Goisis 2018. All Rights Reserved)

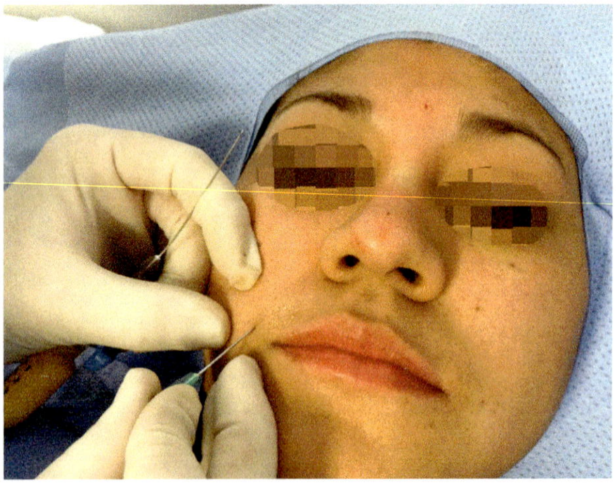

Fig. 17.7 An opening is created with a 21-G needle at the level of the modiolus. (Published by kind permission of ©Mario Goisis 2018. All Rights Reserved)

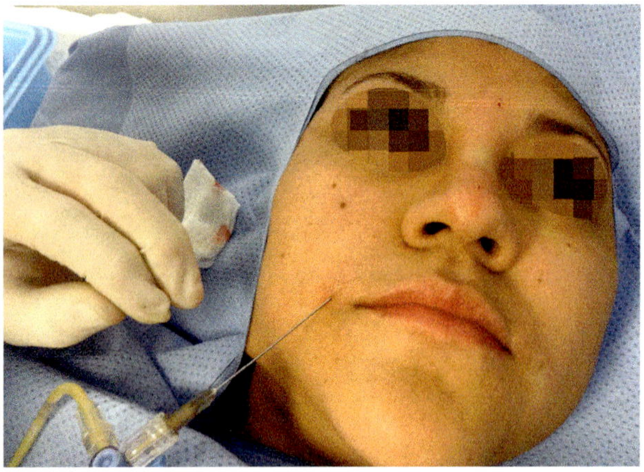

Fig. 17.8 A 22-G blunt-tip cannula is inserted perpendicularly into the surface of the skin, and the cannula is then pivoted parallel to the plane of the skin. (Published by kind permission of ©Mario Goisis 2018. All Rights Reserved)

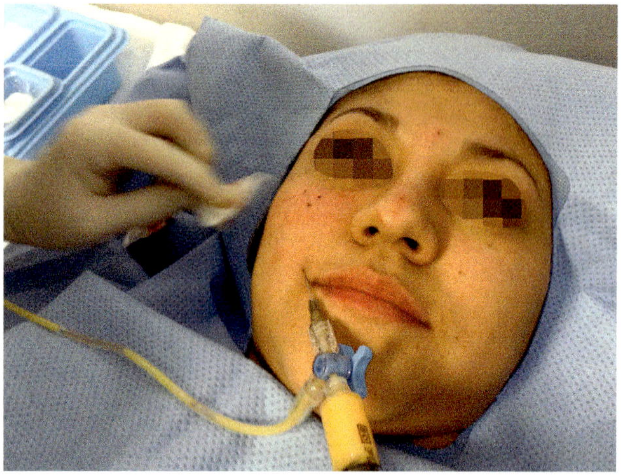

Fig. 17.9 The fat is delivered slowly while the cannula is withdrawn by retrograde injection. The fat is injected into the SMAS, in particular into the zygomaticus major and risorius muscles. (Published by kind permission of ©Mario Goisis 2018. All Rights Reserved)

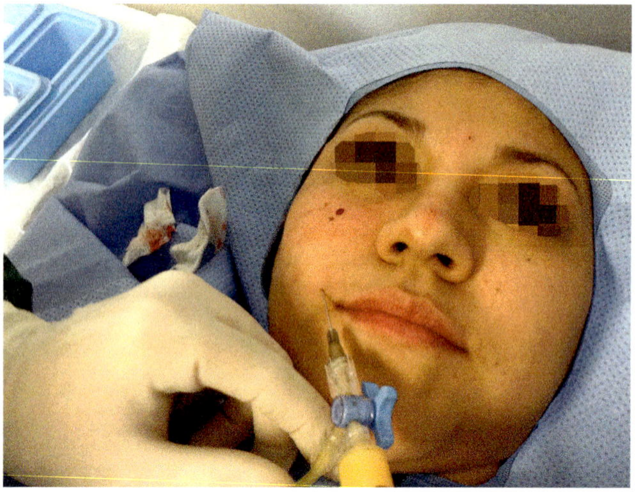

Fig. 17.10 The fat is delivered slowly while the cannula is withdrawn by retrograde injection. The fat is injected into the SMAS, in particular into the zygomaticus major and risorius muscles. (Published by kind permission of ©Mario Goisis 2018. All Rights Reserved)

17.5.7 Cadaver Dissection After Microfat Injection into the Area of the Cheeks (Figs. 17.11, 17.12, 17.13, and 17.14) (Courtesy by of the Doctor's Equipe)

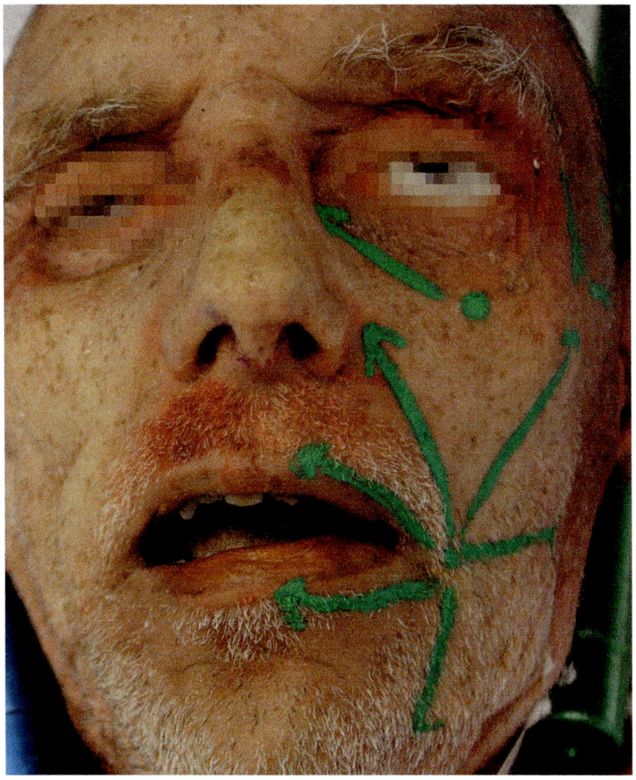

Fig. 17.11 The checks are filled using a single entry point, located 1.5–2 cm laterally to the oral rim, in correspondence to the modiolus. (Published by kind permission of ©Mario Goisis 2018. All Rights Reserved)

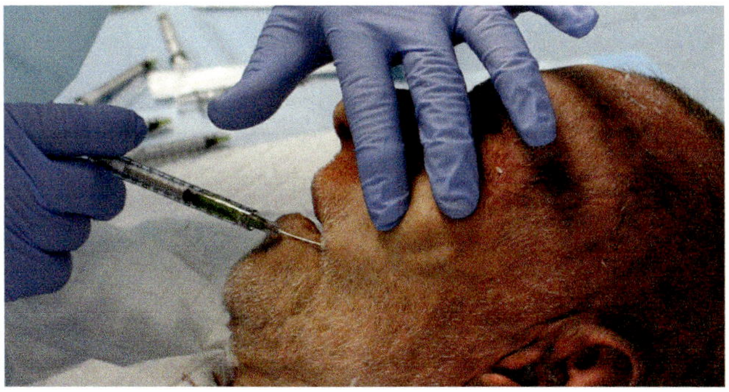

Fig. 17.12 The fat is delivered slowly into the muscular-SMAS plane while the cannula is withdrawn with by retrograde injection. (Published by kind permission of ©Mario Goisis 2018. All Rights Reserved)

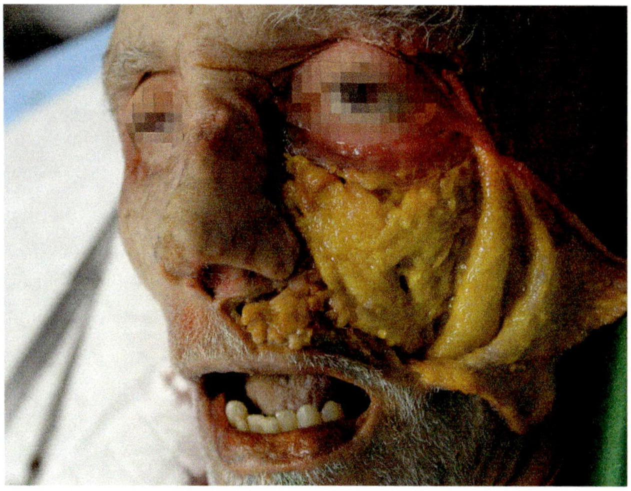

Fig. 17.13 After of the fat, a midfacial dissection is executed starting with a subcillary incision of the lower lid, continuing below the internal cantus following a paranasal route to the labial filter as far as the vermilion border and along its entire length. The subcutaneous plane is thus exposed. No evidence of fat is shown in the subcutaneous plane. (Published with by kind permission of ©Mario Goisis 2018. All Rights Reserved)

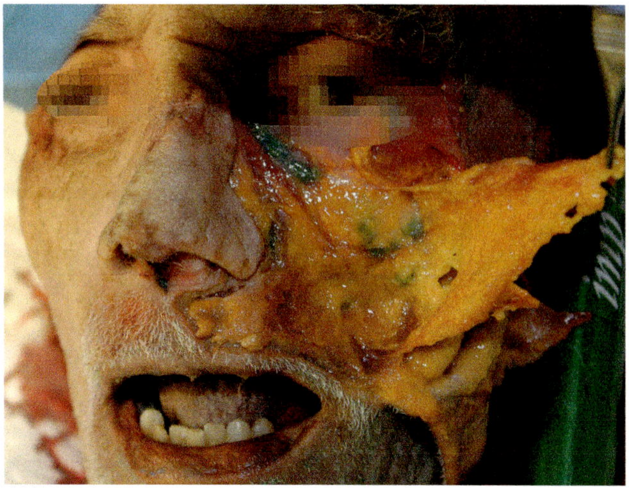

Fig. 17.14 It is possible to retrieve the coloured fat from the aponeurotic plane of the facial muscles and the muscolar plane itself. (Published by kind permission of ©Mario Goisis 2018. All Rights Reserved)

17.6 Amelioration of the Region of the Cheek with PRP and a Blunt-Tip Cannula

17.6.1 Indications

Amelioration of small wrinkles and acne scars in the cheeks. The use of a blunt-tip cannula permits atraumatic dissection of the tissue placement of the PRP into the subcutaneous plane, as well as the creation of fewer needle entry marks and significantly less pain and bruising.

17.6.2 Contraindications

- The PRP should not be injected into areas that lack sufficient blood supply or suffering from infection or inflammation.
- No injection should be performed if the cheek has been previously treated with liquid silicone or other permanent fillers because new injections might lead to inflammation or infection of the implants.

17.6.3 Operating Time

The procedure usually takes from 10 to 15 min, once the blood sample has been taken.

Plane of injection: dermis, superficial fat compartments

17.6.4 Materials

Bandages and antiseptic solution.

0.2 cc of local anesthetic (2% lidocaine or 2% mepivacaine) with epinephrine 1:100000.

A 1 -cc luer -lock syringe.

A 26-G needle.

A 27-G blunt cannula.

1–2 cc of PRP.

Tubes for PRP preparation, empty and with anticoagulant (www.microfat.com)

17.6.5 Methods

The procedure is described in Figs. 17.15, 17.16, 17.17, 17.18, 17.19, 17.20, 17.21, 17.29, 17.30, 17.31, and 17.32.

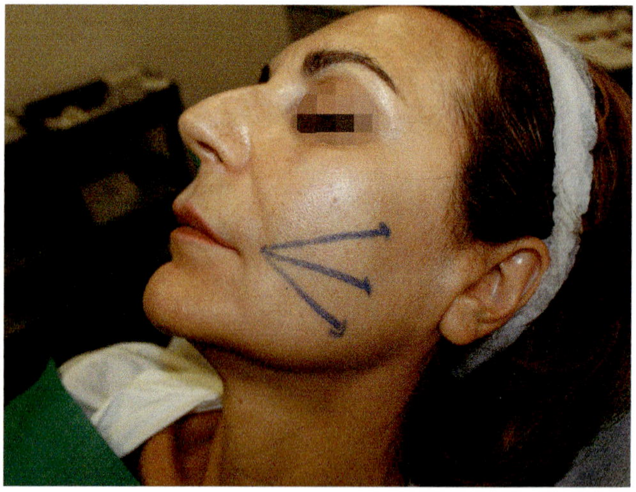

Fig. 17.15 Graphic superficial representation of the route of the cannula. (Published by kind permission of ©Mario Goisis 2018. All Rights Reserved)

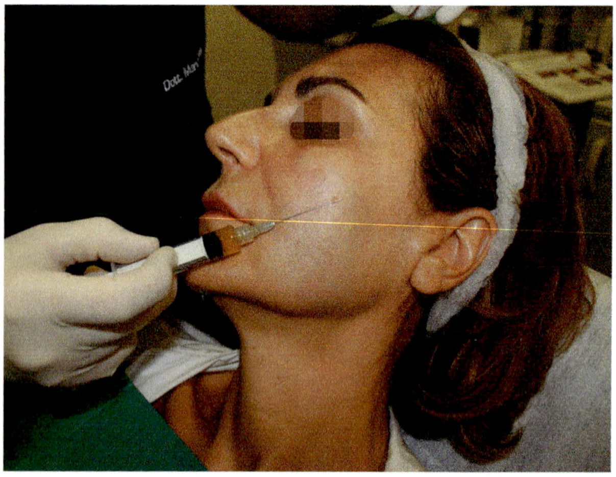

Fig. 17.16 Graphic superficial representation of the route of the cannula. (Published by kind permission of ©Mario Goisis 2018. All Rights Reserved)

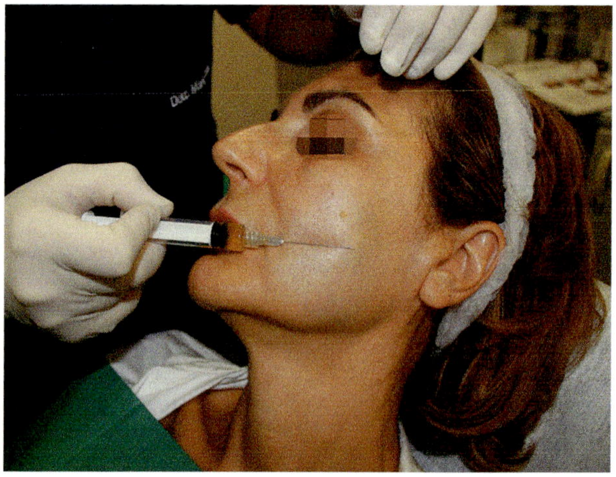

Fig. 17.17 Graphic superficial representation of the route of the cannula. (Published by kind permission of ©Mario Goisis 2018. All Rights Reserved)

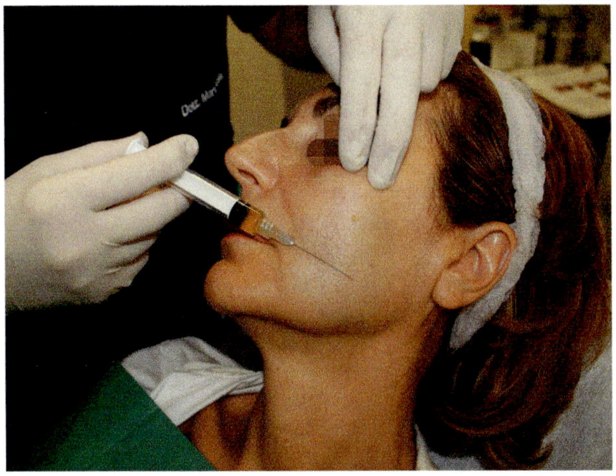

Fig. 17.18 Graphic superficial representation of the route of the cannula. (Published by kind permission of ©Mario Goisis 2018. All Rights Reserved)

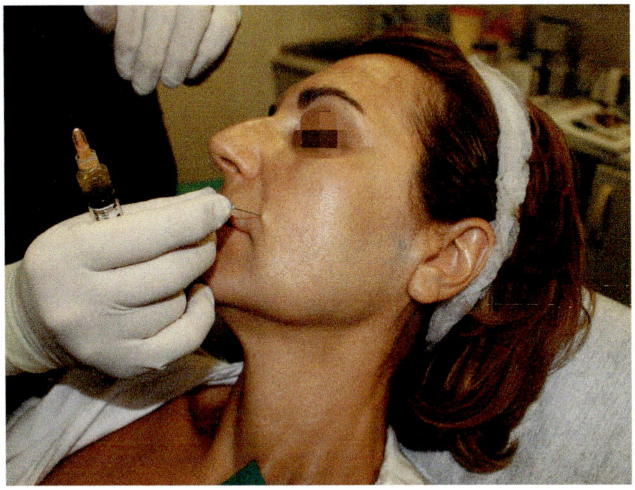

Fig. 17.19 After local anaesthesia, an opening is created inserting a 25-G needle at the base of the level of the modiolus. (Published by kind permission of ©Mario Goisis 2018. All Rights Reserved)

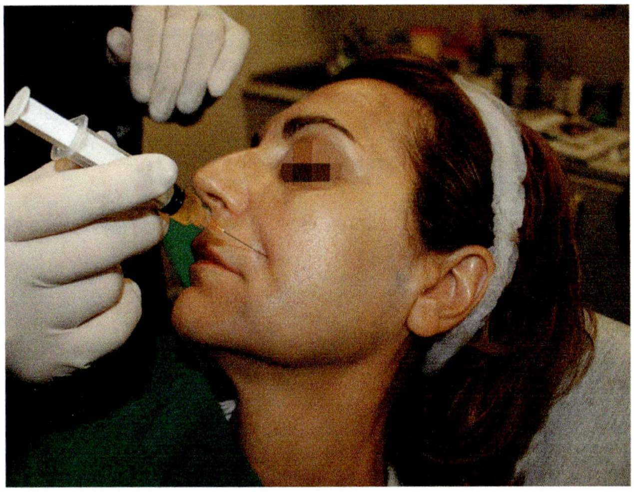

Fig. 17.20 A 27-G blunt-tip cannula is inserted perpendicularly into skin's surface. (Published by kind permission of ©Mario Goisis 2018. All Rights Reserved)

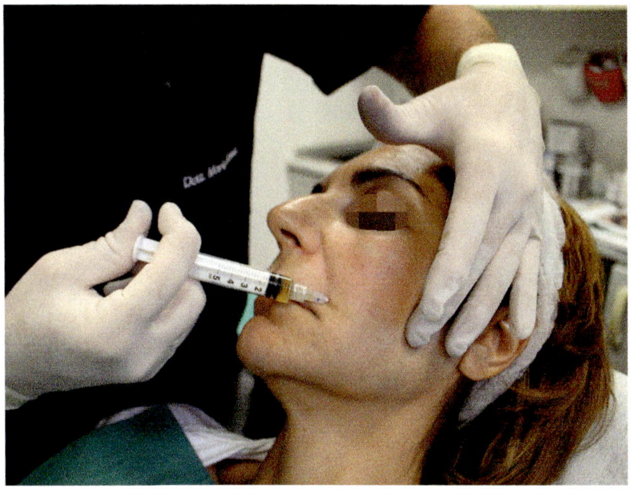

Fig. 17.21 The cannula is then pivoted parallel to the plane of the skin, and the PRP is delivered slowly while the cannula is withdrawn by retrograde injection. (Published by kind permission of ©Mario Goisis 2018. All Rights Reserved)

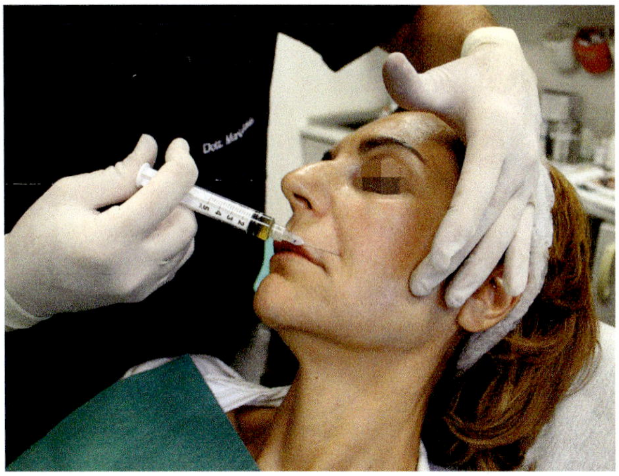

Fig. 17.22 The cannula is then pivoted parallel to plane of the skin, and the PRP is delivered slowly while the cannula is withdrawn by retrograde injection. (Published by kind permission of ©Mario Goisis 2018. All Rights Reserved)

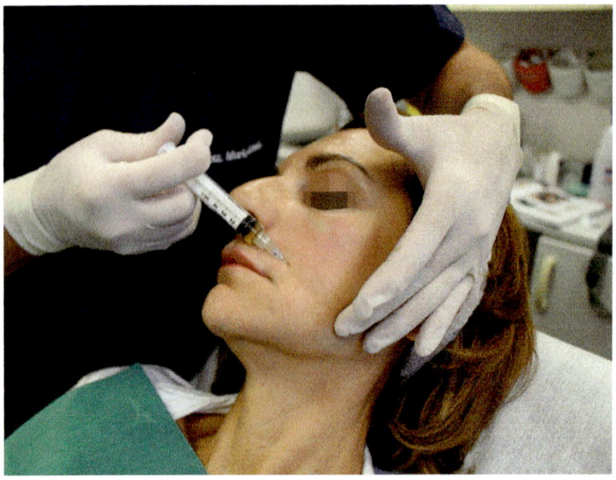

Fig. 17.23 The cannula is then pivoted parallel to plane of the skin, and the PRP is delivered slowly while the cannula is withdrawn by retrograde injection. (Published by kind permission of ©Mario Goisis 2018. All Rights Reserved)

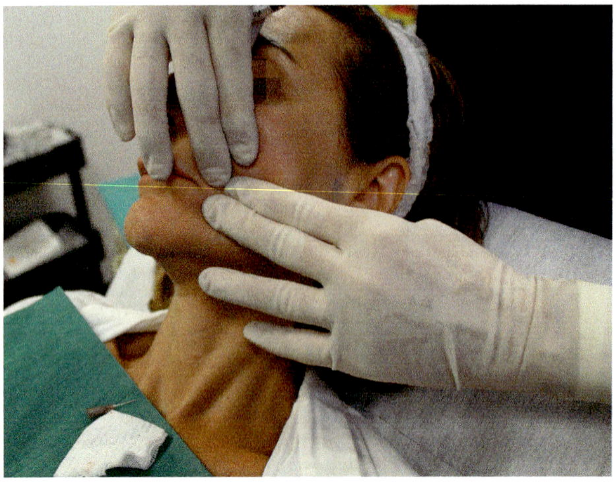

Fig. 17.24 After the treatment, a strong massage is applied to the area. (Published by kind permission of ©Mario Goisis 2018. All Rights Reserved)

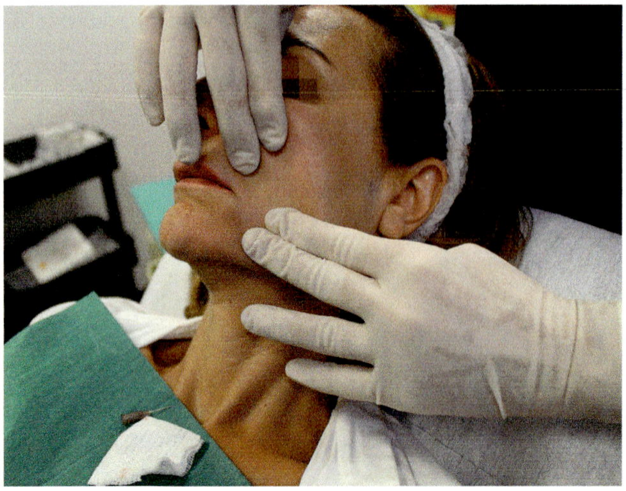

Fig. 17.25 After the treatment, a strong massage is applied to the area. (Published by kind permission of ©Mario Goisis 2018. All Rights Reserved)

17.7 Amelioration of the Cheek using Nanofat

17.7.1 Indications

Amelioration of small wrinkles and laxity of the cheeks. The use of a blunt-tip cannula permits atraumatic dissection of the tissue with placement of the PRP into the subcutaneous plane, as well as the creation of fewer needle entry marks and significantly less pain and bruising.

17.7.2 Contraindications

- The nanofat should not be injected into areas that lack sufficient blood supply or affected by infection or inflammation.
- No injection should be carried out if the area has been previously treated with liquid silicone or other permanent fillers because new injections might lead to inflammation or infection of the implants.

17.7.3 Operating Time

The procedure usually takes from 10 to 15 min, once the nanofat has been produced.

Plane of injection: hypodermis-superficial fat compartment

17.7.4 Indications

Amelioration of small wrinkles and laxness of the cheeks. The use of a blunt-tip cannula permits atraumatic dissection of the tissue with placement of the PRP into the subcutaneous plane, as well as the creation of fewer needle entry marks and significantly less pain and bruising.

17.7.5 Contraindications

- The nanofat should not be injected into areas lacking sufficient blood supply or affected by infection or inflammation.
- No injection should be carried out if the area has been treated previously with liquid silicone or other permanent fillers because new injections might lead to inflammation or infection of the nanofat.

17.7.6 Materials

- *1–2 cc of nanofat on each side for injection of nanofat: 1-2 cc of nanofat for injection into both sides*
  - *A 26-gauge needle.*
  - *A 27-gauge 3.7-cm blunt cannula.*

A standard system for producing nanofat is used, in particular:

- A nanofat system (www.microfat.com), composed of a connector with a closed system for emulsion of microfat and filtration.
- 2 10-cc syringes.

To harvest and process microfat
A standard system is used, in particular:

- A microfat box (www.microfat.com), composed of a ramp with a closed system for washing and filtration.
- 4 60-cc syringes.
- 2 10-cc syringes.
- One 1-cc syringe.
- A 30-gauge needle.
- A 16-gauge needle.
- A 2-mm diameter, 10-cm long Goisis cannula for harvesting the fat.
- A chlorhexidine-alcohol solution (2% chlorhexidine gluconate and 70% isopropyl alcohol), sterile drapes, or towels.
- Ice packs.
- Sterile 2 cm × 2-cm gauze squares.
- Occlusive dressing cover.

Medications include:

100 cc of cold saline solution.
120 cc of cold Klein solution.
1 litre of Klein solution is composed of 800 mg of lidocaine, 1 mg of epinephrine, 40 MEq of sodium bicarbonate, and 1000 cc of saline solution.

Location: The microfat harvesting can be carried out in a small operating theatre/physician's surgery. The oxygen, pulse oximetry, and a crash cart/box should be present.

Assistance: An assistant can prove useful when transferring items to the procedure field in a sterile manner during the first part stage of the procedure. Nevertheless, a single doctor can execute all easily perform the entire procedure the procedure alone.

17.7.7 Methods

Method is shown in Figs. 17.26, 17.27, 17.28, 17.29, 17.30, 17.31, 17.32, 17.33, 17.34, and 17.35.

17.7.8 Cadaver Dissection After an Injection of Nanofat into the Cheeks (Courtesy of the Doctor's Equipe) (Figs. 17.36, 17.37, and 17.38)

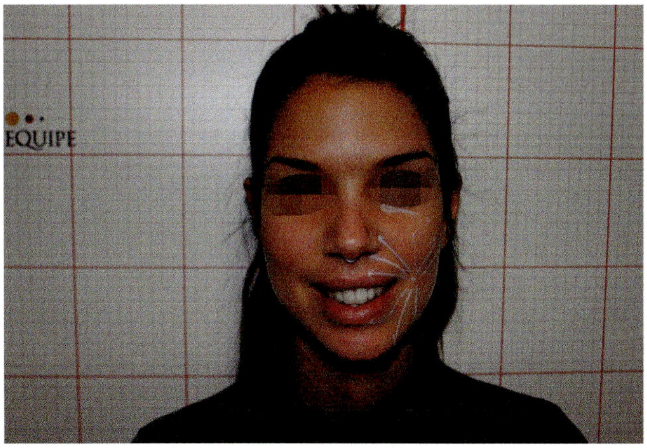

Fig. 17.26 The route of the cannula is drawn on the patient's cheek. (Published by kind permission of ©Mario Goisis 2018. All Rights Reserved)

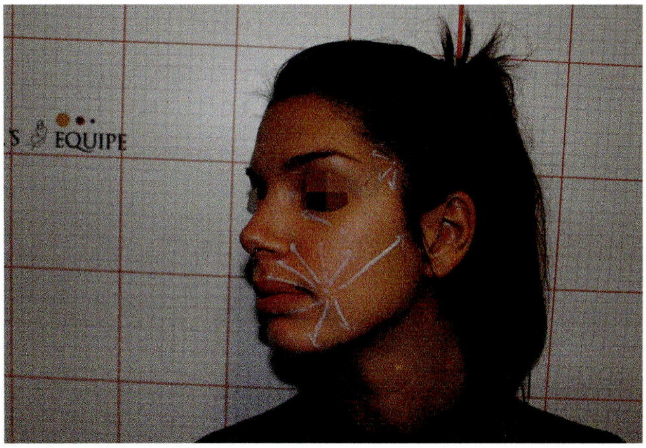

Fig. 17.27 The route of the cannula is drawn on the patient's cheek. (Published by kind permission of ©Mario Goisis 2018. All Rights Reserved)

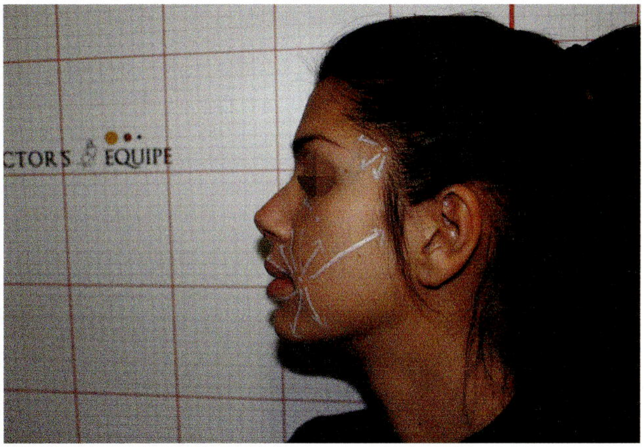

Fig. 17.28 The route of the cannula is drawn on the patient's cheek. (Published by kind permission of ©Mario Goisis 2018. All Rights Reserved)

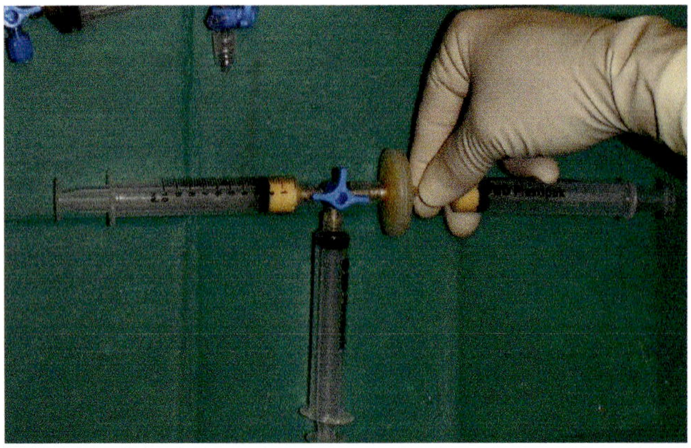

Fig. 17.29 The nanofat is produced using a nanofat kit (www.nanofat.com). (Published by kind permission of ©Mario Goisis 2018. All Rights Reserved)

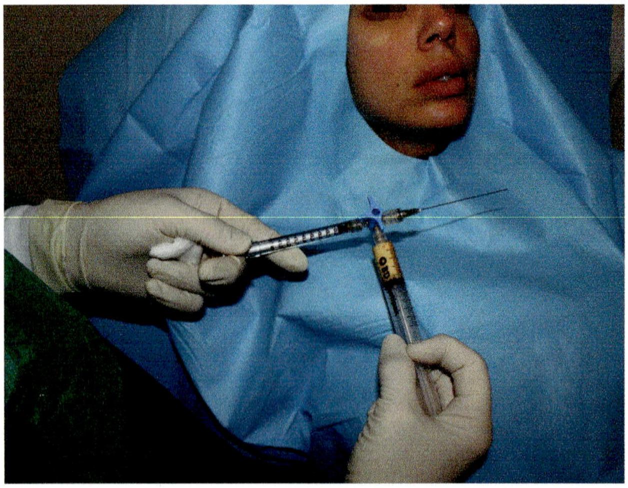

Fig. 17.30 The 10 cc -syringe, filled with nanofat, is connected to a 1 cc syringe. (Published by kind permission of ©Mario Goisis 2018. All Rights Reserved)

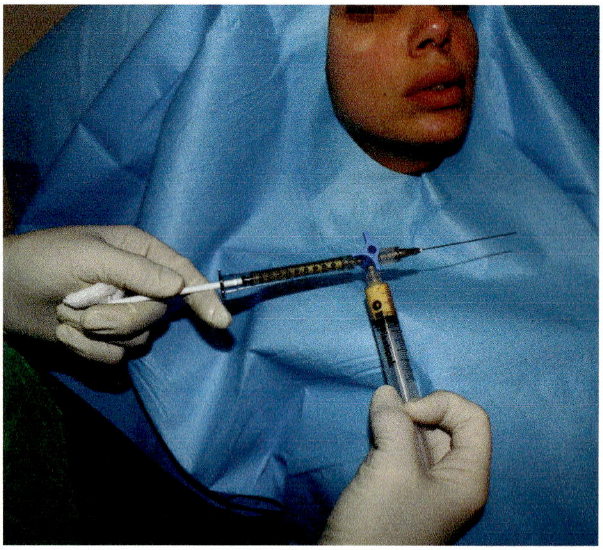

Fig. 17.31 The 1-cc syringe is used to inject the nanofat. (Published by kind permission of ©Mario Goisis 2018. All Rights Reserved)

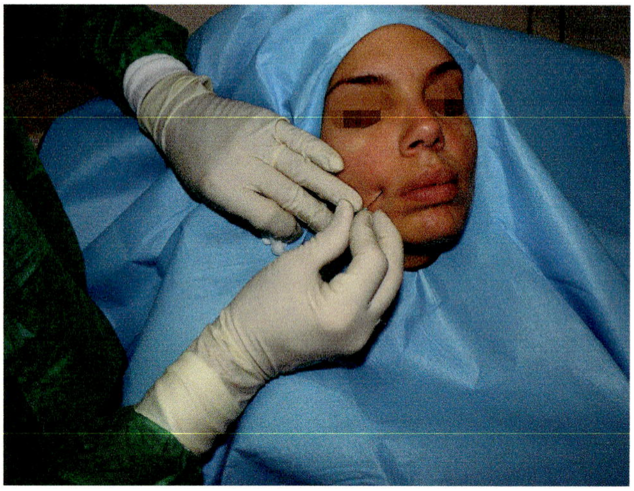

Fig. 17.32 An opening is created at the base of the nasolabial fold using a 25-G needle. (Published by kind permission of ©Mario Goisis 2018. All Rights Reserved)

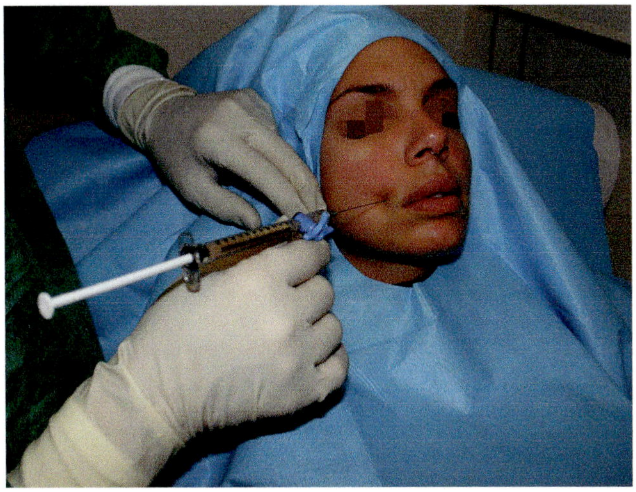

Fig. 17.33 A 27-G blunt-tip cannula is inserted perpendicularly into the skin's surface. (Published by kind permission of ©Mario Goisis 2018. All Rights Reserved)

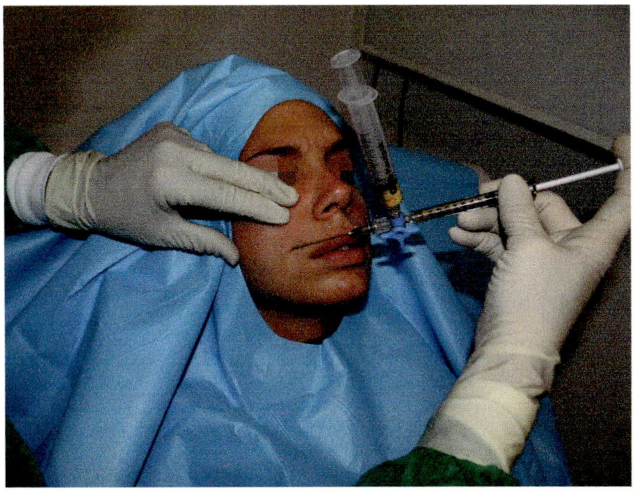

Fig. 17.34 The cannula is then pivoted parallel to the plane of the skin, and the cellular matrix is delivered slowly while the cannula is withdrawn by retrograde injection. (Published by kind permission of ©Mario Goisis 2018. All Rights Reserved)

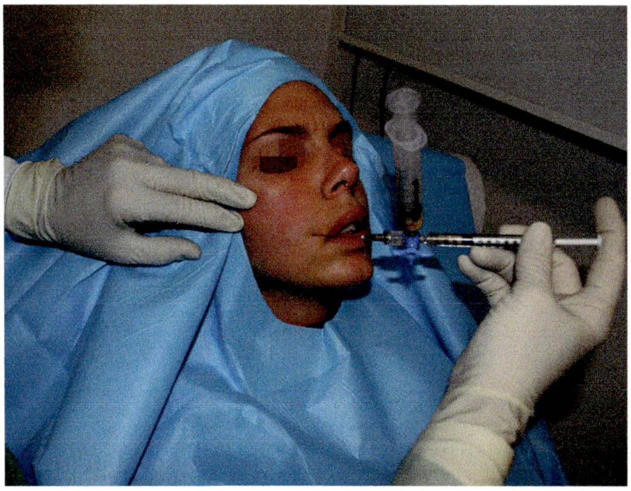

Fig. 17.35 The cannula is then pivoted parallel to the plane of the skin, and the cellular matrix is delivered slowly while the cannula is withdrawn by retrograde injection. (Published by kind permission of ©Mario Goisis 2018. All Rights Reserved)

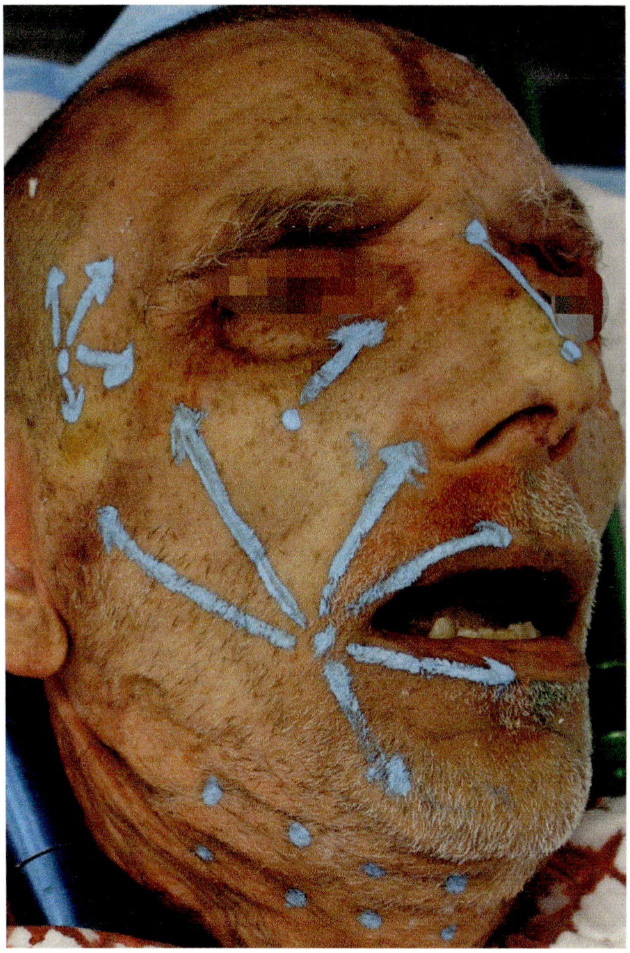

Fig. 17.36 The cheeks are filled with nanofat using a single injection -point localised at the base of the nasolabial folds. (Published by kind permission of ©Mario Goisis 2018. All Rights Reserved)

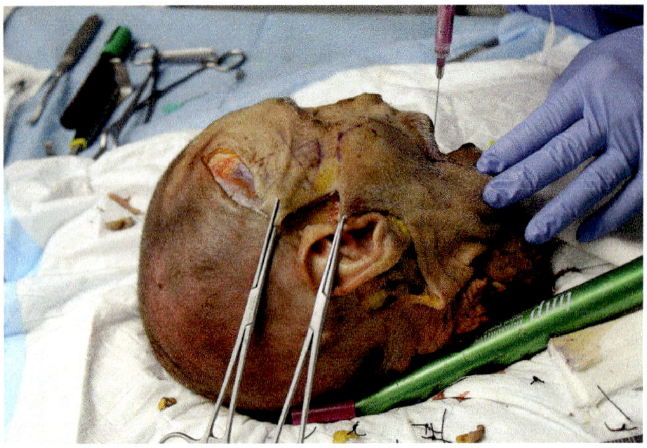

Fig. 17.37 An opening is created using a 25-G needle. A blunt-tip 27-Gcannula is inserted perpendicularly into the skin's surface through the hole created ad hoc. (Published by kind permission of ©Mario Goisis 2018. All Rights Reserved)

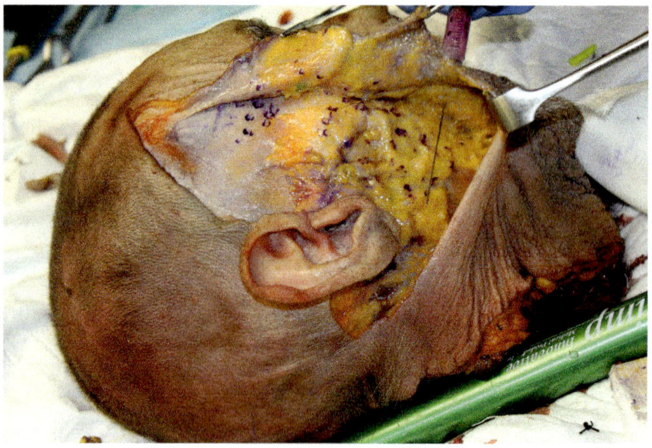

Fig. 17.38 After injection of the nanofat, a midfacial dissection is executed, and the subcutaneous plane is exposed. The presence of the injected cellular matrix is shown in depths in this plane. (Published by kind permission of ©Mario Goisis 2018. All Rights Reserved)

18 The Lips

Mario Goisis, Sara Izzo, and Giovanni Francesco Nicoletti

The lips are a tactile organ which play a vital role in human anatomy and life. Aesthetically, they contribute considerably towards what we perceive as a beautiful face.

18.1 Anatomy

The upper lip extends between the nasolabial folds from the free edge of the vermilion border below the base of the nose. The lower lip extends between the oral commissures from the mandible below the upper free vermilion edge. The vermilion border is composed of nonkeratinized squamous epithelium covering numerous capillaries, which provide the vermilion with its characteristic color. All around the border of the vermilion skin, a fine line of whitish skin accentuates the chromatic difference between the vermilion and the surrounding skin.

A midline depression called the philtrum is located between two raised vertical columns of tissue made of fibres of the orbicularis oris. The philtrum is located between the columella and the paramedian elevations of the vermilion. These two paramedian elevating curves of the vermilion form the so-called Cupid's bow (Figs. 18.1 and 18.2).

18.2 Pitfalls

Injecting fat or PRP into the lips can easily activate the dormant herpes simplex virus in those prone to it who should be on antiviral prophylactic medication when undergoing the treatment. Lit injections have to be tailored to suit

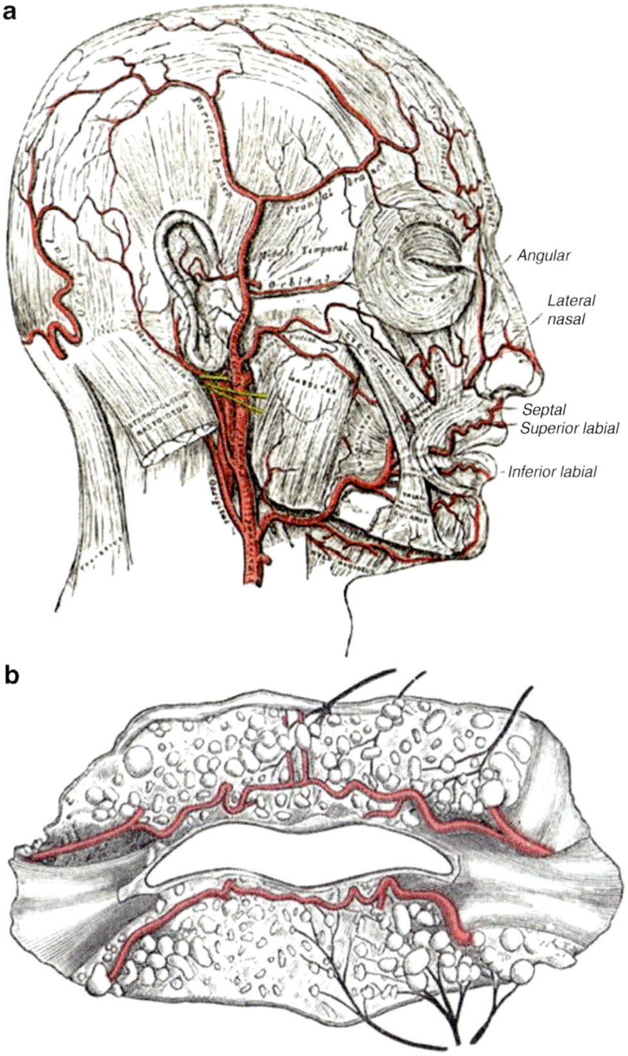

Fig. 18.1 (**a**, **b**) Vascular supply of the lips (Reproduced lithograph plate from Henry Gray, Anatomy: Descriptive and Surgical, in Anatomy of the human body, 20th ed., Lea & Febiger, 1918, Philadelphia, available to Public Domain under Creative Commons CC0 License). (Published by kind permission of ©Mario Goisis 2018. All Rights Reserved)

M. Goisis (✉)
Maxillo-Facial and Aesthetic Surgeon, Go Easy Clinic, Milan, Italy

S. Izzo · G. F. Nicoletti
Department of Plastic Surgery, University of Campania "Luigi Vanvitelli", Naples, Italy
e-mail: giovannif.nicoletti@unicampania.it

M. Goisis (ed.), *Outpatient Regenerative Medicine*, https://doi.org/10.1007/978-3-319-44894-7_18

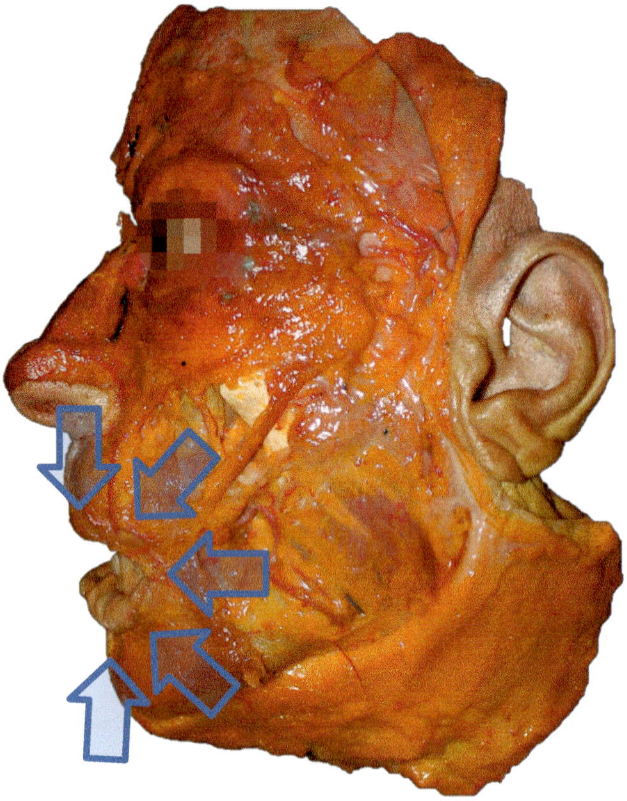

Fig. 18.2 Cadaver dissection shows the orbicularis oris, the main mimic muscle of the lips (blue arrows). The muscle represents the vast majority of the volume of the lips. (Published by kind permission of ©Mario Goisis 2018. All Rights Reserved)

individual patients. Injections along the vermillion border typically enhance the projection of the lip. Injections in the red lip enhance volume. When injecting, it is important to avoid any kind of unnatural look (such as the duckbill look) or unbalanced lips. As regards "central or outer," it is better to inject more centrally than laterally. This is because overzealous lateral injections can make the lips look very unnatural, almost sausage-like. Overfilling or overcorrection of the vermilion border is not recommended. This creates an acute angle at the mucocutaneous junction that appears unnatural.

18.3 Re-shaping the Upper and Lower Lips using Microfat

Lips can be recontoured to retore a youthful appearance by placing microfat into the body of the lips.

18.3.1 Contraindications

- The fat should not be injected in areas that lack sufficient blood supply or that are suffering from an infection or inflammation.
- No injection should be carried out if the lip has been previously treated with liquid silicone or other permanent fillers because new injections might lead to inflammation or infection of the implants.
- Anatomical alterations due to previous trauma or surgical intervention (cleft lip). Scarring often induces retracting scars that can cause asymmetry and unequal filling of the part treated.

18.3.2 Complications and Management

Immediate complications (within 72 h after injection) are transient erythema, oedema, induration, pruritus, and ecchymosis.

Early complications (days to weeks after injection) include overcorrection, local infection, necrosis of the skin, reactivation of herpes, discoloration, and persistent local symptoms (erythema, oedema, induration, pruritus, and hyperpigmentation).

Later or delayed complications include high rates of fat resorption and cyst.

18.3.3 Materials

- *2–4 cc of microfat on each side for injection of microfat: 2–4 cc of microfat per side*
  - *A 21-gauge needle*
  - *A 22-gauge 4 cm blunt cannula*

To harvest and process microfat:

A standard system is used, in particular:

- A microfat box (www.microfat.com), composed of a ramp with a closed system for washing and filtration
- 4 60-cc syringes
- 2 10-cc syringes
- One 1-cc syringe
- A 30-gauge needle
- A 16-gauge needle
- A 2-mm diameter, 10-cm-long Goisis cannula for fat harvesting
- A chlorhexidine-alcohol solution (2% chlorhexidine gluconate and 70% isopropyl alcohol), sterile drapes, or towels
- Ice packs
- Sterile 2 cm × 2 cm gauze squares
- Occlusive dressing cover

Medications include:

100 cc of cold saline solution.
120 cc of cold Klein solution.
1 litre of Klein solution is composed of 800 mg of lidocaine, 1 mg of epinephrine, 40 MEq of sodium bicarbonate, and 1000 cc of saline solution.

Location: Microfat harvesting can be carried out in a small operating theatre/doctor's surgery. The oxygen, pulse oximetry, and a crash cart/box should be present.

Assistance: An assistant can prove useful when transferring items to the procedure field in a sterile manner during the first stage of the procedure. Nevertheless, a doctor can carry out the entire procedure single-handed.

18.3.4 Operating Time

Once the fat has been harvested, the procedure usually takes 10 min.

Plane of injection: intramuscular

18.3.5 Method

The procedure is shown in Figs. 18.3, 18.4, 18.5, 18.6, 18.7, 18.8, 18.9, 18.10, 18.11, 18.12, 18.13, 18.14, 18.15, 18.16, and 18.17 (augmentation of the body of the lips by means of injections of micrograft)

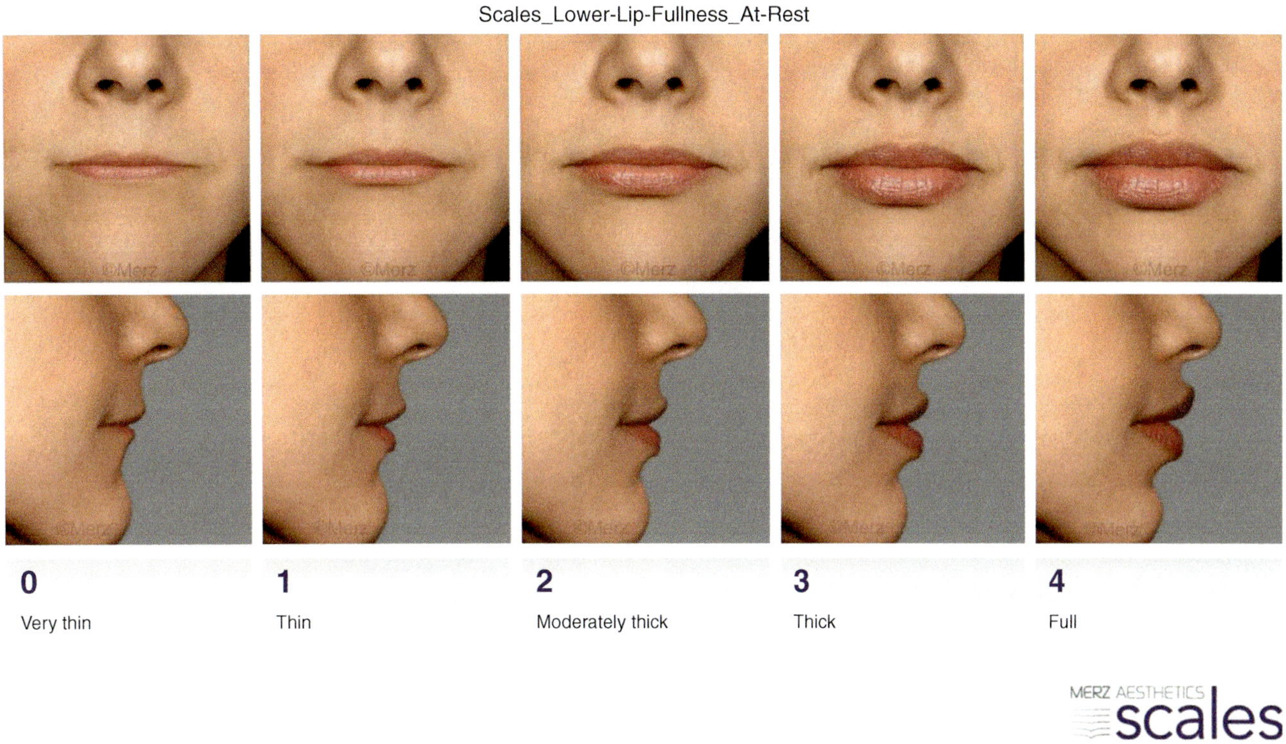

Fig. 18.3 Different dimensions of lip (courtesy by Merz Company). (Published by kind permission of ©Mario Goisis 2018. All Rights Reserved)

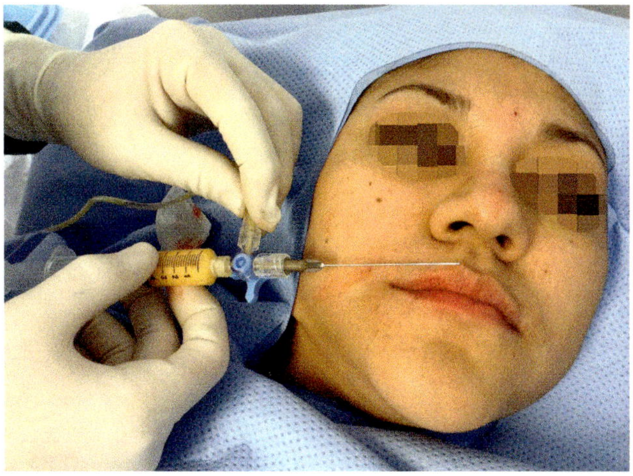

Fig. 18.4 The route of the cannula on the upper lip. (Published by kind permission of ©Mario Goisis 2018. All Rights Reserved)

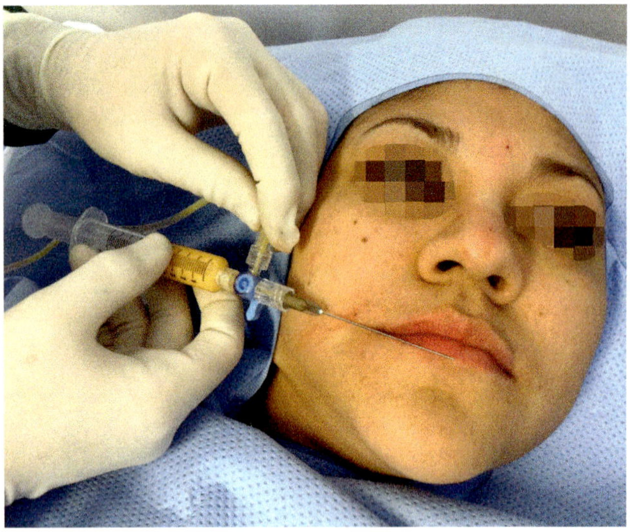

Fig. 18.5 The route of the cannula on the lip. (Published by kind permission of ©Mario Goisis 2018. All Rights Reserved)

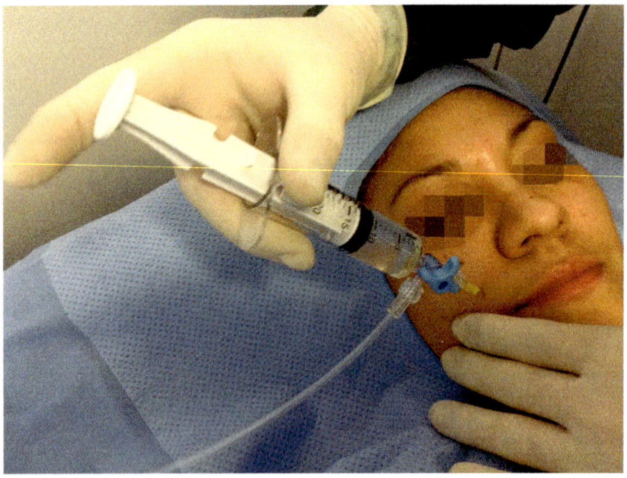

Fig. 18.6 Anesthesia is performed through the entry-point at the base of the nasolabial fold, 1.5–2 cm laterally to the oral rim, with 0.5 cc of Klein solution. (Published by kind permission of ©Mario Goisis 2018. All Rights Reserved)

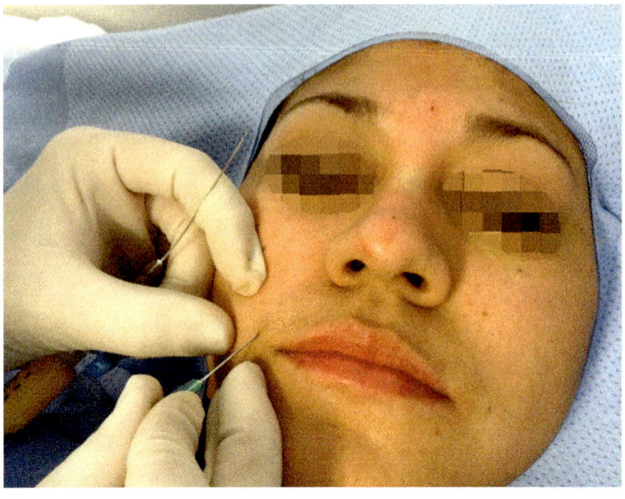

Fig. 18.7 An opening is created using a 21-G needle. (Published by kind permission of ©Mario Goisis 2018. All Rights Reserved)

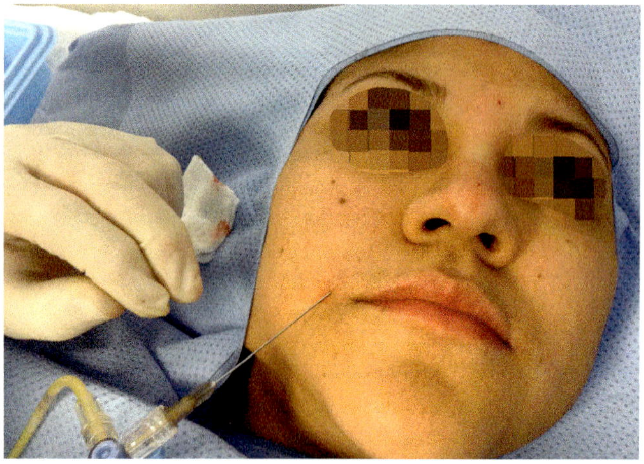

Fig. 18.8 A blunt-tip 22-G cannula is inserted under the plane of the skin through the hole created. (Published by kind permission of ©Mario Goisis 2018. All Rights Reserved)

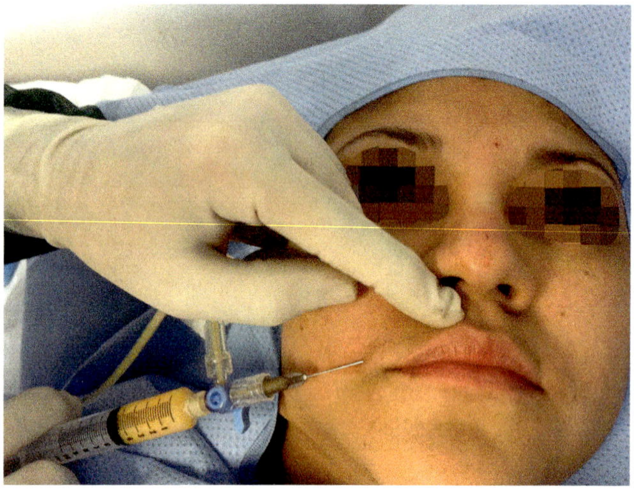

Fig. 18.9 The cannula is then pivoted parallel to the plane of the skin and slid with the utmost precision along and just above the border of the vermilion. (Published by kind permission of ©Mario Goisis 2018. All Rights Reserved)

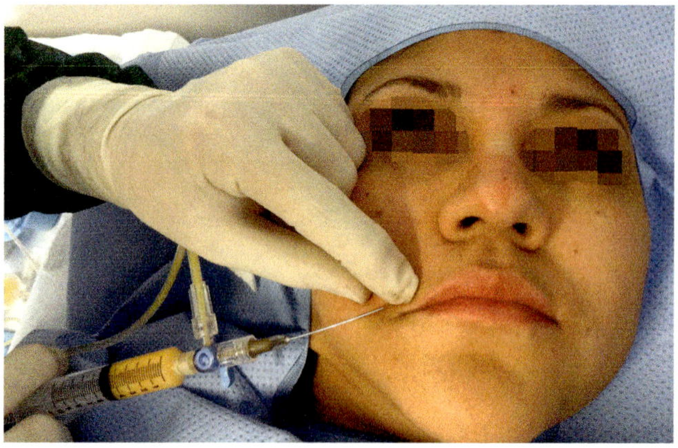

Fig. 18.10 The microfat is released, retrograde fashion, into the body of the upper lip. (Published by kind permission of ©Mario Goisis 2018. All Rights Reserved)

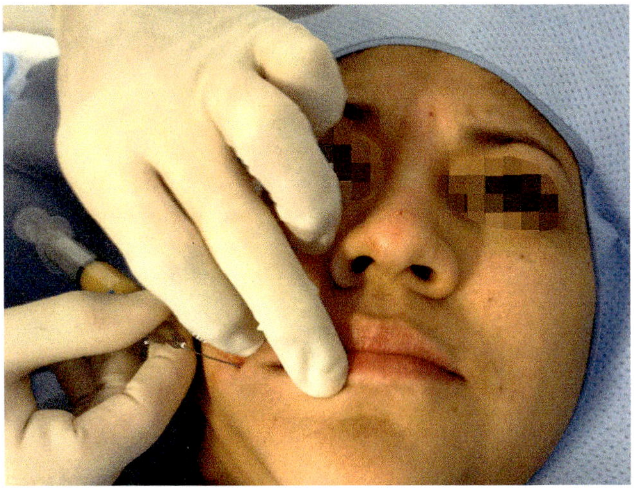

Fig. 18.11 The cannula is slid with the utmost precision along the border of vermilion, just below it. (Published by kind permission of ©Mario Goisis 2018. All Rights Reserved)

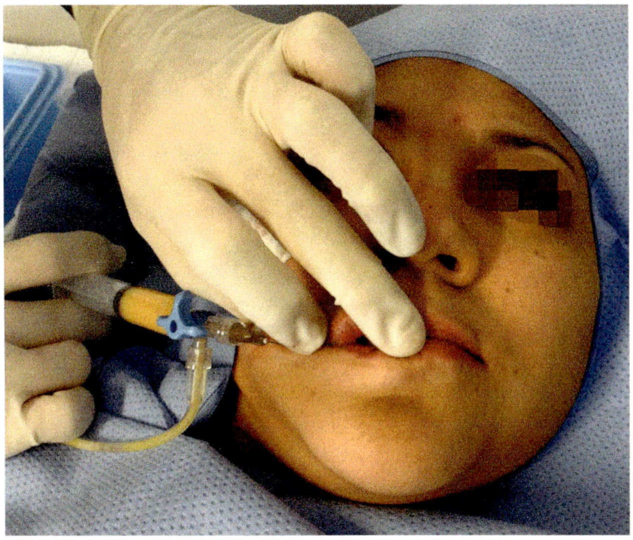

Fig. 18.12 The cannula is slid medially. (Published by kind permission of ©Mario Goisis 2018. All Rights Reserved)

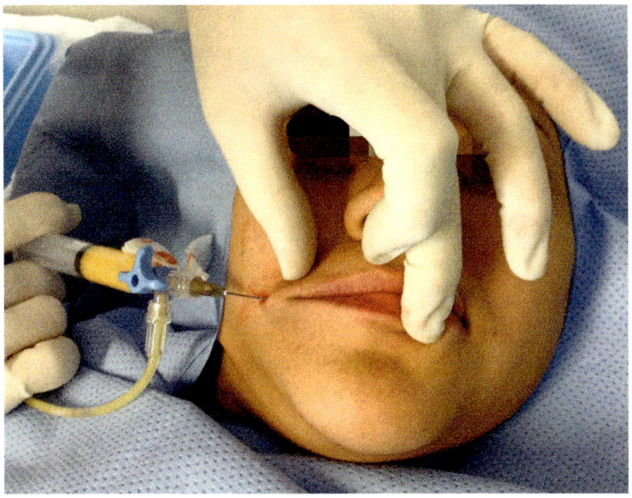

Fig. 18.13 The microfat is released, retrograde fashion, into the body of the lower lip. (Published by kind permission of ©Mario Goisis 2018. All Rights Reserved)

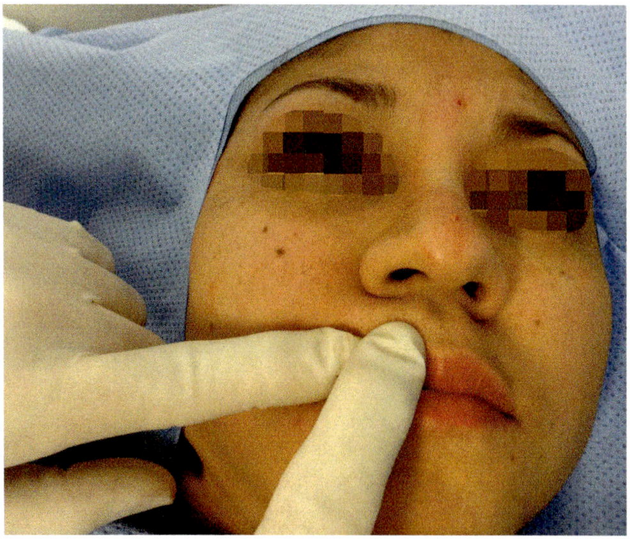

Fig. 18.14 After the treatment, the upper lip is massaged. (Published by kind permission of ©Mario Goisis 2018. All Rights Reserved)

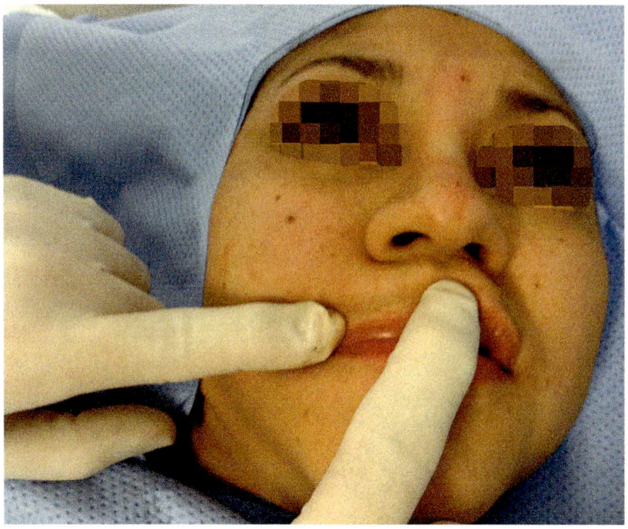

Fig. 18.15 Upper lip massage

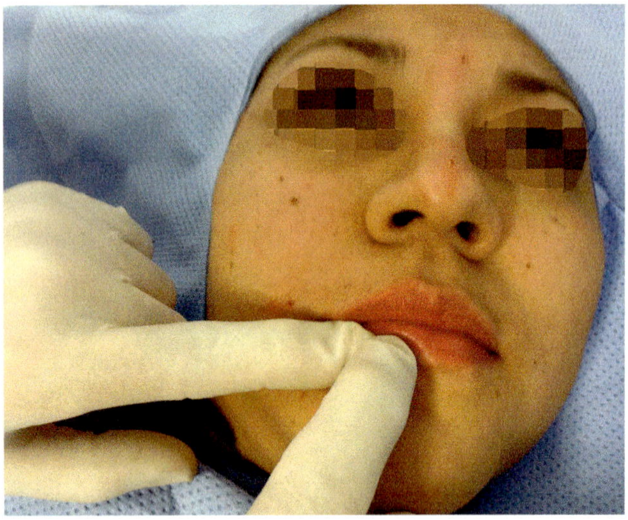

Fig. 18.16 After the treatment, the lower lip is massaged. (Published by kind permission of ©Mario Goisis 2018. All Rights Reserved)

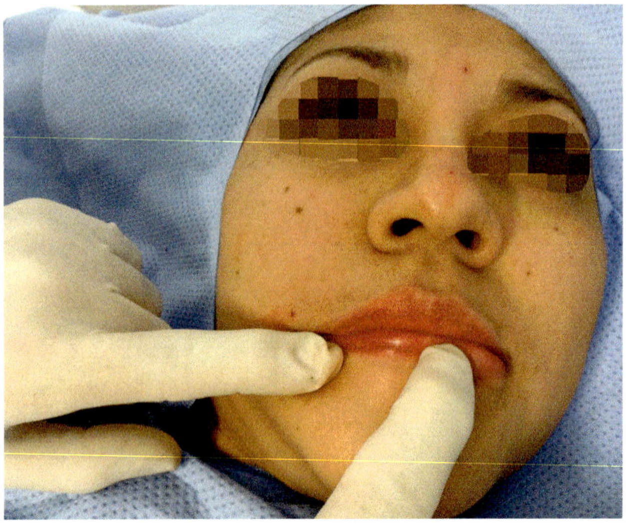

Fig. 18.17 Massage. (Published by kind permission of ©Mario Goisis 2018. All Rights Reserved)

18.3.6 Cadaver Dissection After Lip Augmentation using Microfat (Courtesy of the Doctor's Equipe) (Figs. 18.18, 18.19, 18.20, 18.21, and 18.22)

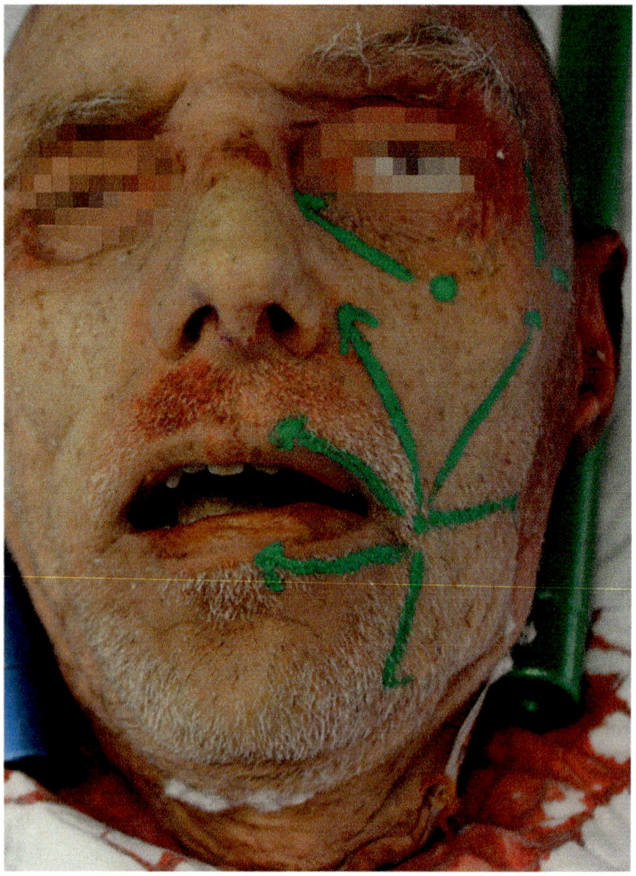

Fig. 18.18 Lips are augmented using a single entry-point located 1.5–2 cm laterally to the oral rim (courtesy of the Doctor's Equipe). (Published by kind permission of ©Mario Goisis 2018. All Rights Reserved)

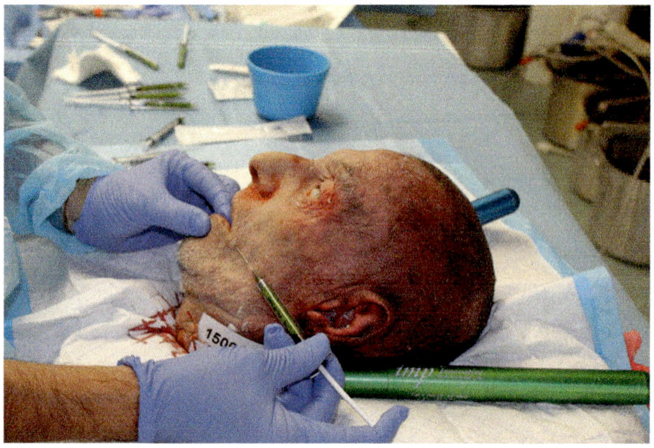

Fig. 18.19 The cannula is pivoted and colored fat-graft injected in the cadaver lip. (Published by kind permission of ©Mario Goisis 2018. All Rights Reserved)

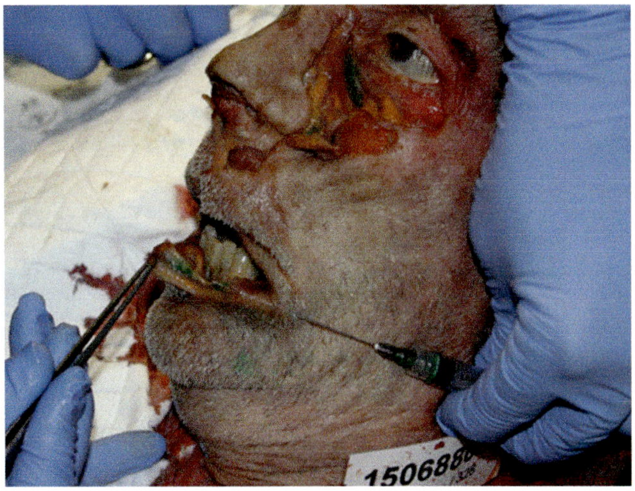

Fig. 18.20 Full-thickness dissection of the lower lip shows the relationship between the tip of the cannula and the lip's muscular plane. (Published by kind permission of ©Mario Goisis 2018. All Rights Reserved)

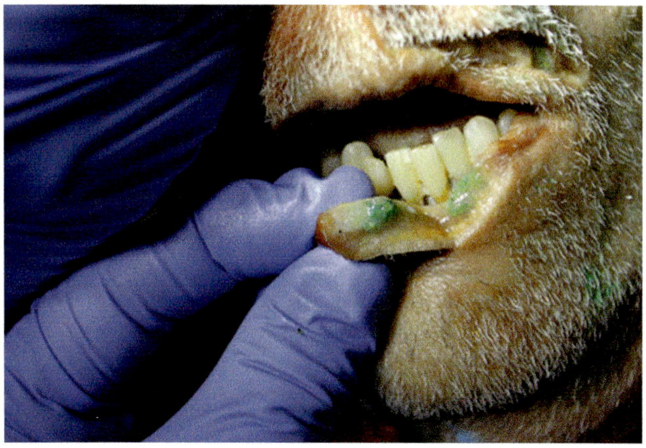

Fig. 18.22 The colored fat appears inside the deep muscular plane. (Published by kind permission of ©Mario Goisis 2018. All Rights Reserved)

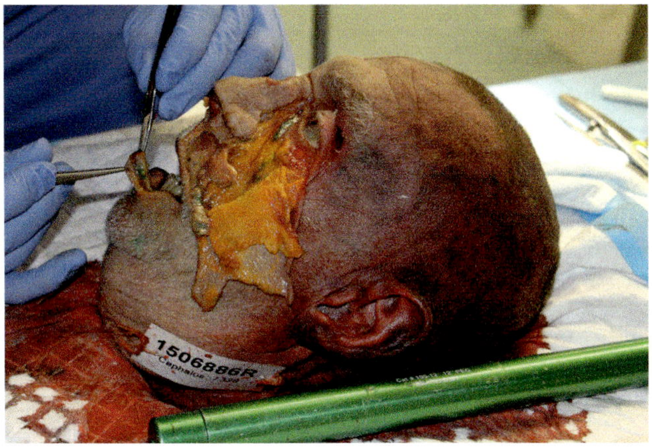

Fig. 18.21 Upon closer inspection, the colored fat appears inside the deep muscular plane, near the mucosal layer. (Published by kind permission of ©Mario Goisis 2018. All Rights Reserved)

18.4 Recontouring of the Lip using Nanofat

Lips can be recontoured to restore a youthful appearance by placing nanofat along their borders (vermillion). Redefinition of this edge with fat produces a more youthful and appealing appearance.

18.4.1 Contraindications

- The nanofat should not be injected in areas that lack sufficient blood supply or suffering from infection or inflammation.
- No injection should be per formed if the lip has been previously treated with liquid silicone or other permanent fillers because new injections might lead to inflammation or infection of the implants.
- Anatomical alterations due to previous trauma or surgical intervention (cleft lip). Scarring often induces retracting scars that can cause asymmetry and unequal filling of the part treated.

18.4.2 Materials

- *1–2 cc of nanofat on each side for injection of nanofat: [1–2 cc of nanofat for injection on both sides]*
  - *A 26-gauge needle*
  - *A blunt 27-gauge, 3.7-cm [blunt] cannula*

A standard system for producing nanofat is used, in particular:

- The Nanofat system (www.microfat.com), composed of a connector with a closed system for emulsion of microfat and filtration
- 2 10-cc syringes

To harvest and process microfat:
A standard system for microfat is used, in particular:

- A Microfat box (www.microfat.com), composed of a ramp with a closed system for washing and filtration
- 4 60-cc syringes
- 2 10-cc syringes
- One 1-cc syringe
- A 30-gauge needle
- A 16-gauge needle
- A 2-mm diameter, 10-cm-long Goisis cannula for fat harvesting
- A chlorhexidine-alcohol solution (2% chlorhexidine gluconate and 70% isopropyl alcohol), sterile drapes, or towels
- Ice packs
- Sterile 2 cm × 2 cm gauze squares
- Occlusive dressing cover

Medications include:

100 cc of cold saline solution.
120 cc of cold Klein solution.
1 litre of Klein solution is composed of 800 mg of lidocaine, 1 mg of epinephrine, 40 MEq of sodium bicarbonate, and 1000 cc of saline solution.

Location: The microfat harvesting can be carried out in a small/medical-consultancy operating theatre. The oxygen, pulse oximetry, and a crash cart/box should be present.

Assistance: An assistant can prove of use when transferring items to the procedure field in a sterile manner during the first stage of the procedure. Nonetheless, a single doctor can the entire procedure alone.

18.4.3 Operating Time

Once the fat has been harvested, the procedure usually takes 10 min.

18.4.4 Method

18.5 Correction of the "Bar Code" using Nanofat (Figs. 18.23, 18.24, 18.25, 18.26, 18.27, 18.28, 18.29, 18.30, 18.31, 18.32)

The so-called "Bar code" can be ameliorated by placing nanofat into the subcutaneous plane. Redefinition of the bar code produces a more youthful and appealing appearance.

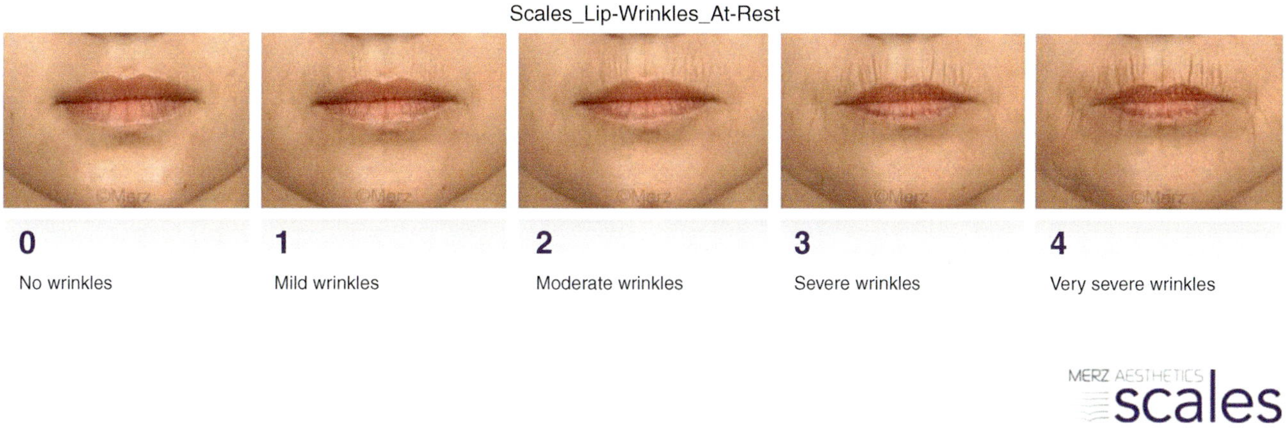

Fig. 18.23 Lip wrinkle ("bar code") classification (courtesy of the Merz company). (Published by kind permission of ©Mario Goisis 2018. All Rights Reserved)

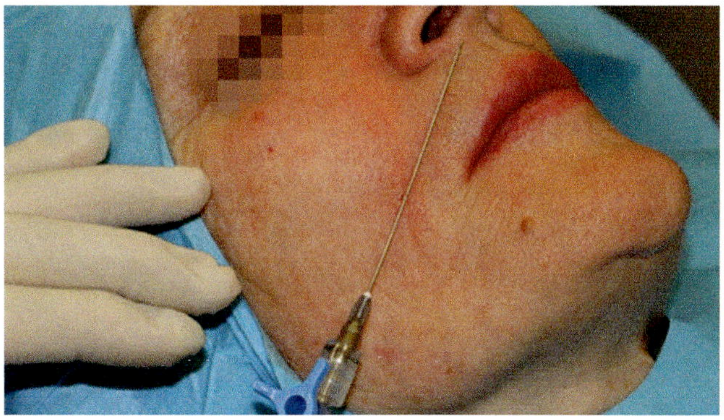

Fig. 18.24 The route of the cannula along the upper lip. (Published by kind permission of ©Mario Goisis 2018. All Rights Reserved)

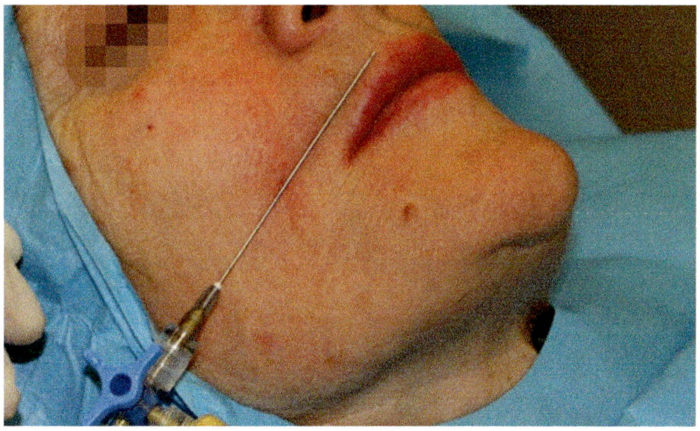

Fig. 18.25 The route of the cannula. (Published by kind permission of ©Mario Goisis 2018. All Rights Reserved)

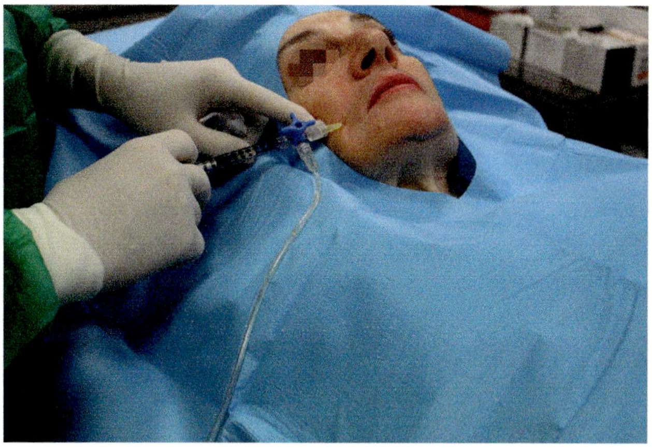

Fig. 18.26 Anesthesia is injected into the entry-point at the level of the modiolus, with 0.2 cc of local anesthetic (lidocaine, mepivacaine) with adrenaline. (Published by kind permission of ©Mario Goisis 2018. All Rights Reserved)

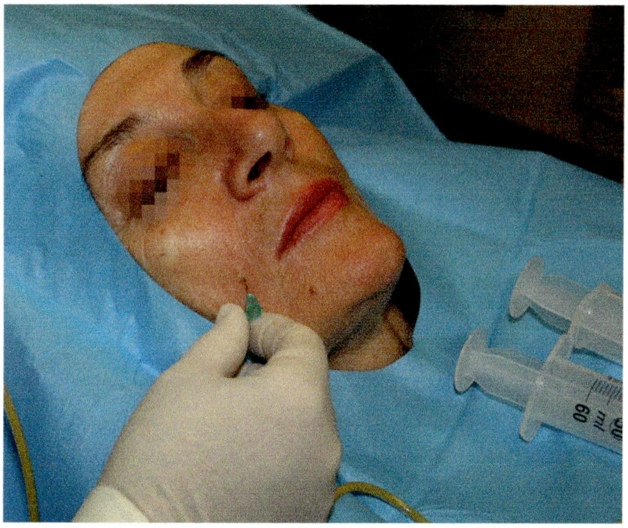

Fig. 18.27 An opening is created using a 21-G needle. (Published by kind permission of ©Mario Goisis 2018. All Rights Reserved)

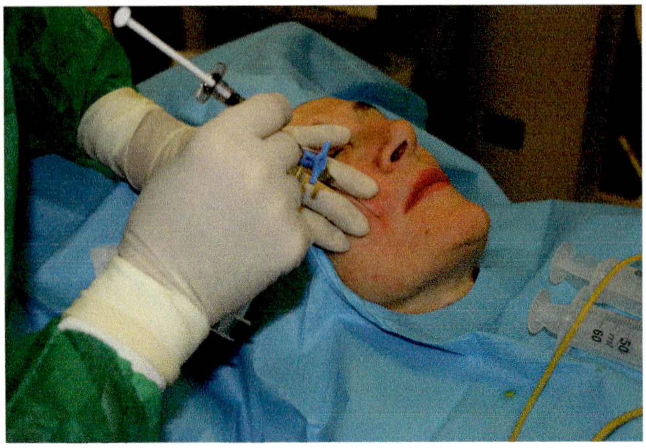

Fig. 18.28 A 22-G, blunt-tip cannula is inserted perpendicularly to the plane of the skin through the hole created for that purpose. (Published by kind permission of ©Mario Goisis 2018. All Rights Reserved)

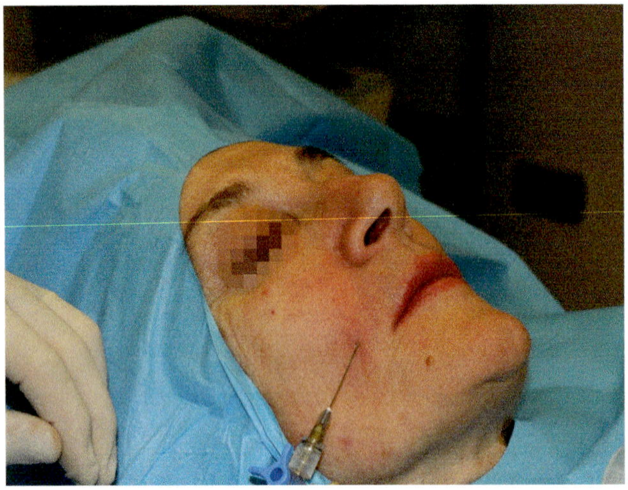

Fig. 18.29 The cannula is then pivoted parallel to the plane of the skin and slid with the utmost precision along the subcutaneous plane (Published by kind permission of ©Mario Goisis 2018. All Rights Reserved)

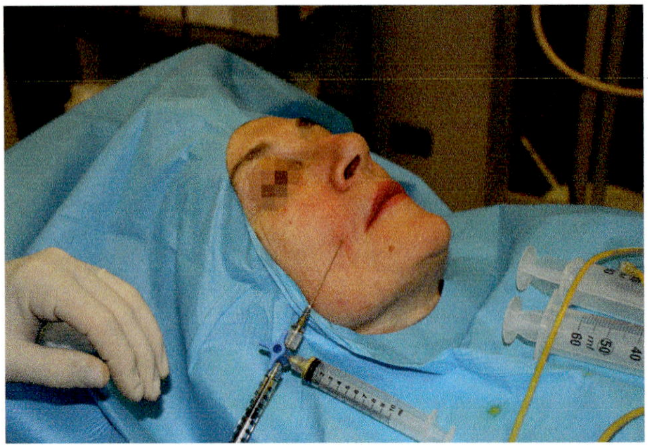

Fig. 18.30 The nanofat is released, retrograde fashion, into the subcutaneous plane. (Published by kind permission of ©Mario Goisis 2018. All Rights Reserved).

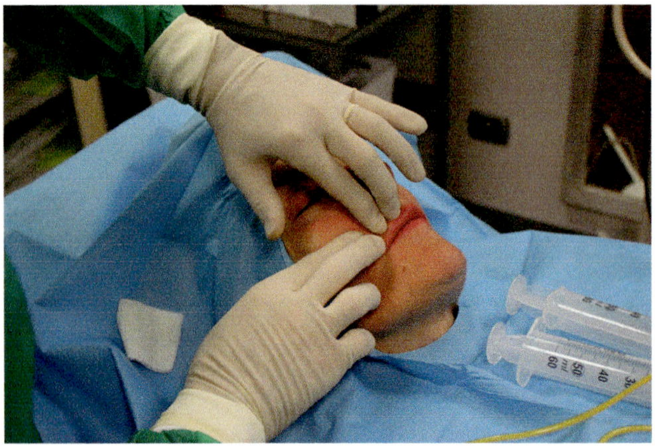

Fig. 18.31 After the treatment the area is massaged. (Published by kind permission of ©Mario Goisis 2018. All Rights Reserved)

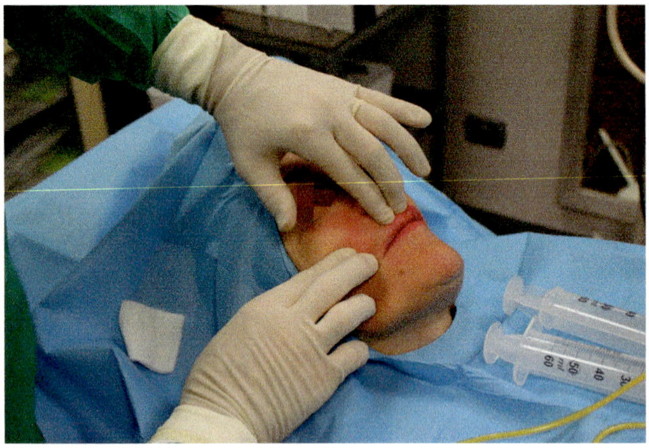

Fig. 18.32 Massage. (Published by kind permission of ©Mario Goisis 2018. All Rights Reserved)

18.5.1 Contraindications

- The nanofat should not be injected in areas that lack sufficient blood supply or suffering from infection or inflammation.
- No injection should performed if the area has been previously treated with liquid silicone or other permanent fillers because new injections might lead to inflammation or infection of the implants.
- Anatomical alterations due to previous trauma or surgical intervention. Scarring often induces retracting scars that can cause asymmetry and unequal filling of the part treated.

18.5.2 Materials

- *1–2 cc of nanofat on each side for injection of nanofat: [1–2 cc of microfat for injection either side]*
  - *A 26-gauge needle*
  - *A 27-gauge 3.7 cm blunt cannula*

A standard system for producing nanofat is used, in particular:

- The Nanofat system (www.microfat.com), composed of a connector with a closed system for emulsion of microfat and filtration
- 2 10-cc syringes

To harvest and process microfat:
A standard system is used, in particular:

- A Microfat box (www.microfat.com), composed of a ramp with a closed system for washing and filtration
- 4 60-cc syringes
- 2 10-cc syringes
- One 1-cc syringe 1 cc
- A 30-gauge needle
- A 16-gauge needle
- A 2-mm-diameter, 10-cm-long Goisis cannula for fat harvesting
- A chlorhexidine-alcohol solution (2% chlorhexidine gluconate and 70% isopropyl alcohol), sterile drapes, or towels
- Ice packs
- Sterile 2 cm × 2cm gauze squares
- Occlusive dressing cover

Medications include:

100 cc of cold saline solution.
120 cc of cold Klein solution.
1 litre of Klein solution is composed of 800 mg of lidocaine, 1 mg of epinephrine, 40 MEq of sodium bicarbonate, and 1000 cc of saline solution.

Location: The microfat may be harvested done in a small/medical-consultancy operating theatre. The oxygen, pulse oximetry, and a crash cart/box should be present.

Assistance: An assistant can prove useful when transferring items to the procedure field in a sterile manner during the first phase of the procedure. Nonetheless, a single doctor can perform the entire procedure alone.

18.5.3 Operating Time

Once the fat has been harvested, the procedure usually takes 10 min.
Plane of injection: subcutaneous

18.5.4 Method

18.6 Recontouring the lips using PRP (Figs. 18.33, 18.34, 18.35, 18.36, 18.37, 18.38, and 18.39)

Lips can be recontoured to restore a youthful look by injecting gel along the borders of the (vermillion). Redefining this edge with natural fillers creates a more youthful and appealing appearance.

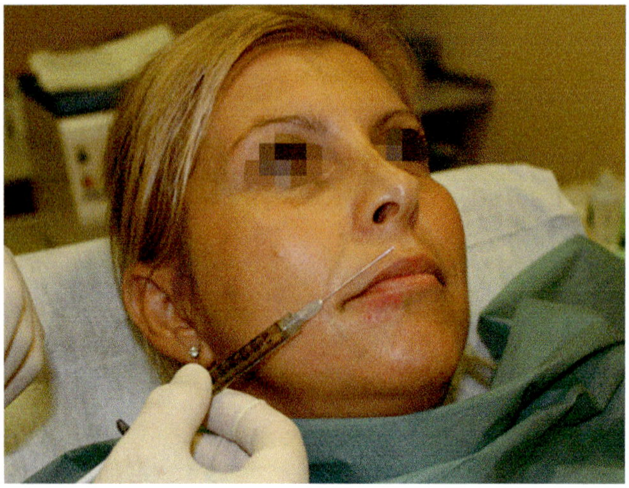

Fig. 18.33 The route of the cannula along the upper lip. (Published by kind permission of ©Mario Goisis 2018. All Rights Reserved)

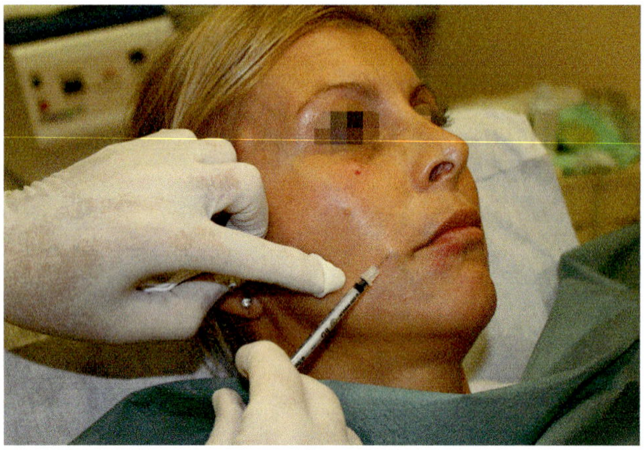

Fig. 18.34 Anaesthesia is injected into the entry-point at the level of the modiolus, with 0.2 cc of local anesthetic (lidocaine, mepivacaine) with adrenaline. (Published by kind permission of ©Mario Goisis 2018. All Rights Reserved)

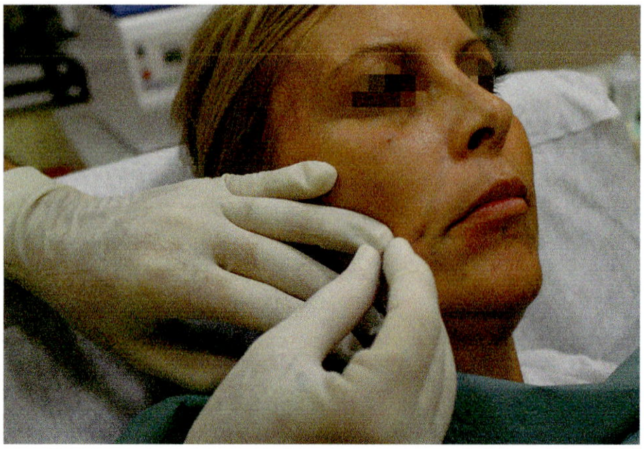

Fig. 18.35 An opening is created using a 26-G needle. (Published by kind permission of ©Mario Goisis 2018. All Rights Reserved)

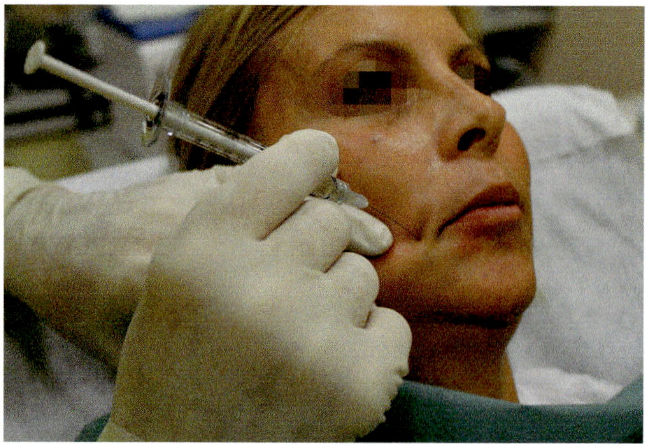

Fig. 18.36 The cannula is then pivoted parallel to the plane of the skin and slid with the utmost precision along the border of vermilion, below it. (Published by kind permission of ©Mario Goisis 2018. All Rights Reserved)

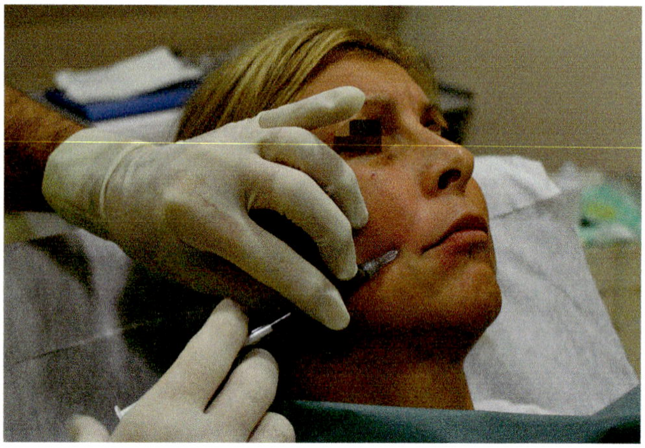

Fig. 18.37 The PRP is delivered slowly. (Published by kind permission of ©Mario Goisis 2018. All Rights Reserved)

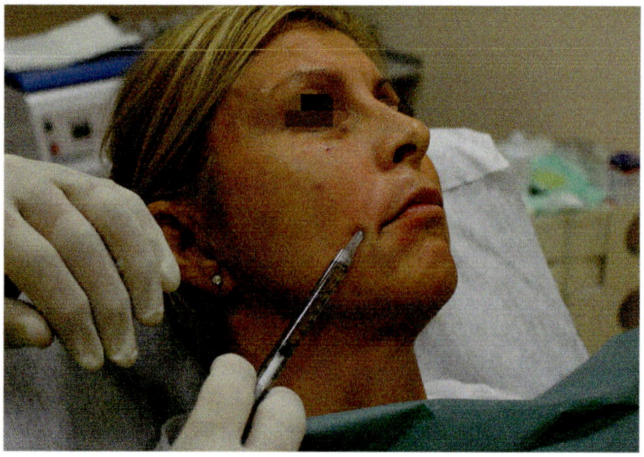

Fig. 18.38 The cannula is withdrawn by retrograde injection. (Published by kind permission of ©Mario Goisis 2018. All Rights Reserved)

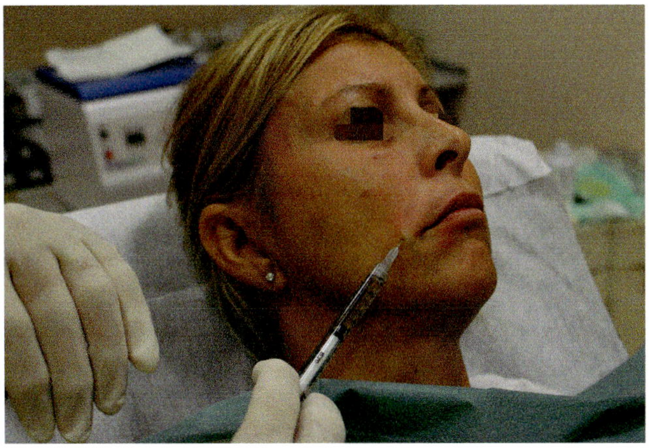

Fig. 18.39 The PRP is delivered. (Published by kind permission of ©Mario Goisis 2018. All Rights Reserved)

18.6.1 Contraindications

- The PRP should not be injected into areas suffering from infection or inflammation.
- No injection should be carried out if the area has been previously treated with liquid silicone or other permanent fillers because new injections might lead to inflammation or infection of the implants.
- Anatomical alterations due to previous trauma or surgical intervention (cleft lip). Scarring often induces retracting scars that can cause asymmetry and unequal filling of the part treated.

18.6.2 Materials

- 1–2 cc of PRP
- A 27-G cannula
- A 26-G needle
- 0.2 cc of local anaesthetic (2% lidocaine, 2% mepivacaine) with epinephrine 1:100 000
- Bandages and antiseptic solution

18.6.3 Operating Time

Once the PRP has been harvested, the procedure usually takes 10 min.

18.6.4 Method

The procedure is shown in.

Chin

19

Mario Goisis, Giuseppe A. Ferraro, Sara Izzo,
Giovanni Francesco Nicoletti, and Rand S. Al Yahya

The dimension and projection of the chin perform a key role in facial aesthetics. Aesthetic medicine plays an important role in the correction of the chin by augmentation and camouflage of the chin's asymmetry.

Ageing of the lower third of the face is associated with increased deepening of marionette lines (Fig. 19.1).

19.1 Anatomy

The chin is the triangular extension of the anterior portion of the mandible situated just below the lower lip. It is formed by the anterior projection of the lower jaw (mandible). The muscle components of the chin are the mentalis, depressor labii inferioris, and depressor anguli oris muscles (Figs. 19.2, 19.3 and 19.4).

19.2 Pitfalls

The noble structures can be preserved using the correct point of injection (safe point). Damage to the mental nerve will lead to loss of sensation in the lower lip. The nerve can easily be identified through palpation of the mental foramen that is situated 1 cm superior to the inferior mandibular border between the first and second premolar teeth (Fig. 19.5). To inject fat or filler into the chin with a sharp needle, we recommend using three injection points: the centre of the mandibular symphysis and, on each side, at a point situated medial to the mental foramen and around 1 cm to the side of the centre of the symphysis.

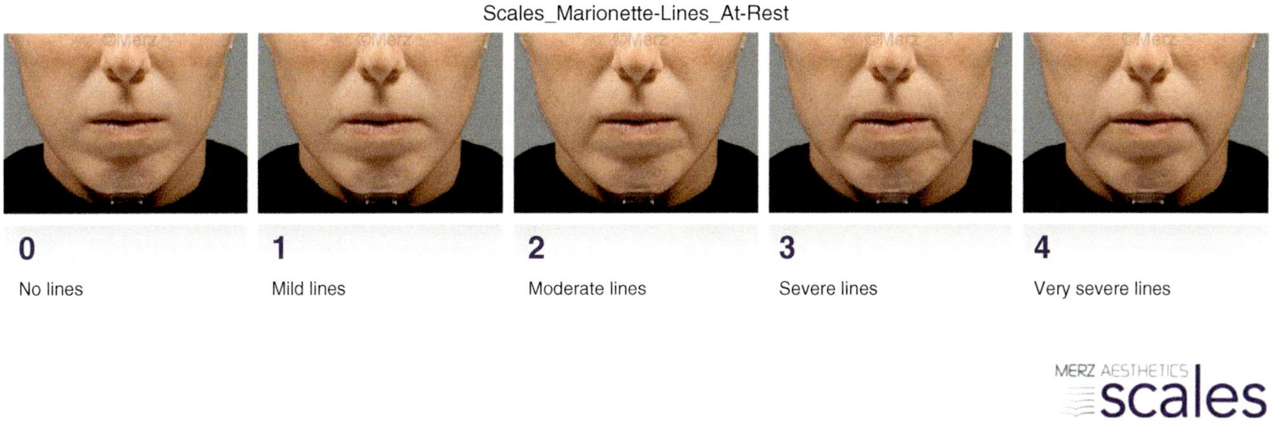

Fig. 19.1 Marionette lines at rest, from none to very severe (courtesy of the Merz company). (Published by kind permission of ©Mario Goisis 2018. All Rights Reserved)

M. Goisis (✉)
Maxillo-Facial and Aesthetic Surgeon, Go Easy Clinic, Milan, Italy

G. A. Ferraro (✉) · S. Izzo · G. F. Nicoletti
Department of Plastic Surgery, University of Campania "Luigi Vanvitelli", Naples, Italy
e-mail: giuseppe.ferraro@unicampania.it; giovannifrancesco.nicoletti@unicampania.it

R. S. Al Yahya
Prince Sattam Bin Abdulaziz University, Al Kharj, Saudi Arabia

M. Goisis (ed.), *Outpatient Regenerative Medicine*, https://doi.org/10.1007/978-3-319-44894-7_19

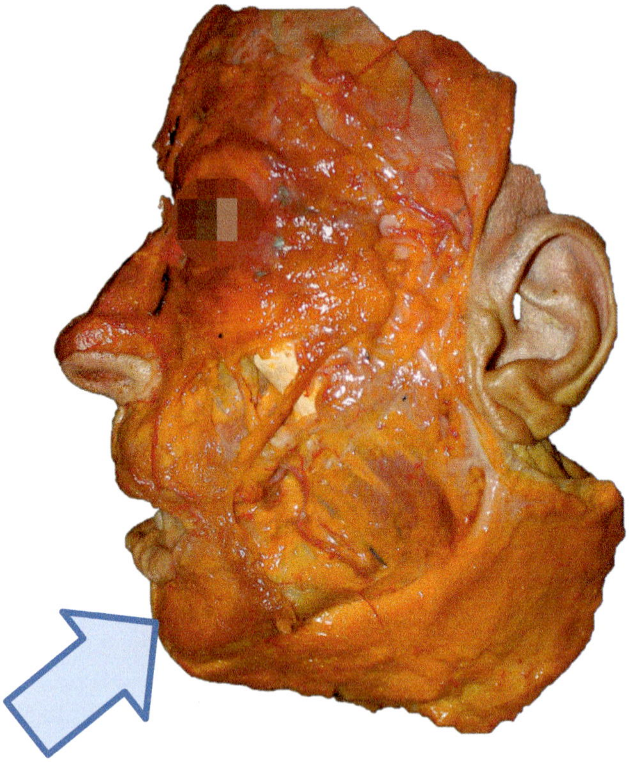

Fig. 19.2 The mentalis is a muscle located at the tip of the chin. It originates from the mentum and is inserted into the chin's soft tissue. (Published by kind permission of ©Mario Goisis 2018. All Rights Reserved)

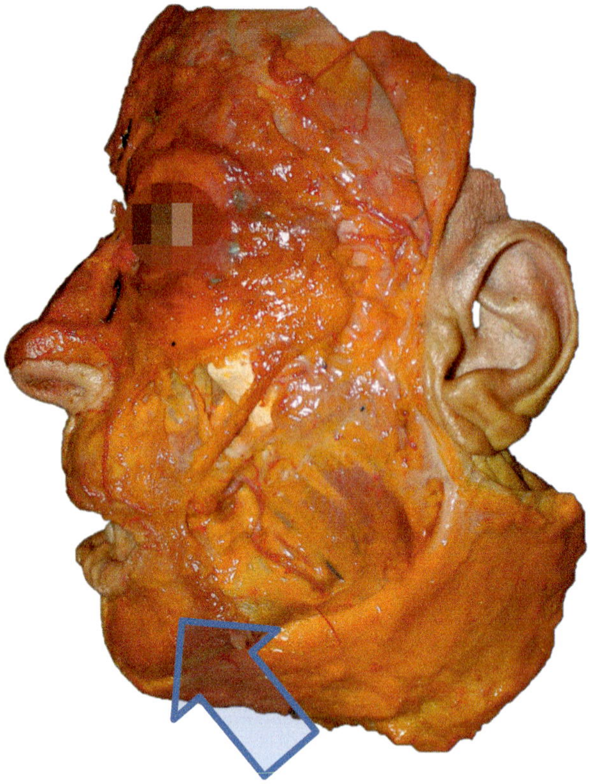

Fig. 19.4 The depressor anguli oris originates from the mandible and inserts into the corner of the mouth (courtesy of the Doctor's Equipe). (Published by kind permission of ©Mario Goisis 2018. All Rights Reserved)

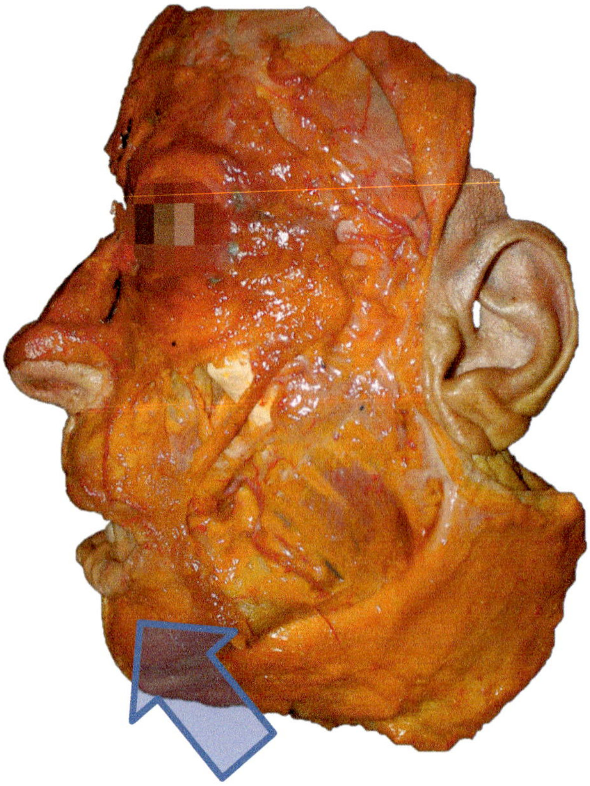

Fig. 19.3 The depressor labii inferioris muscle arises from the oblique line of the mandible, and is inserted into the skin of the lower lip (courtesy of the Doctor's Equipe). (Published by kind permission of ©Mario Goisis 2018. All Rights Reserved)

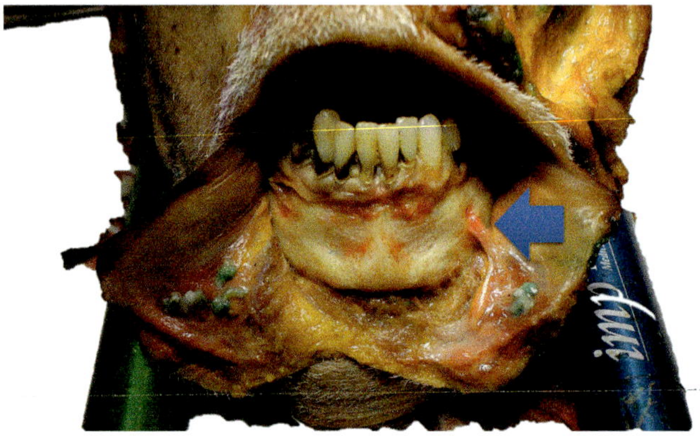

Fig. 19.5 The Mental nerve: The inferior alveolar nerve (sometimes called the inferior dental nerve) is a branch of the mandibular nerve, which is itself the third branch (V3) of the trigeminal nerve (cranial nerve V) (Fig.). Anteriorly, the nerve gives rise to the mental nerve roughly at the level of the 2nd mandibular premolars, which exits the mandible via the mental foramen (supplying sensory branches to the chin and lower lip). (Published by kind permission of ©Mario Goisis 2018. All Rights Reserved)

19.3 Augmentation of the Chin

Augmentation of the chin can lead to substantial improvement in the appearance of the face. It can correct age-related chin reduction, and sagging of the area of the neck below the chin. It is also helpful when seeking to camouflage facial asymmetry, and can also augment the dimension of the lower third of the face [?]. Augmentation of the chin is a simple procedure, which may be carried out in the physician's surgery under local anaesthesia. Few noble structures need to be preserved, but even this can be accomplished simply.

19.4 Augmentation of the Chin with Microfat Mixed with PRP

19.4.1 Indications

Asymmetries, age-related chin reduction, aesthetic purposes.

19.4.2 Contraindications

Anatomical alterations due to precedent trauma or surgical intervention (maxillofacial surgery). In fact, scarring and the presence of internal fixation often induce displacement of the structures that can lead to asymmetry and unequal filling of the part treated. Presence of surgical implants (previous chin augmentation with silicone implants, etc.).

- Because new injection can lead to inflammation or infection of the implants so as that surgery may be necessary to remove them.

19.4.3 Complications and Management

Immediate complications (within 72 h after injection) are transient erythema, oedema, induration, pruritus, and ecchymosis.

Early complications (days to weeks after injection) include hyper correction, local infection, necrosis of the skin, reactivation of herpes, discoloration, and persistent local symptoms (erythema, oedema, induration, pruritus, and hyperpigmentation).

Late complications include high rates of fat resorption and cysts.

19.4.4 Operating Time

Once the fat has been harvested, the procedure usually takes from 10 to 15 min.

19.4.5 Materials

- *2–4 cc of microfat on each side for injection of microfat: [2-4 cc of microfat for injection on both sides]*
  - *21-gauge needle*
  - *22-gauge 4-cm blunt cannula*

For microfat harvesting and processing:
A standard system for microfat is used, in particular:

- Microfat box (www.microfat.com), composed of a ramp with a closed system for washing and filtration
- 4 60-cc syringes
- 2 10-cc syringes
- One 1-cc syringe
- A 30-gauge needle
- A 16-gauge needle
- A 2-mm diameter, 10-cm-long Goisis cannula for fat harvesting
- A chlorhexidine-alcohol solution (2% chlorhexidine gluconate and 70% isopropyl alcohol), sterile drapes or towels
- Ice packs
- Sterile 2 cm × 2 cm gauze squares
- Occlusive dressing cover.

Medications include:

100 cc of cold saline solution.
120 cc of cold Klein solution.
1 litre of Klein solution is composed of 800 mg of lidocaine, 1 mg of epinephrine, 40 MEq of sodium bicarbonate, and 1000 cc of saline solution.

Location: The microfat harvesting may be carried out in a small operating theatre/a medical surgery. Oxygen, pulse oximetry, and a crash cart/box should be present.

Assistance: An assistant can prove useful when transferring items to the procedure field in a sterile manner during the first stage of the procedure. Despite this, a single doctor can perform the entire procedure alone (Figs. 19.6, 19.7, 19.8, 19.9, 19.10 and 19.11).

Plane of injection: intramuscular-SMAS

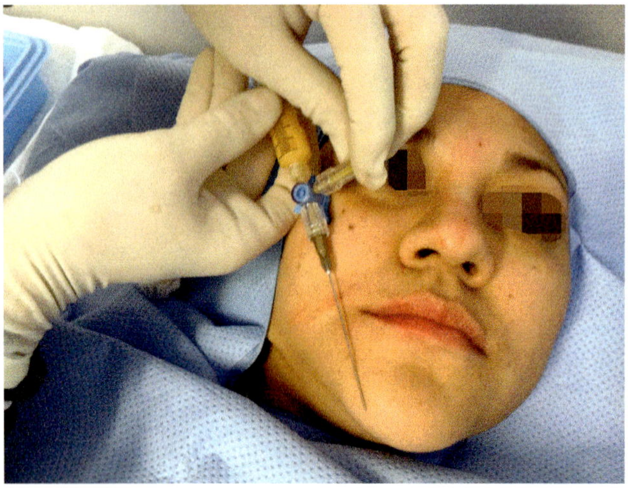

Fig. 19.6 Chin region is approached using a single entry point located 1.5–2 cm laterally to the oral rim. Direction of the cannula is shown. (Published by kind permission of ©Mario Goisis 2018. All Rights Reserved)

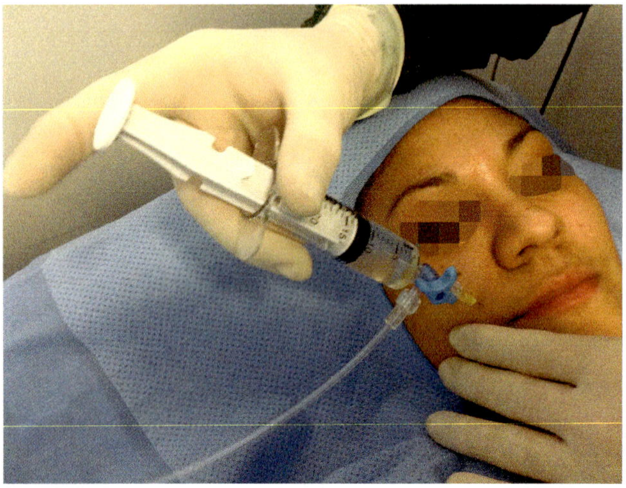

Fig. 19.7 Anaesthesia is performed at the entry point at the level of the modiolus using 0.2 cc of the Klein solution. (Published by kind permission of ©Mario Goisis 2018. All Rights Reserved)

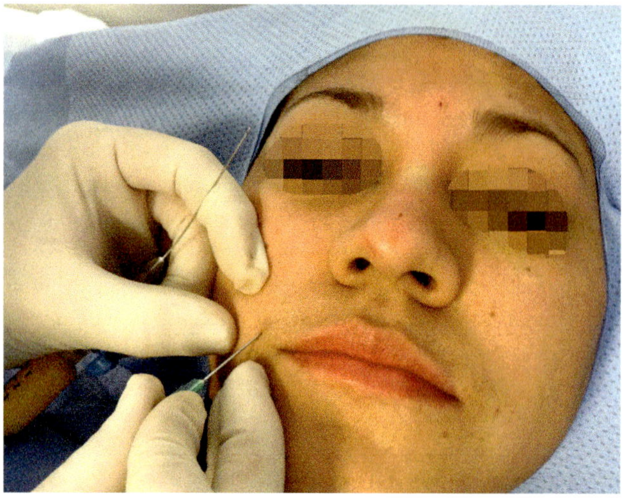

Fig. 19.8 An opening is created with a 21-G needle. (Published my kind permission of ©Mario Goisis 2018. All Rights Reserved)

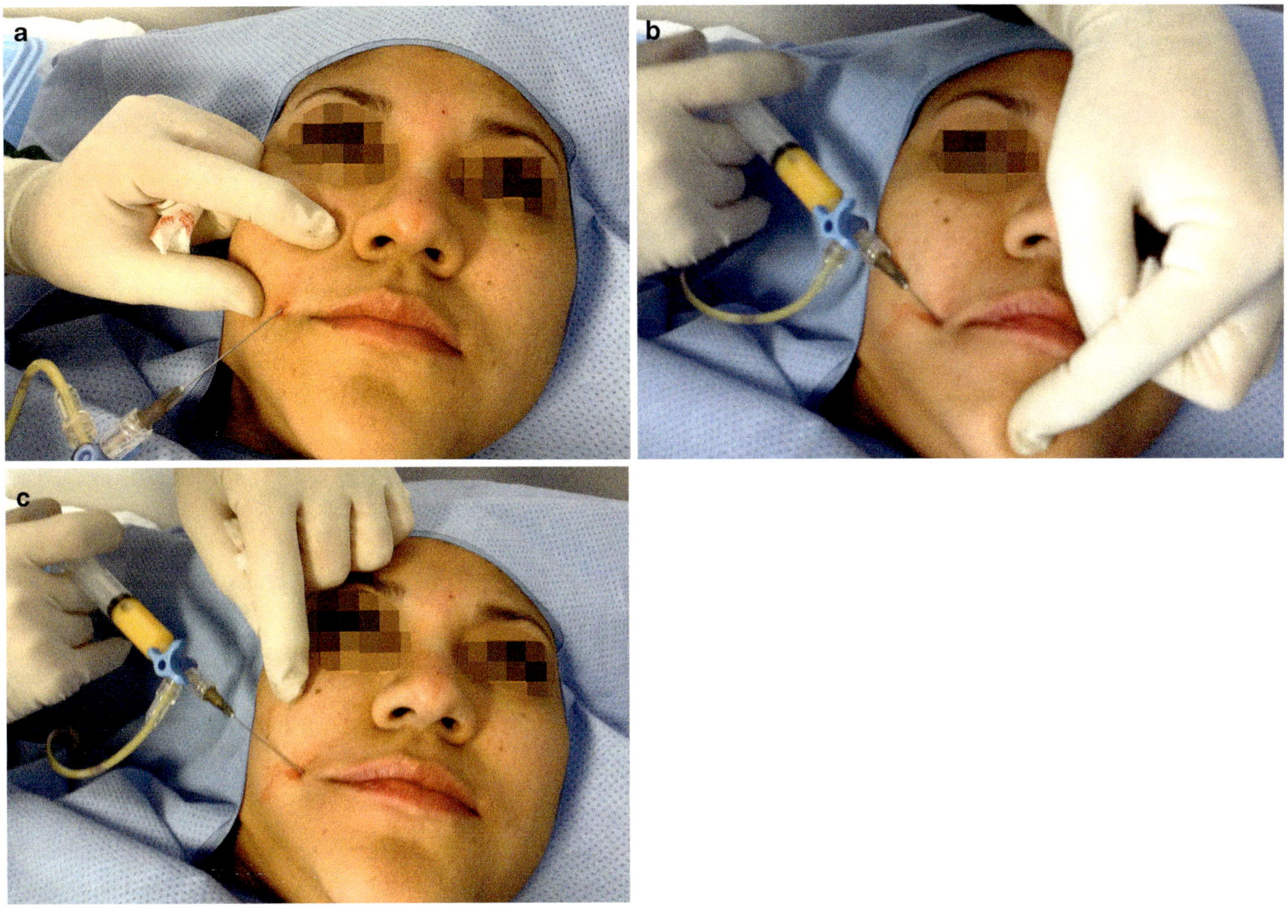

Fig. 19.9 A 22-G blunt-tip cannula is inserted perpendicularly into the skin's surface, and the cannula is then pivoted parallel to the plane of the skin into the muscular plane, and slid in the direction of the the top of the chin. (Published by kind permission of ©Mario Goisis 2018. All Rights Reserved)

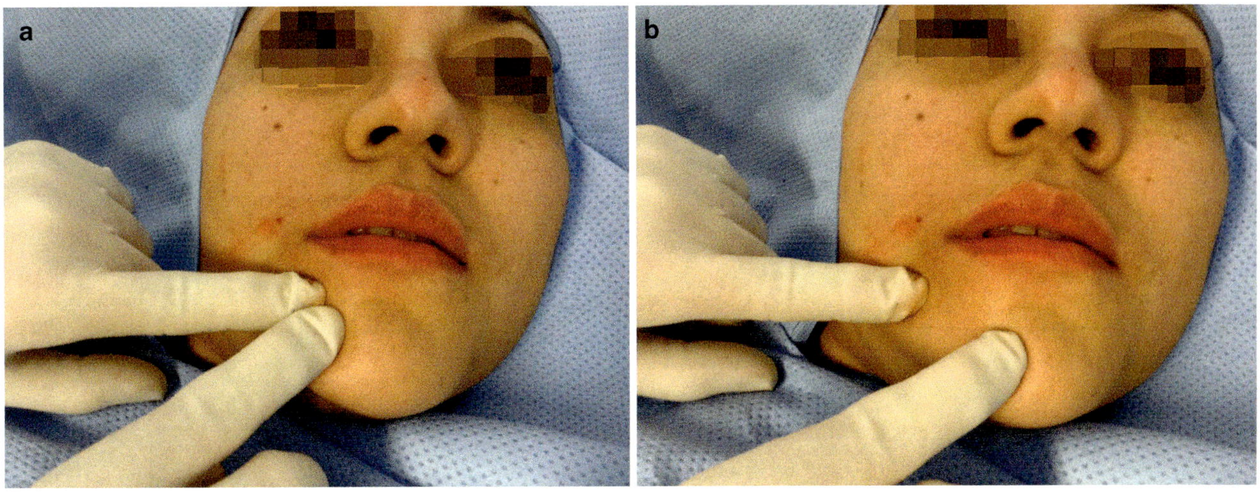

Fig. 19.10 At the end of the treatment, the injected area is injected. (Published by kind permission of ©Mario Goisis 2018. All Rights Reserved)

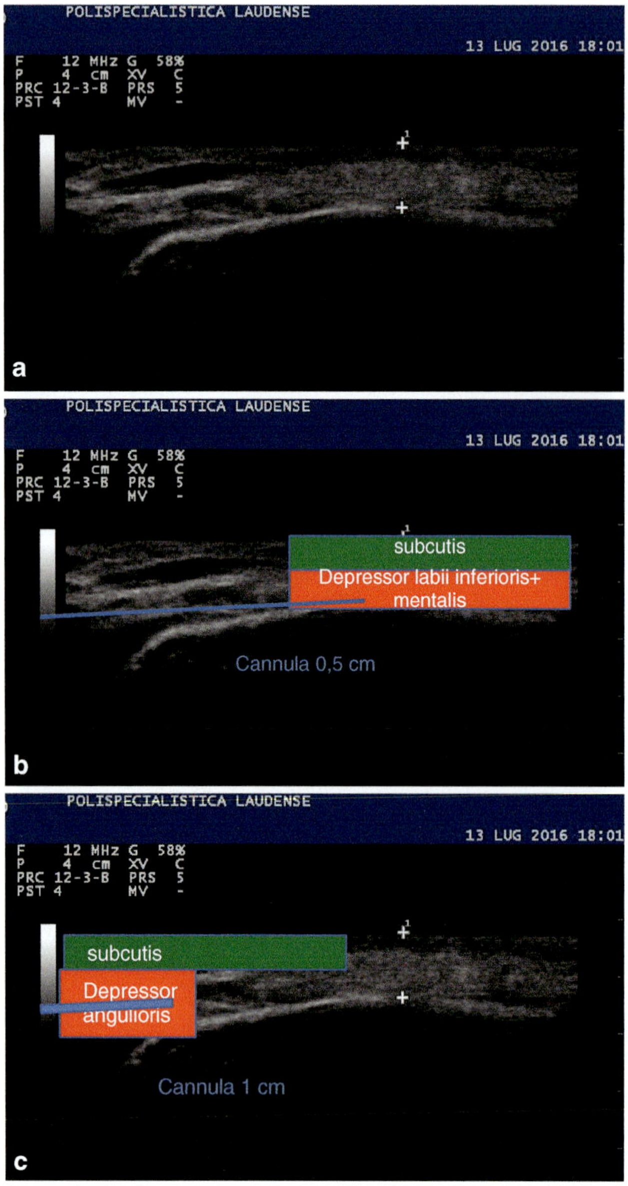

Fig. 19.11 Ultrasound demonstration of the procedure: the cannula is inserted into the muscular plane. The depth reached by the the cannula is 5 mm at the centre of the chin and 10 mm laterally (courtesy of the Doctor's Equipe). (Published by kind permission of ©Mario Goisis 2018. All Rights Reserved)

19.4.6 Cadaver Dissection After Injection of Microfat into the Chin

The cannula crosses the lip depressors and the mentalis muscle and thus contributes to the augmentation of the lip and the correction of the marionette lines. In particular, the fat is injected into the depressor labii inferioris, depressor anguli oris, and mentalis muscles. The fat is delivered slowly, while the cannula is withdrawn by means of retrograde injection (Fig. 19.12, 19.13 and 19.14). (courtesy Doctor's Equipe).

19.5 Amelioration of the Chin Region using PRP

19.5.1 Indications

Acne scars and small wrinkles

19.5.2 Contraindications

– No injection should be carried out if the area has been previously treated with liquid silicone or other permanent fillers.

19.5.3 Operating Time

Once the PRP has been harvested, the procedure usually takes from 10 to 15 min.

19.5.4 Materials

Tubes for PRP preparation, empty and with anticoagulant (www.microfat.com)

- 1–2 cc of PRP
- A 27G cannula, 3.6 cm long
- A 26-G needle
- 0.2 cc of local anesthetic (2% Lidocaine, 2% mepivacaine) with epinephrine 1:100 000
- Bandages and antiseptic solution

Plane of injection: the hypodermis

19.5.5 Methods

The procedure is described in Figs. 19.15, 19.16, 19.17, 19.18 and 19.19.

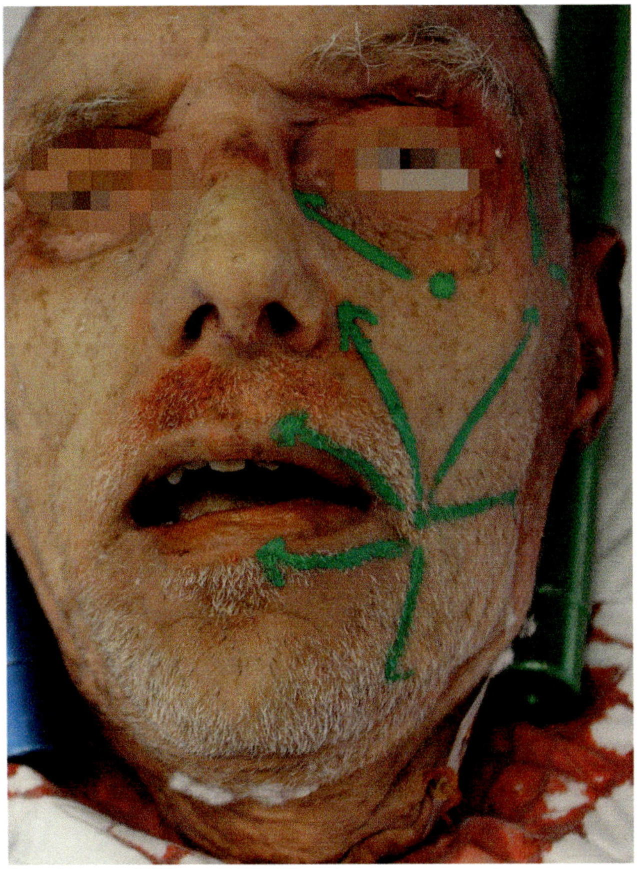

Fig. 19.12 The region of the chin is approached using a single entry point located 1.5–2 cm laterally to the oral rim (courtesy of the Doctor's Equipe). (Published by kind permission of ©Mario Goisis 2018. All Rights Reserved)

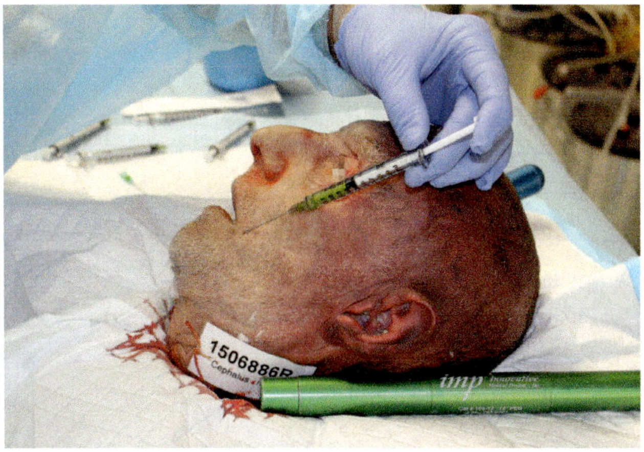

Fig. 19.13 A 22-G, blunt-tip cannula is inserted perpendicularly into the surface of the sking through the ad-hoc hole created. (Published by kind permission of ©Mario Goisis 2018. All Rights Reserved)

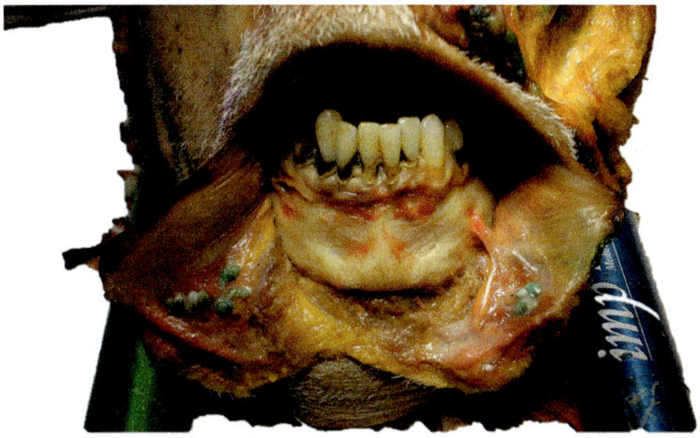

Fig. 19.14 After injection of the fat, dissection of the lower third of the face is executed starting from a middle-line incision of the lower lip. The subperiosteal plane is exposed. No evidence of fat in the subcutaneous plane appears. Considerable evidence of fat is seen in the intramuscular plane (courtesy of the Doctor's Equipe). (Published by kind permission of ©Mario Goisis 2018. All Rights Reserved)

19.6 Cadaver Dissection After PRP Injection of The Chin (Figs. 19.20, 19.21 and 19.22)

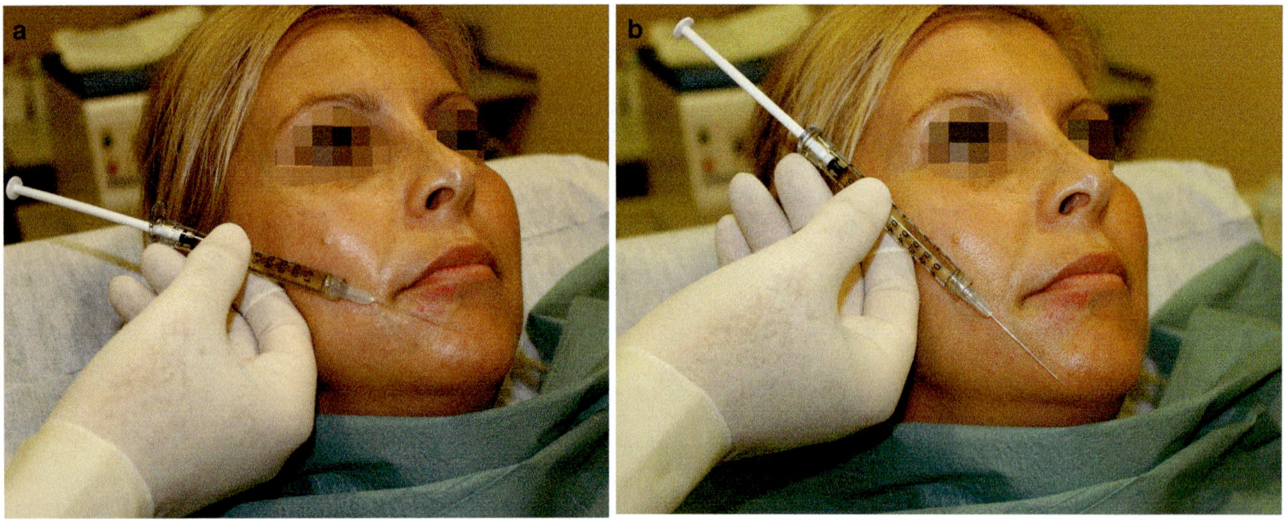

Fig. 19.15 PRP injection the direction of the cannula is indicated (Published by kind permission of ©Mario Goisis 2018. All Rights Reserved)

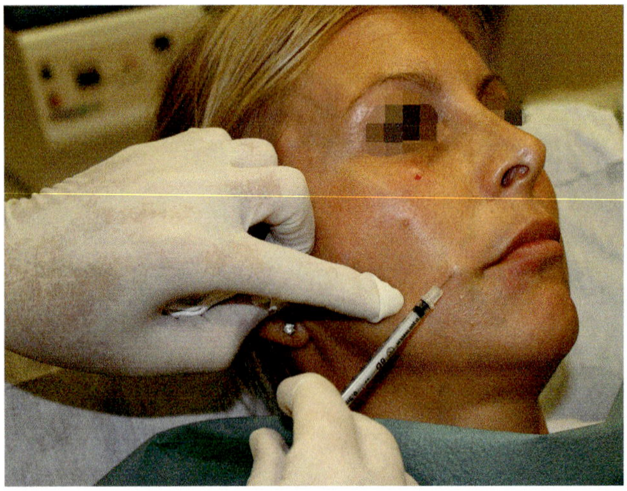

Fig. 19.16 Anaesthesia is performed at the entry-point at the modiolus with 0.2 cc of local anaesthetic (lidocaine, mepivacaine) with adrenaline. (Published by kind permission of ©Mario Goisis 2018. All Rights Reserved)

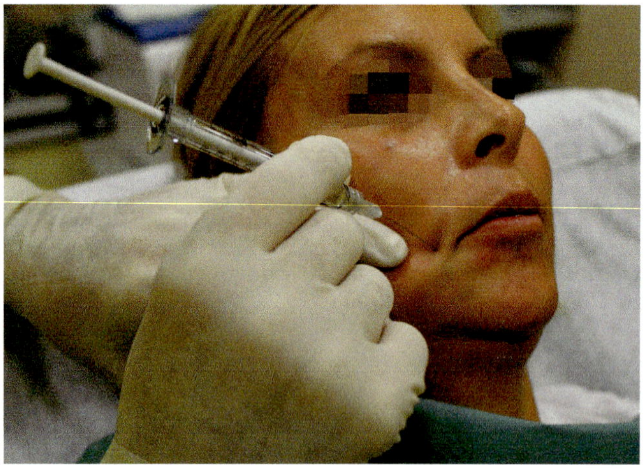

Fig. 19.18 The cannula is then pivoted, parallel to the skin, into the subcutaneous plane, and slid in the direction of the chin. (Published by kind permission of ©Mario Goisis 2018. All Rights Reserved)

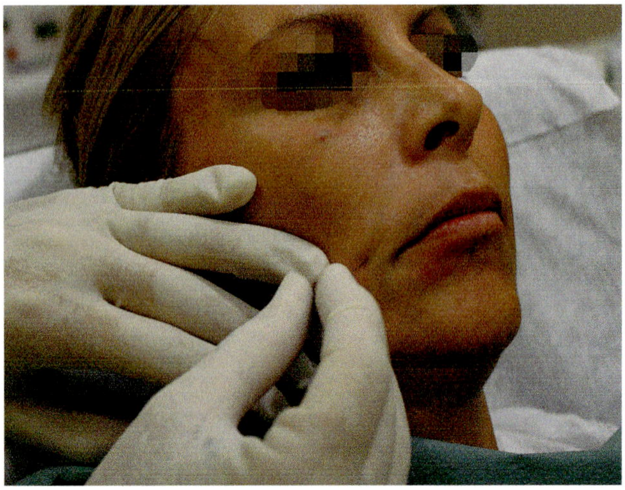

Fig. 19.17 An opening is created with a 26-G needle at the level of the modiolus. (Published by kind permission of ©Mario Goisis 2018. All Rights Reserved)

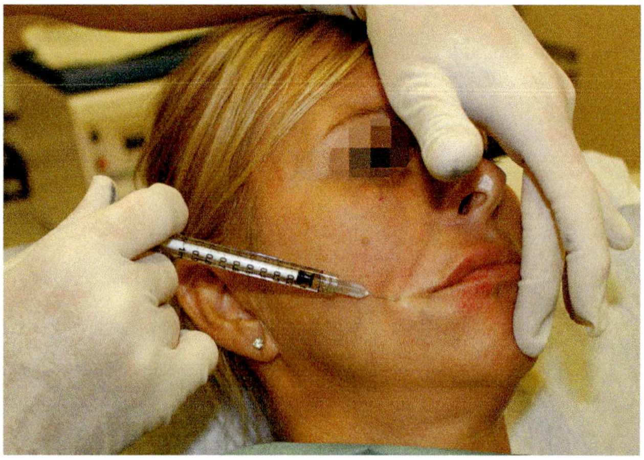

Fig. 19.19 The PRP is delivered slowly, while the cannula is withdrawn with retrograde injection. (Published by kind permission of ©Mario Goisis 2018. All Rights Reserved).

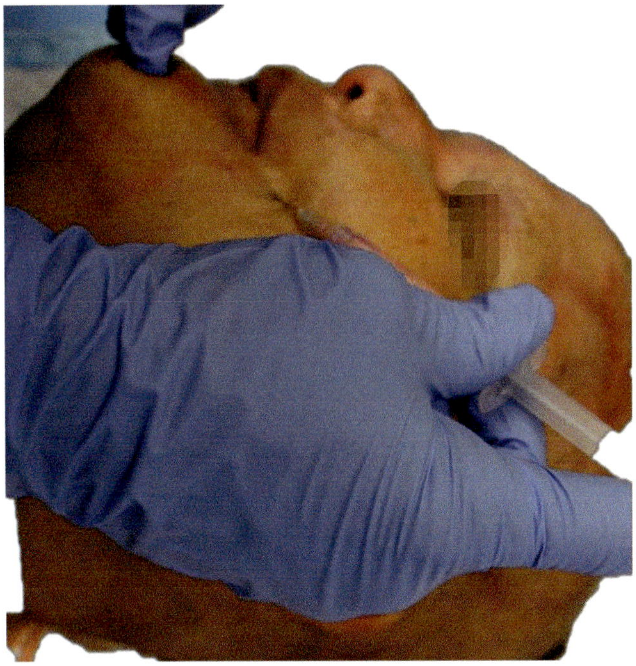

Fig. 19.20 A 27-G, blunt-tip cannula is used to distribute the product in the subcutaneous tissue (courtesy of the Doctor's Equipe). (Published by kind permission of ©Mario Goisis 2018. All Rights Reserved)

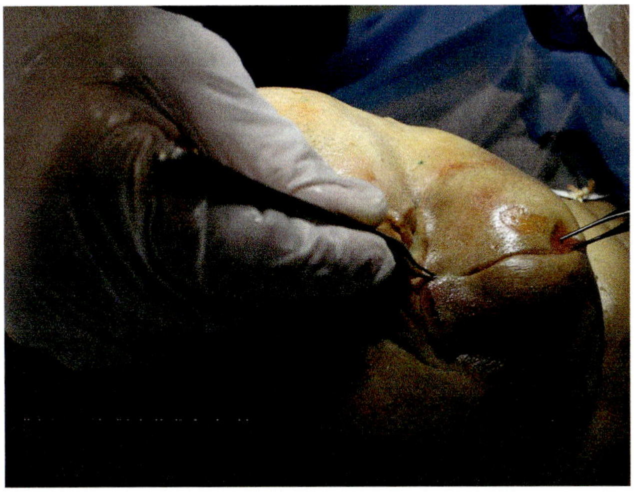

Fig. 19.21 After PRP (purple) injection, lower third of the face dissection is executed starting from a middle-line incision of the lower lip. (courtesy of the Doctor's Equipe). (Published with by kind permission of ©Mario Goisis 2018. All Rights Reserved)

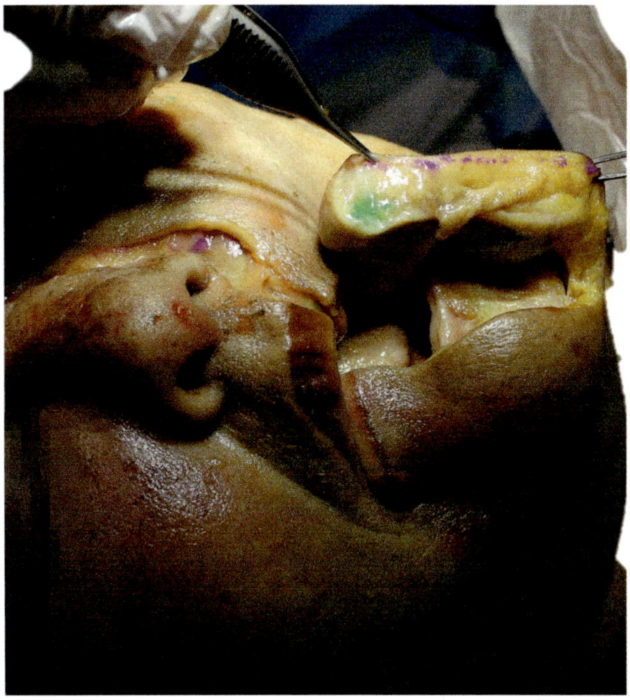

Fig. 19.22 PRP (purple) is located on the subcutaneous plane (courtesy of the Doctor's Equipe). (Published by kind permission of ©Mario Goisis 2018. All Rights Reserved)

The Neck

20

Alessandro Di Petrillo and Mario Goisis

Treatment of the neck and décolleté is an integral part of the procedures aimed at improving the aesthetic appearance of patients. Ageing in these regions is associated with loss of skin elasticity and sagging. Good results can be achieved by treating the neck and décolleté with nanograft injections and even by using autologous material such as PRP.

20.1 Anatomy

The region of the neck region is anatomically very complex. Among the structures present in the area, attention should be paid to the surface vessels. In particular, the external jugular vein which commences in the substance of the parotid gland, at the level of the angle of the mandible, and runs perpendicularly down to the neck in the direction of a line linking the angle of the mandible to the middle of the clavicle on the posterior border of the sternocleidomastoideus, crossing the muscle obliquely.

The anterior jugular vein begins near the hyoid bone and is the result of the confluence of several superficial veins flowing from the submaxillary region. It descends between the median line and the anterior border of the sternocleidomastoideus and, in the lower part of the neck, passes beneath that muscle to open into the termination of the external jugular or, in some instances, into the subclavian vein. It varies considerably in size, usually inversely proportionate to the external jugular; most frequently, there are two anterior jugulars, one right, one left, but sometimes only one (Fig. 20.1).

20.2 Pitfalls

Examination and identification of the major vessels of the neck's surface, of the external and anterior jugular vein, is important to avoid haematomas. The existence of a great anatomic variety makes it mandatory to introduce the needle only a few millimeters beneath the skin's surface.

Avoid overly superficial injections, in particular in the epidermidis: in this case, small lumps might form after a few days.

20.3 Nanograft Injection for the Treatment of the Neck and "Décolleté"

Nanograft can be used to improve atrophism of the skin, the texture, and elasticity of the dermis of every area of the human anatomy but is usually practiced on the skin of the face, neck, décolleté, and hands.

Rejuvenation is particularly indicated in people who smoke and have been exposed to sunlight for long periods of time.

Nanograft can be injected following a combined, alternating 12-month protocol. The standard protocol usually includes:

Nanograft injection at months 4, 8, and 12
Injection of non-low-viscosity hyaluronic acid at months 1, 2,3, 5, 6, 7, 9, 10, and 11

20.3.1 Contraindications

In patients with coagulation issues or on current anticoagulant therapy, the treatment is relatively contraindicated. As with all injections, these subjects are at increasing risk of bleeding and the formation of haematomata.

- The nanofat should not be injected into areas lacking sufficient blood supply or suffering from infection or inflammation.
- No injection should be done if the area has been previously treated with liquid silicone or other permanent

A. Di Petrillo
Doctor's Equipe, Milan, Italy

M. Goisis (✉)
Maxillo-Facial and Aesthetic Surgeon, Go Easy Clinic, Milan, Italy

M. Goisis (ed.), *Outpatient Regenerative Medicine*, https://doi.org/10.1007/978-3-319-44894-7_20

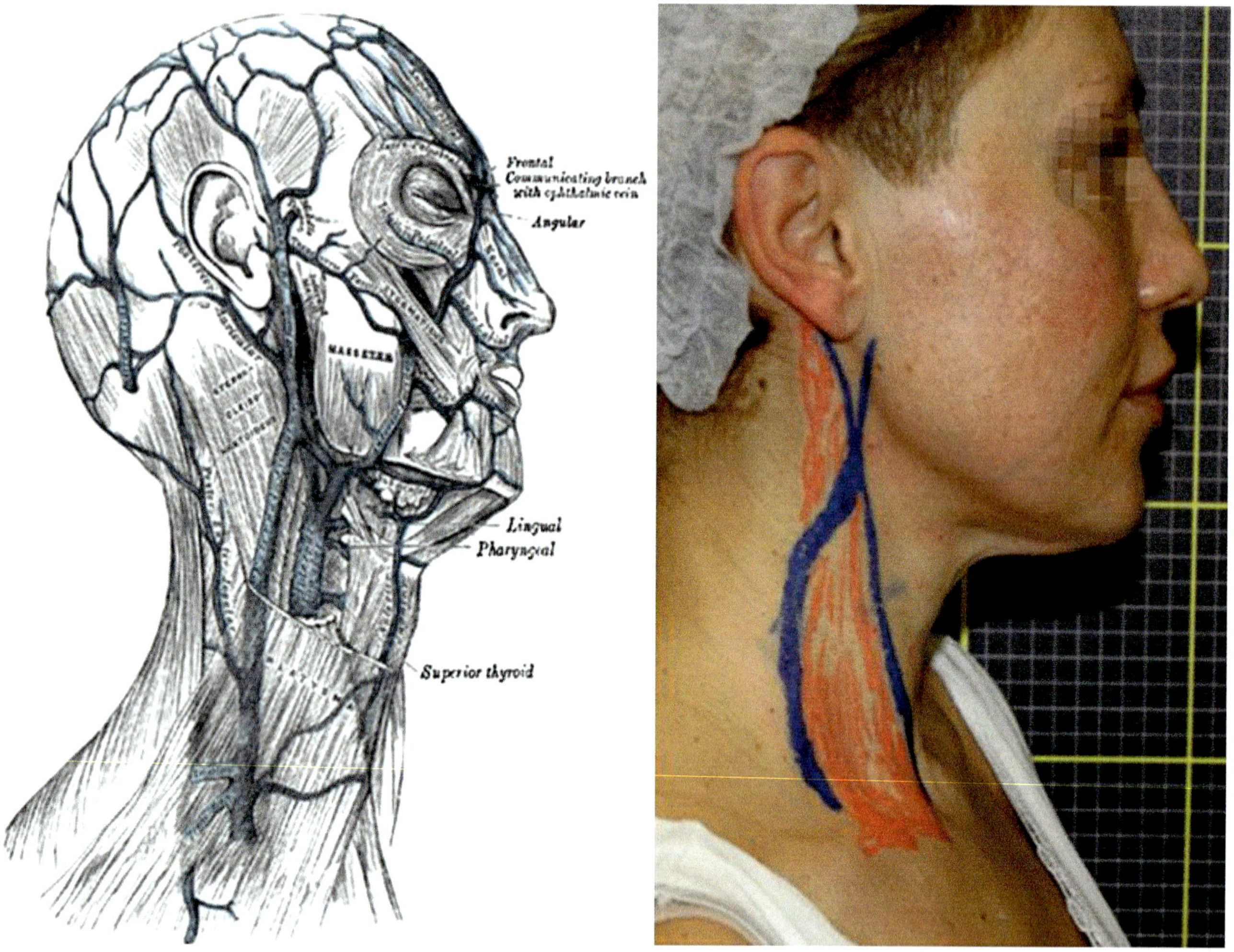

Fig. 20.1 Left, a graphic representation of the veinous system of the head and neck from Gray's Anatomy. Right, the veins and arteries of the neck outlined on the skin (Published by kind permission of ©Mario Goisis 2018. All Rights Reserved)

fillers because a new injections might lead to inflammation or infection of the implants.

Hyperthyroidism due to Graves' disease is a relative contraindication.

20.3.2 Complications and Management

Immediate complications (within 72 h after injection) are transient erythema, oedema, induration, pruritus, and ecchymosis.

Early complications (days to weeks after injection) include hypercorrection, local infection, necrosis of the skin, reactivation of herpes, discoloration, and persistent local symptoms (erythema, oedema, induration, pruritus, and hyperpigmentation).

Later or delayed complications include high rates of fat resorption and cysts.

20.3.3 Operating Time

The procedure usually takes from 5 to 10 min, once the nanofat has been produced.

Plane of injection: dermis-hypodermis

20.3.4 Indications

Amelioration of small wrinkle and laxity of the neck

20.3.5 Materials

- *2–6 cc of nanofat for injection:*
  - *20-gauge needle*

A standard system for producing nanofat is used, in particular:

- The Nanofat system (www.microfat.com), composed a connector with a closed system for emulsion of microfat and filtration
- Two10-cc syringes

To harvest and process the microfat, a standard system is used, in particular:

- A Microfat box (www.microfat.com), composed of a ramp with a closed system for washing and filtration
- 4 60-cc syringes
- 2 10-cc syringes
- One 1-cc syringe
- A 30-gauge needle
- A 16-gauge needle
- A 2-mm-diameter, 10-cm-long Goisis cannula for fat harvesting
- A chlorhexidine-alcohol solution (2% chlorhexidine gluconate and 70% isopropyl alcohol), sterile drapes or towels
- Ice packs
- Sterile 2 cm x 2 cm gauze squares
- Occlusive dressing cover

Medications include:

100 cc of cold saline solution.
120 cc of cold Klein solution.
One litre of Klein solution is composed of 800 mg of lidocaine, 1 mg of epinephrine, 40 MEq of sodium bicarbonate, and 1000 cc of saline solution.

Location: Microfat harvesting can be carried out in a small operating theatre/medical surgery. The oxygen, pulse oximetry, and a crash cart/box should be present.

Assistance: An assistant can prove useful when transferring items to the procedure field in a sterile manner during the first stage of the procedure. In any case, a single doctor can carry out the entire procedure alone.

Plane of injection: subcutaneous-intradermal

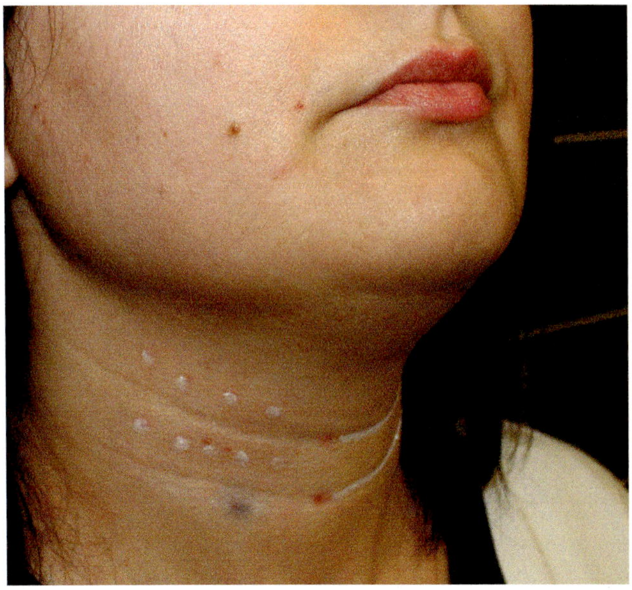

Fig. 20.2 The injection points on the patient's skin are indicated here. No local anaesthesia is needed, except for a mild local anaesthetic gel that may be applied 10–20 min before the treatment. (Published by kind permission of ©Mario Goisis 2018. All Rights Reserved)

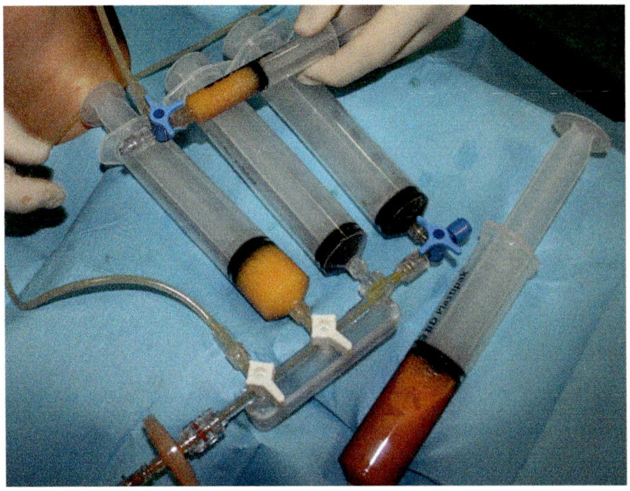

Fig. 20.3 5 cc of microfat is produced using the microfat box (www.microfat.com). (Published by kind permission of ©Mario Goisis 2018. All Rights Reserved)

20.3.6 Methods

The method is illustrated in Figs. 20.2, 20.3, 20.4, 20.5a, b, 20.6a, b, 20.7, 20.8, 20.9a, b, 20.10a, b, and 20.11a, b.

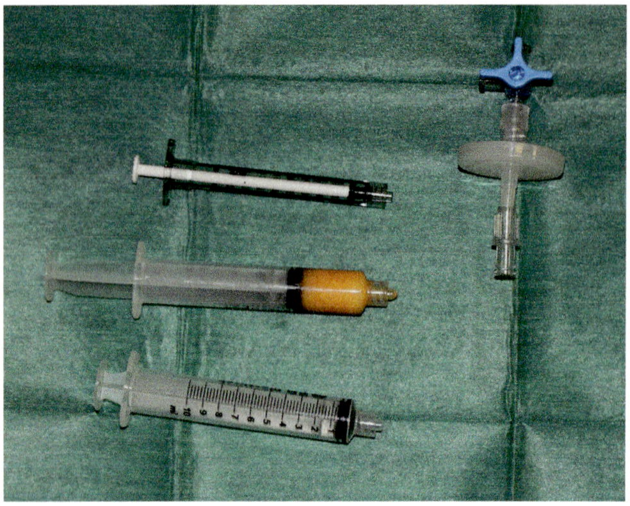

Fig. 20.4 The DE nanofat kit. (Published by kind permission of ©Mario Goisis 2018. All Rights Reserved)

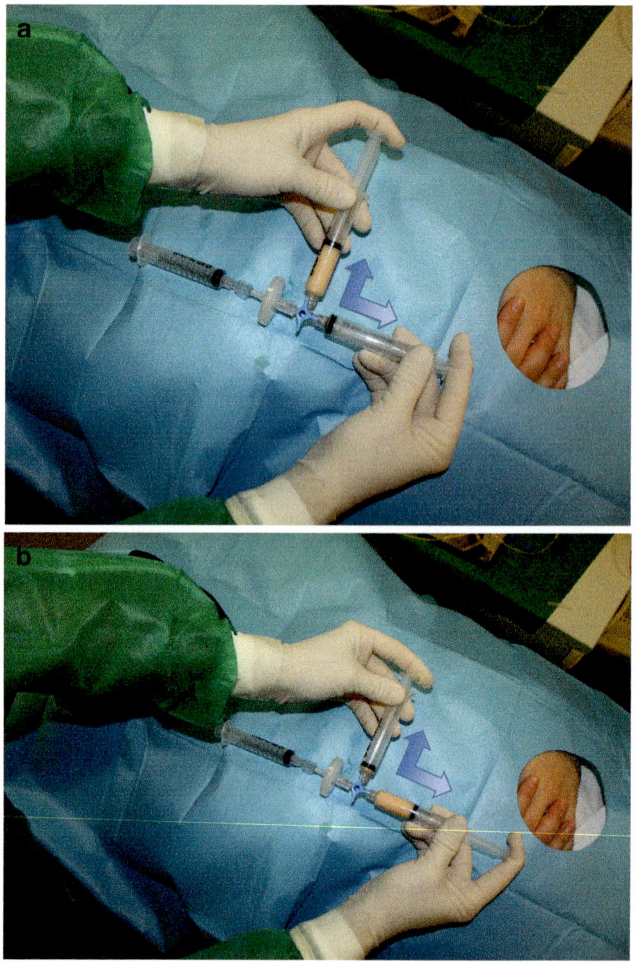

Fig. 20.5 (**a**, **b**) 10-cc syringes are connected to the kit. The fat is moved rapidly between the two syringes 30 times. (Published by kind permission of ©Mario Goisis 2018. All Rights Reserved)

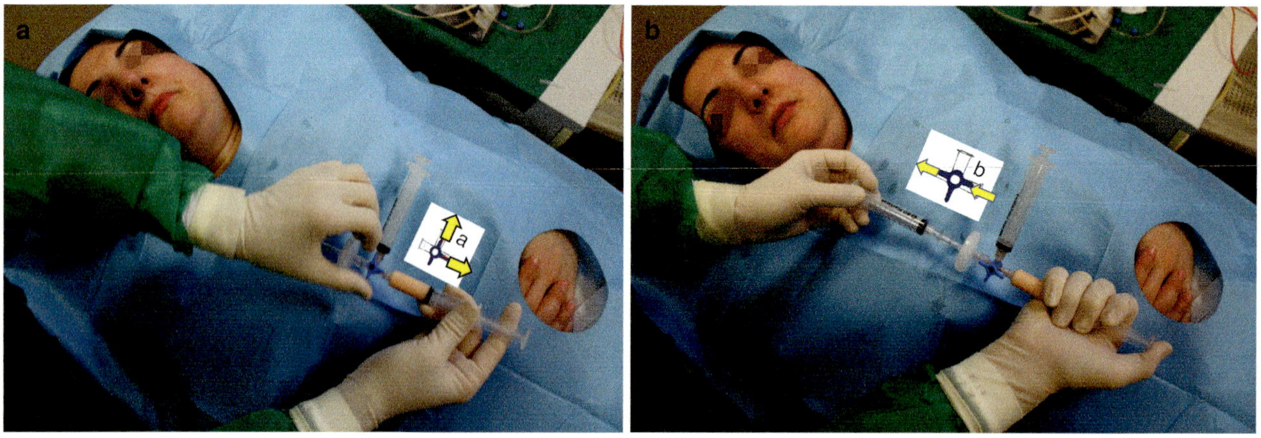

Fig. 20.6 (**a**, **b**) The stopcock is moved from position "a" to position "b". (Published by kind permission of ©Mario Goisis 2018. All Rights Reserved)

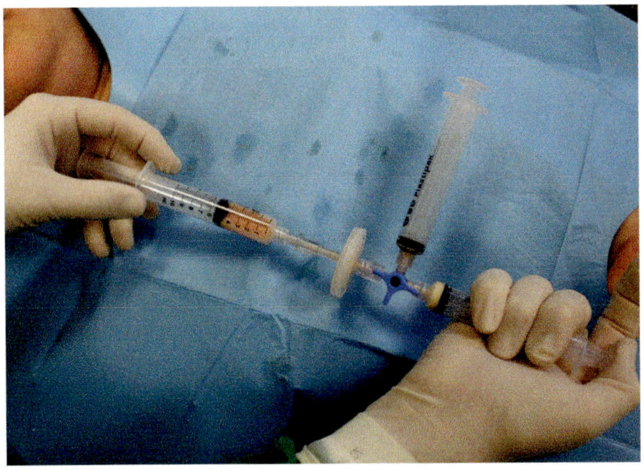

Fig. 20.7 This way, the fat is filtered and transferred directly into the third syringe. (Published by kind permission of ©Mario Goisis 2018. All Rights Reserved)

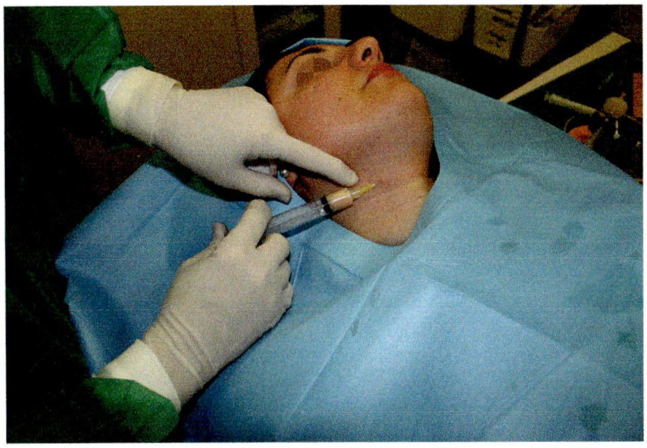

Fig. 20.8 Because of filtration, the fat can be injected directly using a 30-G needle. (Published by kind permission of ©Mario Goisis 2018. All Rights Reserved)

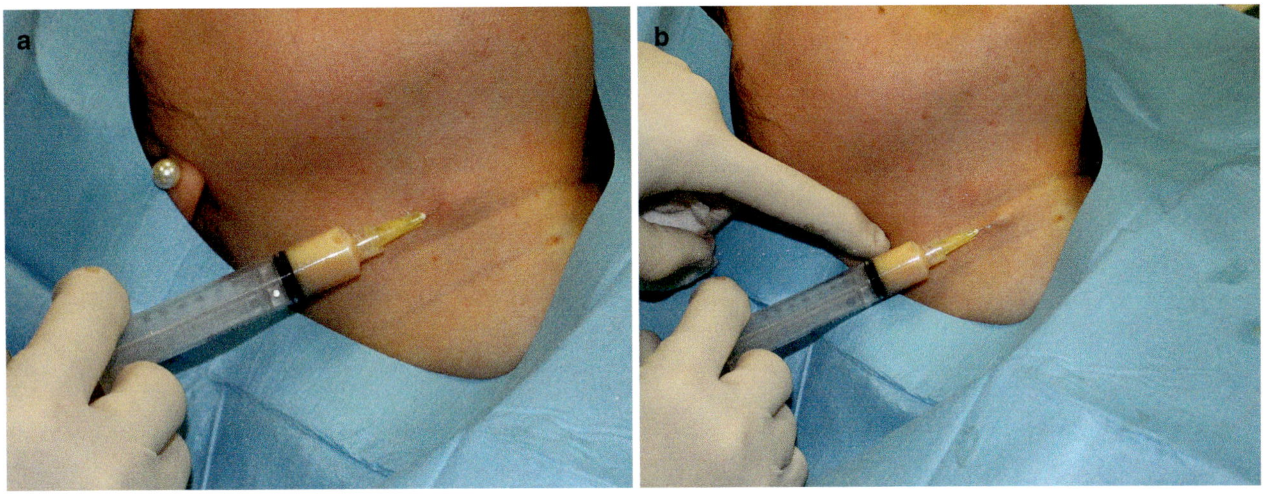

Fig. 20.9 (**a**, **b**) The nanograft is injected into the intradermal and subcutaneous planes of the neck. The needle is inserted for a depth of 2–3 mm; the quantity of product injected is really small, about 0.1 ml or less. (Published by kind permission of ©Mario Goisis 2018. All Rights Reserved)

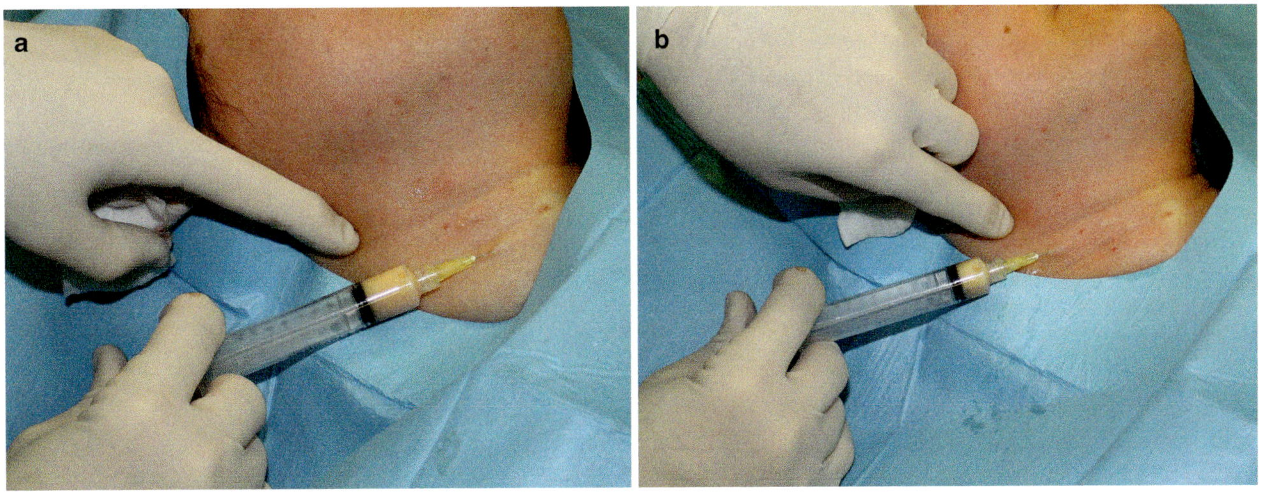

Fig. 20.10 (**a**, **b**) The ideal distance between different inkection-points is 1 cm. (Published by kind permission of ©Mario Goisis 2018. All Rights Reserved)

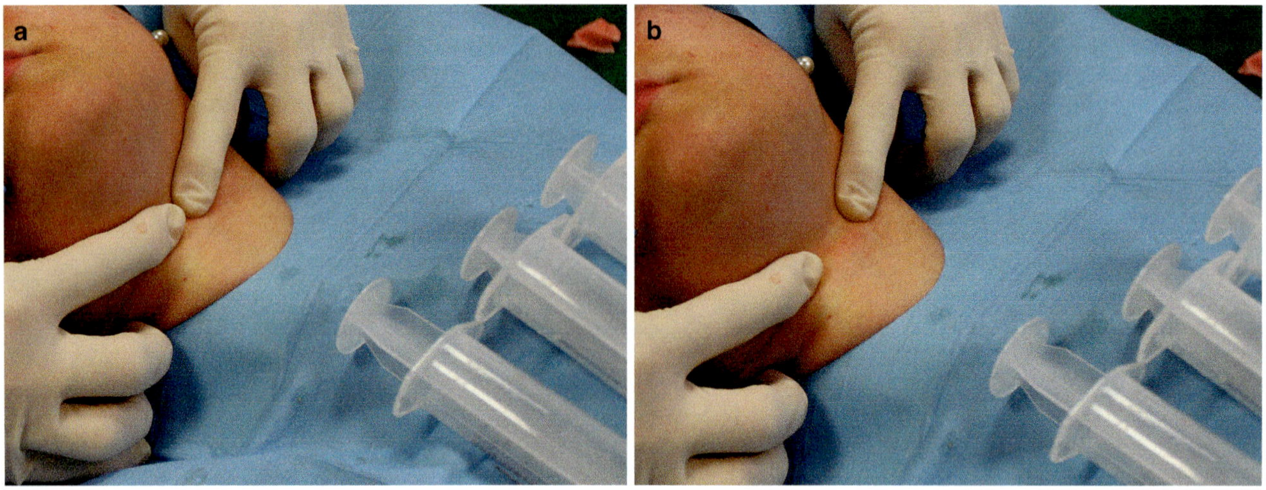

Fig. 20.11 (**a**, **b**) A strong massage is applied to the area after injection. (Published by kind permission of ©Mario Goisis 2018. All Rights Reserved)

20.4 Treatment of the Horizontal Neck Lines using Micrograft

20.4.1 Indications

Horizontal neck lines are usually a part of the natural ageing process. As the skin of the neck loses *collagen and elasticity*, it will no longer be able to return to its normal position after it has stretched. This will inevitably lead to the development of horizontal neck lines. One of the main factors that increase horizontal neck lines is excessive exposure to the sun with no skin protection. Exposure to wind and sun exposure can cause the skin to dry, the which causes a significant amount of damage.

Correction of horizontal neck lines can be obtained with filling the lines with micrograft. The use of a blunt-tip cannula permits atraumatic dissection of the tissue with placement of the microfat superficially along the subcutaneous plane and permits the performance of needle entry marks and causes significantly less pain and bruising.

20.4.2 Contraindications

- The micrograft should not be injected into areas that lack sufficient blood supply or suffering from infection or inflammation.
- No injection should be carried out if the area has been previously treated with liquid silicone or other permanent fillers because new injections might lead to inflammation or infection of the implants.

20.4.3 Complications and Management

Immediate complications (within 72 h after injection) are transient erythema,o edema, induration, pruritus, and ecchymosis.

Early complications (days to weeks after injection) include hypercorrection, local infection, necrosis of the skin, reactivation of herpes, discoloration, and persistent local symptoms (erythema, oedema, induration, pruritus, and hyperpigmentation).

Late complications include high rate of fat resorption and cyst.

20.4.4 Materials

- *2–4 cc pf microfat for injection either side:*
  - *A 21-gauge needle*
  - *A 22-gauge 4-cm blunt cannula*

To harvest and process microfat, a standard system used, in particular:

- A Microfat box (www.microfat.com), composed by a ramp with a closed system for washing and filtration
- 4 60-cc syringes
- 2 10-cc syringes
- One 1-cc syringe
- A 30-gauge needle
- A 16-gauge needle
- A 2-mm-diameter, 10-cm-long Goisis cannula for fat harvesting

- A chlorhexidine-alcohol solution (2% chlorhexidine gluconate and 70% isopropyl alcohol), sterile drapes or towels
- Ice packs
- Sterile 2 cm x 2 cm gauze squares
- Occlusive dressing cover

Medications include:

100 cc of cold saline solution.
120 cc of cold Klein solution.

One litre of Klein solution is composed of 800 mg of lidocaine, 1 mg of epinephrine, 40 MEq of sodium bicarbonate, and 1000 cc of saline solution.

Location: Microfat harvesting can be carried out in a small operating theatre /medical surgery. The oxygen, pulse oximetry, and a crash cart/box should be present.

Assistance: An assistant can prove useful when transferring items to the procedure field in a sterile manner during the first stage of the procedure. Nonetless, a single doctor can perform the entire procedure alone.

Plane of injection: subcutaneous

20.4.5 Operating Time

Once the fat has been harvested, the procedure usually takes from 5 to 15 min.

20.4.6 Methods

The procedure is described in Figs. 20.12, 20.13a, b, 20.14a, b, 20.15, 20.16, 20.17, 20.18a, b, 20.19a, b, and 20.20.

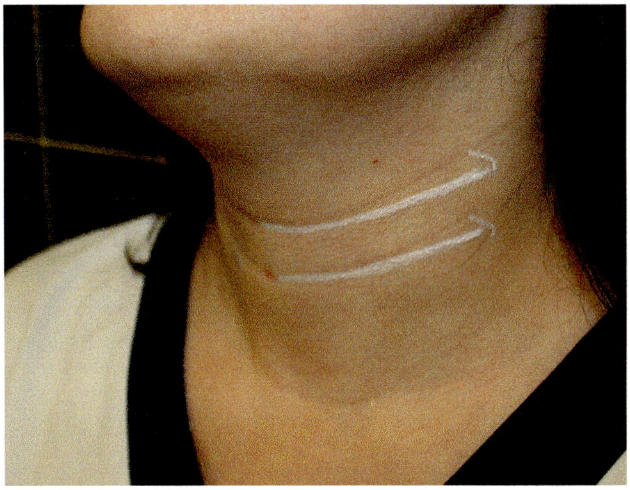

Fig. 20.12 The area of treatment is outlined on the skin. (Published by kind permission of ©Mario Goisis 2018. All Rights Reserved)

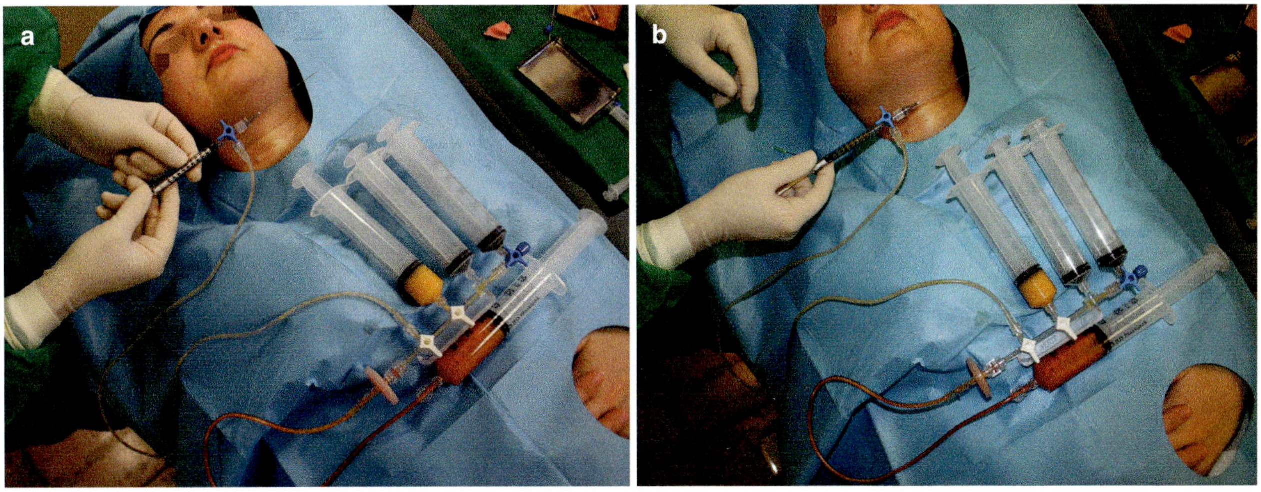

Fig. 20.13 (**a**, **b**) The 1-ml syringe is filled with microfat (www.microfat.com). (Published by kind permission of ©Mario Goisis 2018. All Rights Reserved)

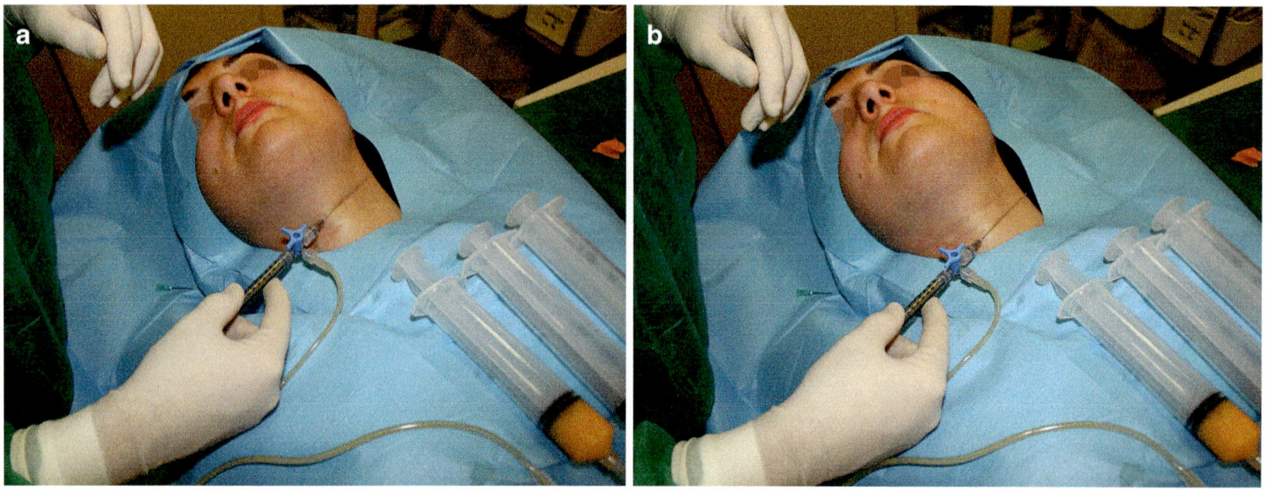

Fig. 20. 14 (**a**, **b**) The route of the cannula. (Published by kind permission of ©Mario Goisis 2018. All Rights Reserved)

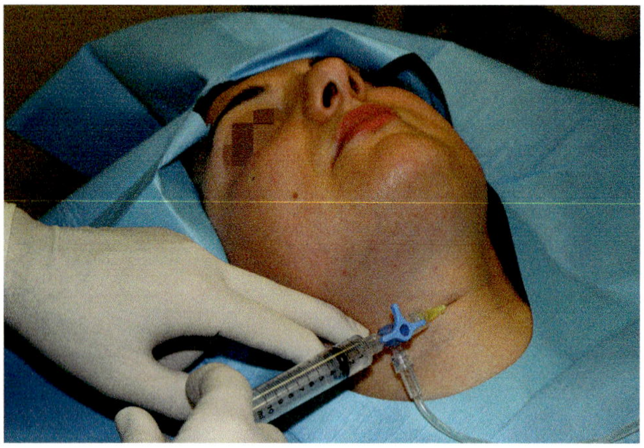

Fig. 20.15 Anaesthesia is performed through the entry-points with 0.2 cc of Klein solution. The entry -points are at the level of the midline, in correspondence to the bigger neck lines. (Published by kind permission of ©Mario Goisis 2018. All Rights Reserved)

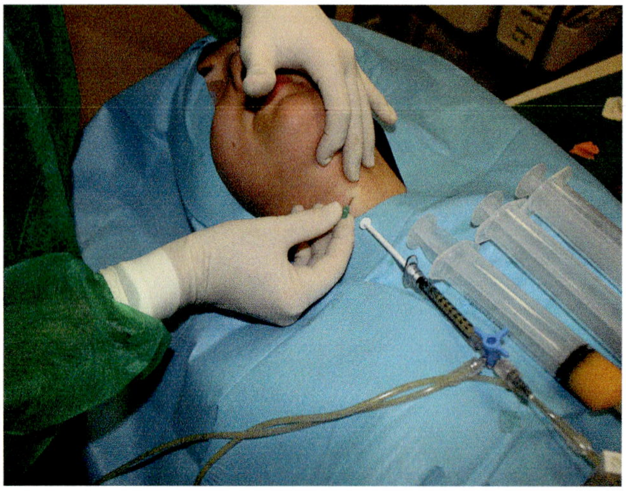

Fig. 20.16 An opening is created using a 21-G needle. (Published by kind permission of ©Mario Goisis 2018. All Rights Reserved)

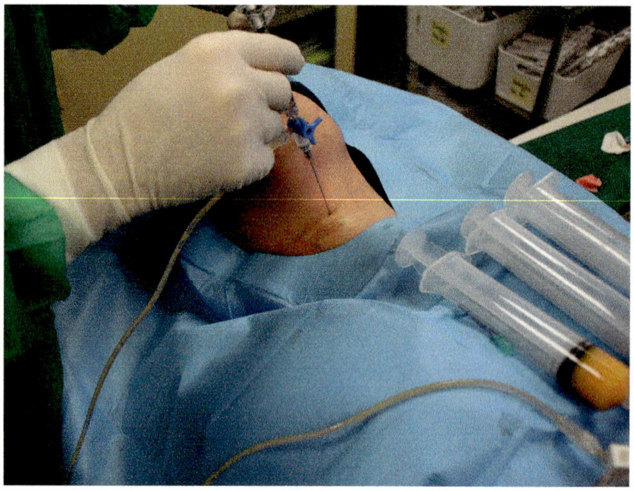

Fig. 20.17 A blunt-tip 22-G cannula is inserted perpendicularly into the surface of the skin, and the cannula is then pivoted parallel to the skin plane. (Published by kind permission of ©Mario Goisis 2018. All Rights Reserved)

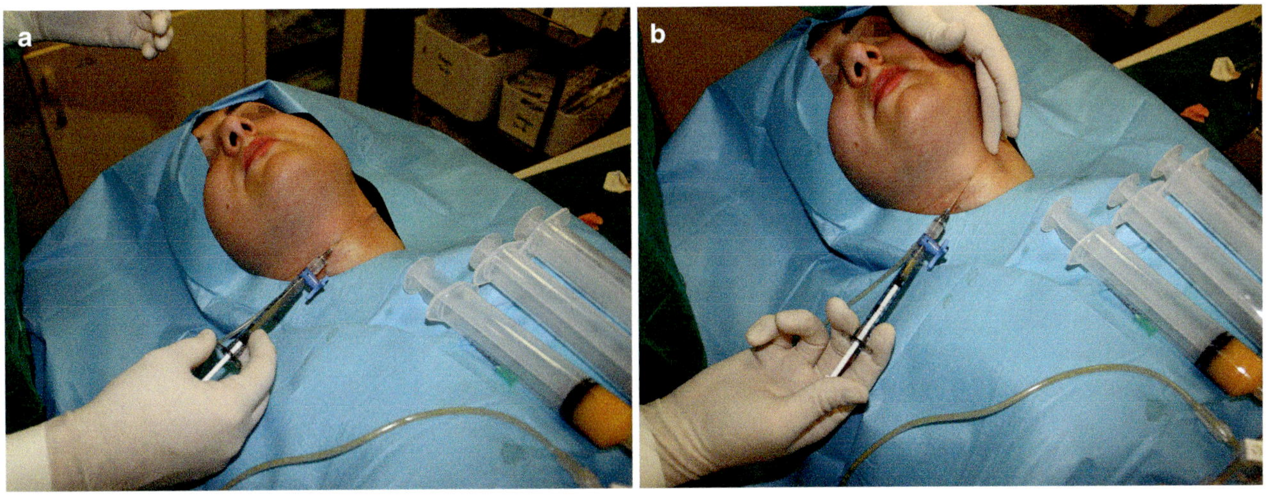

Fig. 20.18 (**a**, **b**) The fat is delivered slowly, while the cannula is withdrawn by retrograde injection. The fat is injected into the subcutaneous plane. (Published by kind permission of ©Mario Goisis 2018. All Rights Reserved)

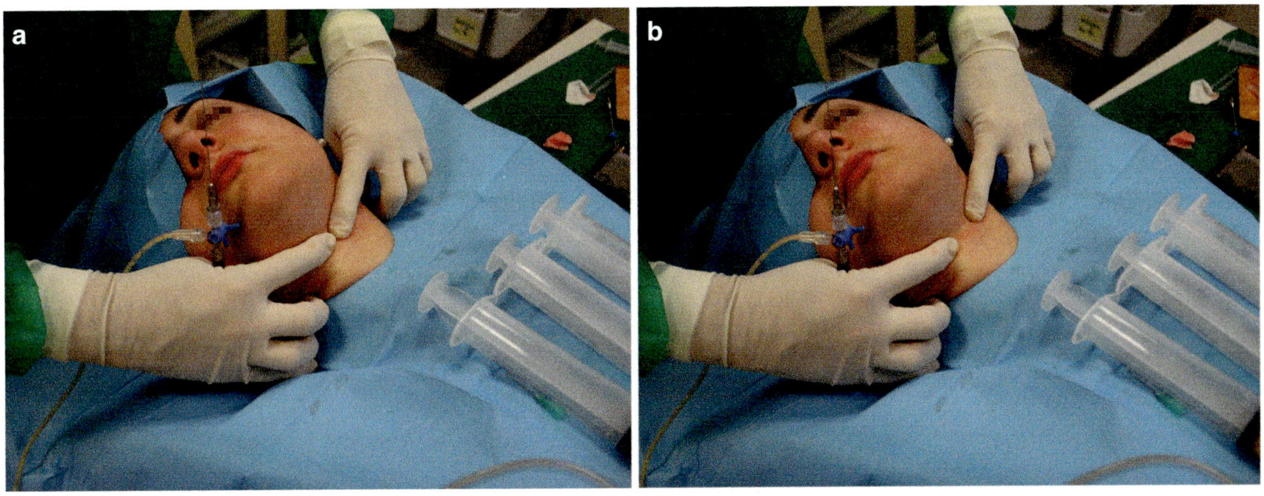

Fig. 20.19 (**a**, **b**) A strong massage is applied to the area. (Published by kind permission of ©Mario Goisis 2018. All Rights Reserved)

Fig. 20.20 The patient during the treatment. The left side of the neck has already been injected. (Published by kind permission of ©Mario Goisis 2018. All Rights Reserved)

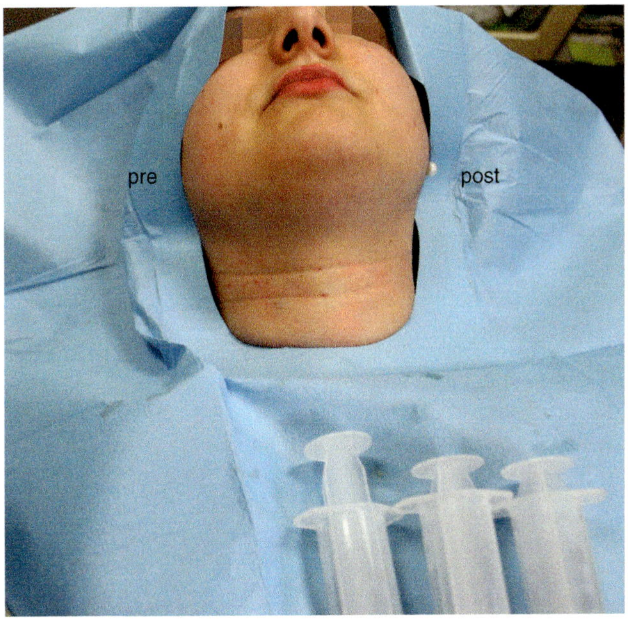

20.5 Bio-rejuvenation Technique for the Treatment of the Neck and "Décolleté"

Bio-rejuvenation is a technique that uses generally low-viscosity hyaluronic acid to stimulate the dermis to produce new matrix and to induce deep hydration of the skin, improving structure and elasticity. The production of endogenous HA declines drastically with age contributing to the formation of wrinkles. Injection of low-viscosity hyaluronic acid into the dermis improves the attraction of fibroblasts, endothelial cells, macrophages, and scavengers of radical-free damaged dermal proteins, thus inducing rejuvenation of the dermal layer (courtesy of Injections in Aesthetic Medicine, Springer).

20.5.1 Indications

Bio-rejuvenation can be used to improve skin trophism, texture, and elasticity of the dermis of every area of the human anatonomy but is usually practiced on the skin of the face, neck, décolleté, and hands.

Low-viscosity hyaluronic acid can be injected follwing a protocol combiniong HA and nanofat over a 12- month period. The standard protocol usually includes:

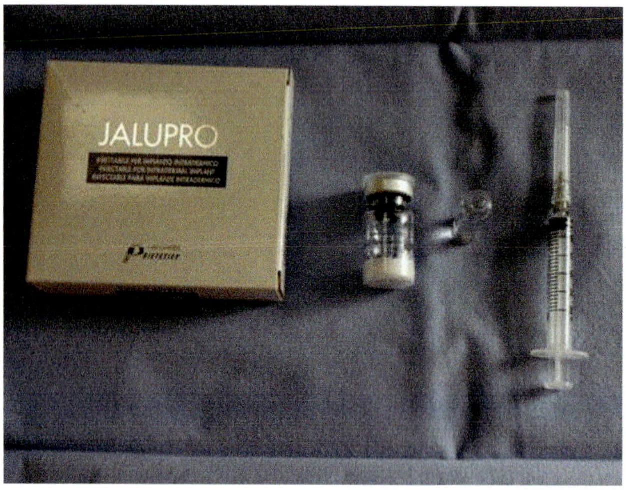

Fig. 20.21 Jalupro (courtesy of Springer, Injections in Aesthetic Medicine). (Published by kind permission of ©Mario Goisis 2018. All Rights Reserved)

Nanograft injection at months 4, 8, and 12
Injection of non-low-viscosity hyaluronic acid at months 1, 2, 3, 5, 6, 7, 9, 10, and 11

20.5.2 Operating Time

The procedure usually takes from 5 to 10 min.

20.5.3 Materials

- 0.8 cc of low-density HA
- 29–30-G needle
- Topical anaesthetic
- Bandages and antiseptic solution

20.5.4 Material Choice

- Jalupro
- Stylage Hydro
- Belotero Soft
- Restylane Vital Light Lidocaine (Figs. 20.21, 20.22a, b, 20.23, 20.24, 20.25, 20.26, and 20.27a, b)

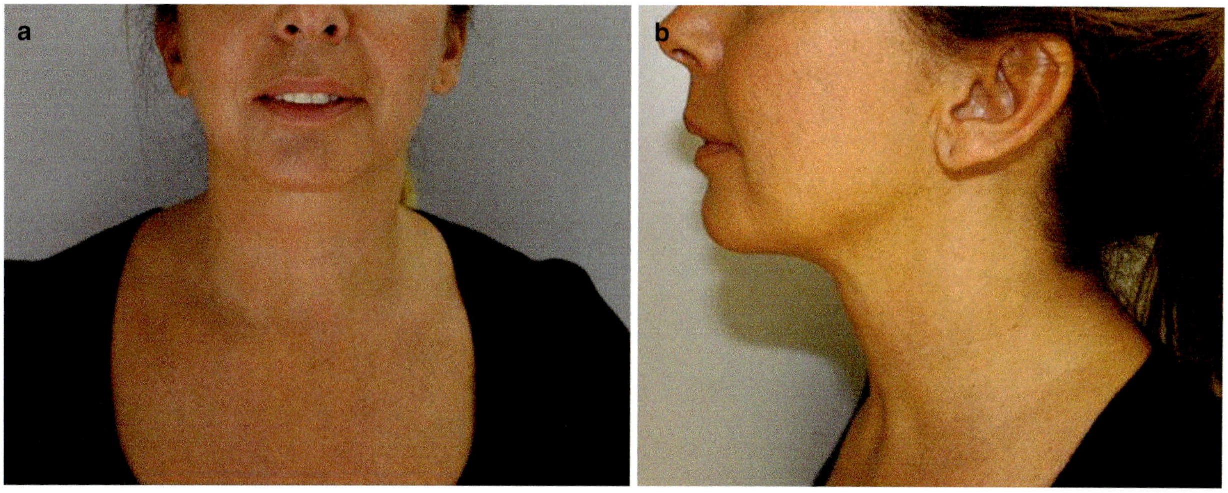

Fig. 20.22 (**a**, **b**) The patient's neck and décolleté before treatment. (Published by kind permission of ©Mario Goisis 2018. All Rights Reserved)

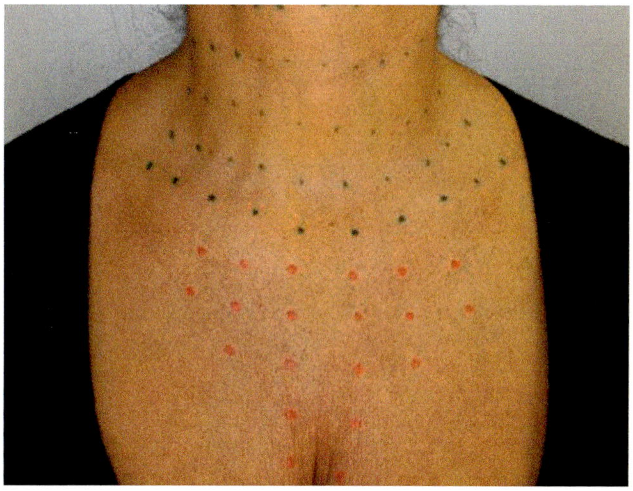

Fig. 20.23 The injection points on the patient's skin are demonstrated. No local anaesthesia is needed, except for a mild local anesthetic gel that may be applied 10–20 min before the treatment. Depending on the product, HA may or may not be mixed with an anaesthetic solution. The presence of the anaesthetic makes the treatment slightly more acceptable for the patient. (Published by kind permission of ©Mario Goisis 2018. All Rights Reserved)

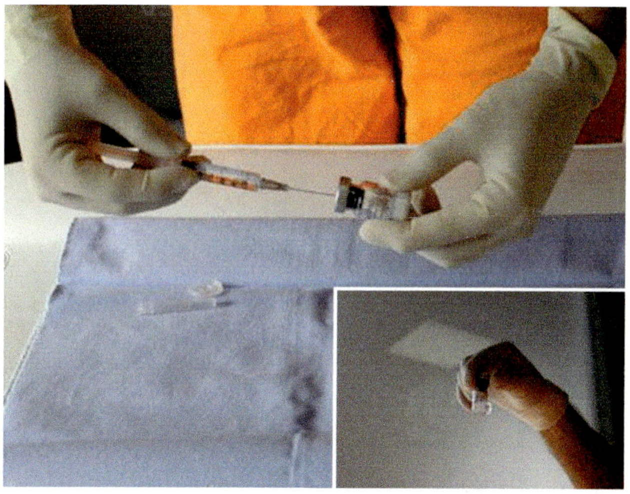

Fig. 20.24 Some products (i.e., Jalupro) are sold as sterile powders and need to be diluted. Here method for dilution of Jalupro is illustrated. The sterile powder is diluted with 2.5 ml of the solvent in the kit. (Published by kind permission of ©Mario Goisis 2018. All Rights Reserved)

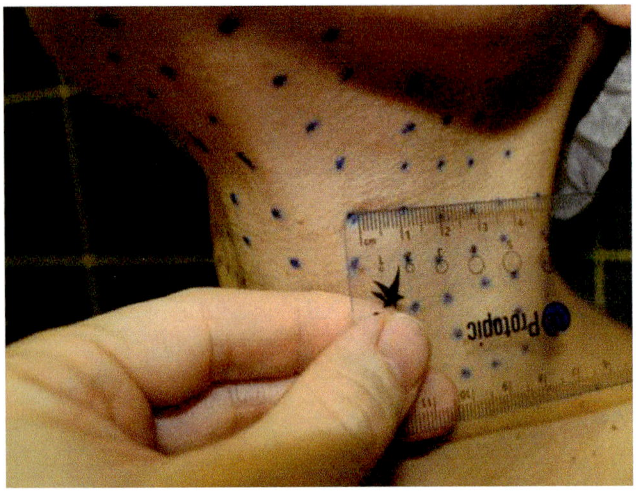

Fig. 20.25 The ideal distance between different injection-points is 1 cm. (Published by kind permission of ©Mario Goisis 2018. All Rights Reserved)

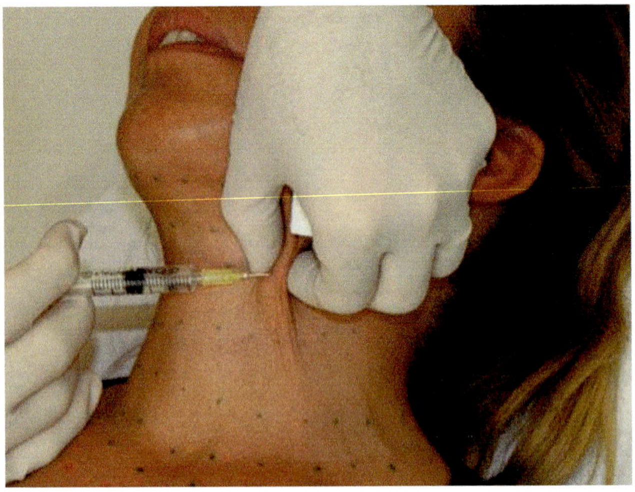

Fig. 20.26 The HA solution is injected into the neck using the picottage technique; pinching the skin between the thumb and index of the free hand permits injection into the correct plane, i.e., the superficial dermis, and reduces the sensation of pain. The needle is inserted for a depth of 2–3 mm; the quantity of product injected is really small, about 0.05 ml or less. (Published by kind permission of ©Mario Goisis 2018. All Rights Reserved)

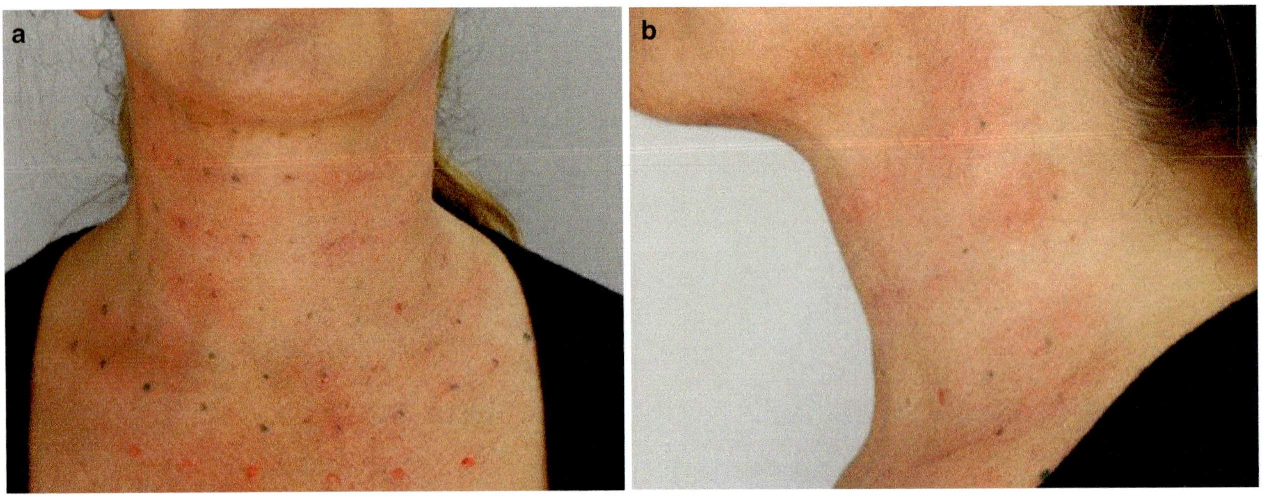

Fig. 20.27 (**a**, **b**) Redness immediately after injection is to be expected. (Published by kind permission of ©Mario Goisis 2018. All Rights Reserved)

20.6 PRP in the Treatment of the Neck and Décolleté

20.6.1 Indications

PRP is not injected into the dermis in order to achieve a volume enhancement such as to fill wrinkles. It is used to obtain fibroblast stimulation. This will lead to production of new collagen and to renewal of the skin.

20.6.2 Contraindications

Platelet dysfunction syndrome

Critical thrombocytopenia

Local infection at the site of the procedure

Consistent use of NSAIDs 48 h prior to the procedure

Corticosteroid injection at treatment site 1 month prior to the procedure

Systemic use of corticosteroids 2 weeks prior to treatment

Cancer (especially hematopoietic or of the bone), HIV, HCV

20.6.3 Operating Time

The procedure usually takes about 45 min.

20.6.4 Materials (Courtesy by Injections in Aesthetic Medicine, Springer)

Tubes for PRP preparation, empty and with anticoagulant (www.microfat.com)

- PRP kit
- Disinfectant alcohol and bandages
- Centrifuge (Figs. 20.28, 20.29, 20.30, and 20.31)

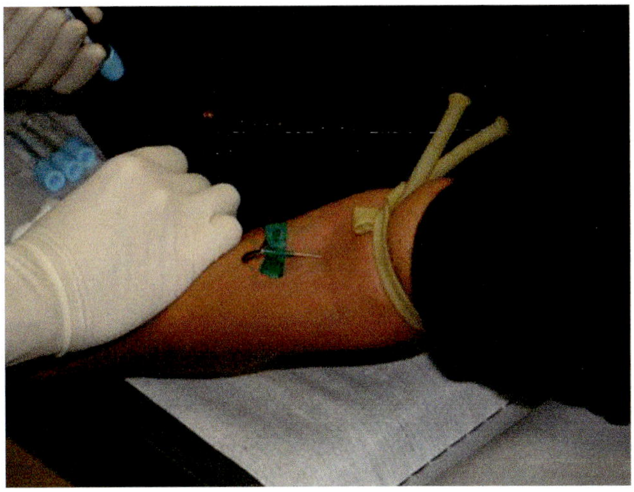

Fig. 20.28 Patient's whole blood is collected. (Published with kind permission of ©Mario Goisis 2018. All Rights Reserved)

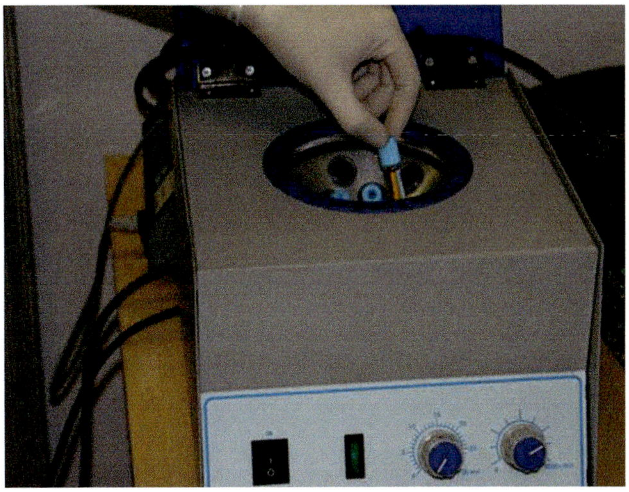

Fig. 20.29 Centrifugation for 5–10 min at 1500 g. (Published by kind permission of ©Mario Goisis 2018. All Rights Reserved)

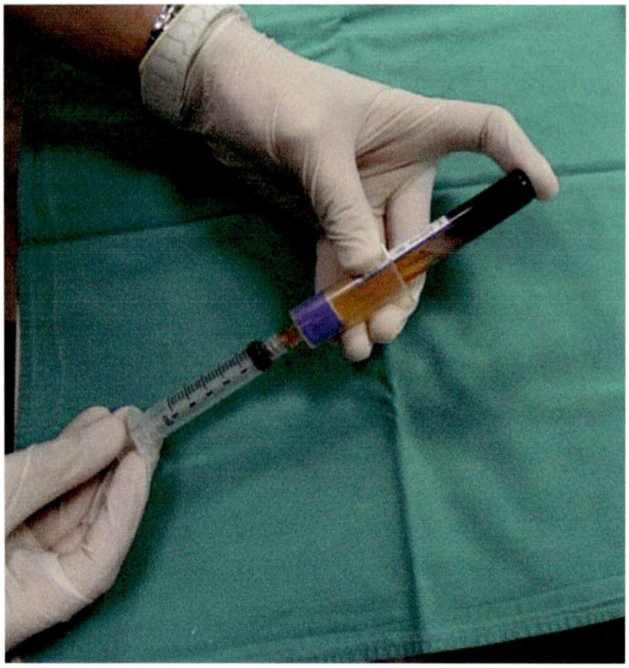

Fig. 20.30 Collection of PRP with a 5-ml luer lock. (Published by kind permission of ©Mario Goisis 2018. All Rights Reserved)

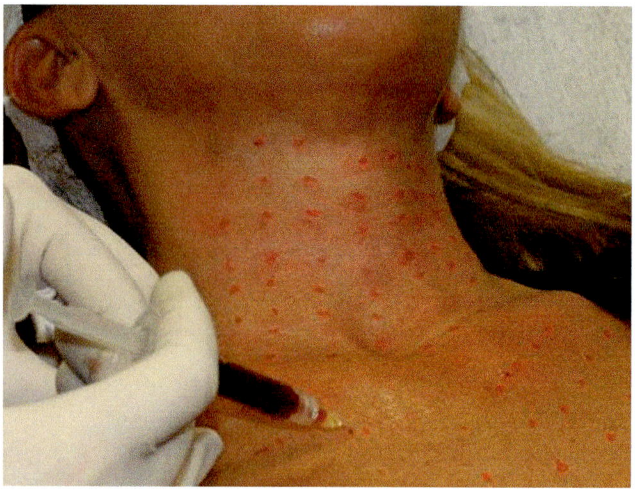

Fig. 20.31 Multiple small injections of 0.1 cc of PRP are injected with 29-/30-G needle (picottage technique) into the neck and décolleté of the patient; the injection should be done into the superficial dermis in each point; the needle should penetrate the skin just 2–3 mm. (Published by kind permission of ©Mario Goisis 2018. All Rights Reserved)

Arms

21

Mario Goisis and Sara Izzo

The ageing process involves the face but does not spare the arms which gradually lose their youthful appearance. Loss of skin elasticity is the principal factor that contributes to the ageing process of the arms.

21.1 Anatomy

The arm extends from the shoulder to the hand and consists of a complex mechanical and functional structure that makes it one of the human body's most useful tools. A fascial layer divides the muscles of the arm into two compartments. The nerve supply is guaranteed by the musculocutaneous and radial nerves. The main artery of the arm is the brachial artery which has an important branch: the profunda brachii. The cephalic and basilic veins are the arm's main veins: the first is located on the medial side of the arm, while the second travels along the lateral side of the arm and ends as the axillary vein. A connection between the two veins is guaranteed by the presence of the medial cubital vein. This vein, which passes through the cubital fossa, is of vital clinical importance for drawing blood (Fig. 21.1).

21.2 Pitfalls

Examination and identification of the major superficial vessels is useful to avoid haematomas.

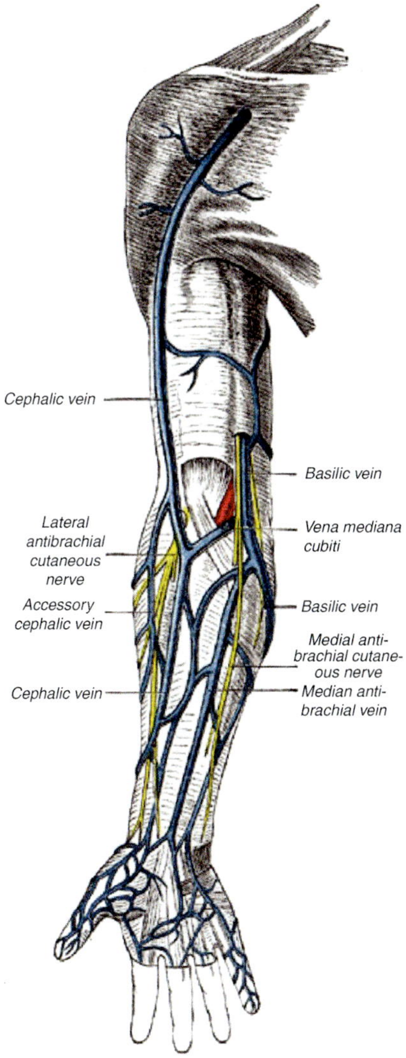

Fig. 21.1 A coloured illustration of the anatomy of the veins of the upper arm. (Published by kind permission of ©Mario Goisis 2018. All Rights Reserved)

M. Goisis (✉)
Maxillo-Facial and Aesthetic Surgeon, Go Easy Clinic, Milan, Italy

S. Izzo
Department of Plastic Surgery, University of Campania "Luigi Vanvitelli", Naples, Italy

M. Goisis (ed.), *Outpatient Regenerative Medicine*, https://doi.org/10.1007/978-3-319-44894-7_21

21.2.1 Improvement of the Arms using Nanofat

Nanograft can be used to improve trophism, texture, and elasticity of the dermis in every area of the body but it is usually injected into the skin of the face, neck, décolleté, and hands.

Rejuvenation is particularly indicated in people who smoke and/or are exposed to sunlight for long periods of time.

21.2.2 Contraindications

In patients with coagulation defects or on current anticoagulant therapy, the treatment is relatively contraindicated. As with all injections, in fact, these subjects are at considerable risk of bleeding and haematoma formation.

- The nanofat should not be injected into areas lacking sufficient blood supply or suffering from infection or inflammation.
- No injection should be carried out if the area has been previously treated with liquid silicone or other permanent fillers because a new injection might lead to inflammation or infection of the implants.

21.2.3 Operating Time

The procedure usually takes from 5 to 10 min, once the nanofat has been produced.

Plane of injection: dermis-hypodermis

21.2.4 Indications

Amelioration of small wrinkles and laxity of the arms

21.2.5 Materials

- *1–2 cc of nanofat on each side for injection of nanofat: [1–2 cc of nanofat for injection into each side]*
  - *26-gauge needle*
  - *27-gauge 3.7 cm blunt cannula*

A standard system for producing nanofat is used, in particular:

- The nanofat system (www.microfat.com), composed of a connector with a closed system for emulsion and filtering of the microfat
- 2 10-cc syringes

To harvest and process the fat, a standard microfat system is used, in particular:

- A microfat box (www.microfat.com), composed of a ramp with a closed system for washing and filtration
- 4 60-cc syringes
- 2 10-cc syringes
- One 1-cc syringe
- 30-gauge needle
- 16-gauge needle
- A 2 mm-diameter, 10 cm-long Goisis cannula for fat harvesting
- A chlorhexidine-alcohol solution (2% chlorhexidine gluconate and 70% isopropyl alcohol), sterile drapes or towels
- Ice packs
- Sterile 2 cm × 2 cm gauze squares
- Occlusive dressing cover

Medications include:

100 cc of cold saline solution.
120 cc of cold Klein solution.
One litre of Klein solution is composed of 800 mg of lidocaine, 1 mg of epinephrine, 40 MEq of sodium bicarbonate, and 1000 cc of saline solution.

Location: The microfat harvesting can be carried out in a small operating theatre/medical surgery. Oxygen, the pulse oximetry, and a crash cart/box should be present.

Assistants: The aid of an assistant can prove useful for the transfer of items to the procedure field in a sterile manner during the first stage of the procedure. In any case, a single doctor may carry out the entire procedure alone.

Plane of injection: subcutaneous-intradermal

21.2.6 Method

The method is illustrated in Figs. 21.2, 21.3, 21.4, 21.5, 21.6, 21.7a, b and 21. 8a, b.

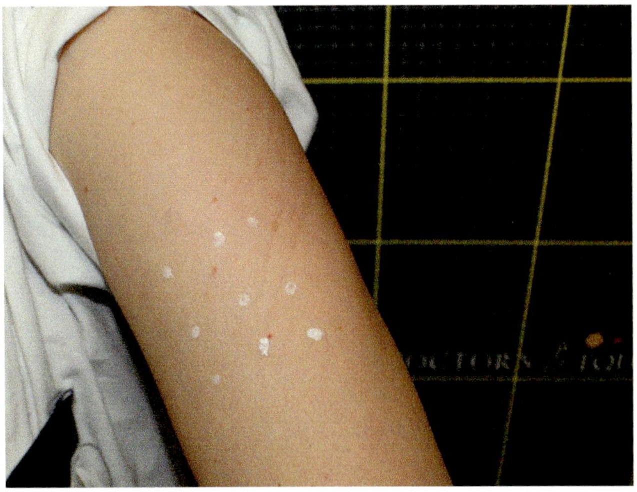

Fig. 21.2 Here the injection points on the patient's skin are shown. No local anesthesia is needed, except for a mild local anesthetic gel which may be applied 10–20 min before the treatment. (Published by kind permission of ©Mario Goisis 2018. All Rights Reserved)

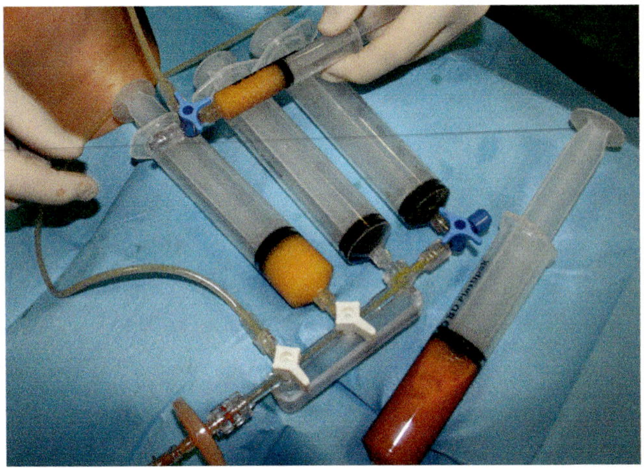

Fig. 21.3 Five cc of microfat is produced using the microfat box (www.microfat.com). (Published by kind permission of ©Mario Goisis 2018. All Rights Reserved)

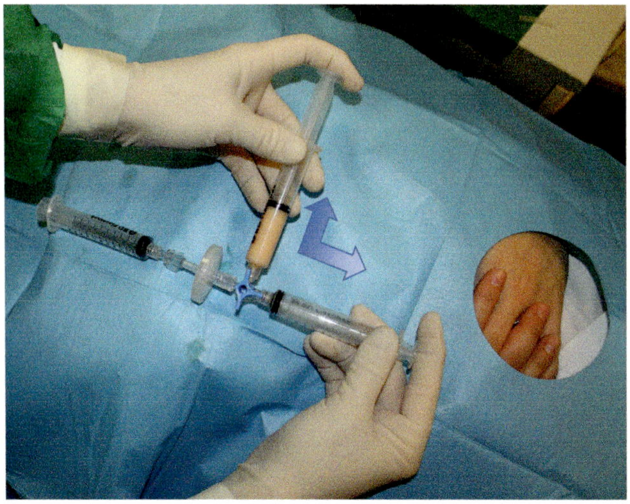

Fig. 21.4 The 10 cc syringes are connected to the DE nanofat kit (www.microfat.com). The fat is moved quickly between the two syringes 30 times. (Published by kind permission of ©Mario Goisis 2018. All Rights Reserved)

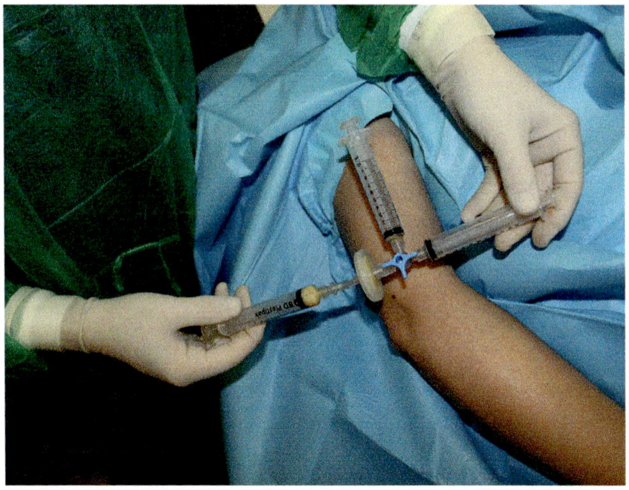

Fig. 21.5 The fat is filtered and transferred directly into the third syringe. (Published by kind permission of ©Mario Goisis 2018. All Rights Reserved)

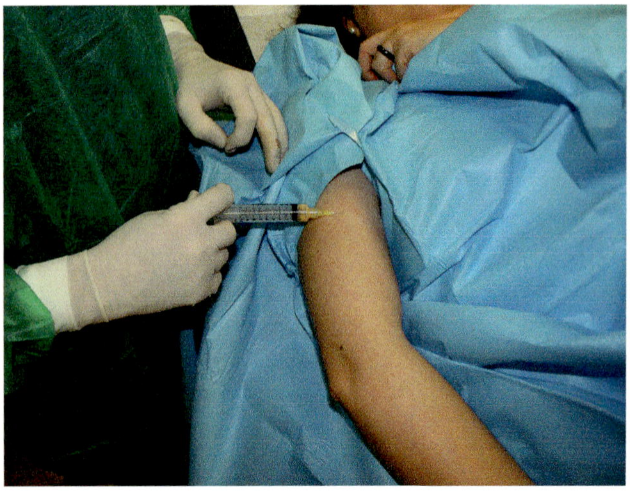

Fig. 21.6 Having been filtered, the nanofat can be injected directly using a 30-G needle. (Published by kind permission of ©Mario Goisis 2018. All Rights Reserved)

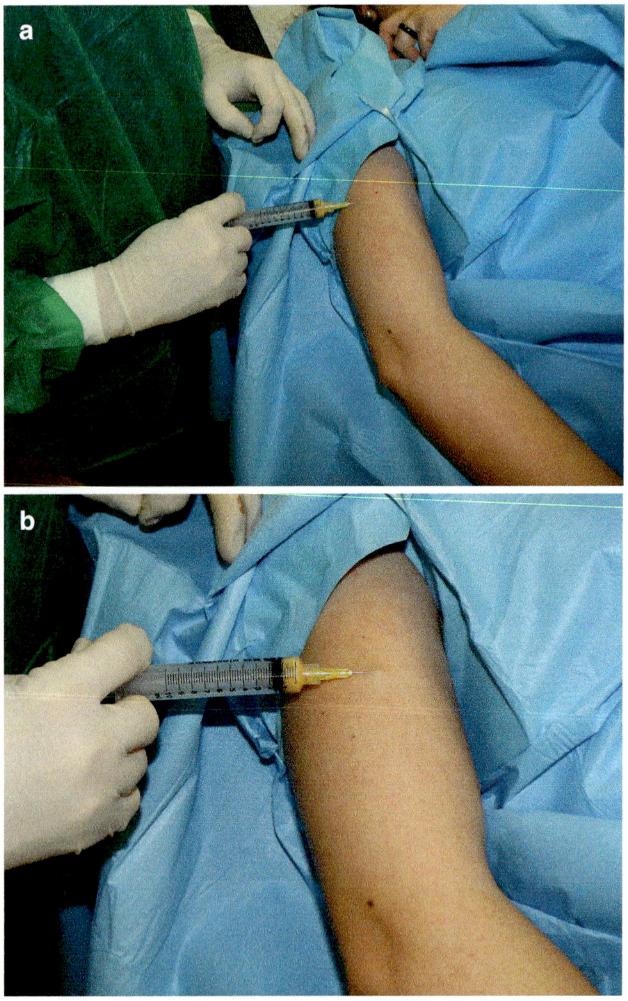

Fig. 21.7 (**a**, **b**) The nanograft is injected into the intradermal/subcutaneous plane of the arms. The needle is inserted for 1–3 mm; the quantity of product injected is really small, about 0.1 ml or less. (Published by kind permission of ©Mario Goisis 2018. All Rights Reserved)

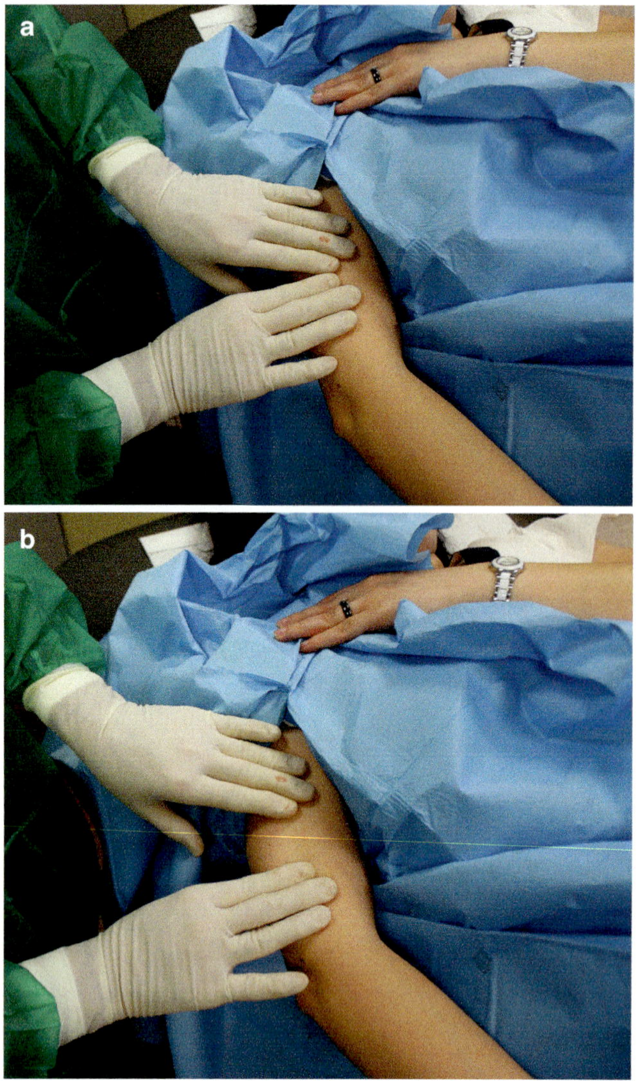

Fig. 21.8 (**a**, **b**) A strong massage is applied to the area after injection. (Published by kind permission of ©Mario Goisis 2018. All Rights Reserved)

Hands

22

Mario Goisis, Sara Izzo, and Claudio Rinna

Hands start showing signs of ageing when they lose volume and the anatomy under the skin becomes noticeably visible. The addition of volume to the hand by injecting fat is a good way to restore its plump fullness and lessen exposure of the joints and veins.

22.1 Anatomy

The dorsal superficial fascia of the hand covers the tendons of the extensor and intrinsic muscles on the dorsal surface of the hand. Between the skin and the superficial dorsal fascia, a network of superficial veins is immersed in a thin layer of subcutaneous tissue.

22.2 Pitfalls

While filling the back of the hand, it is important to insert the needle into the surface of the dorsal fascia, in order to obtain a satisfying aesthetic result. The use of a blunt needle is recommended to minimize the chances of damaging the superficial vein network. Safe and reliable points of injection can be obtained in the gap between each of the tendons distal to the wrist. Irregularities and hypercorrection can be particularly evident in this area and cause significant discomfort to patients who need their hands to perform numerous everyday activities. For this reason, recourse to the injection technique avoids damage to the noble structures of the hand. It is mandatory not to inject too much product at once and it is vital to recommend that the patient massage the treated areas (Figs. 22.1 and 22.2).

M. Goisis (✉)
Maxillo-Facial and Aesthetic Surgeon, Go Easy Clinic, Milan, Italy

S. Izzo
Department of Plastic Surgery, University of Campania "Luigi Vanvitelli", Naples, Italy

C. Rinna
Doctor's Equipe, Milan, Italy

22.3 Augmentation of the Back of the Hand Using a Mix of Micrograft and PRP

22.3.1 Indications

Hands that have lost volume and roundness and whose veings are prominent on the back.

The mix of micrograft and PRP may be used successfully even on the hands of the very elderly.

22.3.2 Contraindications

- Relative contraindications are anatomical alterations due to previous trauma or surgical intervention. Scarring often induces a displacement of the noble structures and can lead to oerforation of the artery perforation or resection of the nerve. It may also induce retracting scars that can cause asymmetry and unequal filling of the part treated.
- The fat should not be injected in areas that lack sufficient blood supply or are suffering from an infection or inflammation.

22.3.3 Complications and Management

Immediate complications (within 72 h after the injection) are transient erythema, oedema, induration, pruritus, and ecchymosis.

Early complications (days to weeks after the injection) include hypercorrection, local infection, necrosis of the skin, reactivation of herpes, discoloration, and persistent local symptoms (erythema, oedema, induration, pruritus, and hyperpigmentation).

Later complications include high rates of fat resorption and cysts.

M. Goisis (ed.), *Outpatient Regenerative Medicine*, https://doi.org/10.1007/978-3-319-44894-7_22

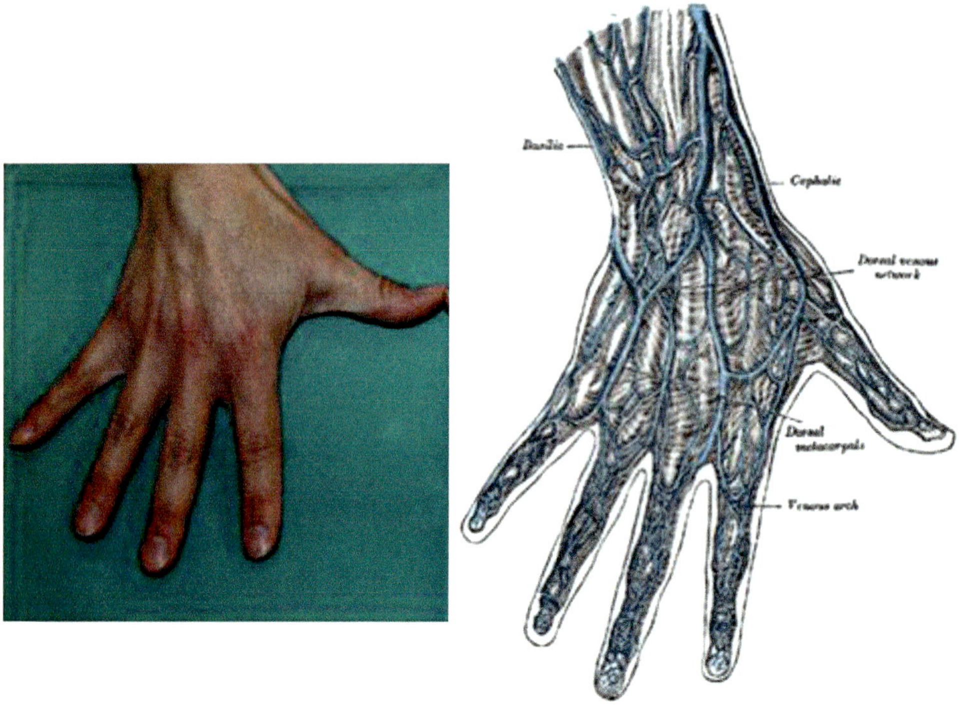

Fig. 22.1 This figure provides two pictures of the hand. The drawing on the right shows the vein plexus of the hand and is a reproduction of a lithographic plate taken from *Gray's Anatomy* (Henry Gray, Anatomy: Descriptive and Surgical). (Published by kind permission of ©Mario Goisis 2018. All Rights Reserved)

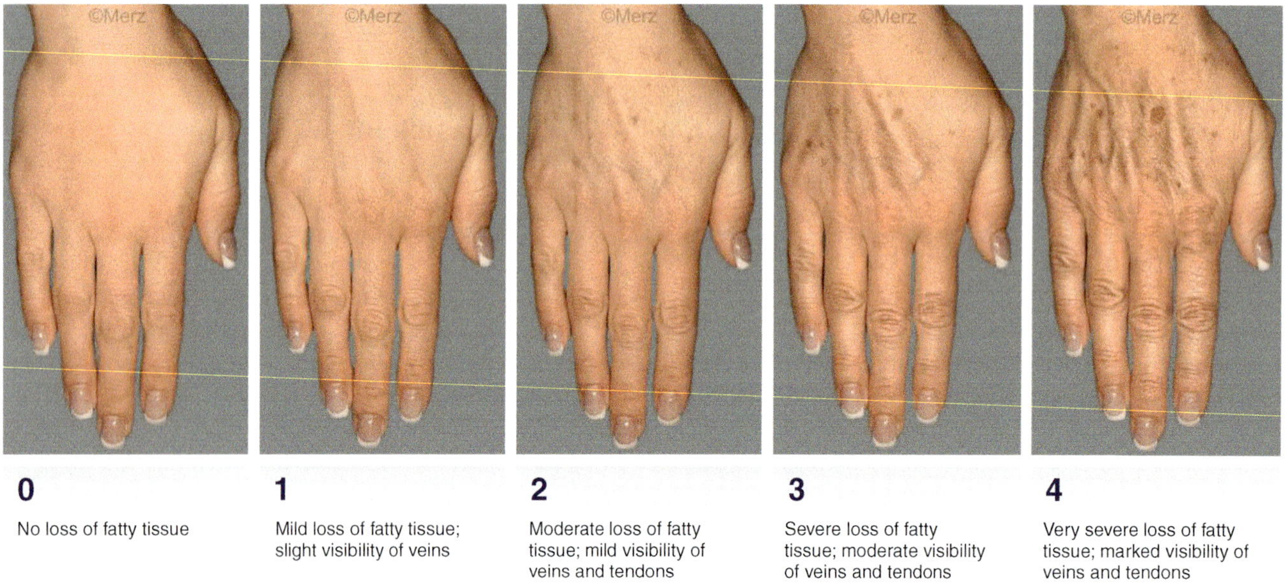

Fig. 22.2 Different degrees of loss of fatty tissue and ageing of the hands (courtesy of the Merz Company). (Published by kind permission of ©Mario Goisis 2018. All Rights Reserved)

22.3.4 Operating Time

The procedure usually takes 5 min, once the fat is harvested.

22.3.5 Materials

- *2–4 cc of microfat on each side for injection of microfat: [2–4 cc of the microfat for injection into both sides]*
  - *21-gauge needle*
  - *22-gauge 4 cm blunt cannula*

To harvest and process the microfat a standard system is used, in particular:

- A microfat box (www.microfat.com), composed of a ramp with a closed system for washing and filtration
- 4 60-cc syringes
- 2 10-cc syringes

- One 1-cc syringe
- 30-gauge needle
- 16-gauge needle
- A 2 mm-diameter, 10 cm-long Goisis cannula for fat harvesting
- A chlorhexidine-alcohol solution (2% chlorhexidine gluconate and 70% isopropyl alcohol), sterile drapes or towels
- Ice packs
- Sterile 2 cm × 2 cm gauze squares
- Occlusive dressing cover

Medications include:

100 cc of cold saline solution.
120 cc of cold Klein solution.
One liter of Klein solution is composed of 800 mg of lidocaine, 1 mg of epinephrine, 40 MEq of sodium bicarbonate, and 1000 cc of saline solution.

Location: Microfat harvesting can be carried out in a small operating theatre/medical surgery. Oxygen, the pulse oximetry, and a crash cart/box should be present.

Assistants: The aid of an assistant can prove useful for the transfer of items into the procedure field in a sterile manner the first part of the procedure. Regardless of this, a single doctor may carry out the entire procedure alone.

22.3.6 The Procedure

The procedure is shown in Figures 22.3, 22.4, 22.5a, b, 22.6, 22.7, 22.8, 22.9, 22.10, 22.11, 22.12, 22.13, 22.14, 22.15, 22.16, 22.17, and 22.18.

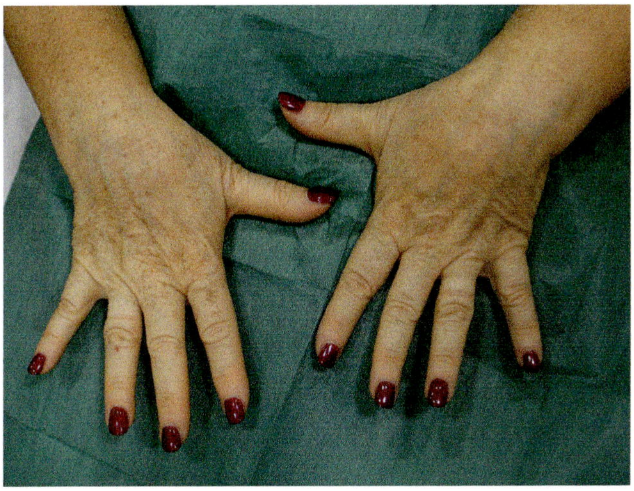

Fig. 22.3 Hands before the treatment. (Published by kind permission of ©Mario Goisis 2018. All Rights Reserved)

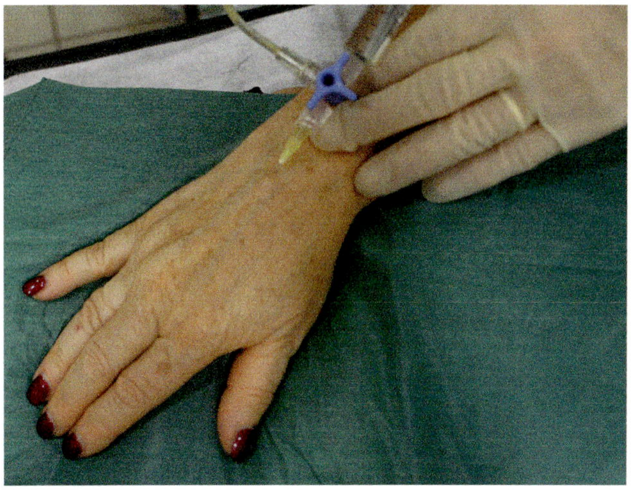

Fig. 22.4 0.5 cc of Klein solution is injected at a single entry point located between the third and fourth metacarpal bones. This precautionary measure ensures that the treatment with the blunt-tip cannula cause the patient no pain. (Published by kind permission of ©Mario Goisis 2018. All Rights Reserved)

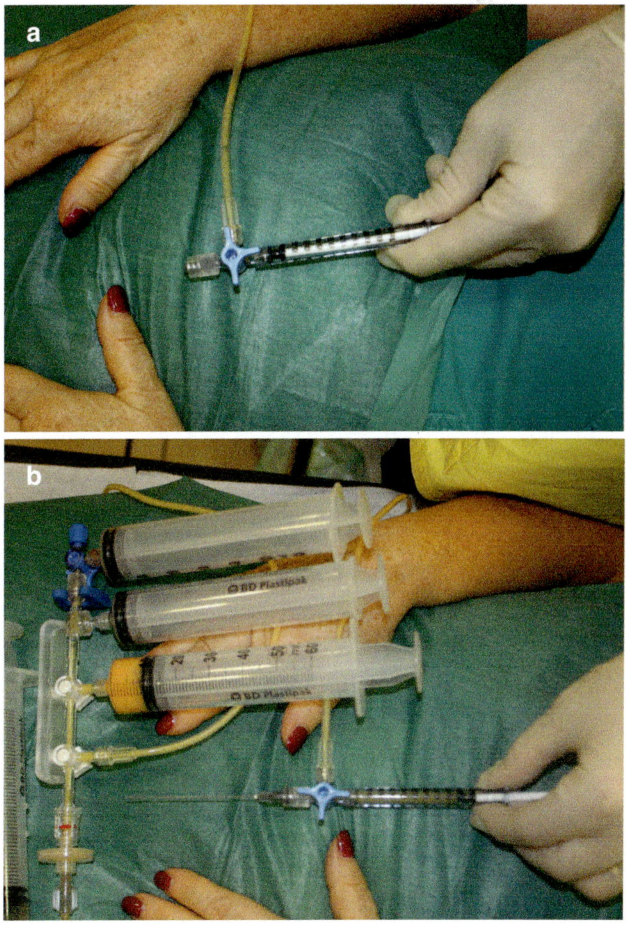

Fig. 22.5 The 1-cc syringe is connected with to the micrograft box is filled with microfat plus PRP. (Published by kind permission of ©Mario Goisis 2018. All Rights Reserved)

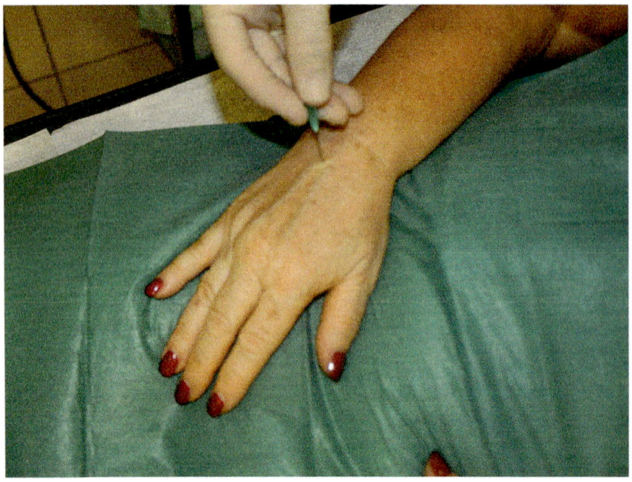

Fig. 22.6 A small hole is made on the border between the hand and wrist, to permit the cannula to enter the subcutaneous plane. A 21-G needle is used for this purpose. (Published by kind permission of ©Mario Goisis 2018. All Rights Reserved)

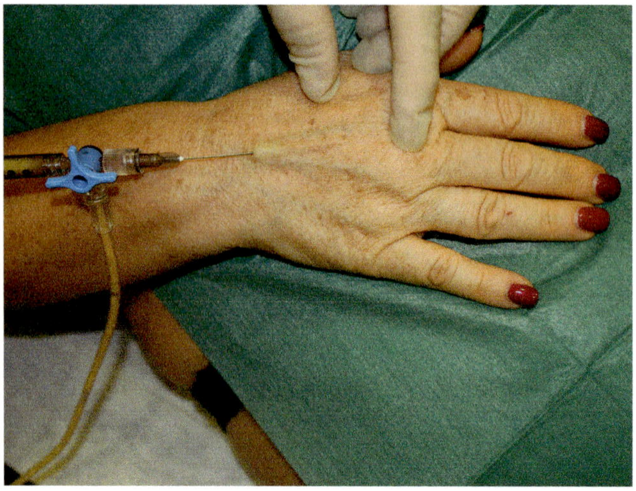

Fig. 22.8 The fat is released, retrograde fashion, onto the subcutaneous plane and into the spaces between the metacarpal bones. (Published by kind permission of ©Mario Goisis 2018. All Rights Reserved)

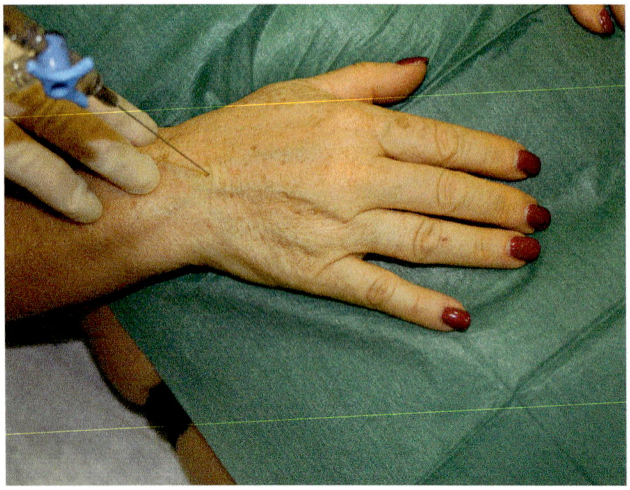

Fig. 22.7 Perpendicular insertion of a 22-G blunt-tip cannula. The cannula is plunged deep into the skin while attention is paid to remaining superficial to the dorsal superficial fascia. The tip of the cannula is then directed up to the level of the finger joints. (Published by kind permission of ©Mario Goisis 2018. All Rights Reserved)

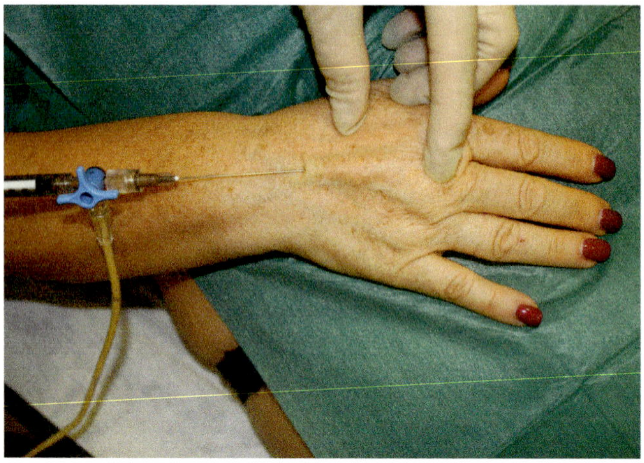

Fig. 22.9 The fat is released, retrograde fashion, onto the subcutaneous plane and into the spaces between the metacarpal bones. (Published by kind permission of ©Mario Goisis 2018. All Rights Reserved)

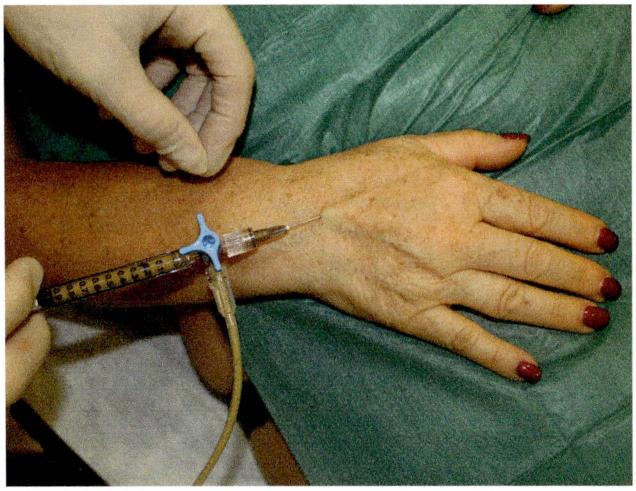

Fig. 22.10 The fat is released, retrograde fashion, onto the subcutaneous plane and into the spaces between the metacarpal bones. (Published by kind permission of ©Mario Goisis 2018. All Rights Reserved)

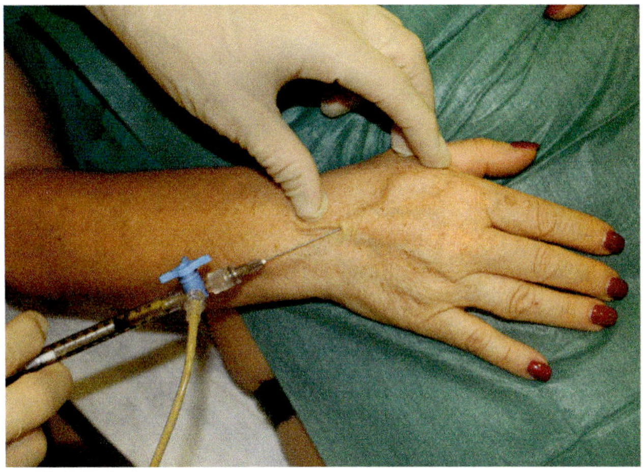

Fig. 22.11 The fat is released, retrograde fashion, onto the subcutaneous plane and into the spaces between the metacarpal bones. (Published by kind permission of ©Mario Goisis 2018. All Rights Reserved)

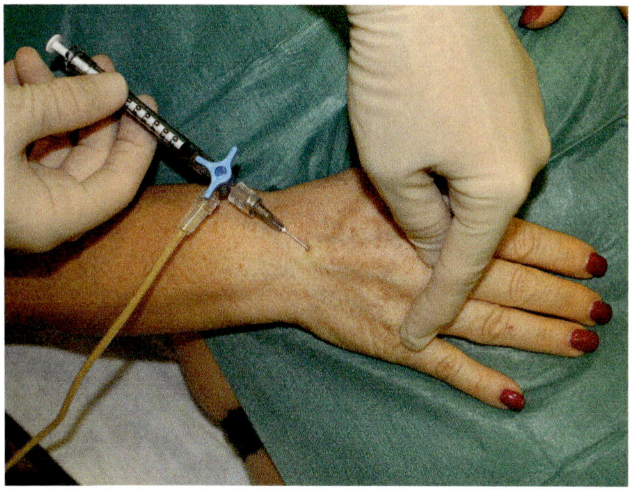

Fig. 22.12 The fat is released, retrograde fashion, onto the subcutaneous plane and into the spaces between the metacarpal bones. (Published by kind permission of ©Mario Goisis 2018. All Rights Reserved)

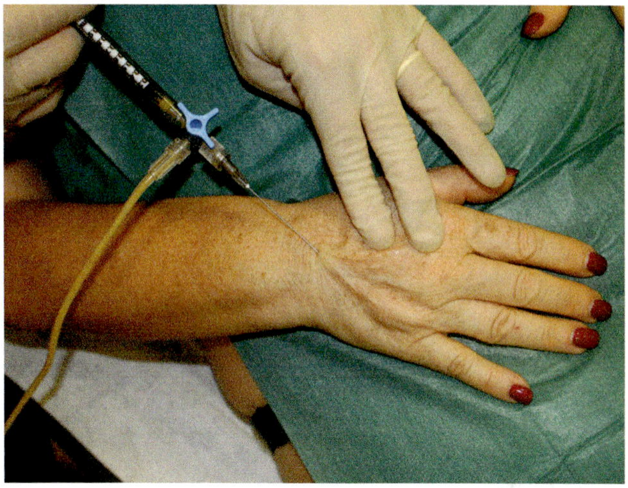

Fig. 22.13 The fat is released, retrograde fashion, onto the subcutaneous plane and into the spaces between the metacarpal bones. (Published by kind permission of ©Mario Goisis 2018. All Rights Reserved)

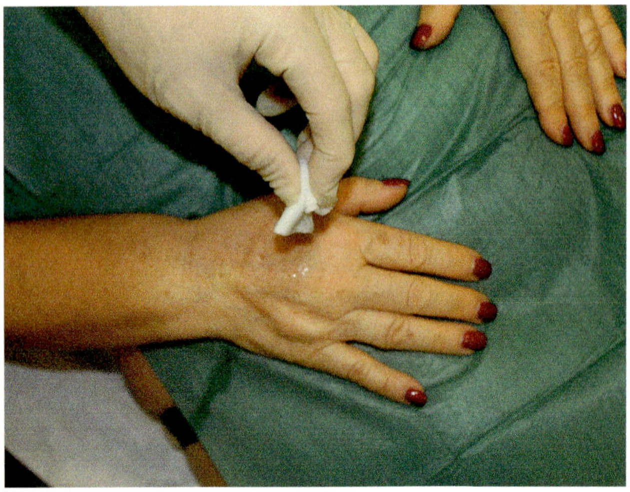

Fig. 22.14 After the injection, a strong massage is applied to the back of the hand. A wet gauze can make it easier to spread the fat. (Published by kind permission of ©Mario Goisis 2018. All Rights Reserved)

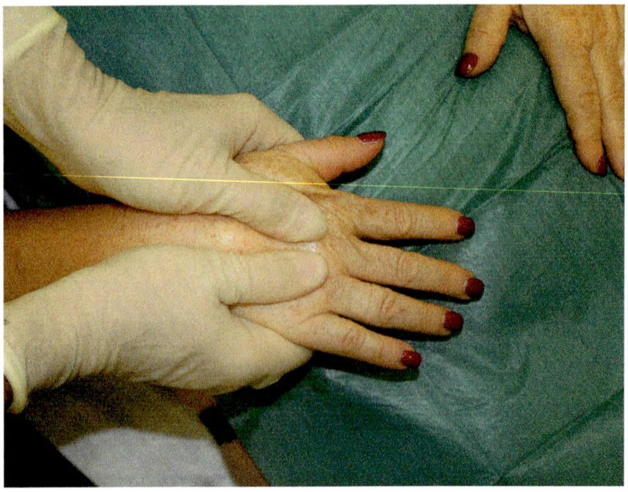

Fig. 22.15 After the injection, a strong massage is applied on the back of the hand. A wet gauze can make it easier to spread the fat. (Published by kind permission of ©Mario Goisis 2018. All Rights Reserved)

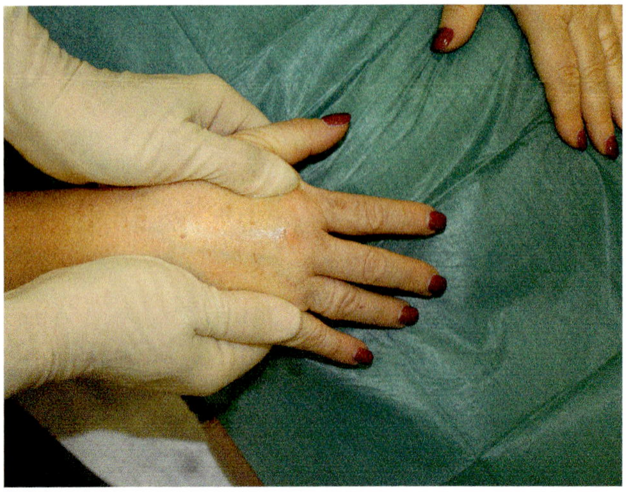

Fig. 22.16 After the injection, a strong massage is applied to the back of the hand. A wet gauze can make it easier to spread the fat. (Published by kind permission of ©Mario Goisis 2018. All Rights Reserved)

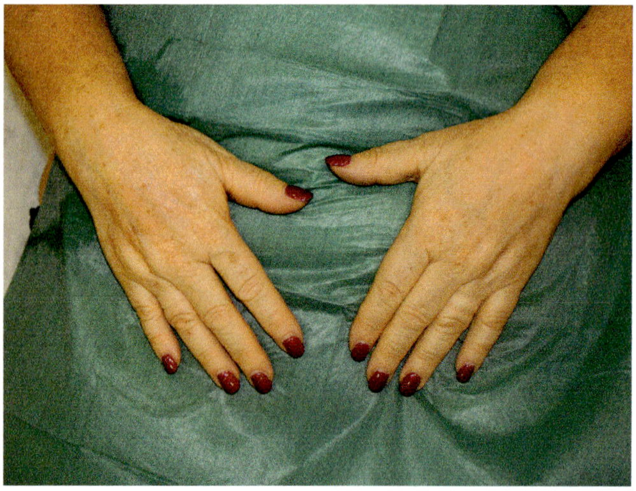

Fig. 22.17 The hands after the treatment. (Published by kind permission of ©Mario Goisis 2018. All Rights Reserved)

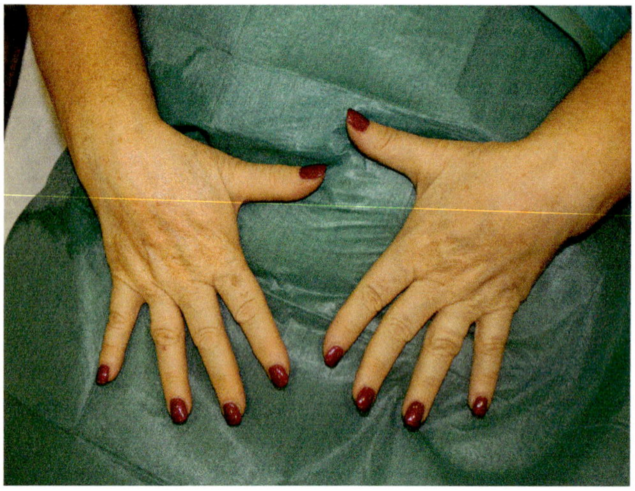

Fig. 22.18 The hands after the treatment. (Published by kind permission of ©Mario Goisis 2018. All Rights Reserved)

Augmentation of the Pectoralis Muscle Using Injections of Microfat

23

Mario Goisis, Sara Izzo, and Claudio Rinna

23.1 Anatomy

The pectoralis major is one of the muscles of the chest. It comprises the bulk of the chest muscles in the male (Fig. 23.1). The pectoralis minor, a triangular muscle, is located underneath the pectoralis major.

23.1.1 Indications

Pectoral enlargement is indicated when seeking to achieve a more athletic figure.

In case of malformation, these methods help restore the symmetry of the thorax.

23.1.2 Contraindications

The fat should not be injected into areas that lack sufficient blood supply or that are suffering from infection or inflammation. No injection should be carried out if the chest has been previously treated with liquid silicone or other permanent fillers because a new injection might lead to inflammation or infection of the implants.

23.1.3 Operating Time

The procedure usually takes 20 min, once the fat has been harvested.

Plane of injection: the intramuscular-submuscular plane

M. Goisis (✉)
Maxillo-Facial and Aesthetic Surgeon, Go Easy Clinic, Milan, Italy

S. Izzo
Department of Plastic Surgery, University of Campania "Luigi Vanvitelli", Naples, Italy

C. Rinna
Doctor's Equipe, Milan, Italy

23.1.4 Materials

- 20–60 cc of microfat for injection into both sides
- 1.5 mm × 150 mm, filling cannula

To harvest and process the microfat, a standard system is used, in particular:

- A microfat box (www.microfat.com), composed of a ramp with a closed system for washing and filtration
- 4 60-cc syringes
- 2 10-cc syringes
- One 1-cc syringe
- 30-gauge needle
- 16-gauge needle
- A 2 mm-diameter, 10 cm-long Goisis cannula for fat harvesting
- A chlorhexidine-alcohol solution (2% chlorhexidine gluconate and 70% isopropyl alcohol), sterile drapes or towels
- Ice packs
- Sterile 2 cm × 2 cm gauze squares
- Occlusive dressing cover

Medications include:

- 200 cc of cold saline solution.
- 500 cc of cold Klein solution.
- One liter of Klein solution is composed of 800 mg of lidocaine, 1 mg of epinephrine, 40 MEq of sodium bicarbonate, and 1000 cc of saline solution.

Location: Harvesting of the microfat can be carried out in a small operating theatre/medical surgery. Oxygen, the pulse oximetry, and a crash cart/box should be present.

Assistants: The aid of an assistant can prove useful when transferring items to the procedure field in a sterile manner during the first stage of the procedure. Nevertheless, a single doctor can carry out the entire procedure alone.

M. Goisis (ed.), *Outpatient Regenerative Medicine*, https://doi.org/10.1007/978-3-319-44894-7_23

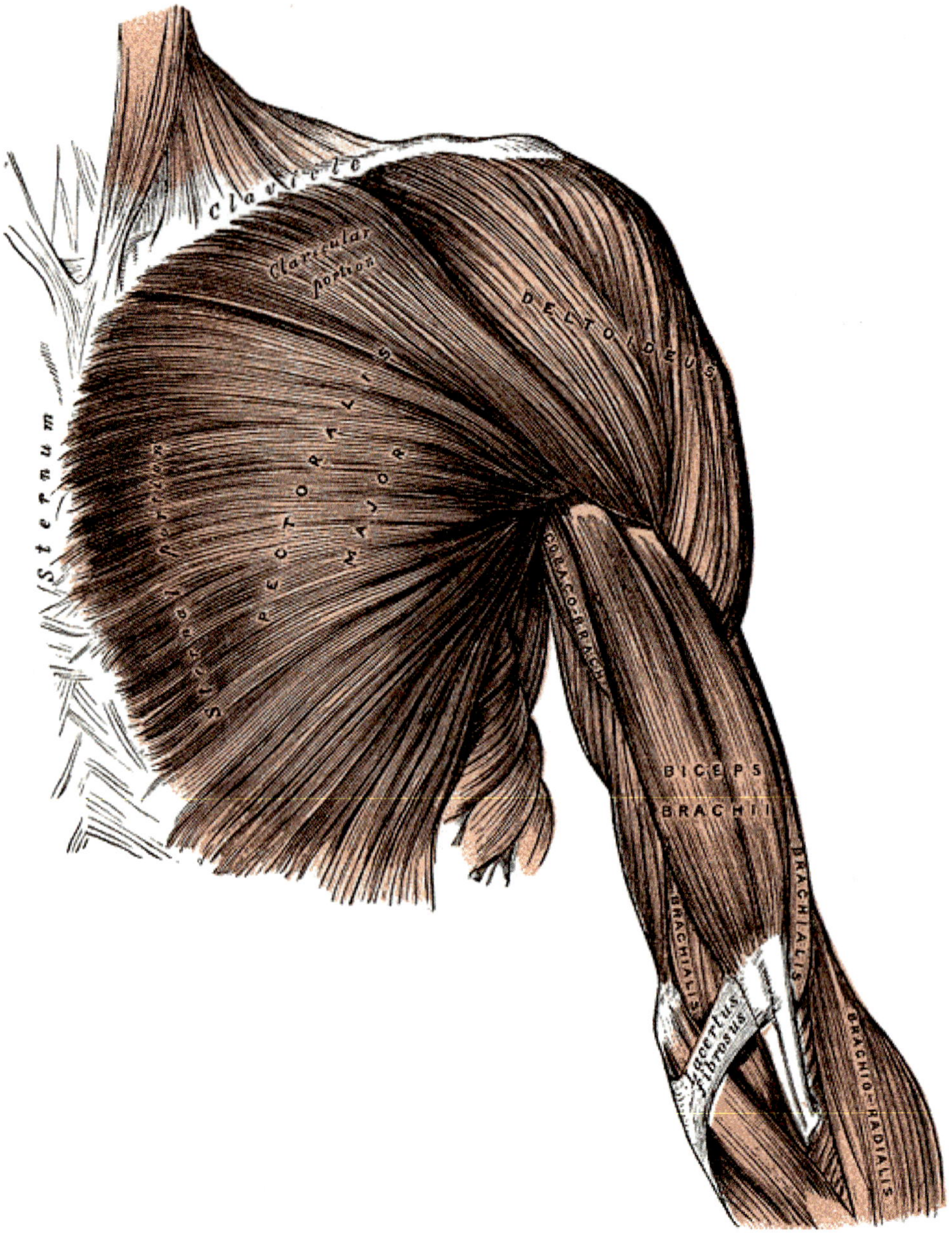

Fig. 23.1 The pectoralis muscles (Gray's Anatomy, 1918). (Published by kind permission of ©Mario Goisis 2018. All Rights Reserved)

23.1.5 The Procedure

The procedure is illustrated in figures 23.2a–d, 23.3, 23.4, 23.5a–d, and 23.6a, b below.

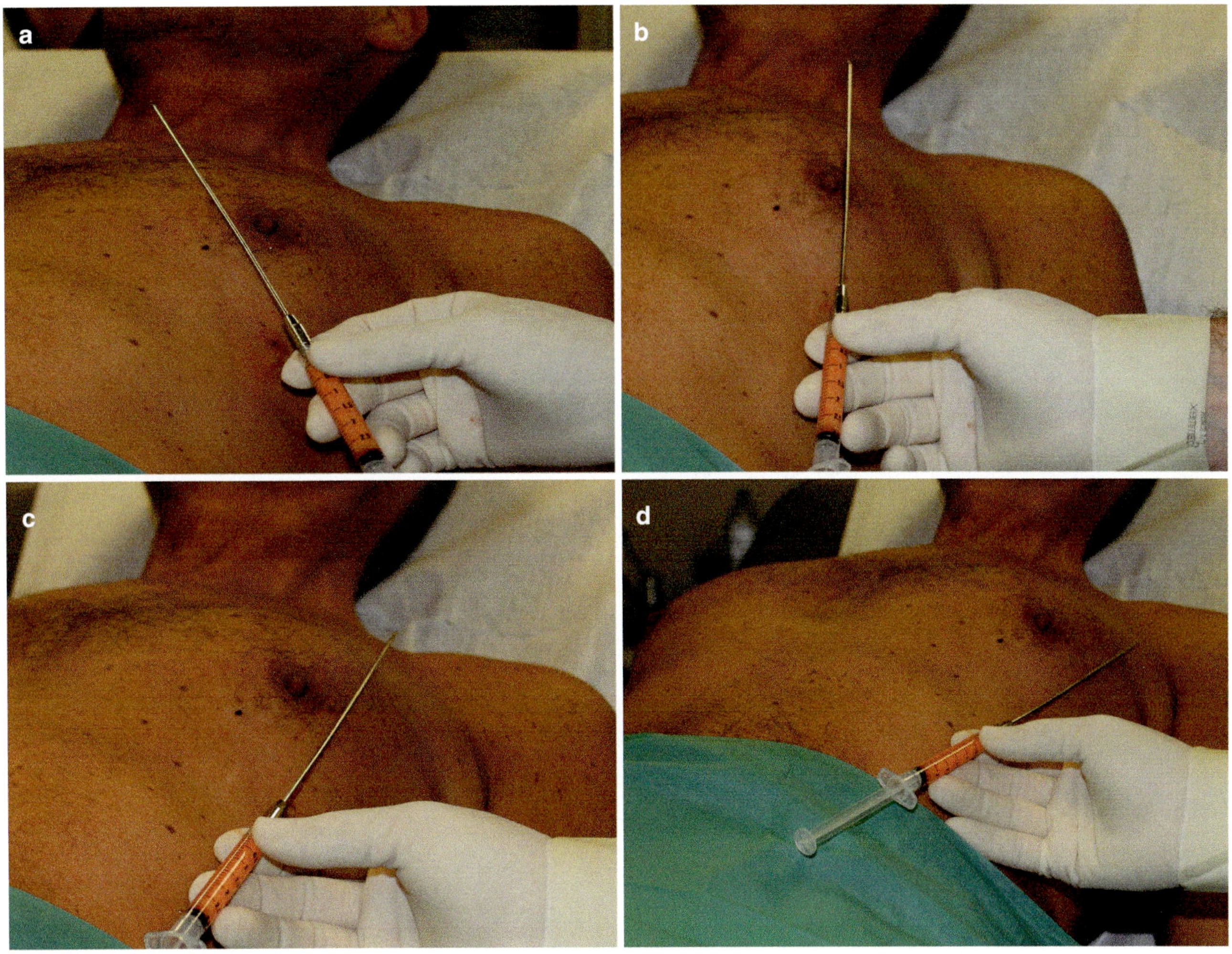

Fig. 23.2 (**a**–**d**) The route of the cannula is demonstrated as well as the fanlike distribution of the microfat. (Published by kind permission of ©Mario Goisis 2018. All Rights Reserved)

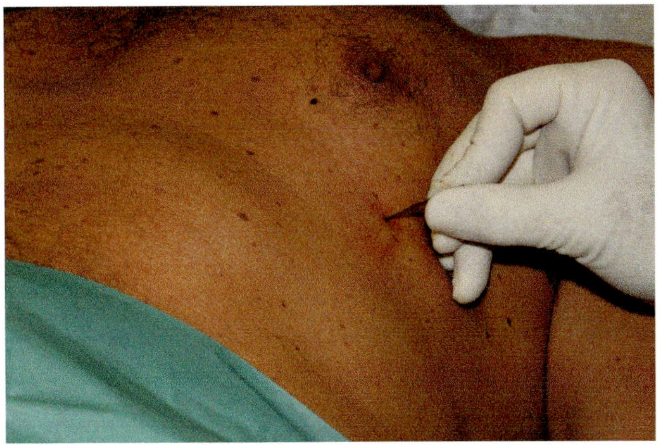

Fig. 23.3 The entry point 1 cm under the inframammary fold is created using eleven blades. (Published by kind permission of ©Mario Goisis 2018. All Rights Reserved)

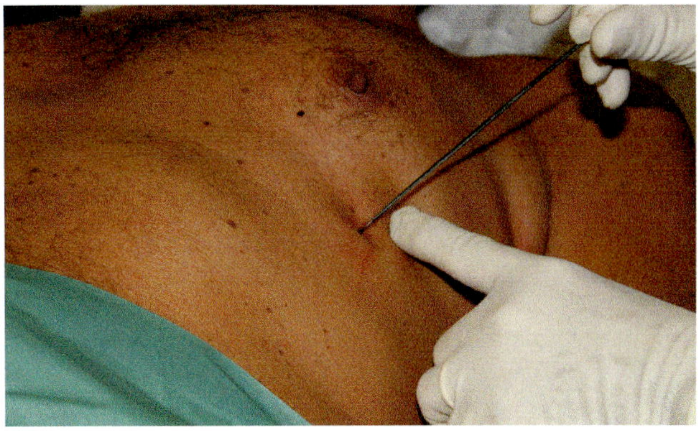

Fig. 23.4 Perpendicular insertion of a 1.5 mm blunt-tip cannula. The cannula is plunged in depth into the pectoralis major muscle. (Published by kind permission of ©Mario Goisis 2018. All Rights Reserved)

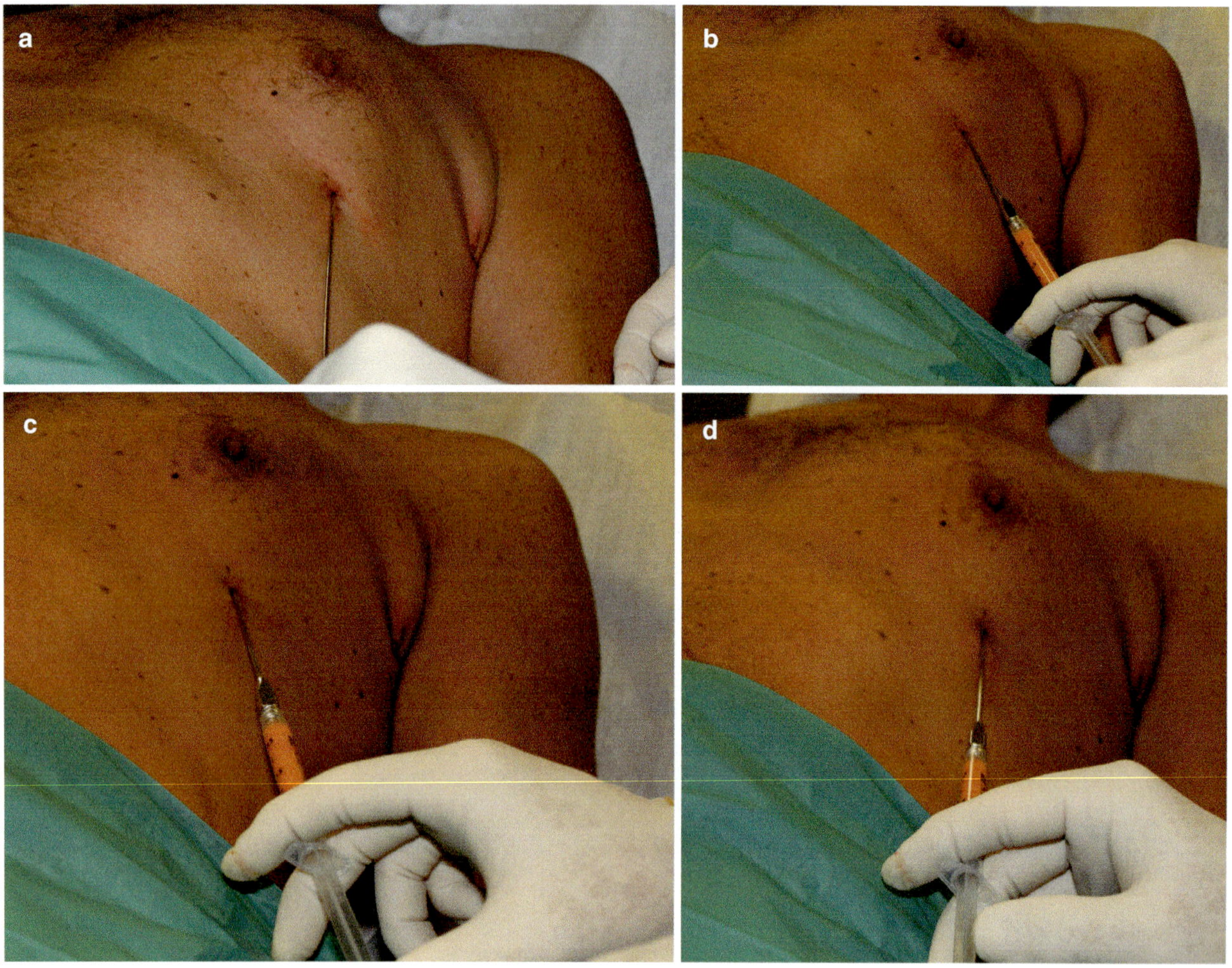

Fig. 23.5 (**a–d**) The cannula is then pivoted to the different parts of the quadrants, as planned before the injection, and the fat is released, retrograde fashion, into the intramuscular-submuscular plane. (Published by kind permission of ©Mario Goisis 2018. All Rights Reserved)

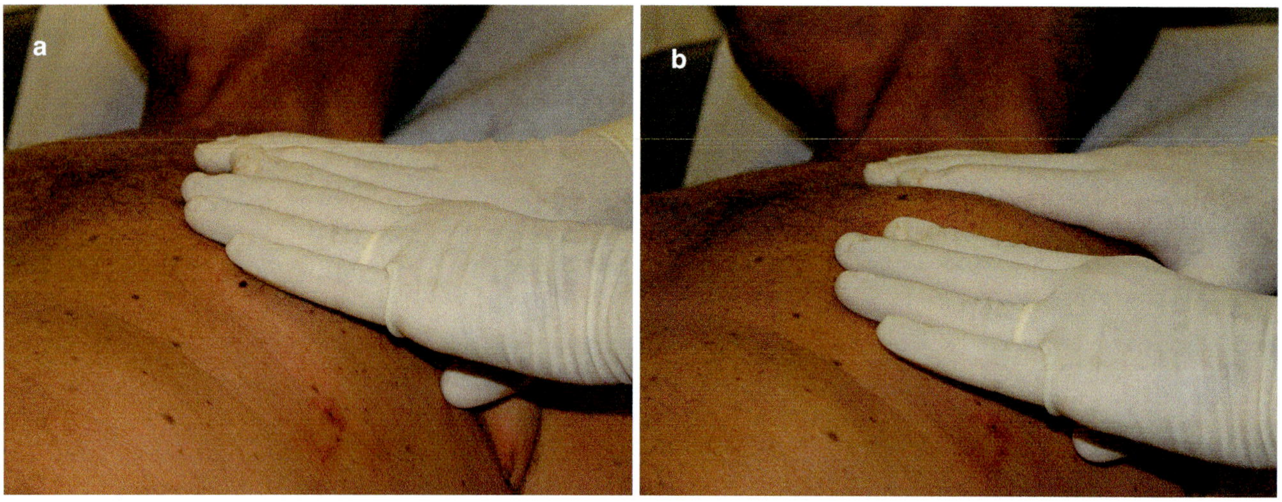

Fig. 23.6 (**a**, **b**) A strong massage is applied to the area after injection. (Published by kind permission of ©Mario Goisis 2018. All Rights Reserved)

Breast

24

Mario Goisis and Sara Izzo

24.1 Anatomy

The breasts are cones with their apex at the nipple and their base at the wall of the chest. The subcutaneous envelope of the breast's surface is the superficial fascia, which is found in the subcutis in practically every area of the body. The superficial fascia is separated from the skin envelope by 0.5–3 cm of subcutaneous fat (adipose tissue). The adult glandular part of the breast encloses lactiferous lobes that converge on the nipple, through the milk ducts (Figs. 24.1 and 24.2).

24.2 Augmentation of the Breast by Injection of Microfat Injected into the Intramuscular-Submuscular Plane

24.2.1 Indications

Augmentation of the volume of the breast

24.2.2 Contraindications

The fat should not be injected into areas lacking sufficient blood supply or which are suffering from an infection or inflammation. No injection should be carried out if the breast has been previously treated with liquid silicone or other permanent fillers, because a new injection might lead to inflammation or infection of the implants.

M. Goisis (✉)
Maxillo-Facial and Aesthetic Surgeon, Go Easy Clinic, Milan, Italy

S. Izzo
Department of Plastic Surgery, University of Campania "Luigi Vanvitelli", Naples, Italy

24.2.3 Complications and Management

Immediate complications (within 72 h after the injection) are transient erythema, oedema, induration, pruritus, and ecchymosis.

Early complications (days to weeks after the injection) include hypercorrection, local infection, necrosis of the skin, reactivation of herpes, discoloration, and persistent local symptoms (erythema, oedema, induration, pruritus, and hyperpigmentation).

Later complications include high rates of fat resorption and cysts.

There is an on-going debate regarding the oncological safety and risks of fat grafting.

De Decker et al. carried out a systematic review of the literature regarding the issue published between 1995 and 2016. The review involved a total of 2,419 patients who had undergone autologous fat grafting of the breast after cancer. Lipofilling emerges as a safe technique with a low oncological morbidity rate [1].

Another debate concerns the impact of fat grafting on radiological evaluation and detection of cancer. Recently, Lindegren et al. published a cohort study which holds that fat grafting does not impair ultrasound and mammogram assessment of patients with a history of breast-cancer surgery or prophylactic mastectomy [2].

24.2.4 Operating Time

The procedure usually takes 20 min, once the fat has been harvested.

24.2.5 Materials

- 20–100 cc of microfat for injection on both sides
- 1.5 mm × 150 mm, filling cannula

M. Goisis (ed.), *Outpatient Regenerative Medicine*, https://doi.org/10.1007/978-3-319-44894-7_24

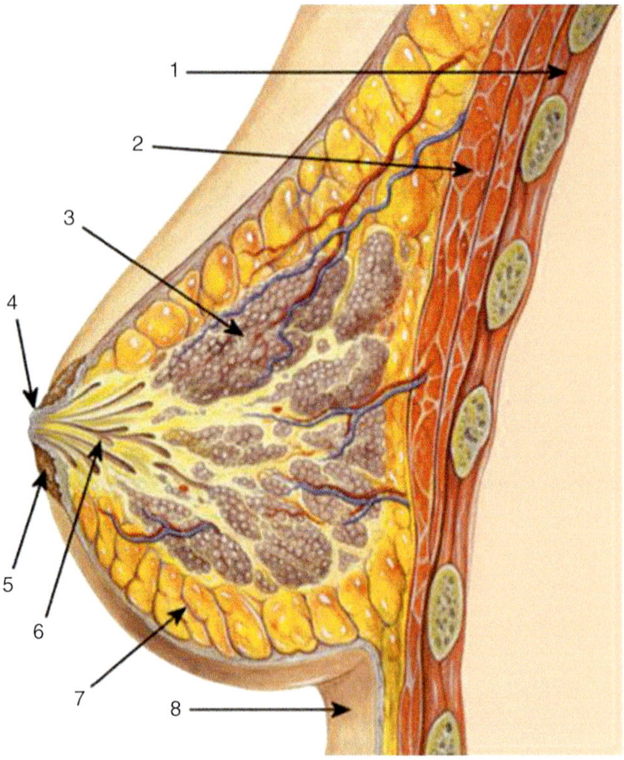

Fig. 24.1 The anatomy of the breast: (1) the chest wall, (2) the pectoralis muscles, (3) the lobules, (4) the nipple, (5) the areola, (6) the milk duct, (7) fatty tissue, (8) skin. (Published by kind permission of ©Mario Goisis 2018. All Rights Reserved)

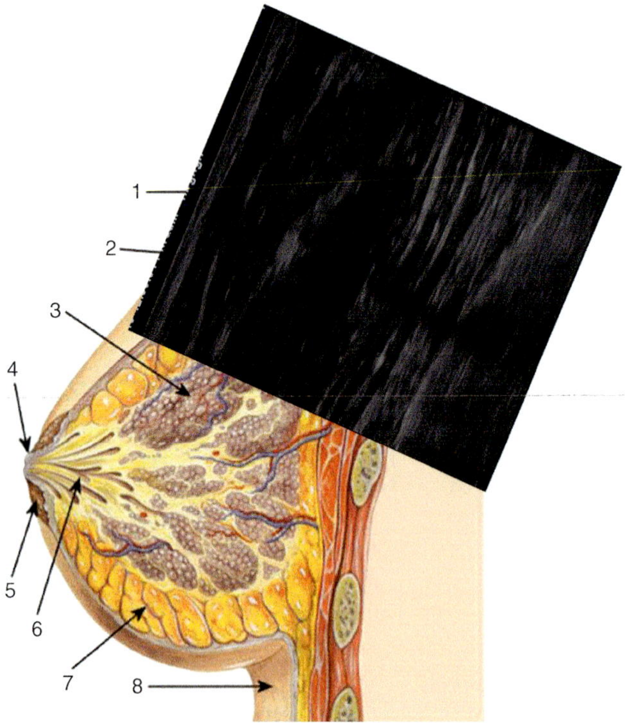

Fig. 24.2 Ultrasound images of different planes. (Published by kind permission of ©Mario Goisis 2018. All Rights Reserved)

To harvest and process the microfat, a dedicated standard system is used, in particular:

- A microfat box (www.microfat.com), composed of a ramp with a closed system for washing and filtration
- 4 60-cc syringes
- 2 10-cc syringes
- One 1-cc syringe
- 30-gauge needle
- 16-gauge needle
- A 2 mm-diameter, 10 cm-long Goisis cannula for fat harvesting
- A chlorhexidine-alcohol solution (2% chlorhexidine gluconate and 70% isopropyl alcohol), sterile drapes or towels
- Ice packs
- Sterile 2 cm × 2 cm gauze squares
- Occlusive dressing cover

Medications include:

200 cc of cold saline solution.
500 cc of cold Klein solution.
One litre of Klein solution is composed of 800 mg of lidocaine, 1 mg of epinephrine, 40 MEq of sodium bicarbonate, and 1000 cc of saline solution.

Location: Harvesting of the microfat can be carried out in a small operating theatre/medical surgery. Oxygen, the pulse oximetry, and a crash cart/box should be present.

Assistants: An assistant is useful for the transfer of items into the procedure field in a sterile manner during the first stage of the procedure. Despite this, a single doctor may carry out the entire procedure alone.

24.2.6 The Procedure

The procedure is illustrated in figures 24.3, 24.4a–c, 24.5, 24.6, 24.7a–c, 24.8a, b, 24.9a, b, 24.10a, b, and 24.11 below.

24.3 Augmentation of the Breast by Injection of Microfat into the Intramuscular-Submuscular Plane

24.3.1 Indications

Augmentation of the the volume of the breast by intraglandular injection of microfat

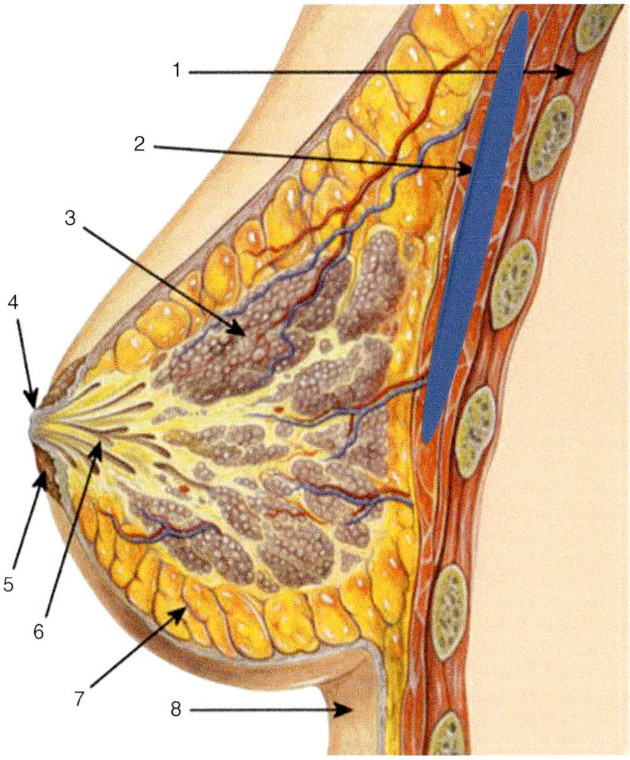

Fig. 24.3 The area of the injection is illustrated. (Published by kind permission of ©Mario Goisis 2018. All Rights Reserved)

24.3.2 Contraindications

Breast diseases (neoplasms, fibrocystic breast, inflammations) are among the absolute and relative contraindications. The fat should not be injected into areas lacking sufficient blood supply or that are suffering from an infection or inflammation. No injection should be carried out if the breast has been previously treated with liquid silicone or other permanent fillers, because new injections might cause inflammation or infection of the implants.

24.3.3 Operating Time

The procedure usually takes 20 min, once the fat has been harvested.

24.3.4 Materials

- 20–100 cc of microfat for injection into each side:
- A cannula, 1 mm in diameter and 10 cm in length

To harvest and process the microfat, a dedicated standard system is used, in particular:

- A microfat box (www.microfat.com), composed of a ramp with a closed system for washing and filtration
- 4 60-cc syringes
- 2 10-cc syringes
- One 1-cc syringe
- 30-gauge needle
- 16-gauge needle
- A 2 mm-diameter, 10 cm-long Goisis cannula for fat harvesting
- A chlorhexidine-alcohol solution (2% chlorhexidine gluconate and 70% isopropyl alcohol), sterile drapes or towels
- Ice packs
- Sterile 2 cm × 2 cm gauze squares
- Occlusive dressing cover

Medications include:

- 200 cc of cold saline solution.
- 500 cc of cold Klein solution.
- One litre of Klein solution is composed of 800 mg of lidocaine, 1 mg of epinephrine, 40 MEq of sodium bicarbonate, and 1000 cc of saline solution.

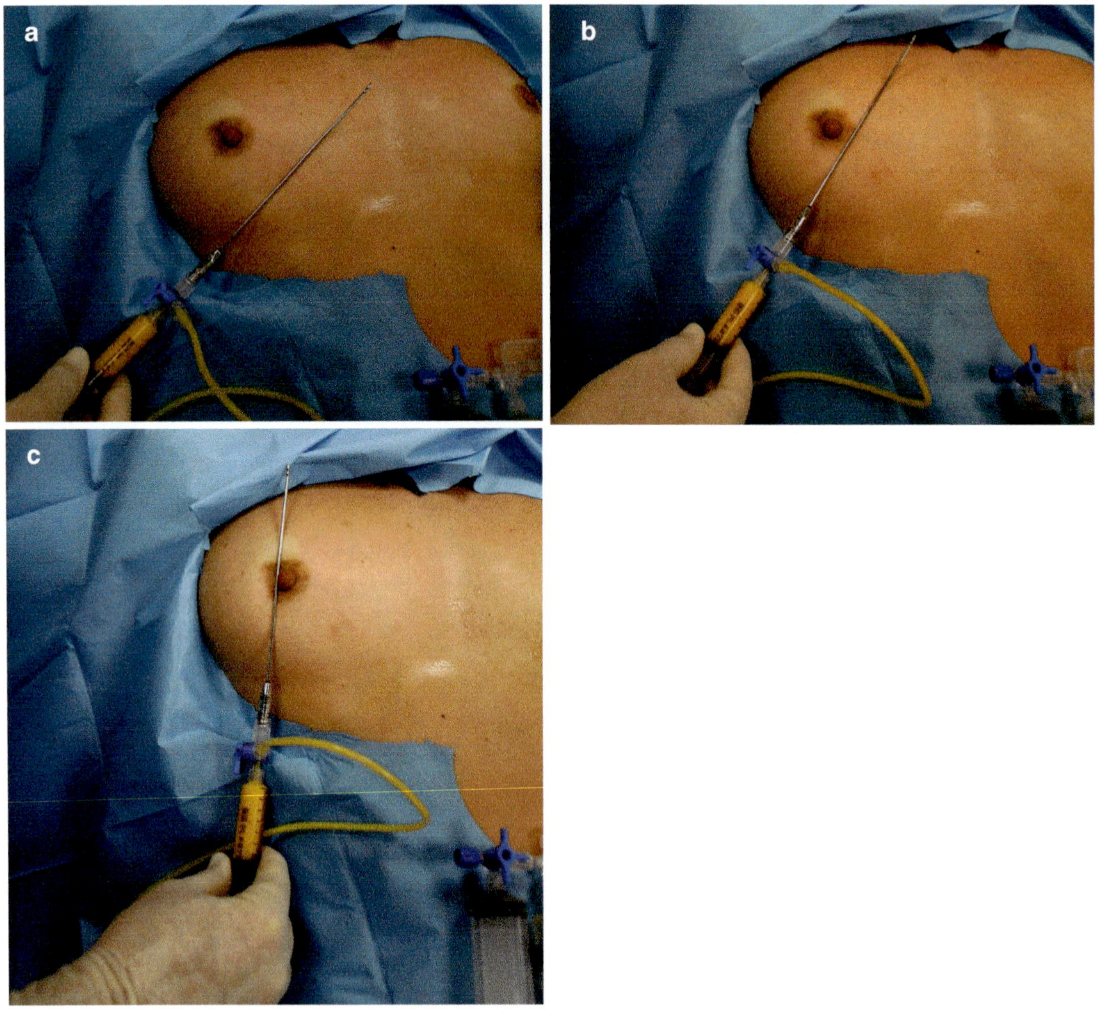

Fig. 24.4 (a–c) The route of the cannula. (Published by kind permission of ©Mario Goisis 2018. All Rights Reserved)

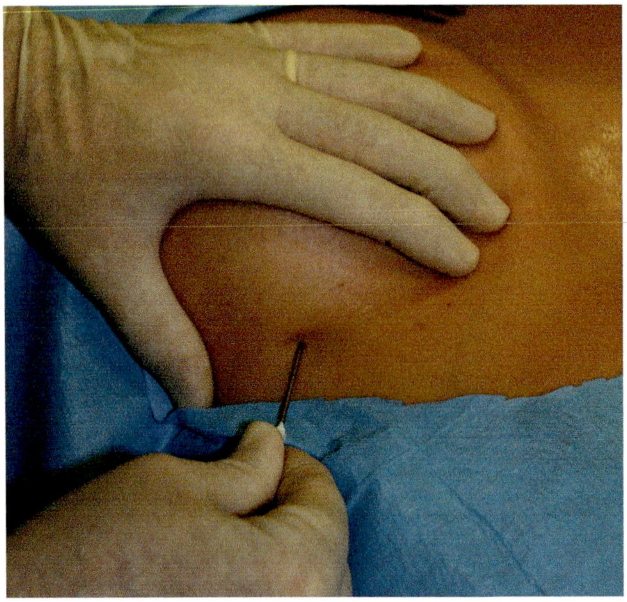

Fig. 24.5 The entry point 1 cm under the inframammary fold is created using a sharp 16-G needle. (Published by kind permission of ©Mario Goisis 2018. All Rights Reserved)

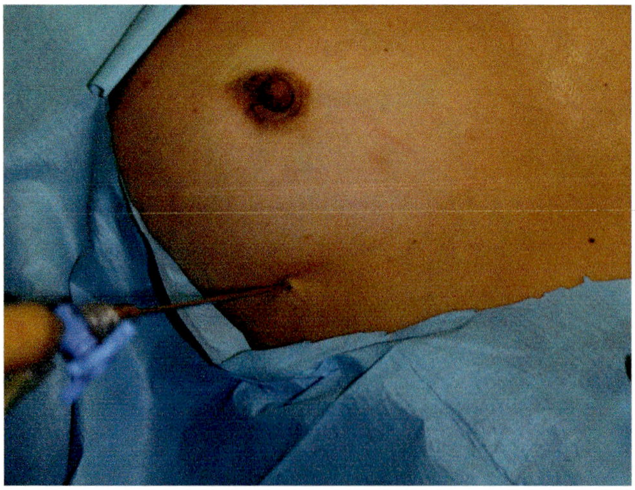

Fig. 24.6 The perpendicular insertion of a 1.5 mm blunt-tip cannula. The cannula is plunged deep into the muscle, paying attention to remain deep within the mammal fascia. (Published by kind permission of ©Mario Goisis 2018. All Rights Reserved)

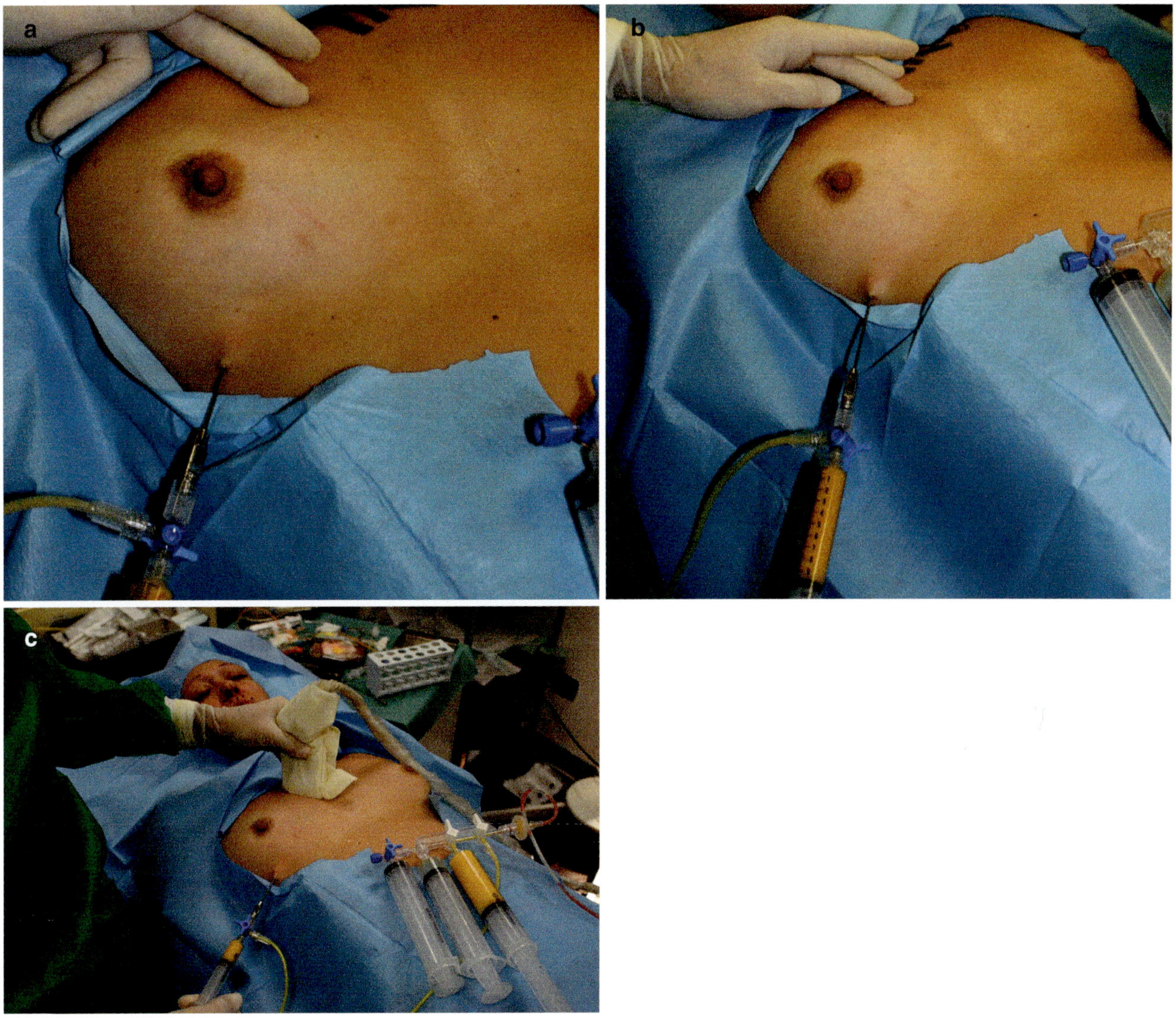

Fig. 24.7 (a–c) The cannula is then pivoted into the different parts of the quadrants, as planned before the injection, and the fat is released, retrograde fashion, into the intramuscular-submuscular plane. (Published by kind permission of ©Mario Goisis 2018. All Rights Reserved)

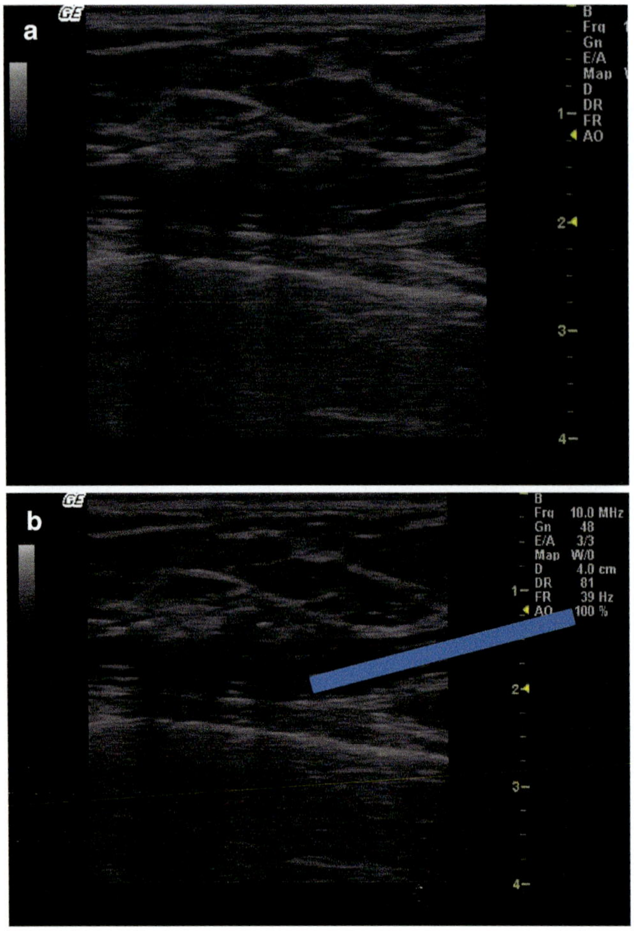

Fig. 24.8 (**a**, **b**) Ultrasound images of the position of the cannula. (Published by kind permission of ©Mario Goisis 2018. All Rights Reserved)

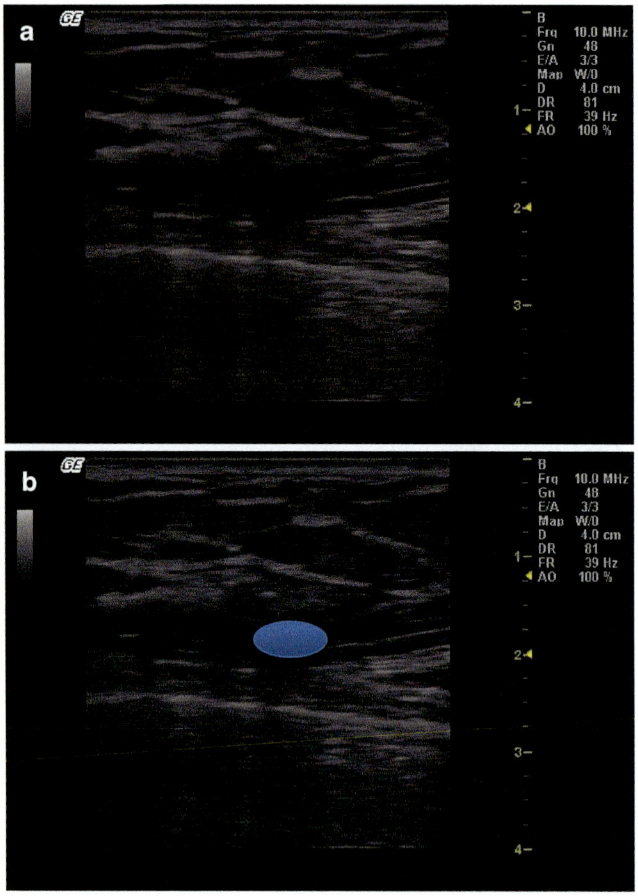

Fig. 24.9 (**a**, **b**) Ultrasound images of the injected fat. (Published by kind permission of ©Mario Goisis 2018. All Rights Reserved)

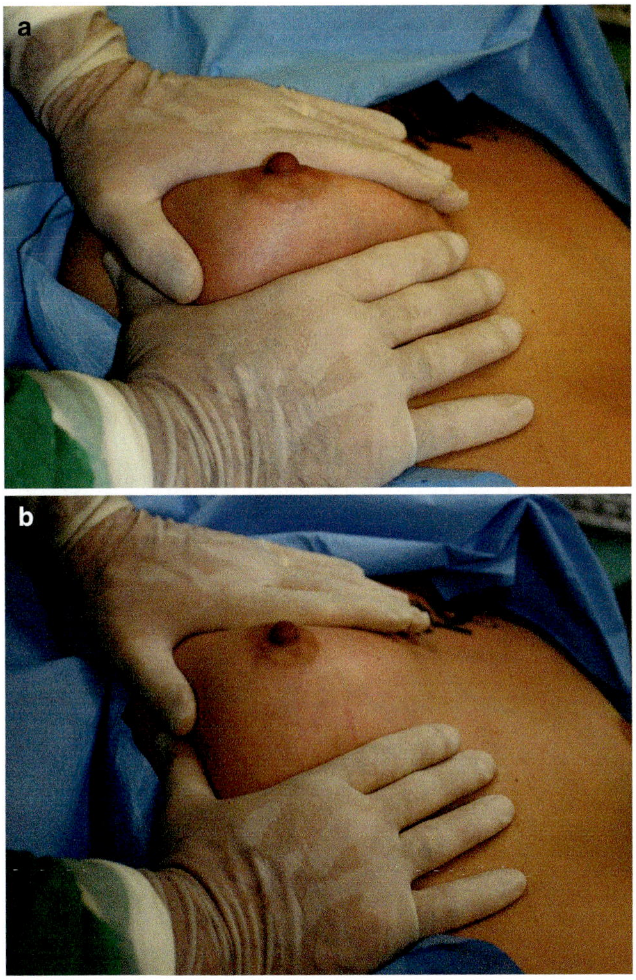

Fig. 24.10 (**a**, **b**) A strong massage is applied to the area after injection. (Published by kind permission of ©Mario Goisis 2018. All Rights Reserved)

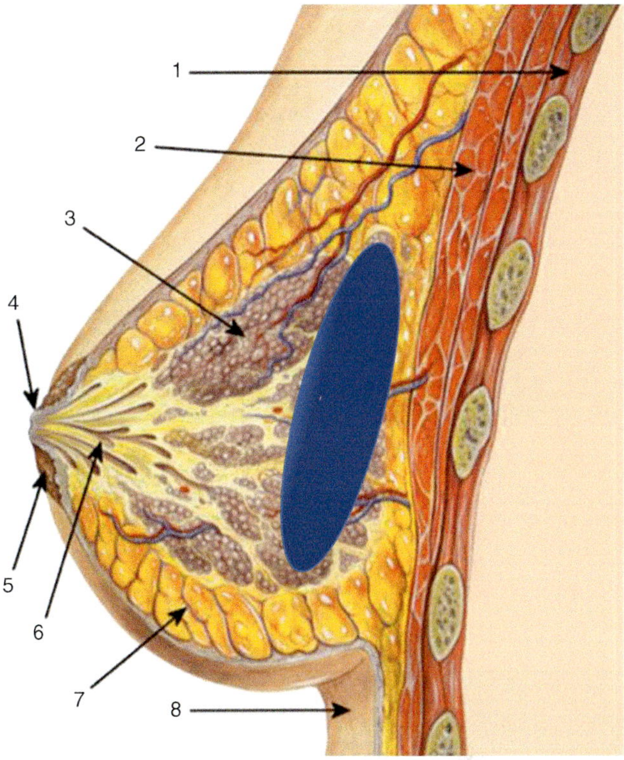

Fig. 24.11 A coloured cross-section illustration of the injection area. (Published by kind permission of ©Mario Goisis 2018. All Rights Reserved)

Location: Harvesting of the microfat may be carried out in a small operating theatre/medical surgery. Oxygen, the pulse oximetry, and a crash cart/box should be present.

Assistants: The help of an assistant can prove useful for the transfer items into the procedure field in a sterile manner during the first stage of the procedure. In any case, a single doctor can perform the entire procedure alone.

24.3.5 The Procedure

The procedure is illustrated in figures 24.12, 24.13, 24.14a–d, 24.15a, b, 24.16a, b, and 24.17a, b below.

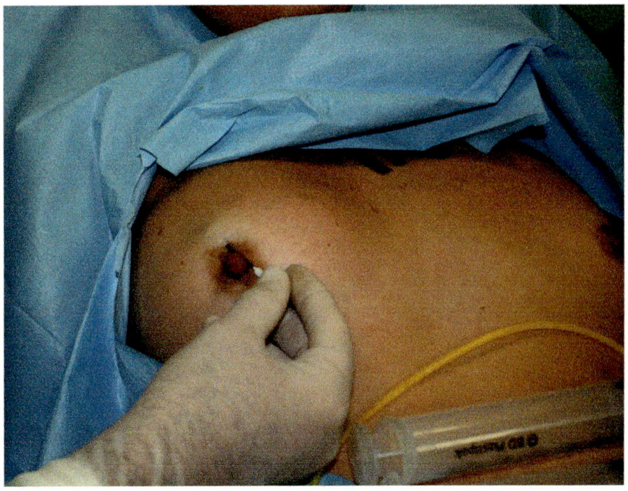

Fig. 24.12 The entry point at the level of the nipple is created using a sharp 16-G needle. (Published by kind permission of ©Mario Goisis 2018. All Rights Reserved)

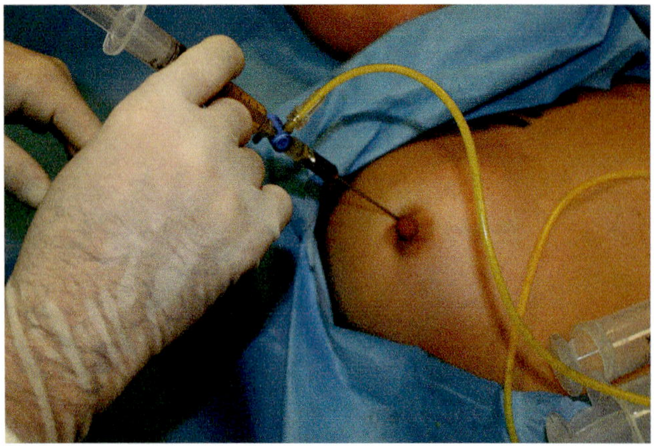

Fig. 24.13 Perpendicular insertion of a 1 mm blunt-tip cannula. The cannula is plunged deep into the glandular tissue, paying attention to remain deep within the superficial mammal fascia. (Published by kind permission of ©Mario Goisis 2018. All Rights Reserved)

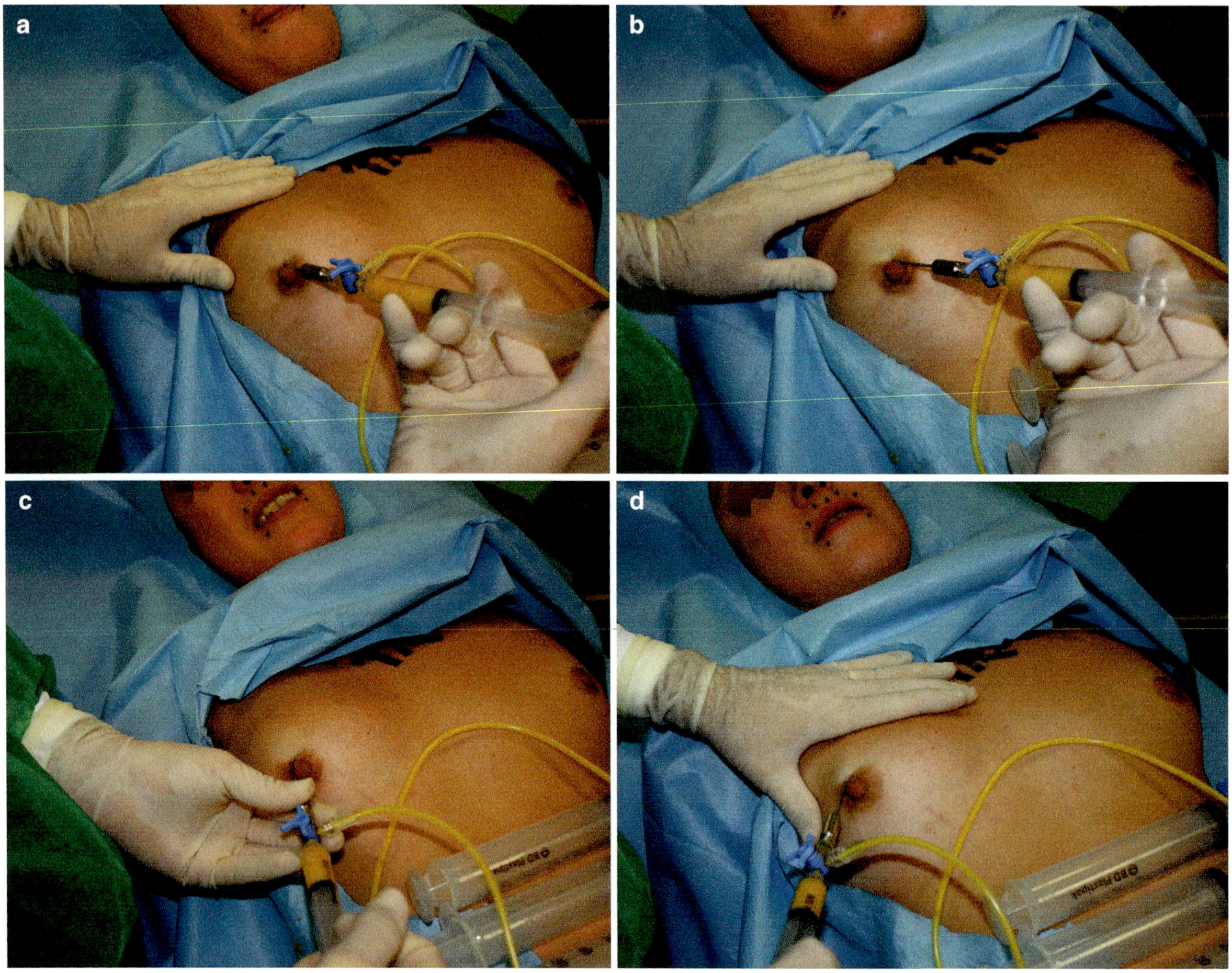

Fig. 24.14 (**a**–**d**) The cannula is then pivoted into the different parts of the quadrants, as planned before the injection, and the fat is released, retrograde fashion, into the intraglandular plane. (Published by kind permission of ©Mario Goisis 2018. All Rights Reserved)

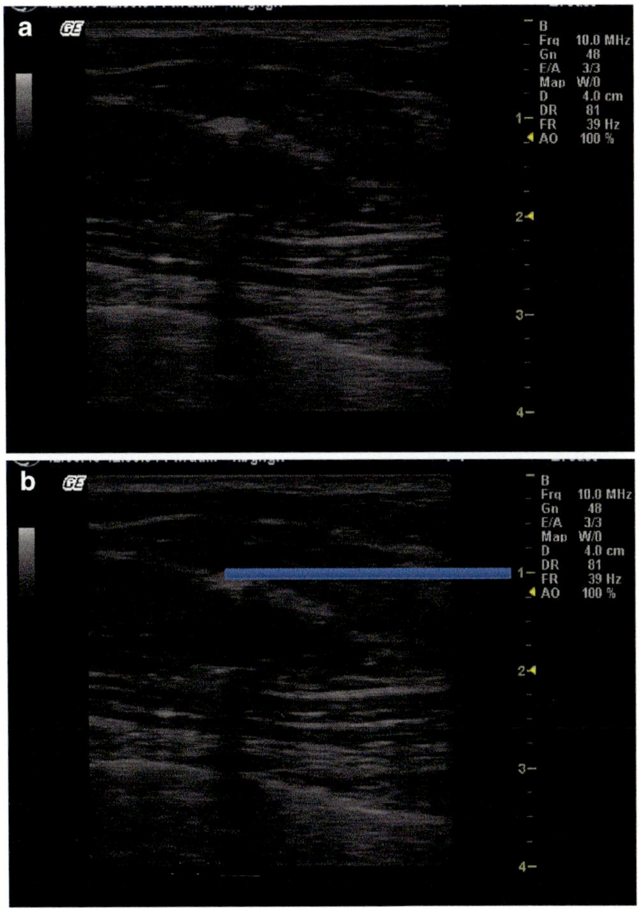

Fig. 24.15 (**a**, **b**) Ultrasound images of the position of the cannula. (Published by kind permission of ©Mario Goisis 2018. All Rights Reserved)

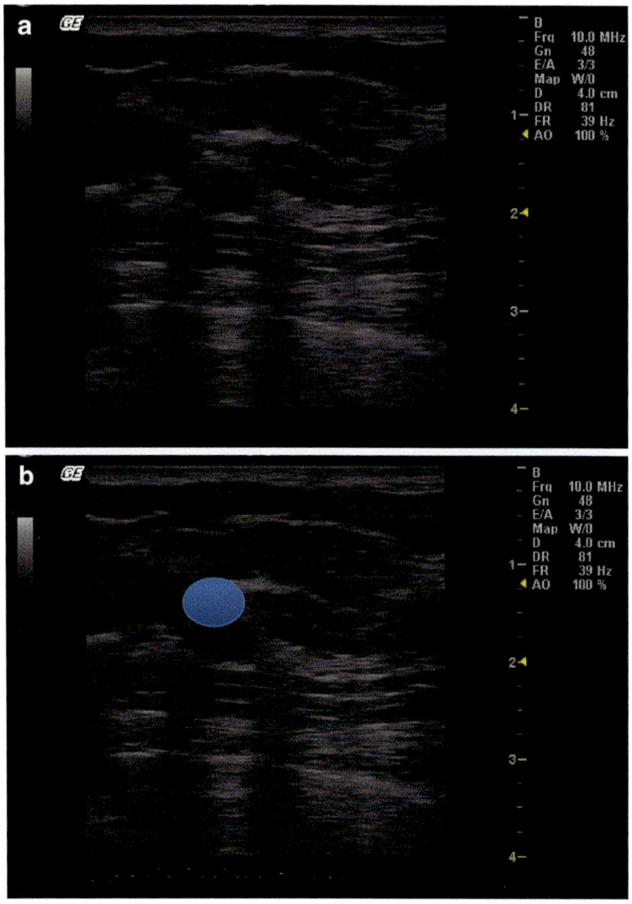

Fig. 24.16 (**a**, **b**) Ultrasound images of the injected fat. (Published by kind permission of ©Mario Goisis 2018. All Rights Reserved)

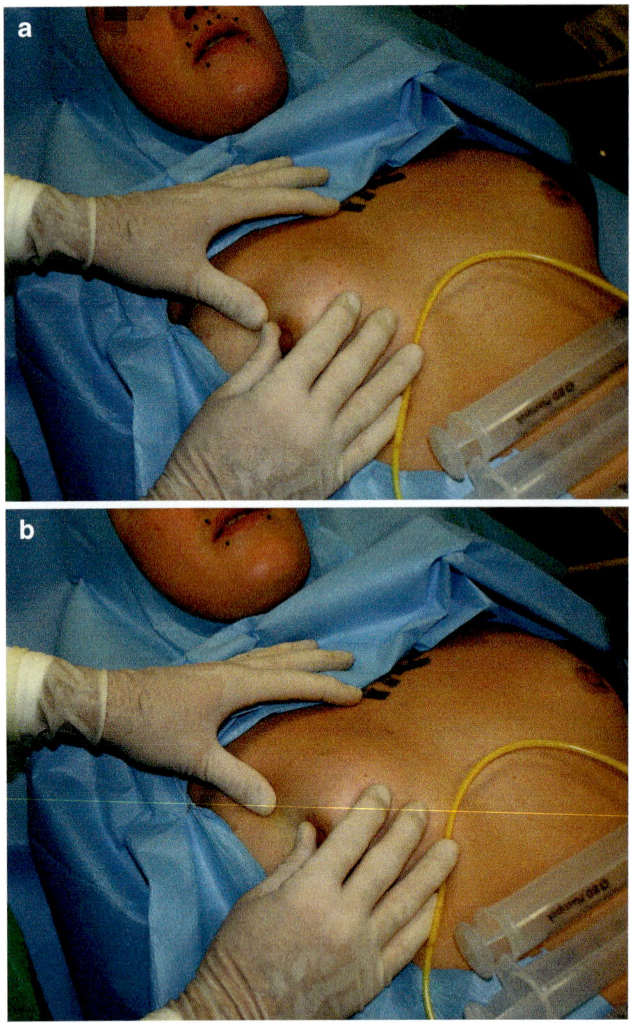

Fig. 24.17 (**a**, **b**) A strong massage is applied to the area after injection. (Published by kind permission of ©Mario Goisis 2018. All Rights Reserved)

24.4 Augmentation of the Breast by Injecting Microfat into the Subcutaneous Plane

24.4.1 Indications

Amelioration of the shape of the breast

24.4.2 Contraindications

Breast diseases (neoplasms, fibrocystic breast, inflammations) are among the absolute and relative contraindications. The fat should not be injected into areas lacking sufficient blood supply or suffering from an infection or inflammation. No injection should be carried out if the breast has been previously treated with liquid silicone or other permanent fillers because a new injection might cause inflammation or infection of the implants.

24.4.3 Operating Time

The procedure usually takes 20 min, once the fat is harvested.

24.4.4 Materials

- 20–40 cc of microfat on each side for injection of microfat:
- A 3.6-metre-long 22-G cannula

To harvest and process the microfat, a standard system for microfat is used, in particular:

- A microfat box (www.microfat.com), composed of a ramp with a closed system for washing and filtration
- 4 60-cc syringes
- 2 10-cc syringes
- One 1-cc syringe
- 30-gauge needle
- 16-gauge needle
- A 2 mm-diameter, 10 cm-long Goisis cannula for fat harvesting
- A chlorhexidine-alcohol solution (2% chlorhexidine gluconate and 70% isopropyl alcohol), sterile drapes or towels
- Ice packs
- Sterile 2 cm × 2 cm gauze squares
- Occlusive dressing cover

Medications include:

- 200 cc of cold saline solution.
- 500 cc of cold Klein solution.
- One litre of Klein solution is composed of 800 mg of lidocaine, 1 mg of epinephrine, 40 MEq of sodium bicarbonate, and 1000 cc of saline solution.

Location: The microfat harvesting may be carried out in a small operating theatre/medical surgery. Oxygen, the pulse oximetry, and a crash cart/box should be present.

Assistants: The help of an assistant may prove useful for the transfer of items into the procedure field in a sterile manner during the first stage of the procedure. However a single doctor may perform the entire procedure alone.

24.4.5 Procedure

Procedure is shown in figures 24.18, 24.19a–c, 24.20, 24.21a, b, 24.22a–d, 24.23a, b, and 24.24a, b below.

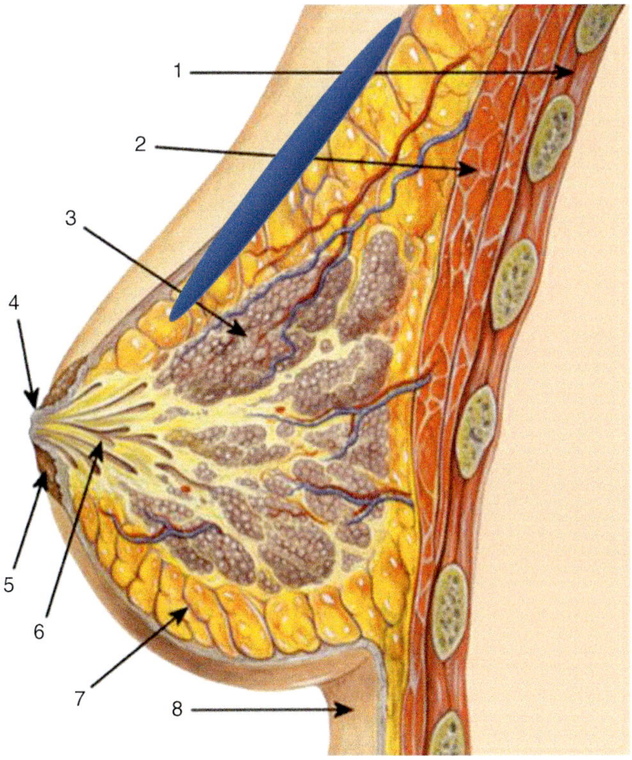

Fig. 24.18 Area of the injection. (Published by kind permission of ©Mario Goisis 2018. All Rights Reserved)

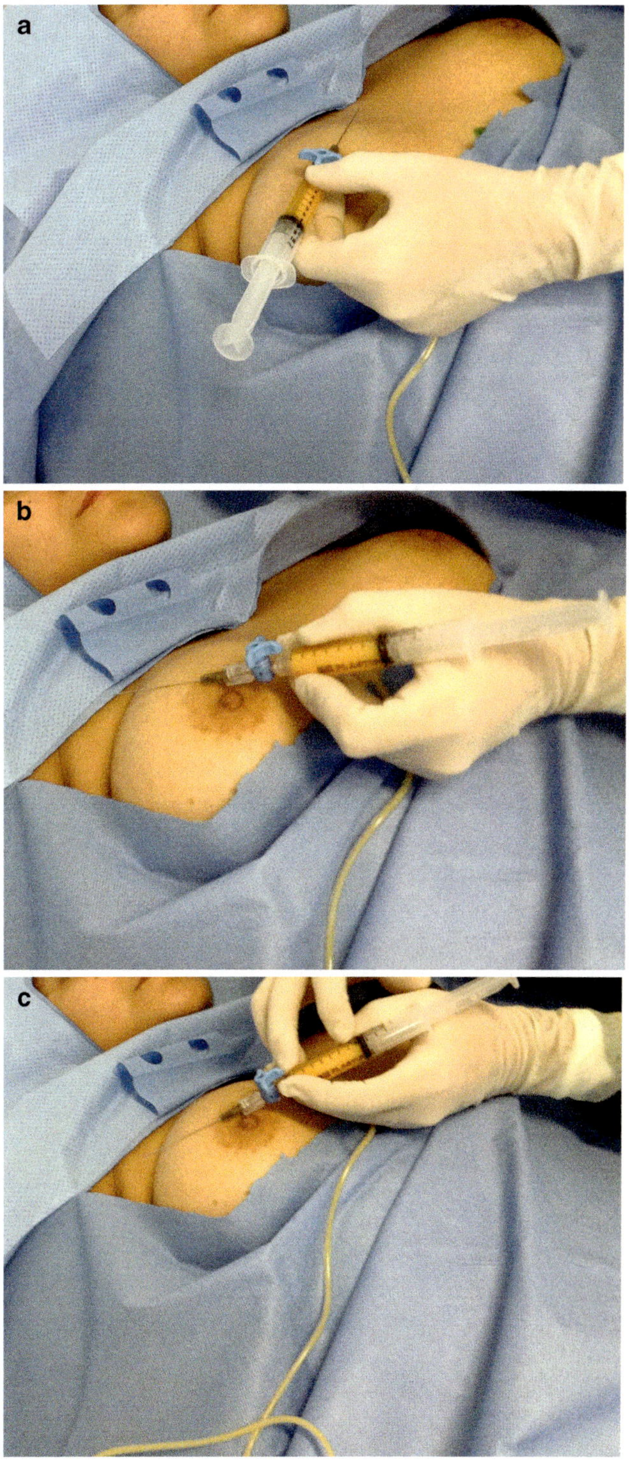

Fig. 24.19 (a–c) The route of the cannula is shown here. (Published by kind permission of ©Mario Goisis 2018. All Rights Reserved)

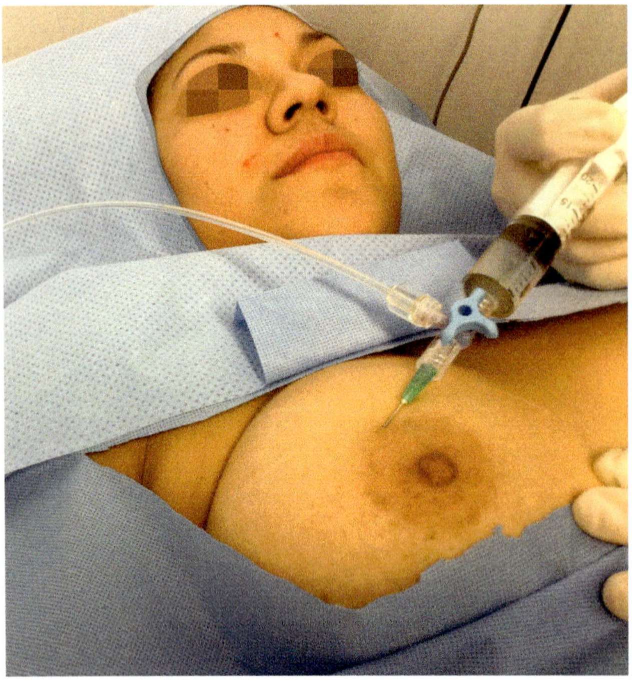

Fig. 24.20 Two cc of local anesthetic (Klein solution) need to be injected into the entry point, at the upper border of the breast's areola. By taking this precaution, the treatment with the blunt-tip cannula will not cause the patient any pain. A small hole is made to permit the cannula to enter the subcutaneous plane. A 21-G needle is used for this purpose. (Published by kind permission of ©Mario Goisis 2018. All Rights Reserved)

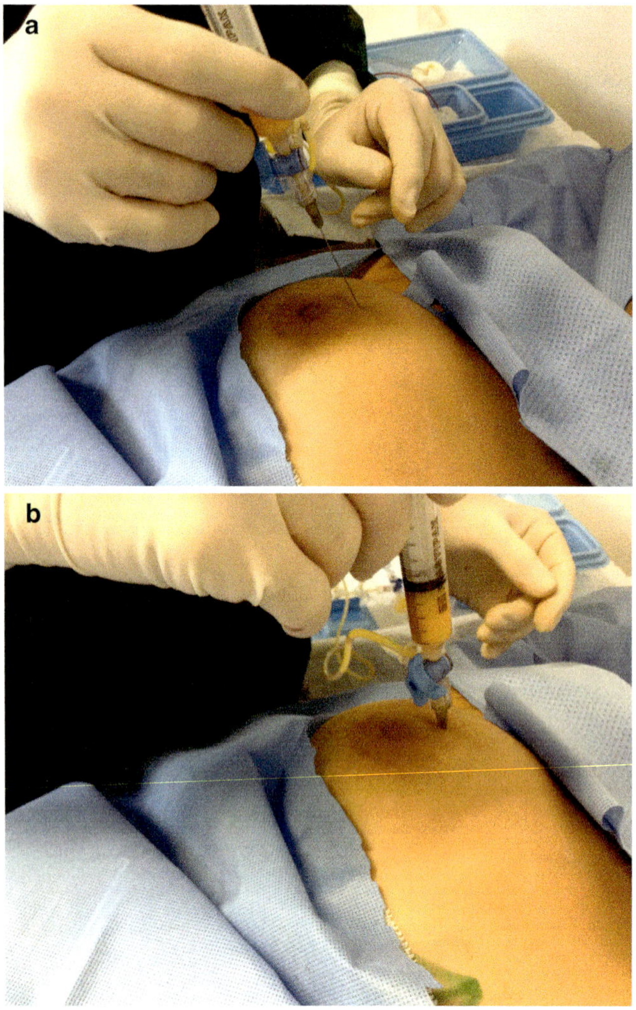

Fig. 24.21 (**a**, **b**) Perpendicular insertion of a 22-G blunt-tip cannula. The cannula is plunged deep into the skin, paying attention to remain superficial with regard to the mammary gland. (Published by kind permission of ©Mario Goisis 2018. All Rights Reserved)

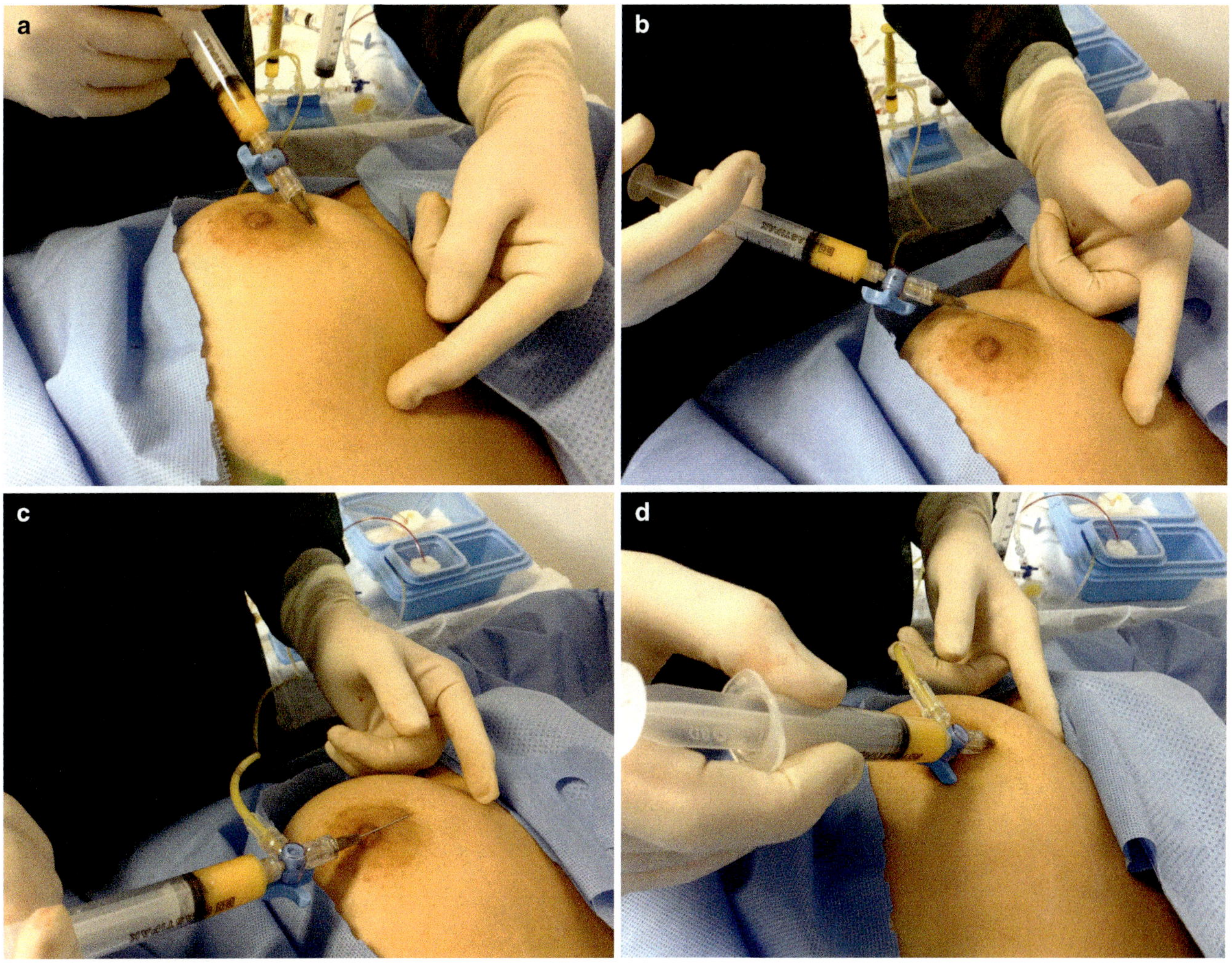

Fig. 24.22 (**a**–**d**) The cannula is then pivoted to the different parts of the upper quadrants, as planned before the injection then the fat is released, retrograde fashion, into the subcutaneous plane. (Published by kind permission of ©Mario Goisis 2018. All Rights Reserved)

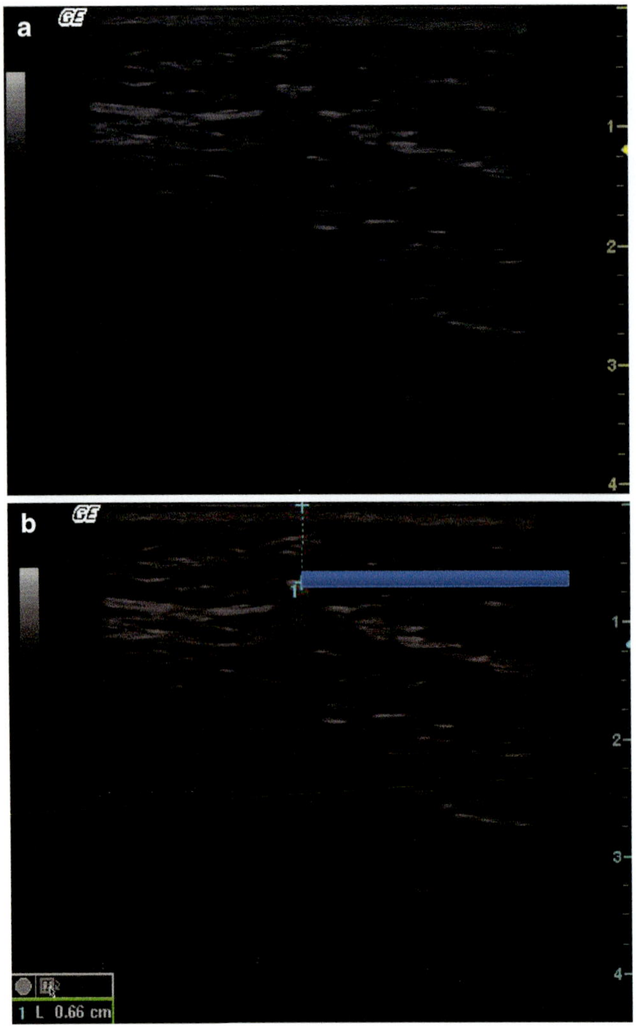

Fig. 24.23 (**a**, **b**) Ultrasound images of the position of the cannula. (Published by kind permission of ©Mario Goisis 2018. All Rights Reserved)

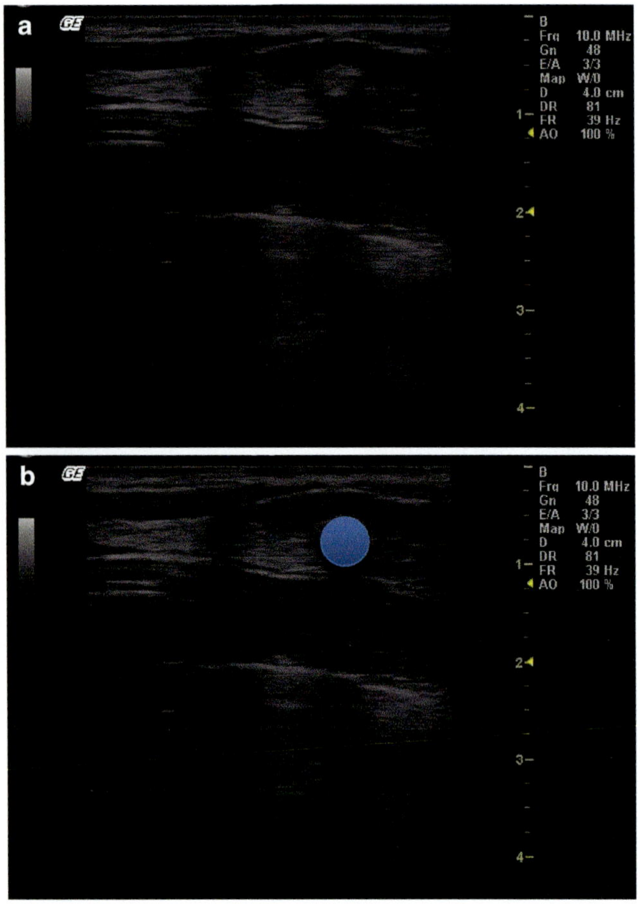

Fig. 24.24 (**a**, **b**) Ultrasound images of the injected fat. (Published by kind permission of ©Mario Goisis 2018. All Rights Reserved)

References

1. De Decker M, De Schrijver L, Thiessen F, Tondu T, Van Goethem M, Tjalma WA. Breast cancer and fat grafting: efficacy, safety and complications-a systematic review. Eur J Obstet Gynecol Reprod Biol. 2016;207:100–8.
2. Lindegren A, Chantereau MW, Bygdeson M, Azavedo E, Schultz I. Autologous fat transplantation to the reconstructed breast does not hinder assessment of mammography and ultrasound: a cohort study. World J Surg. 2016;40(5):1104–11.

Gluteal Augmentation and Remodelling

25

Sara Izzo, Mario Goisis, and Rand S. Al Yahya

25.1 Anatomy

The sciatic nerve begins in the lower back and runs through the buttock and down to the lower limb. Going from the top of the leg to the foot, it is the longest and widest single nerve in the human body. The sciatic innervates the muscles of the posterior compartment of the thigh and all the muscles of the leg and foot and nearly the whole of the skin of the leg. The superior gluteal nerve originates in the pelvis and innervates the tensor fasciae latae muscles and the gluteus medius and minimus. The inferior gluteal nerve is mainly responsible for motor innervation of the gluteus maximus muscle. It extends the thigh to execute activities such as climbing stairs. All the cited nerves are placed deeply into the gluteus maximus. The superficial branch of the superior gluteal artery enters the deep surface of the gluteus maximus and supplies the muscle anastomosing with the inferior gluteal artery. Numerous terminal branches perforate its tendinous origin to supply the superficial tissues covering the posterior surface of the sacrum. The inferior branch of the gluteal artery descends in the gap between the greater trochanter of the femur and tuberosity of the ischium and is continued down to the back of the thigh, supplying the skin. It anastomoses with branches of the perforating arteries (Figs. 25.1 and 25.2).

25.2 Pitfalls

Accidental injuries to the nerve and vessel of gluteal region can be avoided by introducing the injecting cannula in the subcutaneous layer, keeping the hedge superficial to the muscularis fascia of the gluteus.

25.3 Gluteal Augmentation by Means of Microfat

25.3.1 Indications

Gluteal augmentation and remodeling are generally sought by patients who desire their buttock to be rounder and full. Gluteal contour defects are common and may be related to a deficiency in gluteal mass, loss of fat in the buttock area, or loss of curvature of the lower spine.

25.3.2 Contraindications

The fat should not be injected in areas that lack sufficient blood supply or that have an infection or inflammation. No injection should be done if the area has been previously treated with liquid silicone or other permanent fillers because new injection could lead to inflammation or infection of the implants. Vascular problems as arterial or venous occlusion are relative contraindications that must be evaluated by a specialist before treatment.

25.3.3 Operating Time

The procedure usually takes 20 min, once the fat is harvested.

S. Izzo
Doctor's Equipe, Milan, Italy

M. Goisis (✉)
Maxillo-Facial and Aesthetic Surgeon, Go Easy Clinic, Milan, Italy

R. S. Al Yahya
Prince Sattam Bin Abdulaziz University, Al Kharj, Saudi Arabia

M. Goisis (ed.), *Outpatient Regenerative Medicine*, https://doi.org/10.1007/978-3-319-44894-7_25

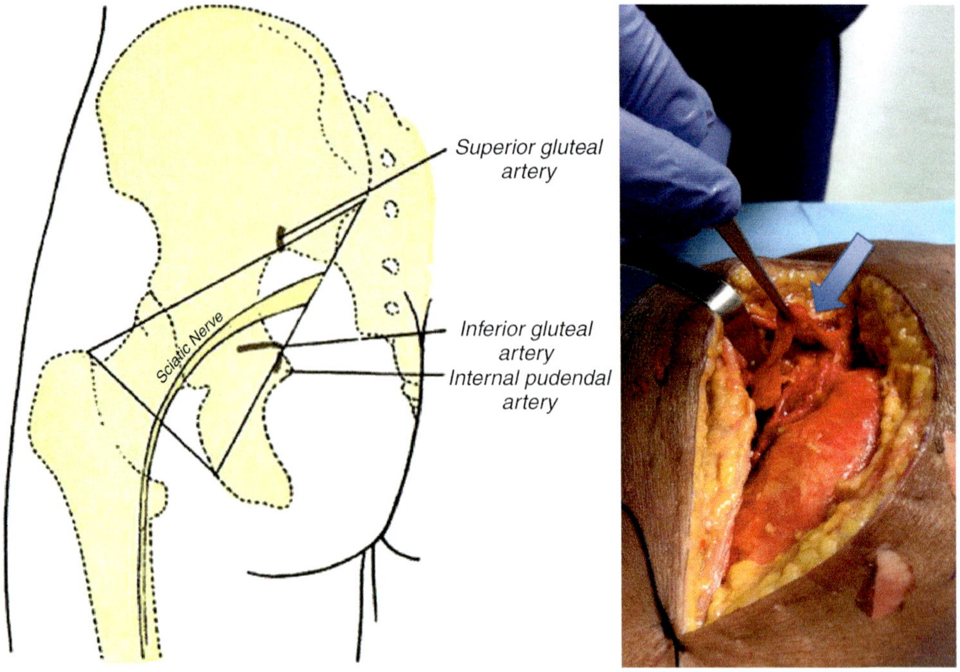

Fig. 25.1 Sciatic nerve anatomy. Reproduction of a lithograph plate from *Gray's Anatomy* (Henry Gray, Anatomy: Descriptive and Surgical, 1918) and dissection of the sciatic nerve (blue arrow, courtesy of Doctor's Equipe). (Published with kind permission of ©Mario Goisis 2018. All Rights Reserved)

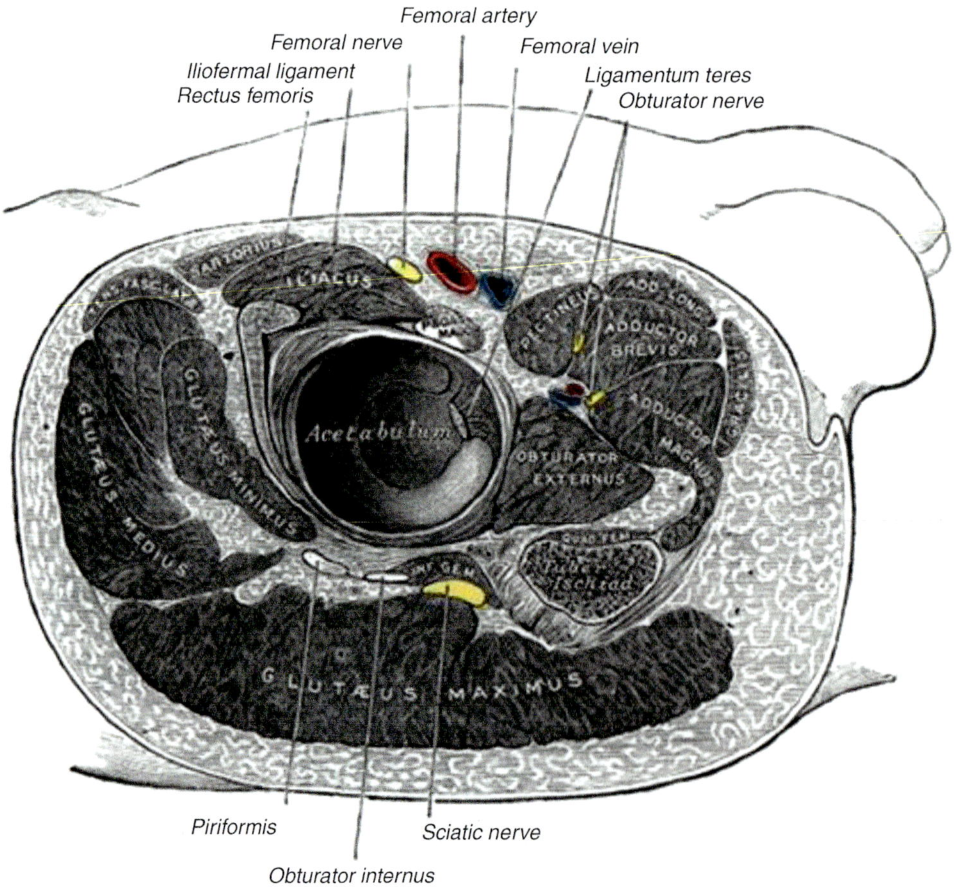

Fig. 25.2 The sciatic nerve is located in a deep plane. Reproduction of a lithograph plate from *Gray's Anatomy* (Henry Gray, Anatomy: Descriptive and Surgical, 1918). (Published with kind permission of ©Mario Goisis 2018. All Rights Reserved)

25.3.4 Materials

- *30–80 cc of microfat on each side for injection of microfat*
- 1.5 mm × 150 mm, filling cannula

For microfat harvesting and processing, a standard system for microfat is used, in particular:

- Microfat box (www.microfat.com), composed of a ramp with a closed system for washing and filtration
- 4 60-cc syringes
- 2 10-cc syringes
- One 1-cc syringe
- 30-gauge needle
- 16-gauge needle
- A 2 mm-diameter, 10 cm-long Goisis cannula for fat harvesting
- A chlorhexidine-alcohol solution (2% chlorhexidine gluconate and 70% isopropyl alcohol), sterile drapes or towels
- Ice packs

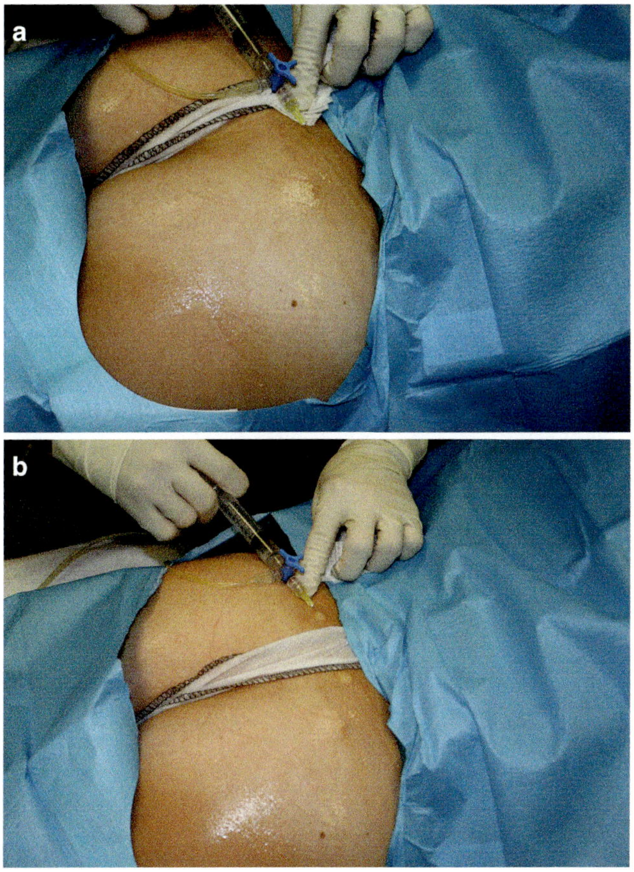

Fig. 25.3 1 cc of Klein solution is injected into the point of injection and in the subcutaneous area in every buttock. (Published with kind permission of ©Mario Goisis 2018. All Rights Reserved)

- Sterile 2 cm for 2 cm gauze squares
- Occlusive dressing cover

Medications include:

200 cc of cold saline solution.
500 cc of cold Klein solution.
One liter of Klein solution is composed of 800 mg of lidocaine, 1 mg of epinephrine, 40 MEq of sodium bicarbonate, and 1000 cc of saline solution.

Location: The microfat harvesting can be done in a small/office operating room. The oxygen, the pulse oximetry, and a crash cart/box should be present.

Assistants: An assistant is useful to transfer items to the procedure field in a sterile manner in the first part of the procedure. Despite that, a single doctor can execute all the procedure.

25.3.5 Procedure

Procedure is shown in Figs. 25.3, 25.4, 25.5, 25.6, 25.7, 25.8, 25.9, 25.10, and 25.11.

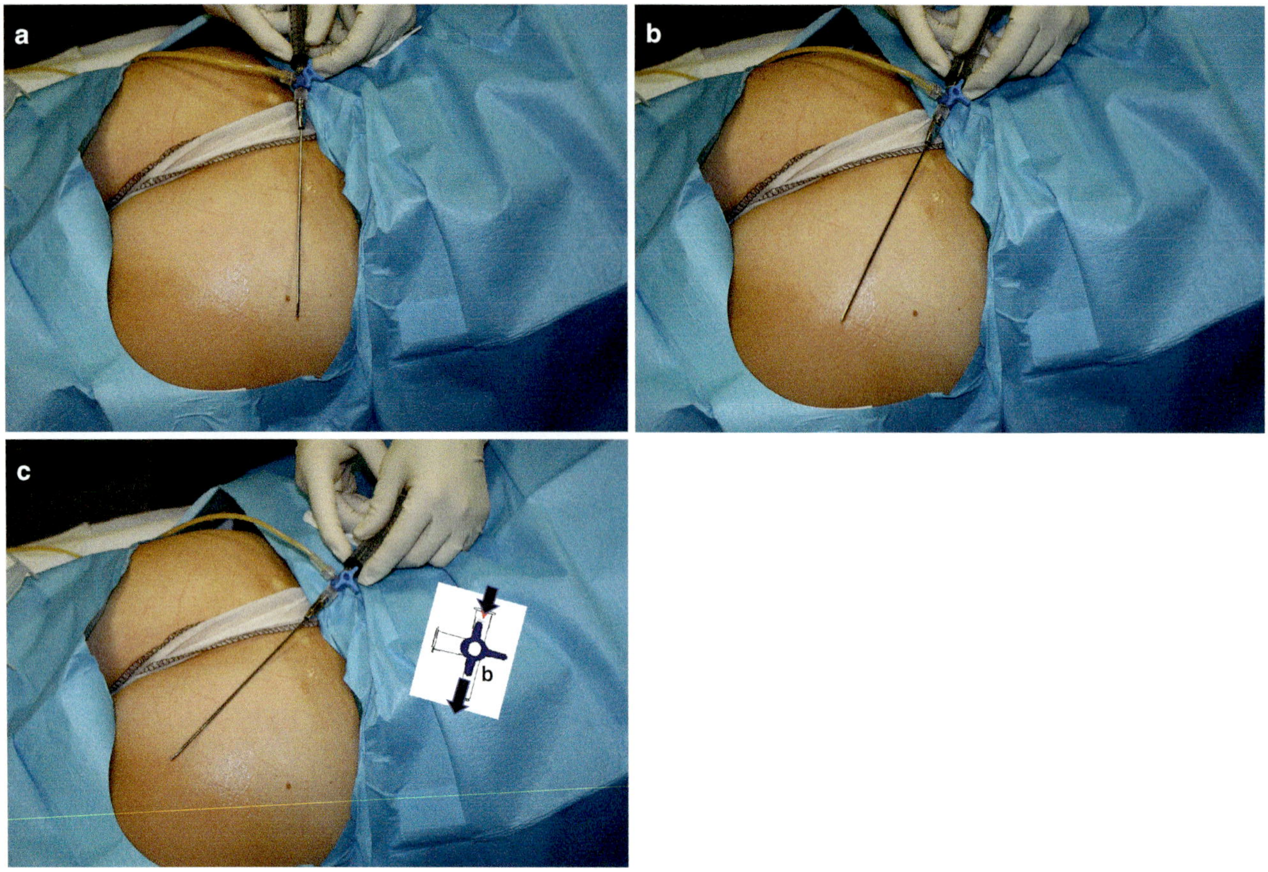

Fig. 25.4 Route of the cannula. (Published with kind permission of ©Mario Goisis 2018. All Rights Reserved)

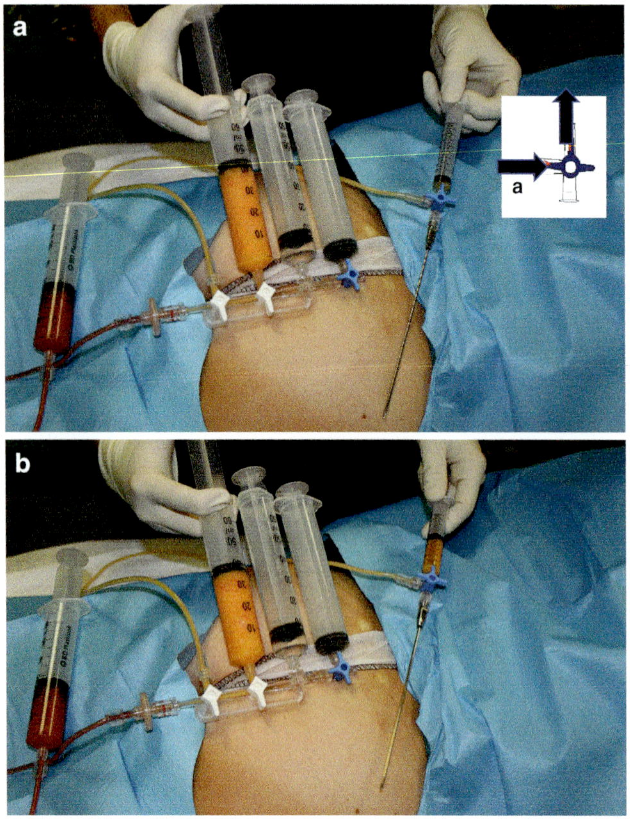

Fig. 25.5 The 10 cc syringe is filled by microfat. (Published with kind permission of ©Mario Goisis 2018. All Rights Reserved)

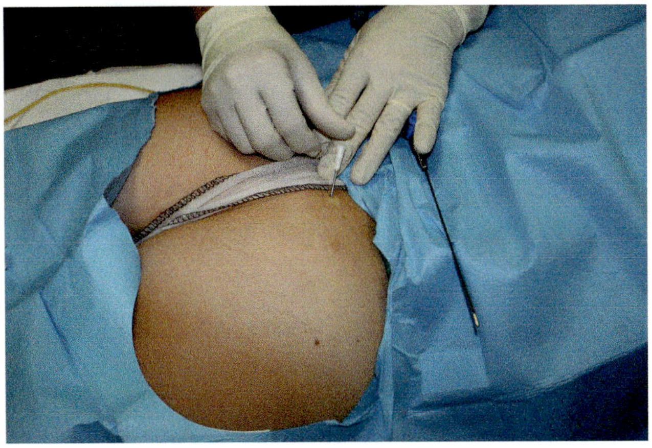

Fig. 25.6 An opening is created with a 16-G needle. (Published with kind permission of ©Mario Goisis 2018. All Rights Reserved)

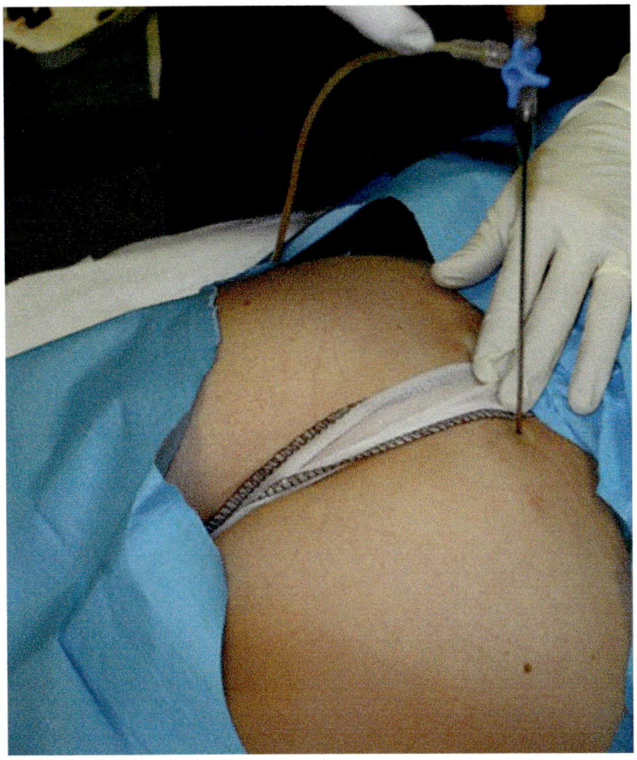

Fig. 25.7 The injecting cannula is inserted under the skin plane in a perpendicular fashion through the hole created. (Published with kind permission of ©Mario Goisis 2018. All Rights Reserved)

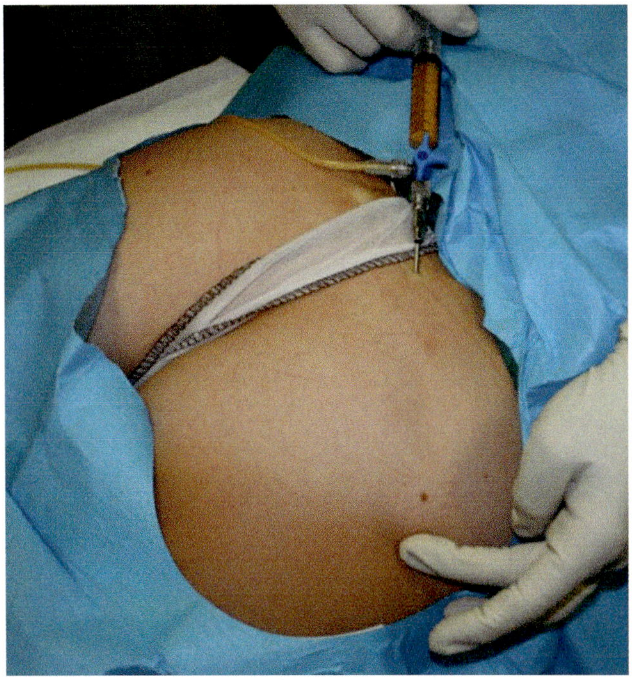

Fig. 25.8 The cannula is then pivoted parallel to the skin plane and is ready for injecting the fat. (Published with kind permission of ©Mario Goisis 2018. All Rights Reserved)

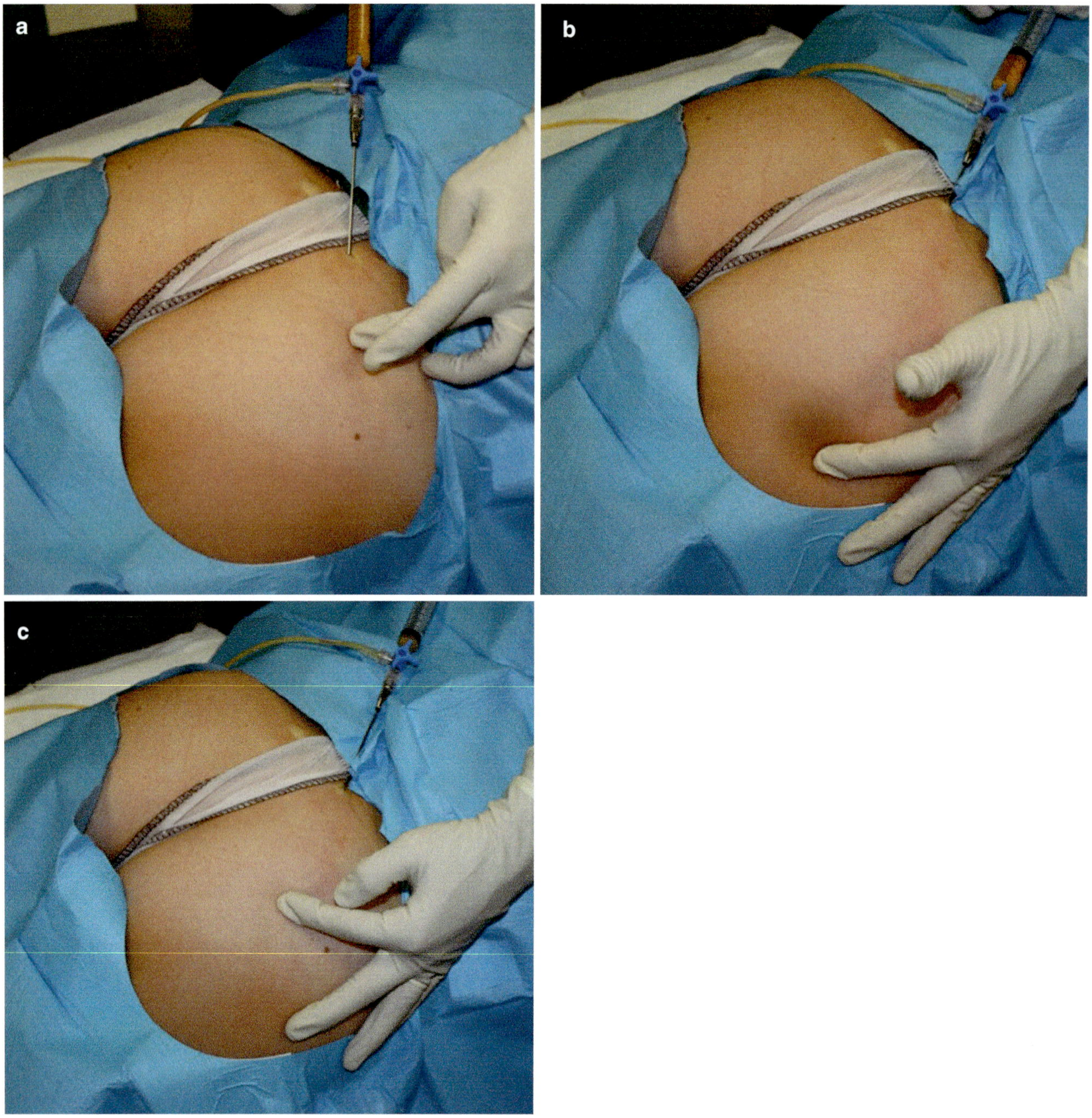

Fig. 25.9

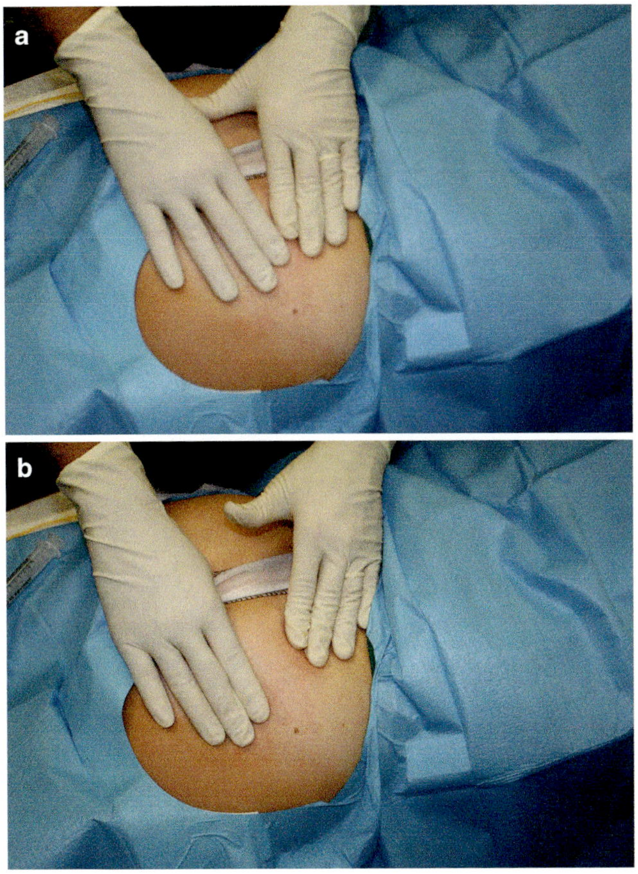

Fig. 25.10

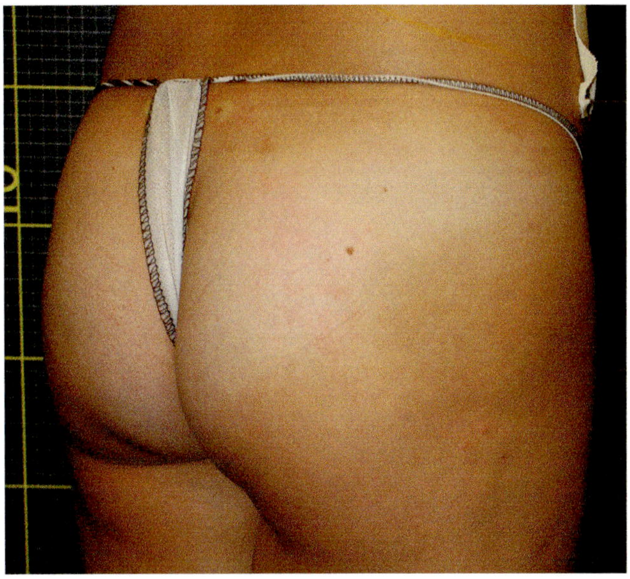

Fig. 25.11 The buttocks immediately after the treatment. (Published with kind permission of ©Mario Goisis 2018. All Rights Reserved)

Vulva

26

Mario Goisis and Sara Izzo

The *labia majora* form the lips of the vulva together with the labia minora.

The labia majora extend downward and backward from the mons pubis as far as the perineum.

The Bulbospongiosus muscle is one of the surface muscles of the perineum. It covers the vestibular bulb. It contributes to clitoral erection and the contractions of orgasm and closes the vagina.

26.1 Labia Majora Augmentation using Microfat

26.1.1 Indications

Loss of volume in the vulva (of the labia majora) is a common issue in women as they age, especially as they reach menopause. Augmentation of the labia majora using microfat is a very simple and effective procedure.

26.1.2 Contraindications

The fat should not be injected into areas that lack sufficient blood supply or are affected by infection or inflammation. No injection should be carried out if the area has been previously treated with liquid silicone or other permanent fillers because new injections might lead to inflammation or infection of the implants.

26.1.3 Operating Time

The procedure usually takes 20 min, once the fat has been harvested.

26.1.4 Materials

- *4–16 cc of microfat for injection:*
  - *A 21-gauge needle*
  - *A 22-gauge, 4-cm blunt cannula*

For harvesting and processing the fat, a standard system for microfat is used, in particular:

- A Microfat box (www.microfat.com), composed of a ramp with a closed system for washing and filtration
- 4 60-cc syringes
- 2 10-cc syringes
- One 1-cc syringe
- A 30-gauge needle
- A 16-gauge needle
- A 2 mm-diameter, 10 cm-long Goisis cannula for fat harvesting
- A chlorhexidine-alcohol solution (2% chlorhexidine gluconate and 70% isopropyl alcohol), sterile drapes or towels
- Ice packs
- Sterile 2 cm × 2 cm gauze squares
- Occlusive dressing cover

Medications include:

- 100 cc of cold saline solution.
- 120 cc of cold Klein solution.
- One litre of Klein solution is composed of 800 mg of lidocaine, 1 mg of epinephrine, 40 MEq of sodium bicarbonate, and 1000 cc of saline solution.

M. Goisis (✉)
Maxillo-Facial and Aesthetic Surgeon, Go Easy Clinic, Milan, Italy

S. Izzo
Department of Plastic Surgery, University of Campania "Luigi Vanvitelli", Naples, Italy

M. Goisis (ed.), *Outpatient Regenerative Medicine*, https://doi.org/10.1007/978-3-319-44894-7_26

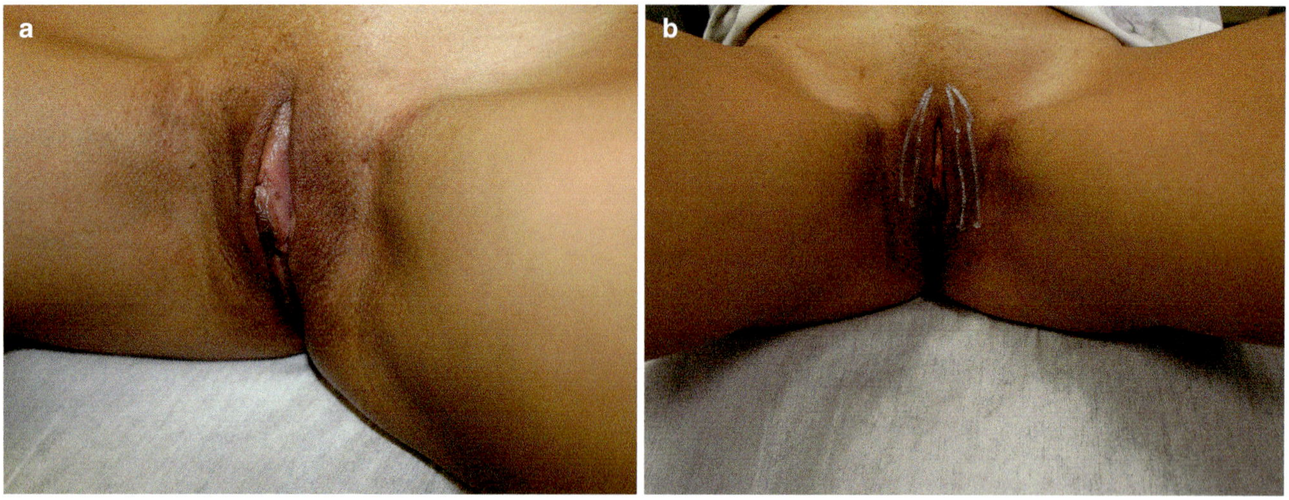

Fig. 26.1 (**a**, **b**) Loss of volume of the labia majora. Pretreatment image. (Published by kind permission of ©Mario Goisis 2018. All Rights Reserved)

Location: Microfat harvesting can be in a small operating theatre/a doctor's surgery. Oxygen, pulse oximetry and a crash cart/box should be present.

Assistance: An assistant can prove useful for the transfer of items to the procedure field in a sterile manner during the first state of the procedure. Nevertheless, a single doctor can perform the entire procedure single-handed.

Plane of injection: subcutaneous

26.1.5 Procedure

The procedure is illustrated in Figs. 26.1, 26.2, 26.3, 26.4, 26.5, 26.6, 26.7, 26.8, 26.9, 26.10, and 26.11.

26.2 The Bio-rejuvenation Technique for the Treatment of the Genital Area

Bio-rejuvenation is a technique that generally avails itself of low-viscosity hyaluronic acid to induce deep hydration of the skin and mucosa and stimulate the dermis to produce new matrix, improving skin structure and elasticity. The production of endogenous HA decreases drastically with age, contributing to wrinkling. Injection of low-viscosity hyaluronic acid to the dermis enhances the attraction of fibroblasts, macrophages, endothelial cells, and scavengers against radical-free damaged dermal proteins, thus inducing rejuvenation of the dermal layer.

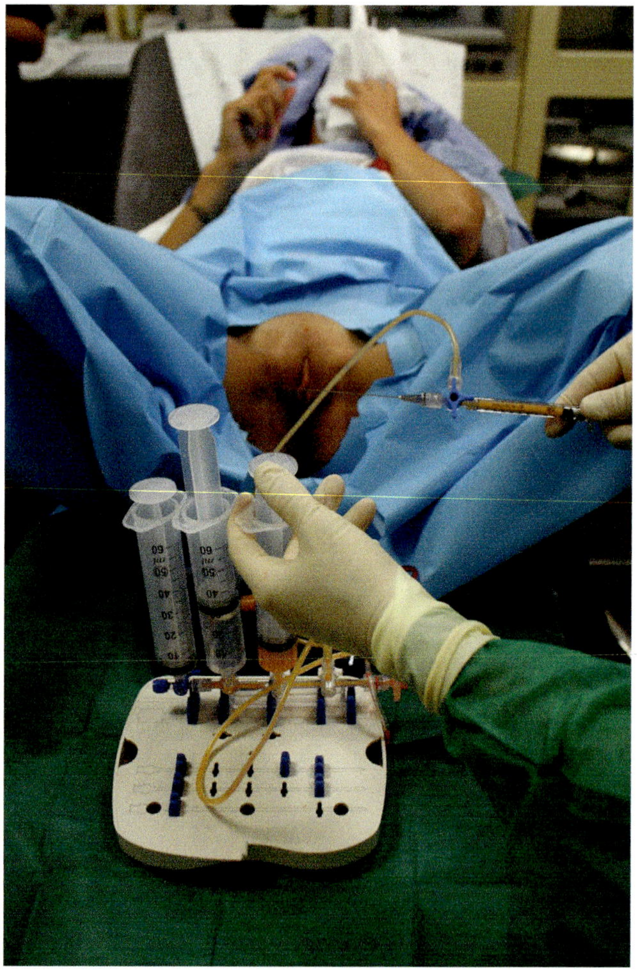

Fig 26.2 20 cc of microfat is harvested using the microfat box (www.microfat.com) and is ready to be injected. (Published by kind permission of ©Mario Goisis 2018. All Rights Reserved)

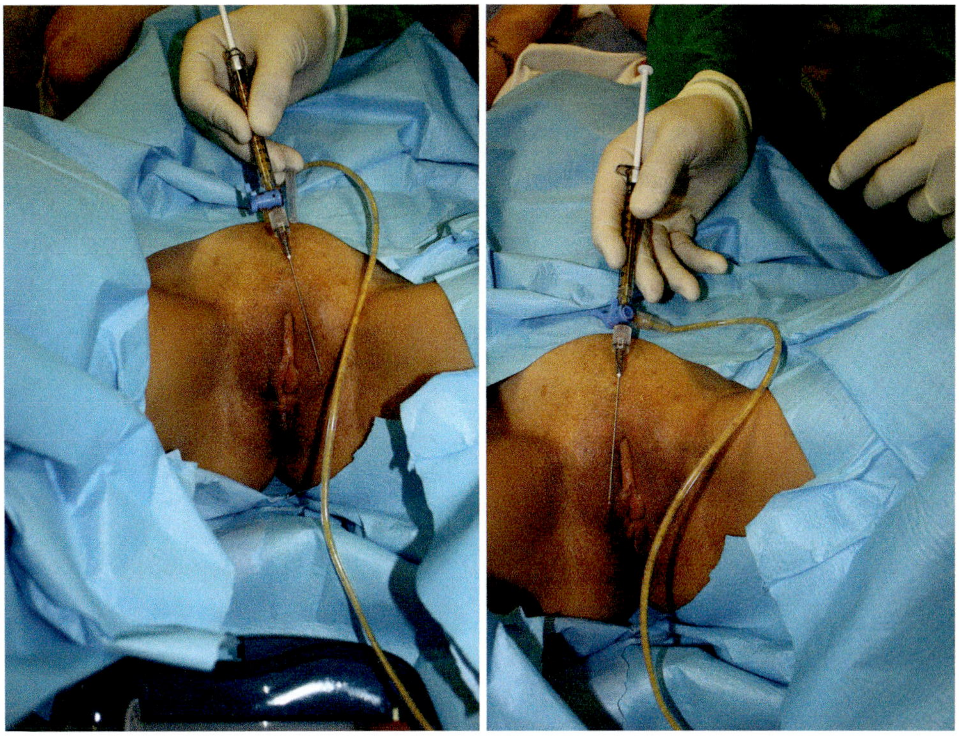

Fig. 26.3 The route of the cannula. (Published by kind permission of ©Mario Goisis 2018. All Rights Reserved)

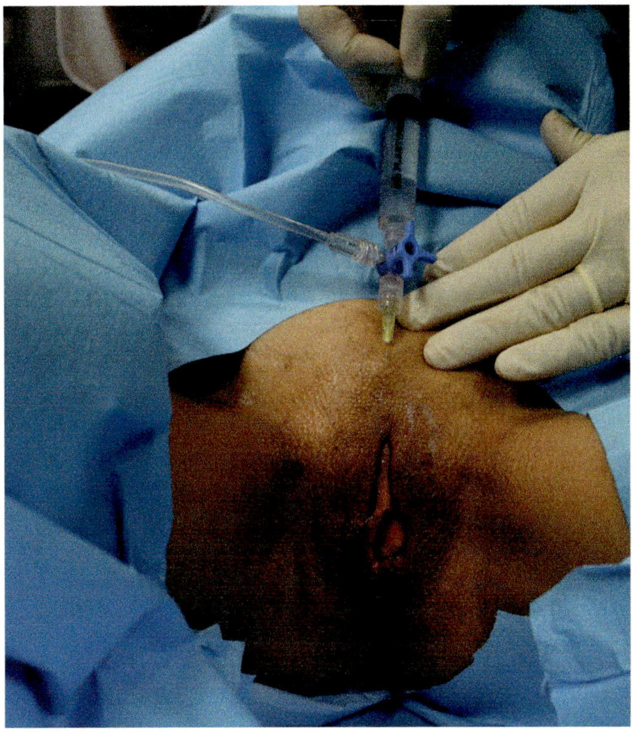

Fig. 26.4 2 cc of local anaesthetic (Klein solution) needs to be injected into the entry point, at the level of the junction between the bulbospongiosus muscles. (Published by kind permission of ©Mario Goisis 2018. All Rights Reserved)

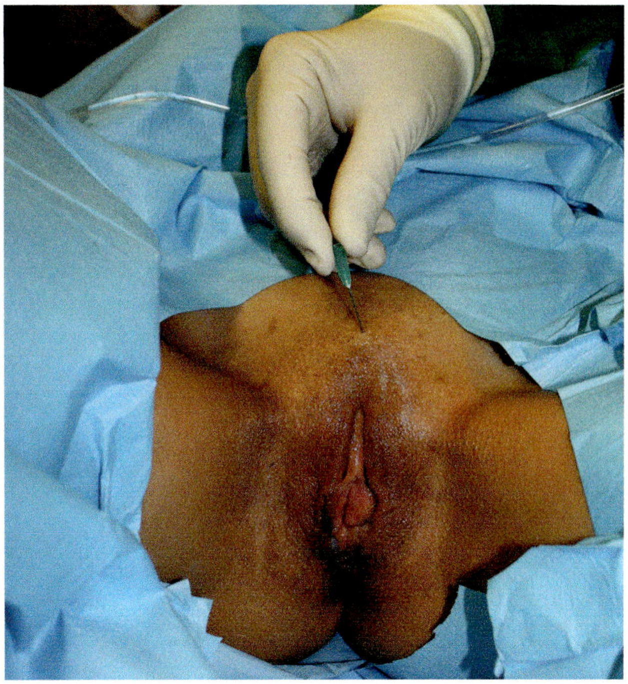

Fig. 26.5 A small hole is created to allow the entrance of the cannula into the subcutaneous plane. A 21-G needle is used for this purpose. (Published by kind permission of ©Mario Goisis 2018. All Rights Reserved)

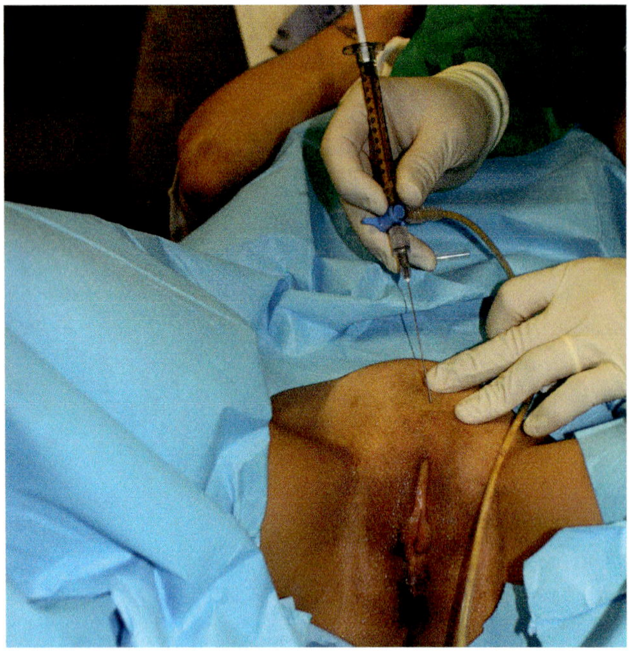

Fig. 26.6 The perpendicular insertion of a 22-G blunt-tip cannula. (Published by kind permission of ©Mario Goisis 2018. All Rights Reserved)

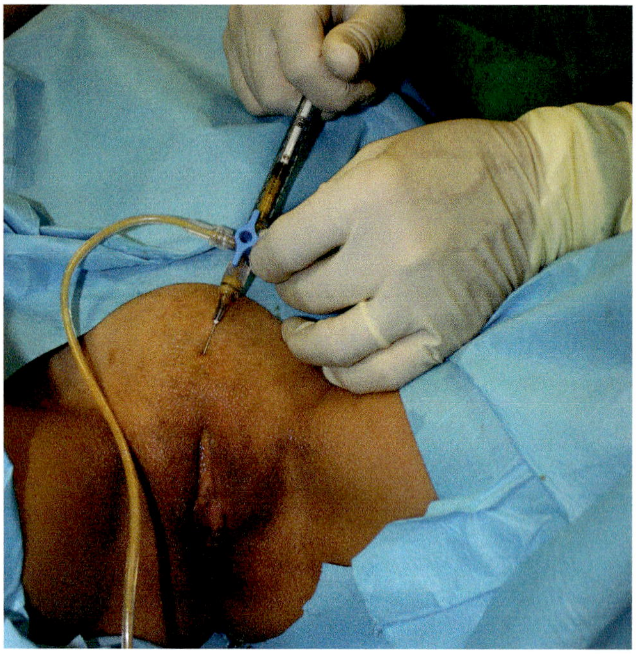

Fig. 26.8 The cannula is then pivoted to the area of the right bulbospongiosus muscle. (Published by kind permission of ©Mario Goisis 2018. All Rights Reserved)

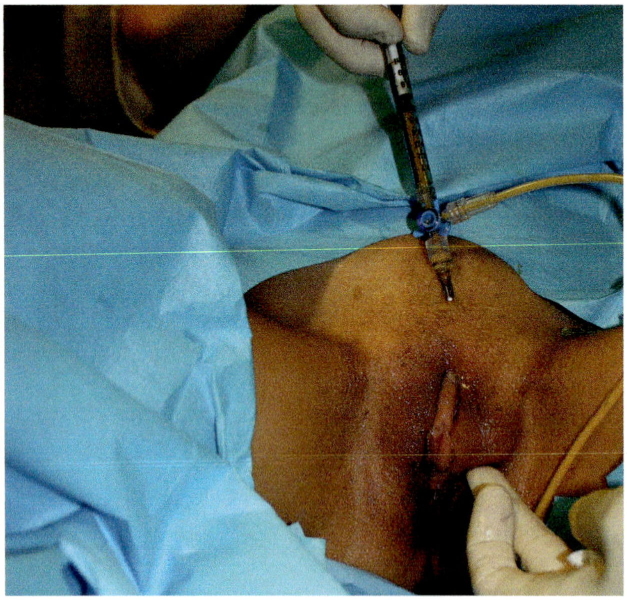

Fig. 26.7 The cannula is plunged inside the subcutaneous area, and the fat is released, retrograde fashion, into the subcutaneous plane. (Published by kind permission of ©Mario Goisis 2018. All Rights Reserved)

26.2.1 Indications

Bio-rejuvenation can be used to improve skin and mucosal trophism, texture, and elasticity of the dermis of every anatomic area but is usually practiced on the skin and mucosa of the genital area.

Low-viscosity hyaluronic acid can be injected, over a period of 12 months, according to standard protocol, in combination with alternated administration of microfat. The standard protocol usually includes:

Microfat injections at months 4, 8, and 12

Injection of not low-viscosity hyaluronic acid at months 1, 2, 3, 5, 6, 7, 9, 10, and 11

26.2.2 Operating Time

The single procedure sessions usually takes from 5 to 10 min.

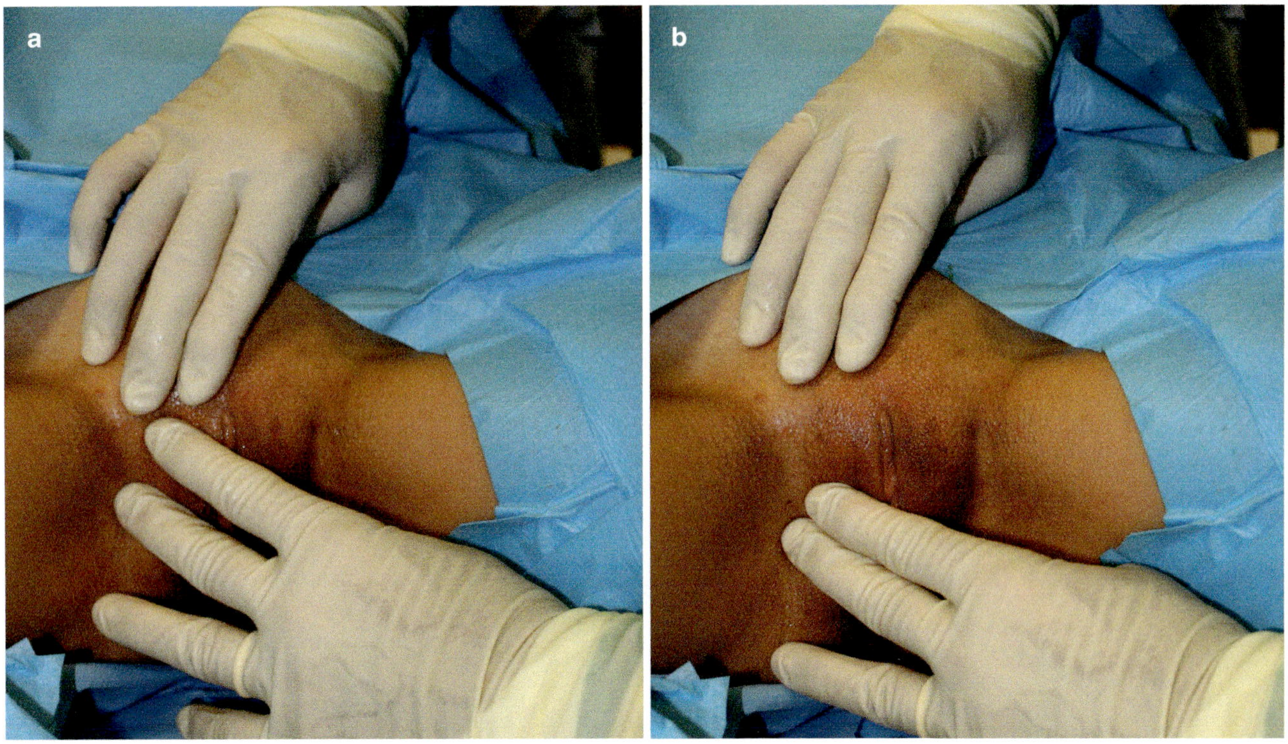

Fig. 26.9 (**a**, **b**) A soft massage of the area is performed after the treatment. (Published by kind permission of ©Mario Goisis 2018. All Rights Reserved)

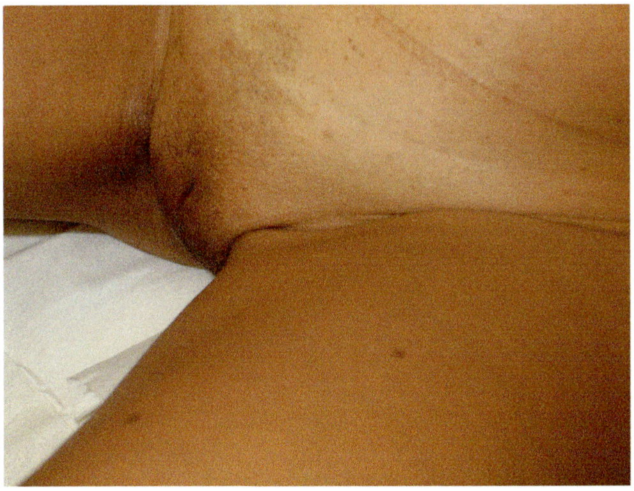

Fig. 26.10 The vulva 9 months after the treatment. (Published by kind permission of ©Mario Goisis 2018. All Rights Reserved)

26.2.3 Materials

- 0.8 cc of low density HA
- 29–30-G needle
- Topical local anaesthetic
- Bandages and antiseptic solution

26.2.4 Choice of Materials

- Jalupro
- Stylage Hydro
- Belotero Soft
- Restylane Vital Light Lidocaine (Figs. 26.12, 26.13, 26.14, 26.15, and 26.16)

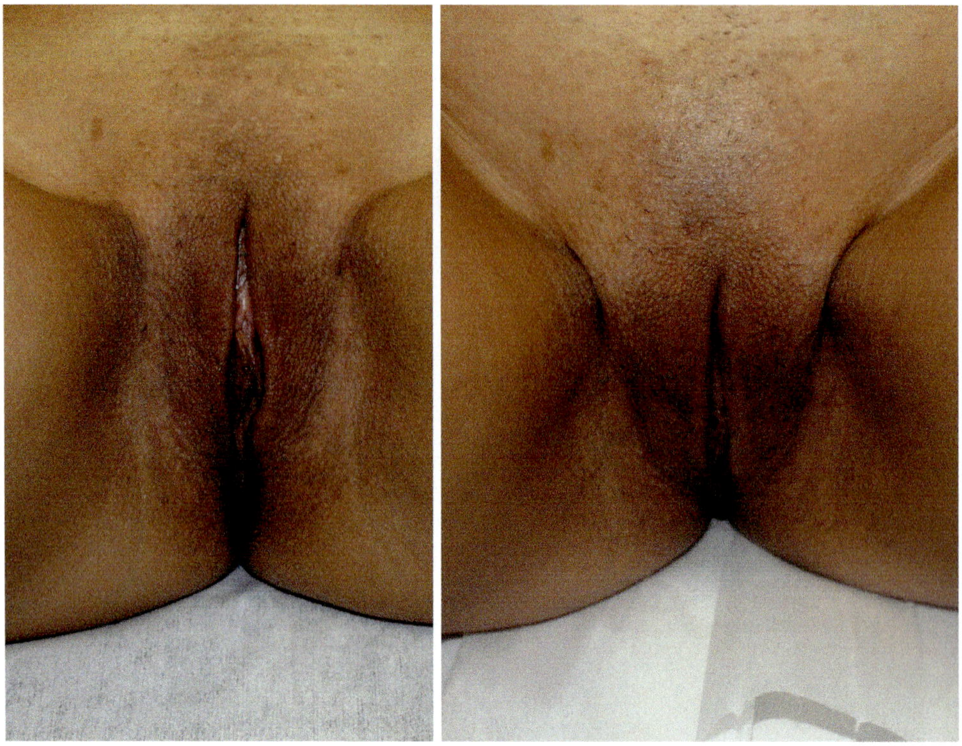

Fig. 26.11 The vulva before treatment and 9 months after. (Published by kind permission of ©Mario Goisis 2018. All Rights Reserved)

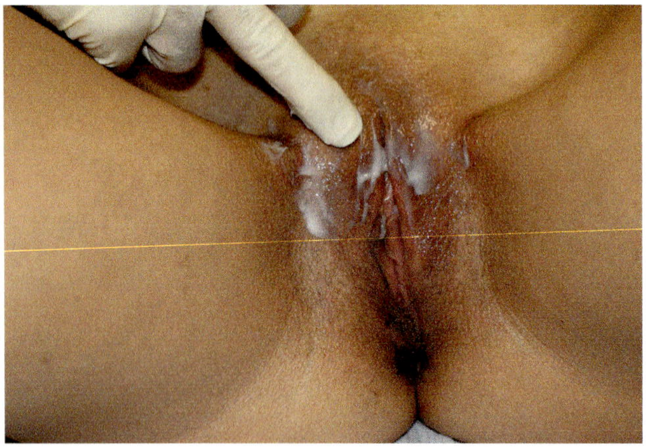

Fig. 26.12 Application of the topical local anaesthesia. (Published by kind permission of ©Mario Goisis 2018. All Rights Reserved)

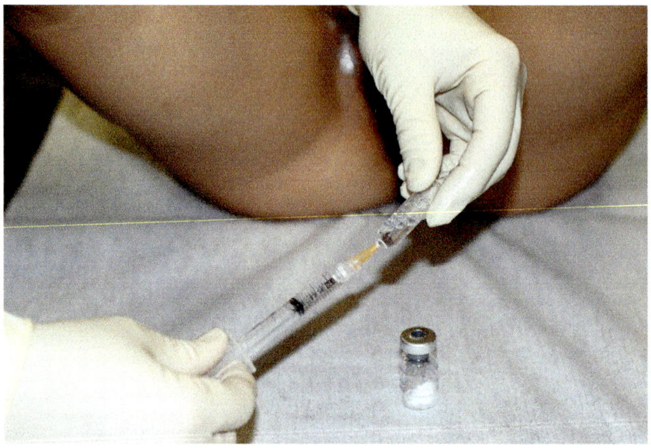

Fig. 26.13 Some products (i.e., Jalupro) are sold as sterile powders and need to be diluted. Here the dilution method of Jalupro is shown. The sterile powder is diluted in 2.5 ml of the solvent included with the powder. (Published by kind permission of ©Mario Goisis 2018. All Rights Reserved)

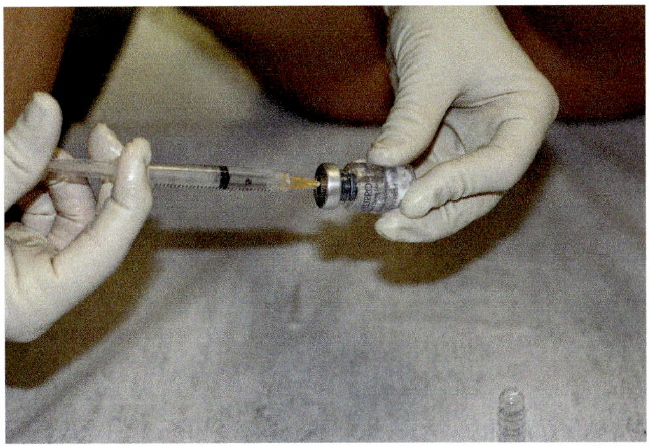

Fig. 26.14 Here dilution method of Jalupro is shown. The sterile powder is diluted in 2.5 ml of the solvent included with the powder. (Published by kind permission of ©Mario Goisis 2018. All Rights Reserved)

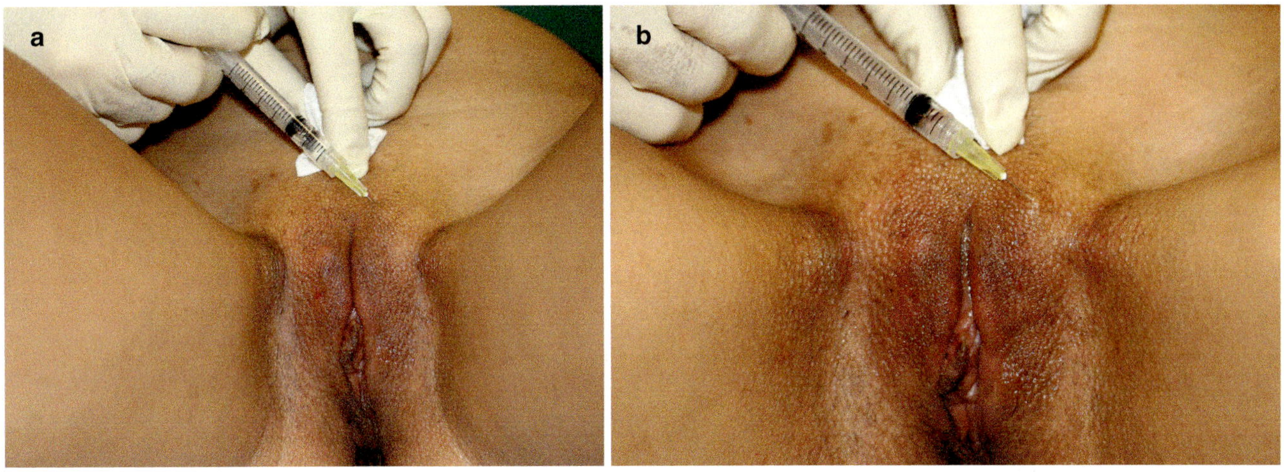

Fig. 26.15 (**a**, **b**) The HA solution is injected into the mucosa using the picottage technique. The needle is inserted for a depth of 2–3 mm; the quantity of product injected is really small, about 0.05 ml or less. (Published by kind permission of ©Mario Goisis 2018. All Rights Reserved)

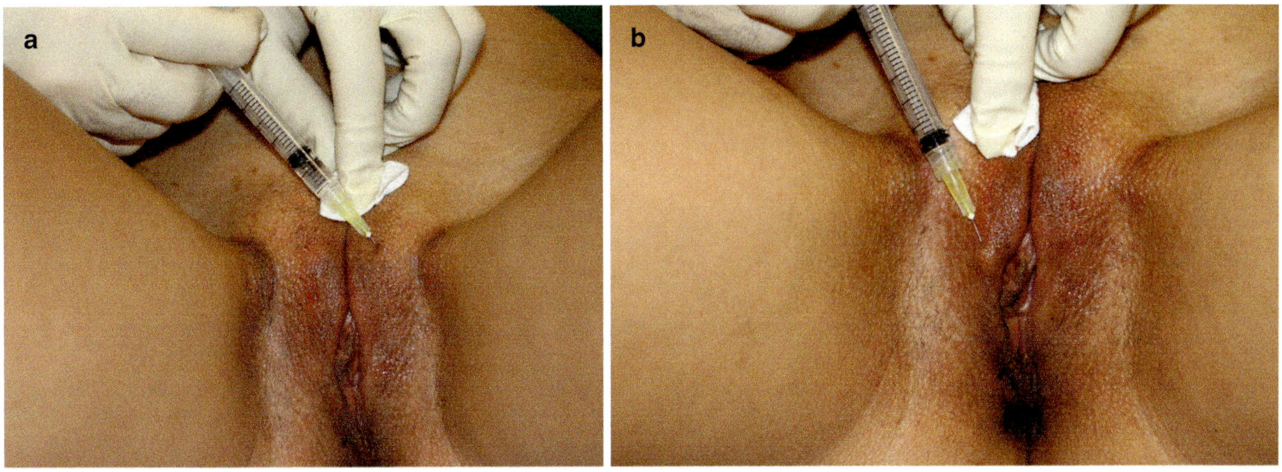

Fig. 26.16 (**a**, **b**) The ideal distance between the different injection points is 1 cm. (Published by kind permission of ©Mario Goisis 2018. All Rights Reserved)

Calves

27

Mario Goisis, Sara Izzo, and Claudio Rinna

Calf enlargement (calf augmentation) is often taken into consideration by patients whose calves are excessively slight (in extreme cases, they may be described as "stork legs") due to insufficient muscular mass, fat atrophy, or illness such as clubfoot, spastic paralysis, spina bifida, and poliomyelitis.

27.1 Anatomy

The great saphenous vein, also called the long saphenous vein, is the large, subcutaneous, superficial vein of the leg and thigh which originates from where the dorsal vein of the first digit (the big toe) merges with the dorsal venous arch of the foot. After passing in front of the medial malleolus (where it can often be seen and palpated), it runs up the medial side of the leg. At the knee, it crosses the posterior border of the medial epicondyle of the femur. The small saphenous vein is a relatively large vein of the surface of the back of the leg. Its originates where the dorsal vein of the fifth digit (smallest toe) merges with the dorsal venous arch of the foot, which flows into the great saphenous vein. It is considered a superficial vein and is subcutaneous (just under the skin). From its source, it proceeds around the lateral area of the foot (inferior and posterior to the lateral malleolus), runs along the posterior area of the leg, passes between the heads of the gastrocnemius muscle, and usually flows into the popliteal vein, approximately at or above the level of the knee joint. Accidental injury to saphenous veins leads to noticeable haematomas and blood infarction of the implant with possible infection (Fig. 27.1).

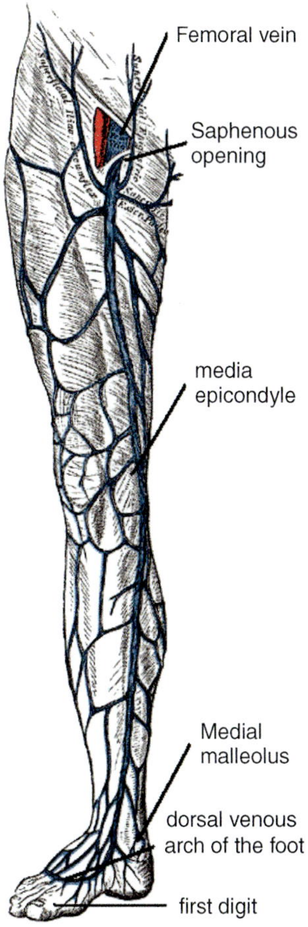

Fig. 27.1 Anatomy of the great saphenous vein. Reproduction of a lithograph plate from *Gray's Anatomy* (Henry Gray, Anatomy: Descriptive and Surgical). (Published by kind permission of ©Mario Goisis 2018. All Rights Reserved)

27.2 Pitfalls

Identification of the saphenous veins by visual, tactile and echographic examinations, must be carried out prior to injecting the fat. The injecting cannula must be directed into the subcutaneous layer, keeping the edge superficial to the muscularis fascia of the gastrocnemius (Figs. 27.2, 27.3, and 27.4).

M. Goisis (✉)
Maxillo-Facial and Aesthetic Surgeon, Go Easy Clinic, Milan, Italy

S. Izzo
Department of Plastic Surgery, University of Campania "Luigi Vanvitelli", Naples, Italy

C. Rinna
Doctor's Equipe, Milan, Italy

M. Goisis (ed.), *Outpatient Regenerative Medicine*, https://doi.org/10.1007/978-3-319-44894-7_27

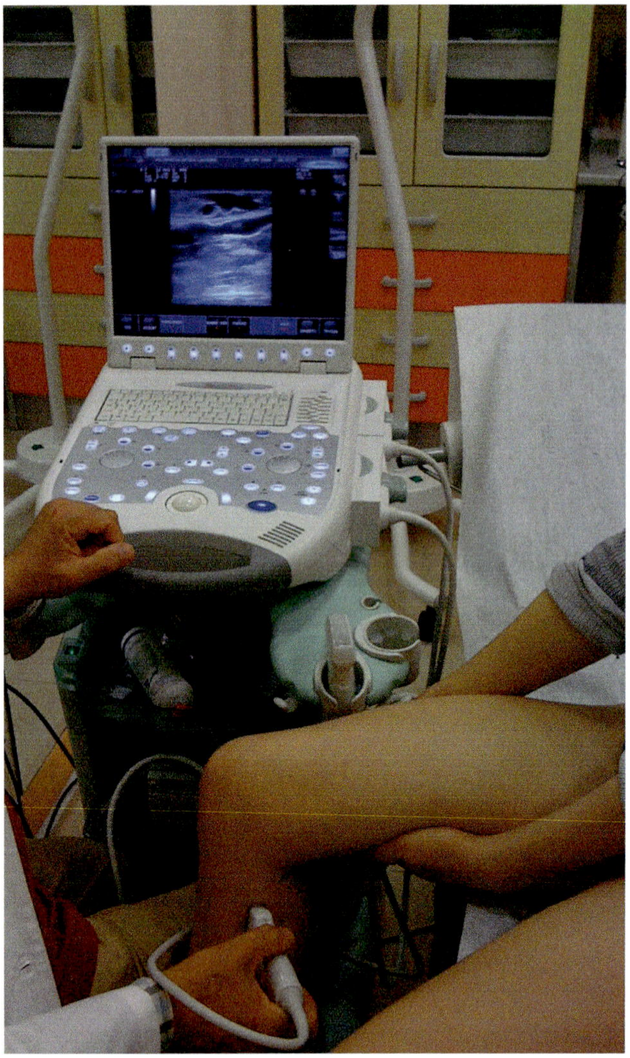

Fig. 27.2 An ultrasound examination is performed in order to trace the course of the saphenous vein (courtesy of Injection in Aesthetic Medicine, Springer). (Published by kind permission of ©Mario Goisis 2018. All Rights Reserved)

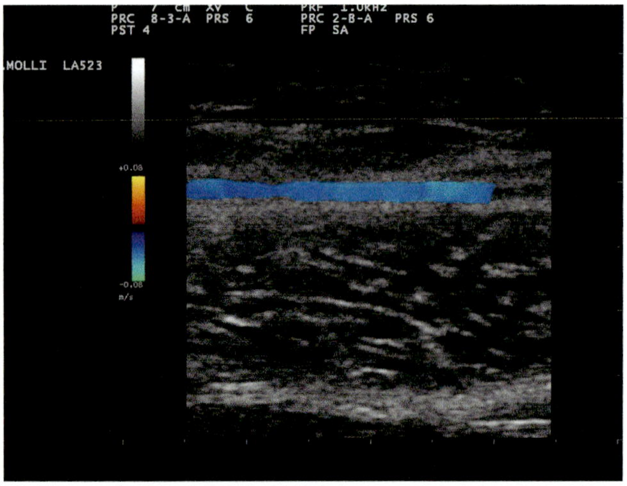

Fig. 27.3 An ultrasound Doppler image of the saphenous vein (courtesy of Injection in Aesthetic Medicine, Springer). (Published by kind permission of ©Mario Goisis 2018. All Rights Reserved)

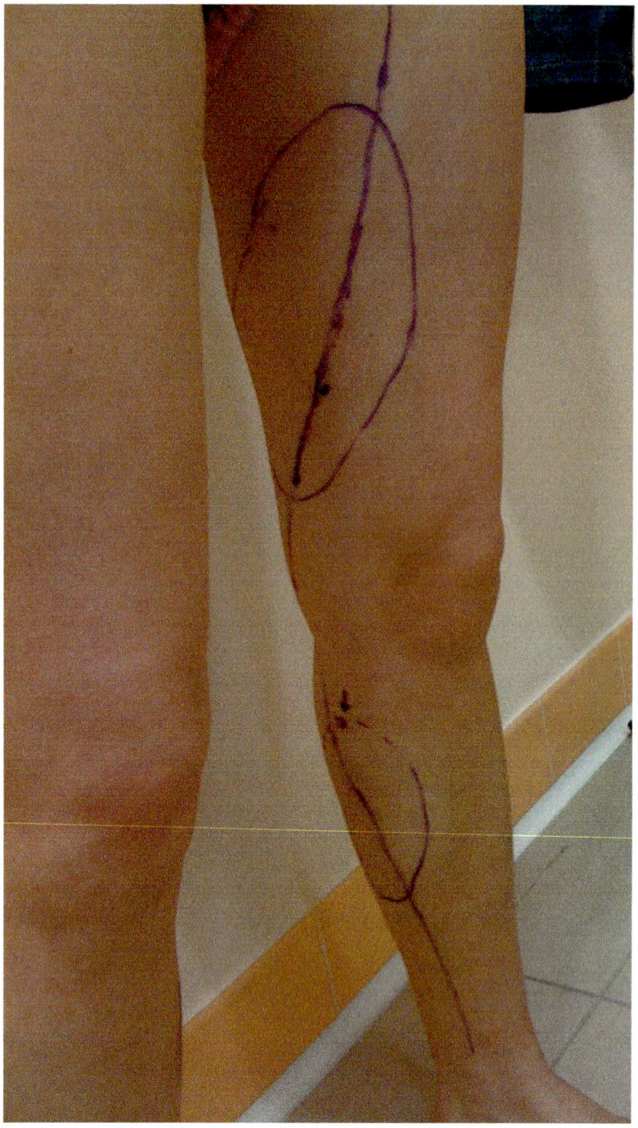

Fig. 27.4 The outline of the course of the saphenous vein drawn on the patient's leg (courtesy of Injection in Aesthetic Medicine, Springer). (Published with kind permission of ©Mario Goisis 2018. All Rights Reserved)

27.3 Calf Augmentation using Microfat

27.3.1 Indications

Augmentation of the calves to improve the harmonic aesthetics of the legs.

27.3.2 Contraindications

The fat should not be injected into areas that lack sufficient blood supply or that are suffering from infection or inflammation. No injection should be carried out if the calf has been previously treated with liquid silicone or other permanent fillers because new injections might lead to inflammation or infection of the implants. Vascular problems such as arterial or venous occlusion are relative contraindications that need to be evaluated by a specialist before treatment.

27.3.3 Operating Time

The procedure usually takes 20 min, once the fat has been harvested.

27.3.4 Materials

- *20–60 cc of micromat for injection on both sides*
- A 1.5 mm × 150 mm, filling cannula

To harvest and process the microfat, a standard system is used, in particular:

- A microfat box (www.microfat.com), composed of a ramp with a closed system for washing and filtration
- 4 60-cc syringes
- 2 10-cc syringes
- One-cc syringe
- A 30-gauge needle
- A 16-gauge needle
- A 2 mm-diameter, 10 cm-long Goisis cannula for fat harvesting
- A chlorhexidine-alcohol solution (2% chlorhexidine gluconate and 70% isopropyl alcohol), sterile drapes or towels
- Ice packs
- Sterile 2 cm × 2 cm gauze squares
- Occlusive dressing cover

Medications include:

200 cc of cold saline solution.
500 cc of cold Klein solution.
One litre of Klein solution is composed of 800 mg of lidocaine, 1 mg of epinephrine, 40 MEq of sodium bicarbonate, and 1000 cc of saline solution.

Location: Harvesting may take place in a small operating theatre/a surgery. The oxygen, pulse oximetry, and a crash cart/box should be present.

Assistance: An assistant can be useful when transferring items to the procedure field in a sterile manner during the first phase of the procedure. Nevertheless, a single doctor can carry out the entire procedure alone.

27.3.5 Procedure

The procedure is illustrated in figures 27.5a–c, 27.6a–c, 27.7, 27.8, 27.9a, b, 27.10a, b, 27.11a, b, 27.12a–c, 27.13a, b, 27.14, and 27.15a, b below.

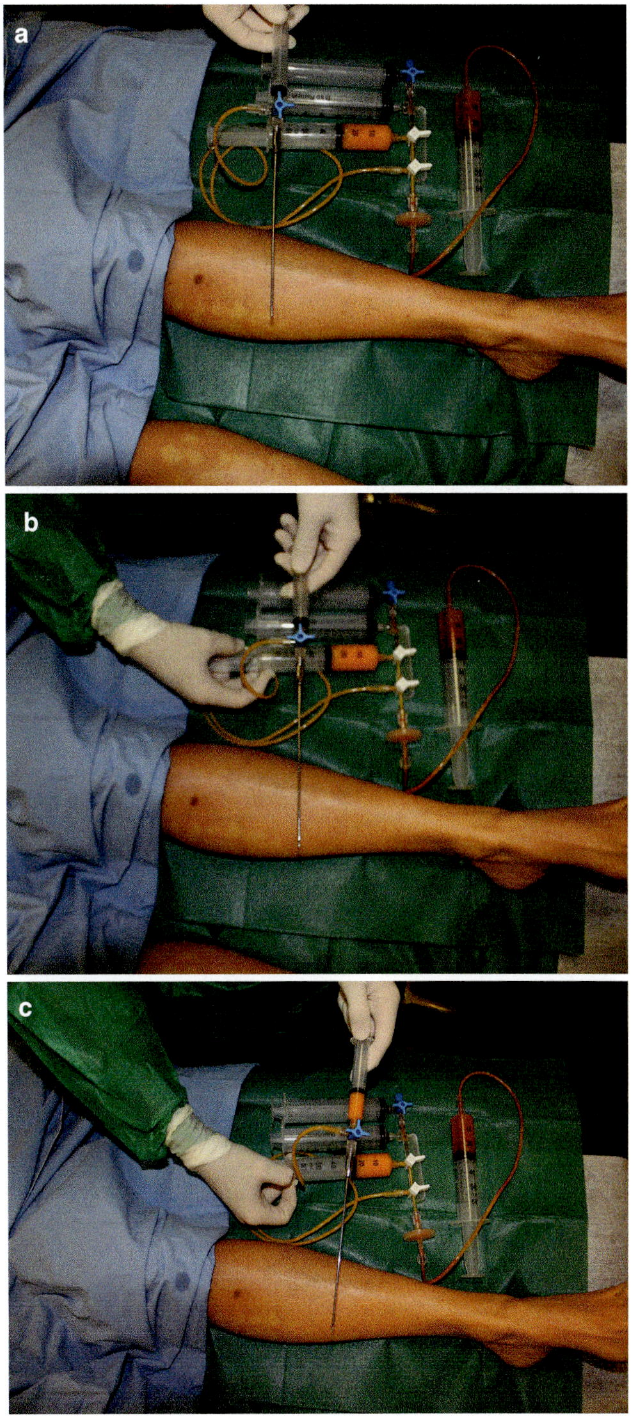

Fig. 27.5 (**a**–**c**) The injection-syringe is filled with microfat. (Published by kind permission of ©Mario Goisis 2018. All Rights Reserved)

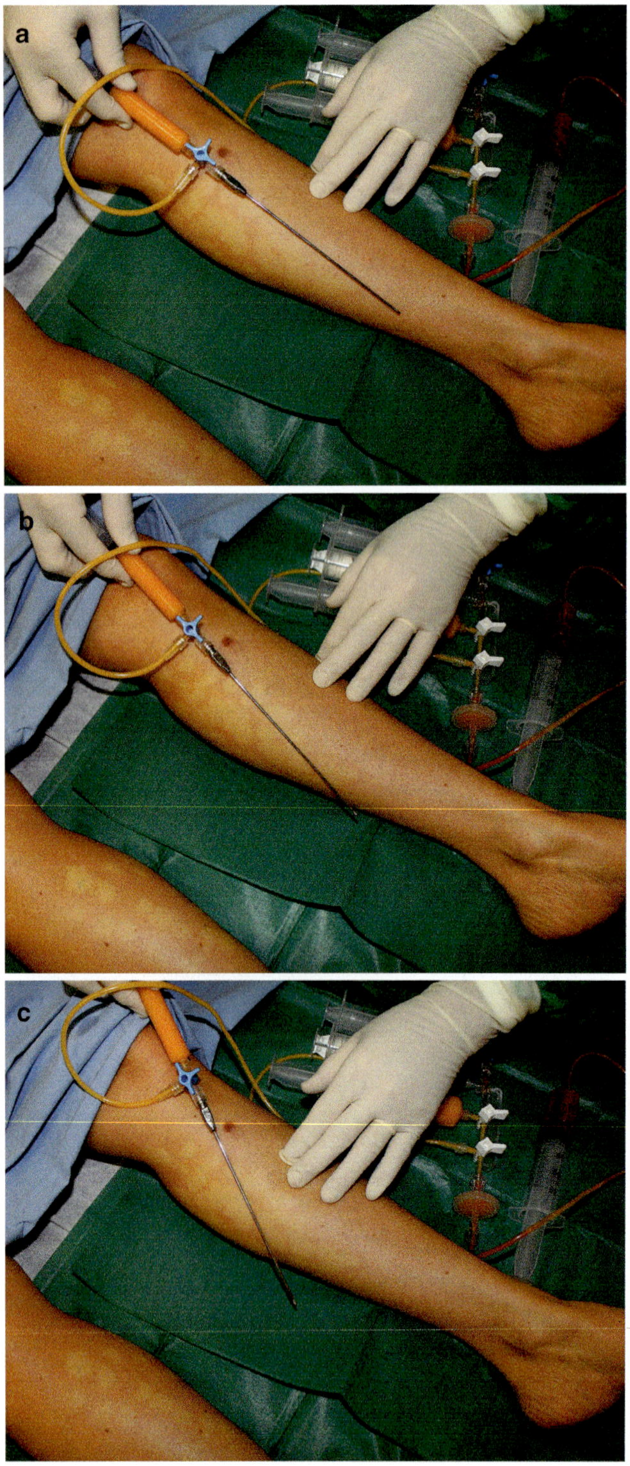

Fig. 27.6 (**a–c**) The route of the cannula entering from a single-entry point is demonstrated here. (Published by kind permission of ©Mario Goisis 2018. All Rights Reserved)

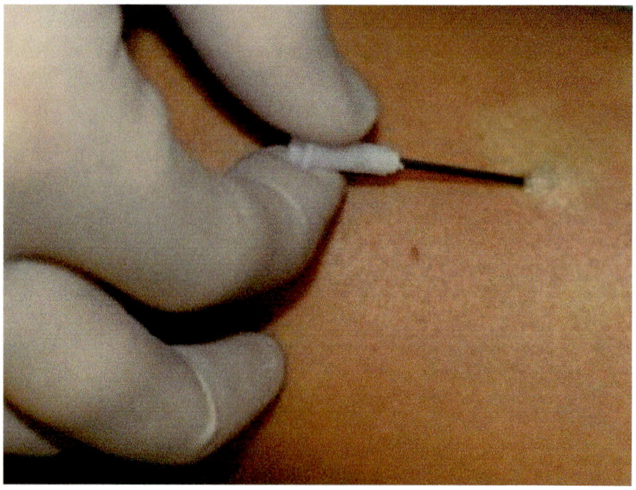

Fig. 27.7 An opening is created using a 16-G needle. (Published by kind permission of ©Mario Goisis 2018. All Rights Reserved)

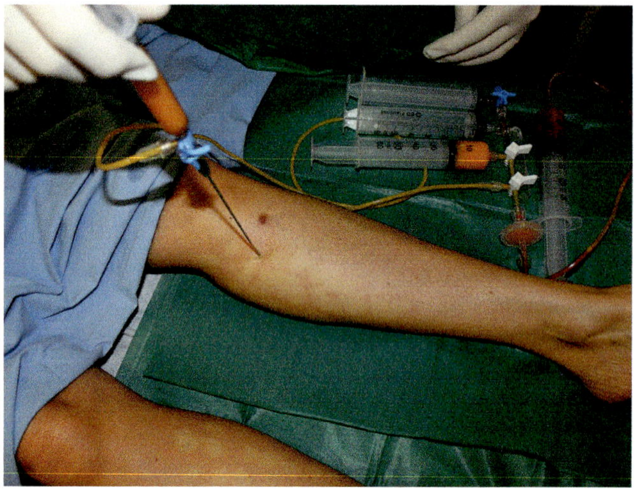

Fig. 27.8 The injecting cannula is inserted under the plane of the skin, perpendicular to it, through the ad-hoc hole. The cannula is then pivoted parallel to the plane of the skin and is then ready for the fat to be injected. (Published by kind permission of ©Mario Goisis 2018. All Rights Reserved)

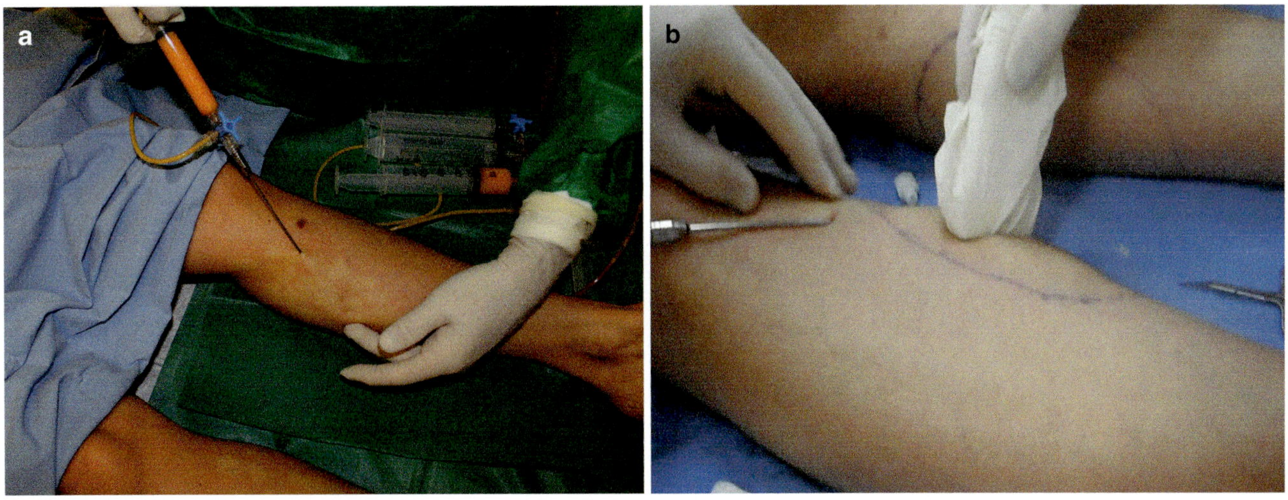

Fig. 27.9 (a, b) The microfat is released, retrograde fashion, into the subcutaneous plane following the route of the cannula as planned. (Published by kind permission of ©Mario Goisis 2018. All Rights Reserved)

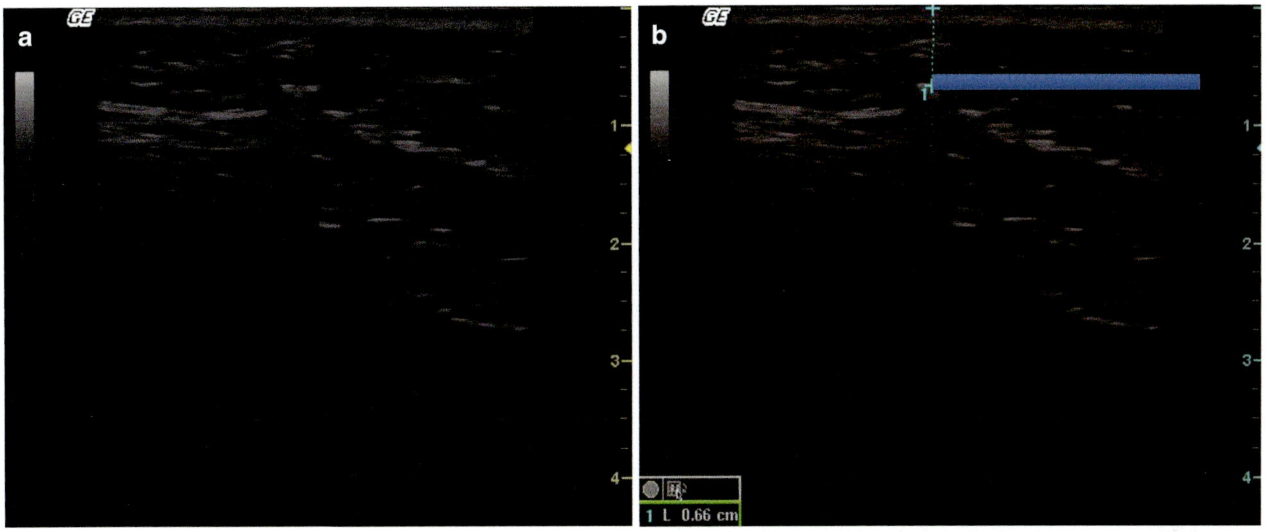

Fig. 27.10 (a, b) An ultrasound image demonstrating the position of the cannula in the subcutaneous plane (N.b. nota1?). (Published by kind permission of ©Mario Goisis 2018. All Rights Reserved)

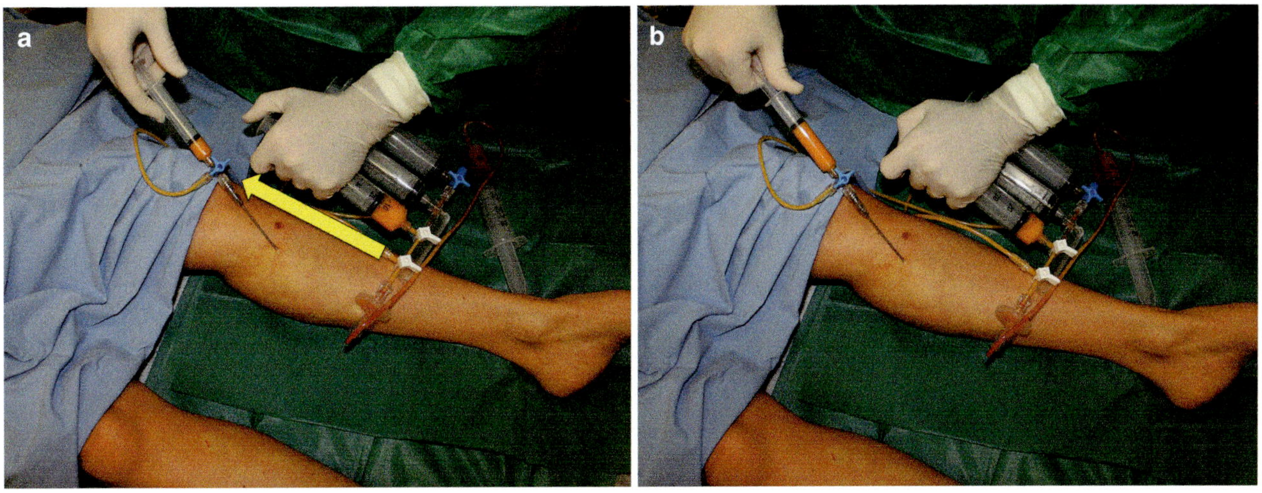

Fig. 27.11 (a, b) The syringe is filled again with microfat. (Published by kind permission of ©Mario Goisis 2018. All Rights Reserved)

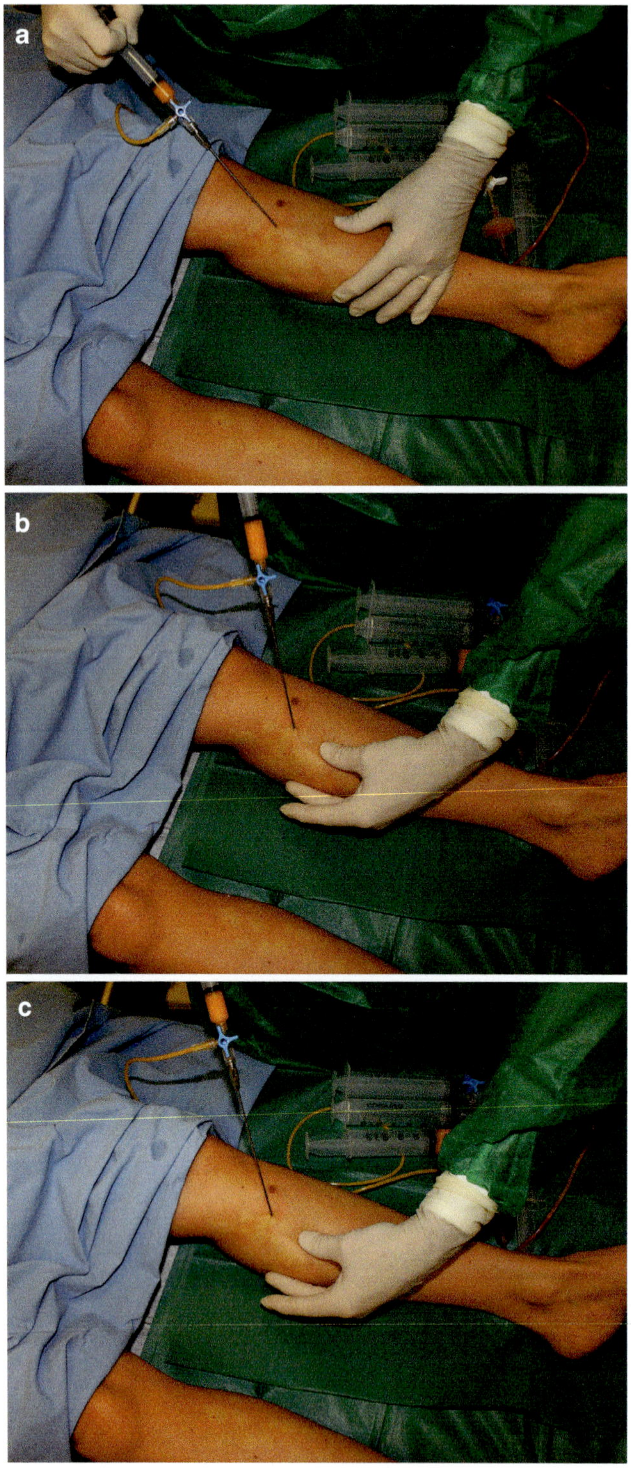

Fig. 27.12 (**a**–**c**) The calf is filled by means of a fan-like distribution of the microfat. (Published by kind permission of ©Mario Goisis 2018. All Rights Reserved)

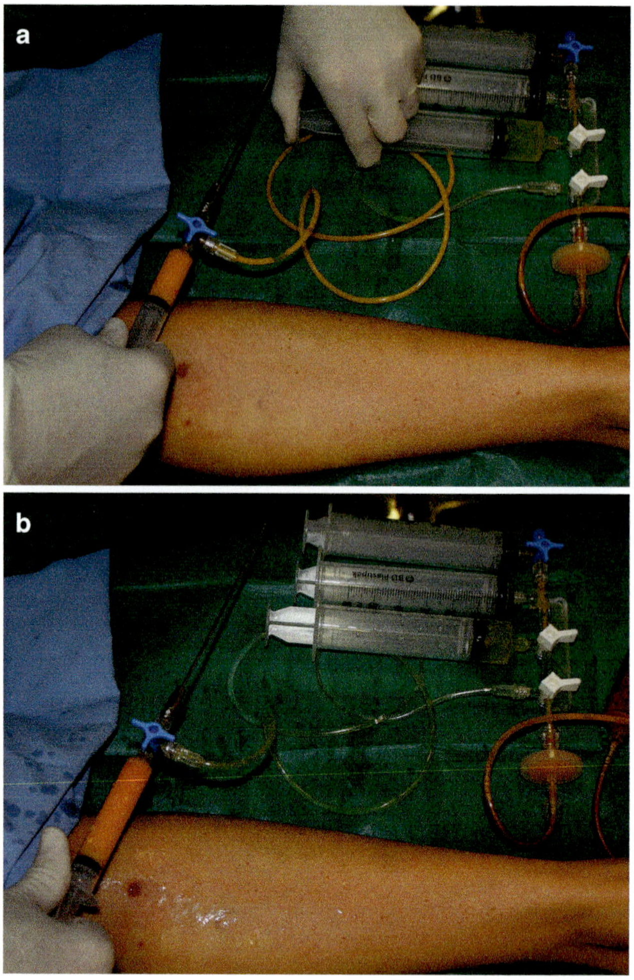

Fig. 27.13 (**a**, **b**) In order to use the microfat contained in the tube, a syringe, filled with saline solution, is connected to the system. This way, all the microfat is transferred into the injection syringe. (Published by kind permission of ©Mario Goisis 2018. All Rights Reserved)

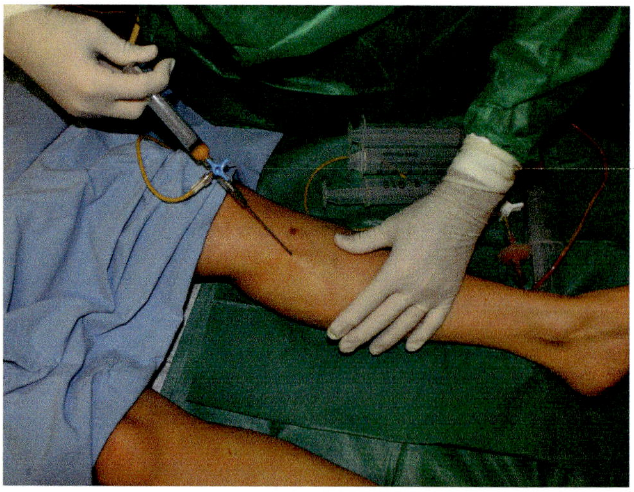

Fig. 27.14 The last syringe of microfat is injected. (Published by kind permission of ©Mario Goisis 2018. All Rights Reserved)

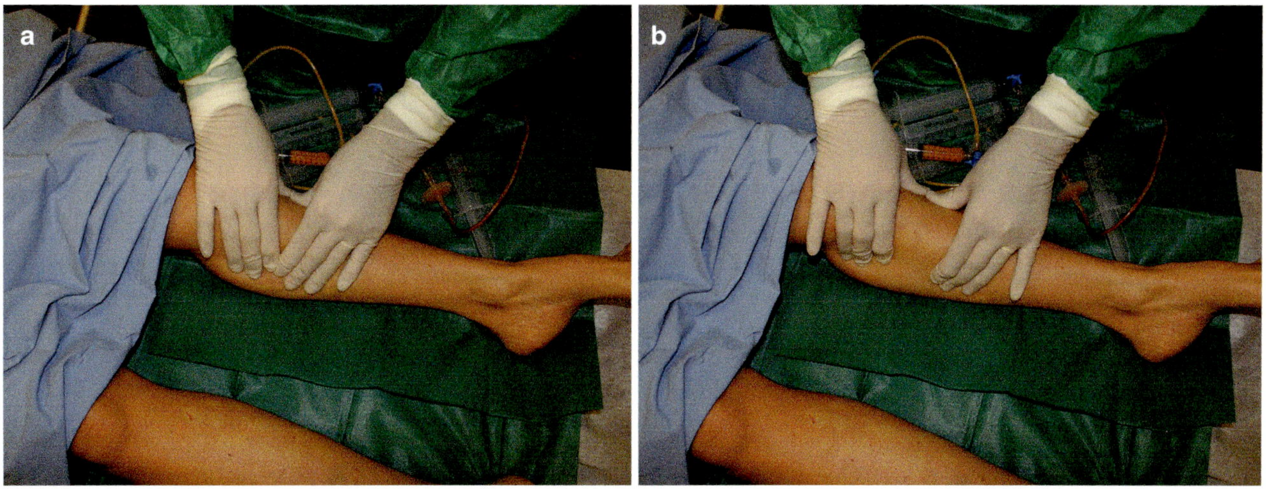

Fig. 27.15 (**a**, **b**) After treatment, the area is massaged vigorously to harmonize the shape of the injected fat. (Published by kind permission of ©Mario Goisis 2018. All Rights Reserved)

The Foot

28

Mario Goisis, Sara Izzo, and Alessandro Di Petrillo

28.1 Anatomy

The human foot is a strong, complex mechanical structure containing 26 bones, 33 joints (20 of which are actively articulated), and more than a hundred muscles, tendons, and ligaments. The muscles acting on the foot can be divided into extrinsic muscles, those originating in the anterior or posterior area of the lower leg, and the intrinsic muscles, originating in the dorsal (top) or plantar (base) area of the foot. The foot is formed by the dorsum and the planum.

To rejuvenate the foot, it is important to have a thorough knowledge of the anatomy of its dorsum, because the regenerative medical techniques aim augmenting the thickness of the dorsum subcutis. Under the subcutaneous tissue on the dorsal face of the foot, there is a system of tendons and an aponeurosis constituted by the extensor muscle of the foot, both extrinsic and intrinsic.

28.2 Augmentation of the Dorsum of the Foot using Microfat

28.2.1 Indications

Augmentation of the dorsum to improve the aesthetics of the foot.

28.2.2 Contraindications

The fat should not be injected into areas that lack a sufficient supply of blood or that are suffering from infection or inflammation. No injection should be carried out if the foot has been previously treated with liquid silicone or other permanent fillers because new injections might lead to inflammation or infection of the implants. Vascular problems such as arterial or venous occlusion are relative contraindications that need to be evaluated by the specialist before treatment.

28.2.3 Operating Time

The procedure usually takes 10 min, once the fat has been harvested.

28.2.4 Materials

- *2–4 cc of microfat to be injected on each side:*
  - *A 21-gauge needle*
  - *A 22-gauge 4-cm blunt cannula*

To harvest and process the microfat, a standard system is used, in particular:

- A microfat box (www.microfat.com), composed of a ramp with a closed a system for washing and filtration
- 4 60-cc syringes
- 2 10-cc syringes
- One 1-cc syringe
- A 30-gauge needle
- A 16-gauge needle
- A 2 mm-diameter, 10 cm-long Goisis cannula for fat harvesting

M. Goisis (✉)
Maxillo-Facial and Aesthetic Surgeon, Go Easy Clinic, Milan, Italy

S. Izzo
Department of Plastic Surgery, University of Campania "Luigi Vanvitelli", Naples, Italy

A. Di Petrillo
Doctor's Equipe, Milan, Italy

M. Goisis (ed.), *Outpatient Regenerative Medicine*, https://doi.org/10.1007/978-3-319-44894-7_28

- A chlorhexidine-alcohol solution (2% chlorhexidine gluconate and 70% isopropyl alcohol), sterile drapes or towels
- Ice packs
- Sterile 2 cm × 2 cm gauze squares
- Occlusive dressing cover

Medications include:

- 100 cc of cold saline solution.
- 120 cc of cold Klein solution.
- One litre of Klein solution is composed of 800 mg of lidocaine, 1 mg of epinephrine, 40 MEq of sodium bicarbonate, and 1000 cc of saline solution.

Location: The microfat harvesting can be carried out in a small operating theatre/medical surgery. Oxygen, the pulse oximetry, and a crash cart/box should be present.

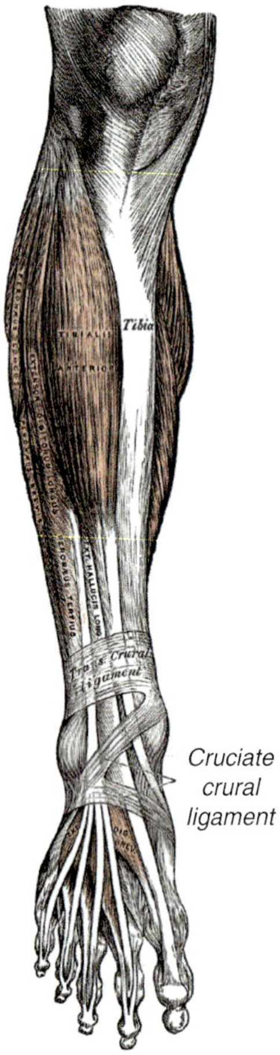

Fig. 28.1 The anatomy of the foot. From *Gray's Anatomy*. (Published by kind permission of ©Mario Goisis 2018. All Rights Reserved)

Assistants: An assistant is useful for the transfer of items to the procedure field in a sterile manner during the first part of the procedure. Despite this, a single doctor may carry out the entire procedure alone.

28.2.5 Procedure

The procedure is shown in Figs. 28.1, 28.2, 28.3, 28.4a, b, 28.5, 28.6, 28.7a–e, 28.8a–c, and 28.9.

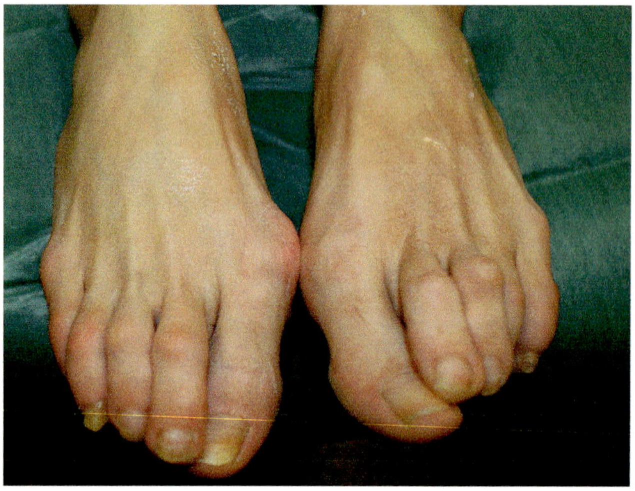

Fig. 28.2 The feet before the treatment. (Published by kind permission of ©Mario Goisis 2018. All Rights Reserved)

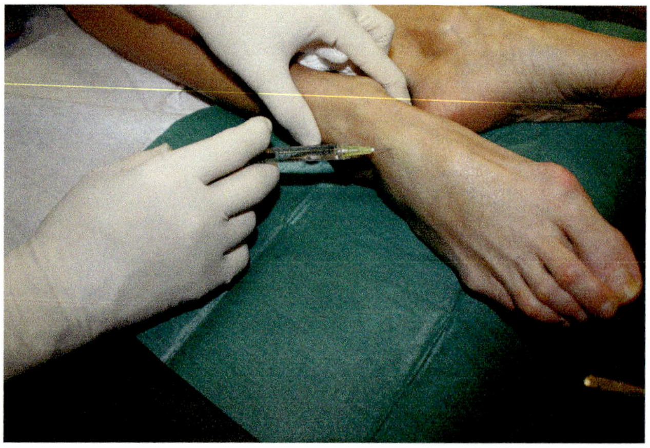

Fig. 28.3 0.5 cc of Klein solution is injected into a single entry-point located between the third and fourth metatarsal bones. This precaution guarantees that treatment with a blunt-tip cannula may cause the patient no pain. (Published by kind permission of ©Mario Goisis 2018. All Rights Reserved)

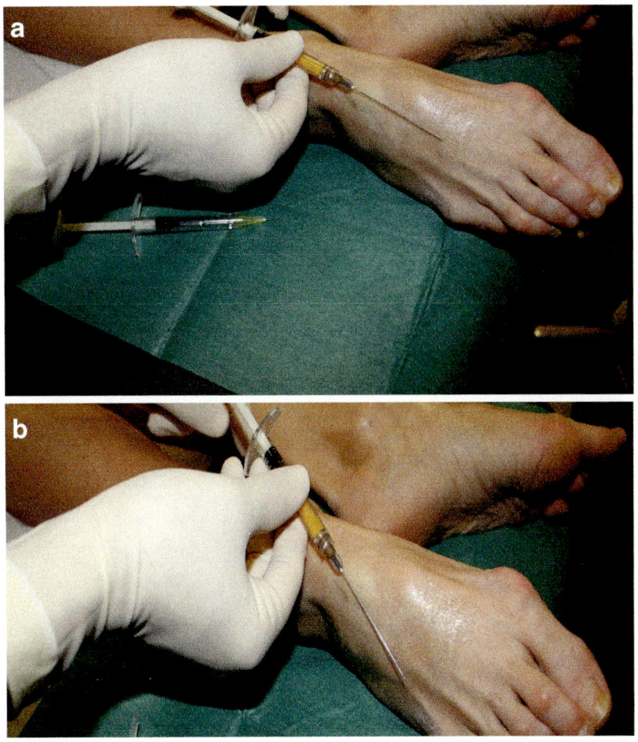

Fig. 28.4 (**a**, **b**) The route of the cannula. (Published by kind permission of ©Mario Goisis 2018. All Rights Reserved)

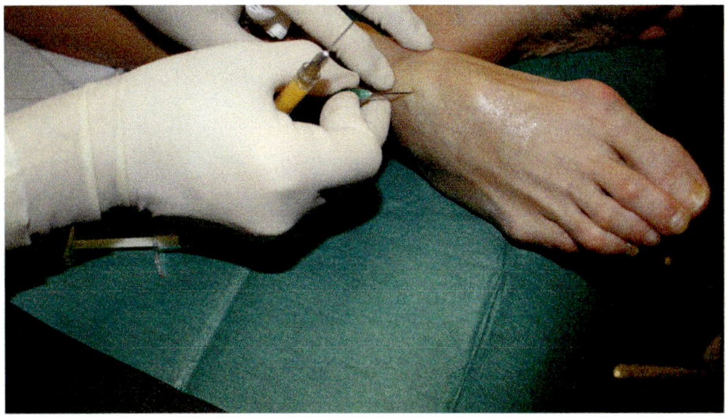

Fig. 28.5 A small hole is created to allow the entrance of the cannula onto the subcutaneous plane. A 21-G needle is used for this purpose. (Published by kind permission of ©Mario Goisis 2018. All Rights Reserved)

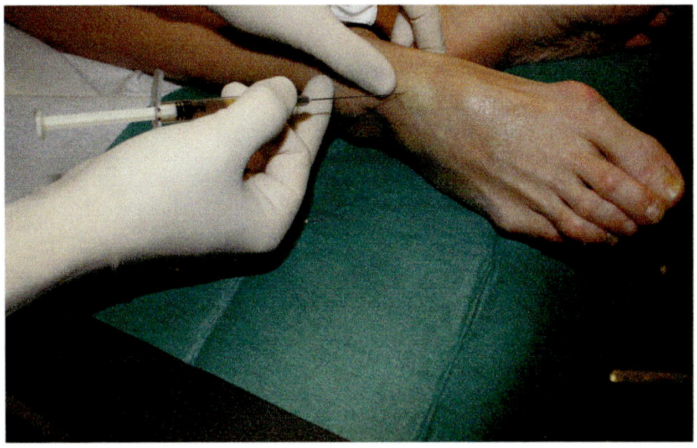

Fig. 28.6 The perpendicular insertion of a 22-G blunt-tip cannula. The cannula is plunged deep into the skin, paying attention to remain above the surface of the dorsal superficial fascia. The tip of the cannula is then directed up to the level of the toe joints. (Published by kind permission of ©Mario Goisis 2018. All Rights Reserved)

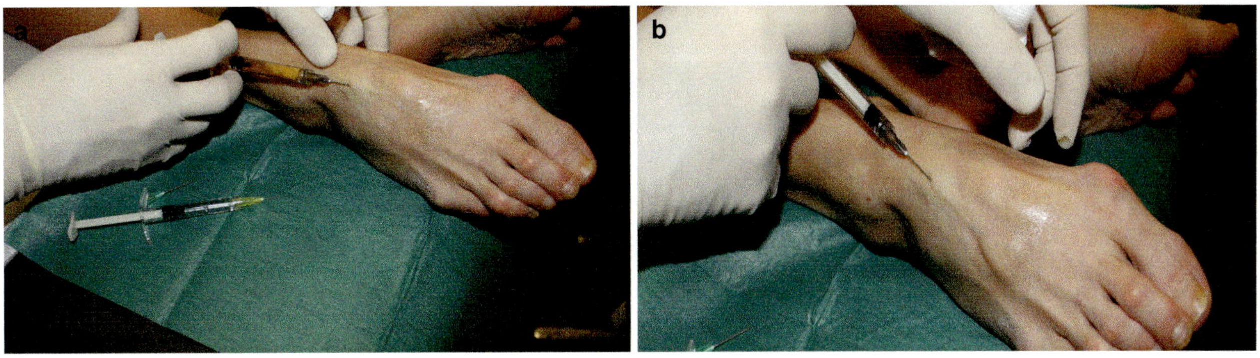

Fig. 28.7 (**a**–**e**) The fat is released, retrograde fashion, onto the subcutaneous plane, into the spaces between the metatarsal bones. (Published by kind permission of ©Mario Goisis 2018. All Rights Reserved)

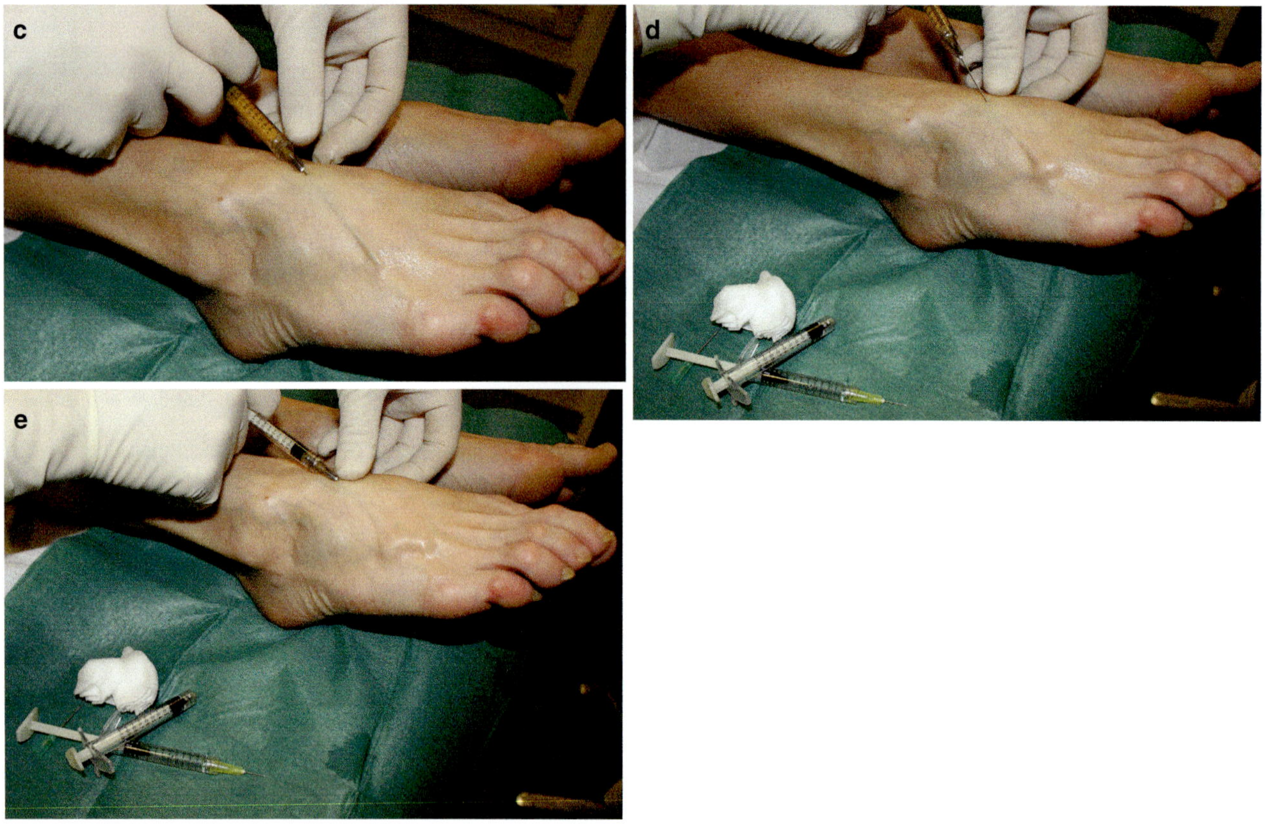

Fig. 28.7 (continued)

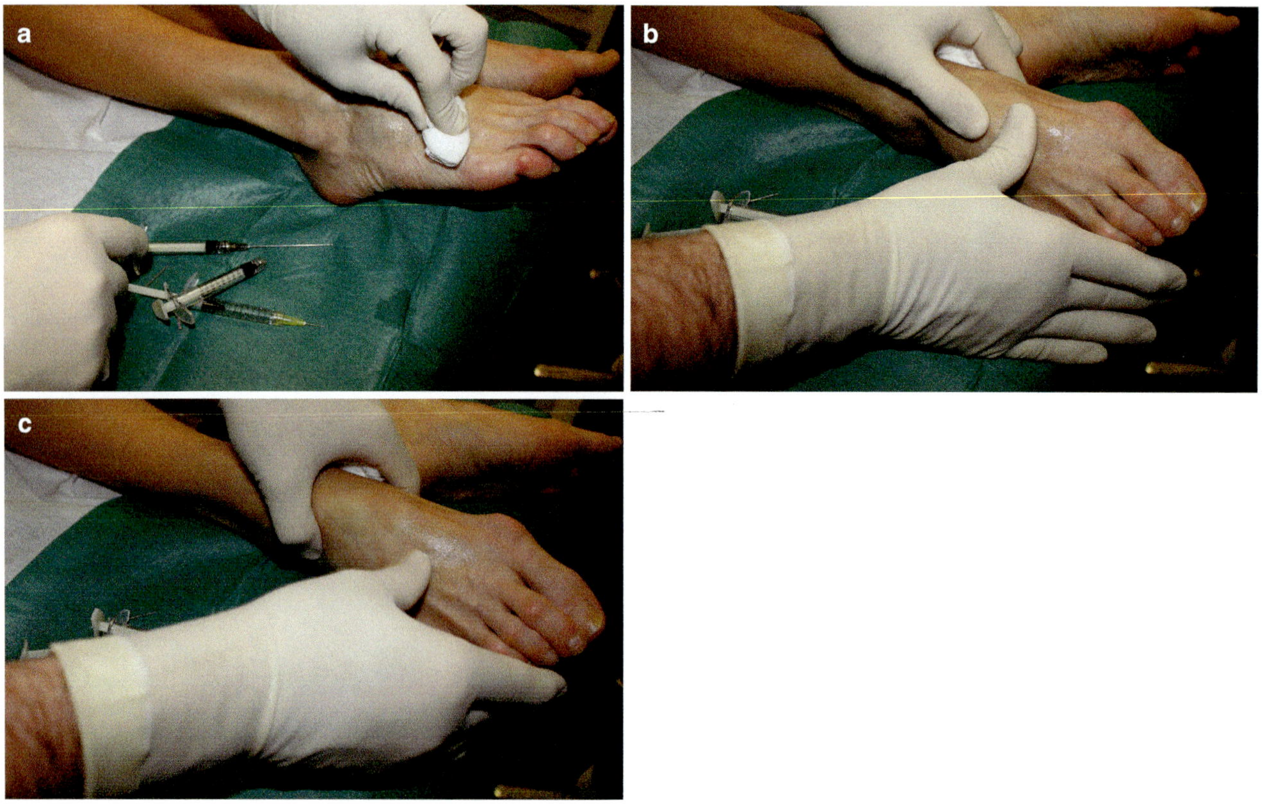

Fig. 28.8 (**a**–**c**) After the injection, a strong massage is applied to the dorsum of the foot. A wet bandage can make it easier to spread the fat evenly. (Published by kind permission of ©Mario Goisis 2018. All Rights Reserved)

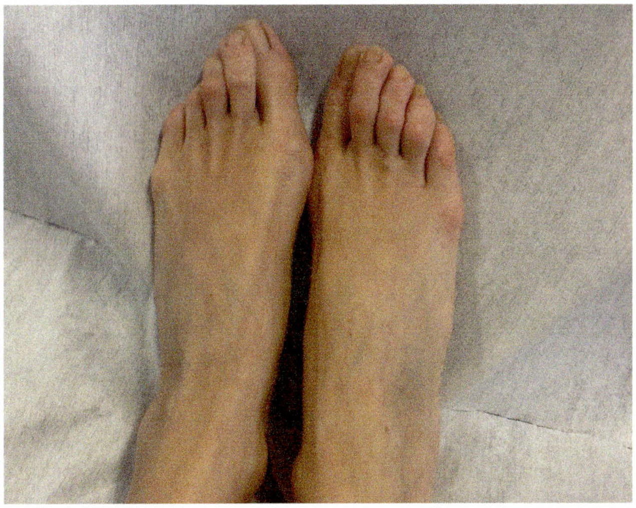

Fig. 28.9 The foot immediately after the treatment. (Published by kind permission of ©Mario Goisis 2018. All Rights Reserved)

Hair and Scalp

29

Margo Gkini, Mario Goisis, and Sara Izzo

29.1 PRP and Androgenic Alopecia

Platelet-rich plasma (PRP) has attracted significant attention in the fields of tissue engineering, wound healing, and angiogenesis over the last decades [1–2]. The regenerative potential of PRP depends on the growth factors (GFs) that are released upon activation of the platelets, which appear to enhance angiogenesis, extracellular matrix remodelling, and cellular effects like cell proliferation and differentiation [1, 3–5]. In 2006, Uebel et al. used PRP during hair transplantation in male patients with androgenetic alopecia [3, 6–8]. After that, further trials followed, evaluating the efficacy of PRP in androgenetic alopecia in both men and women.

29.2 Growth Factors

The main growth factors (GFs) involved in androgenetic alopecia are platelet-derived growth factors (PDGF), transforming growth factors (TGF),vascular endothelial growth factors (VEGF), and insulin-like growth factors (IGF) along with their isoforms [9–12]. After binding with their respective receptors in the bulge area of hair follicle, the GFs trigger interaction between them and different types of cells. In detail, in the bulge area, primitive stem-cells derived from ectoderm which differentiate into epidermis and sebaceous gland cells are found. In the matrix, germinative cells of mesenchymal origin are found in the dermal papilla. These two kinds of cells, along with growth factors, interact and activate the proliferative phase of hair growth, giving rise to the future follicular unit [6].

Various types of cells, such as endothelial cells and keratinocytes, produce PDGF, which is fundamental for cell growth and proliferation. In vitro, cytokines, which are proven to be positive and negative regulators of HF growth activity, modify the expression of PDGF isoforms in HFs [13]. Furthermore, PDGF induces and maintains the anagen phase in mouse hair cycling [14]. PDGF signals are involved in both the epidermis-follicle and dermal-mesenchymal interaction required for hair-canal formation [15].

Androgen-inducible TGF-b1 from balding DP cells is an inhibitory paracrine mediator in androgenetic alopecia. Therefore, it has been established that the progression of androgenetic alopecia (AGA) is associated with androgen and TGF-b1 levels. Vascular endothelial growth factors appear to be a major mediator of HF growth and cycling, providing direct evidence that improved follicle revascularisation promotes hair growth.

Insulin-like growth factor 1 (IGF-I) also appears to play a critical role in promoting hair growth. IGF-I, produced by DP cells, acts on the IGF-I receptor of keratinocytes, promoting hair growth through stimulation of the proliferation of keratinocytes in HFs. In several reports, IGF-I and IGF-II prevented the HF from obtaining catagen-like status, and Sheong et al. showed that IGF-I has a significant effect on the rate of linear hair growth and extends the overall anagen phase [5].

29.3 Androgenetic Alopecia

Androgenetic alopecia is a common chronic hair-loss disorder, affecting both sexes. Its prevalence increases with age, despite the fact that it may start during puberty. Irrespective of age and gender, hair loss leads to a significant impairment of quality of life in patients diagnosed with androgenetic alopecia, as hair is an important feature of image, charm, and self-confidence. Although androgenetic alopecia is a burden for both males and females, it is more distressing for women. Numerous products have been

M. Gkini
Doctor's Equipe, Milan, Italy

M. Goisis (✉)
Maxillo-Facial and Aesthetic Surgeon, Go Easy Clinic, Milan, Italy

S. Izzo
Department of Plastic Surgery, University of Campania "Luigi Vanvitelli", Naples, Italy

M. Goisis (ed.), *Outpatient Regenerative Medicine*, https://doi.org/10.1007/978-3-319-44894-7_29

proposed and used as hair loss therapies. Drug therapies, approved by the Food and Drug Administration (FDA), for treating AGA include minoxidil and finasteride. Both can be used alone or in combination [16]. Despite the therapeutic options available, low levels of patient satisfaction and compliance with treatment as well as the numerous adverse effects, have made the need for research in the field of new AGA new treatment urgent [16, 17].

29.4 Treatment using PRP

Since PRP might serve as a potential treatment for AGA, a protocol using PRP injections, with encouraging results, is proposed here.

29.5 Selection of Patients and Diagnosis

Patients with early stages of alopecia according to the Norwood-Hamilton scale for men and the Ludwig scale for women, are perfect candidates for treatement using PRP. Patients with present or a history of immunosuppression (malignancy, chemotherapy, steroid therapy), dermatological diseases affecting the scalp, autoimmune disorders, haematologic disorders, and the platelet-dysfunction syndrome should be excluded. PRP, due to the fact that it is autologous, may cause an autoimmune reaction in patients with autoimmunity. Nevertheless, it has been proposed as a treatment for alopecia areata with encouraging results. Other exclusion criteria include a tendency towards keloids and anticoagulation treatment. If the patient is taking aspirin or other nonsteroidal anti-inflammatory drugs, he/she is advised to suspend this kind of medication for 7 days before treatment [17].

Diagnosis of androgenetic alopecia in all patients should be based on a detailed medical history (any drugs causing hair loss), a thorough clinical examination, laboratory tests, and trichoscopy. The laboratory tests should include (a) CBC; (b) serum iron, serum ferritin, and TIBC (total iron-binding capacity); (c) folic acid; (d) T3, T4, TSH, fT3, fT4, and anti-TPO; (e) VDRL; and (f), for women, a female hormone profile (DHEA, testosterone, androstenedione, prolactin, follicle-stimulating and luteinizing hormone) should be carried out [18, 19]. Trichoscopic criteria for the diagnosis of androgenetic alopecia include:

(a) Diversity of the diameter of hair, due to miniaturization of hair follicles. Variability of more than 20% in hair shaft diameter is one of the diagnostic indicators of this condition.
(b) Peripilar signs.
(c) Yellow dots.
(d) Predominance of single hairs in follicular ostia, instead of 2–3 hair shafts [19].

In case of differential diagnostic problems, a biopsy is advisaeble.

29.6 Preparation of PRP

According to international bibliography, platelet-rich plasma is produced using different methods for platelet concentration through centrifugation and cell separation. There are several commercially available systems. Differences are also observed in its activation media, with calcium chloride and calcium gluconate as the most common. As a result, different platelet and growth factor concentrations occur, hence leading to different outcomes during trials [5].

It is strongly recommended to use kits approved for the preparation of PRP. Manual preparation might not achieve the desired levels of platelets and might lead to poor, non-reproducible, and noncomparable results.

For the preparation of PRP, the RegenKit BCT-3 (RegenLab SA®, Le Mont-sur-Lausanne, Switzerland) may be used. Initially, whole blood is collected from the patient's antecubital vein (16 ml). The blood is then introduced into two tubes (Regen BCT) and centrifugated for 5 min at 1500 g using a RegenA-PRPCentri laboratory centrifuge. Each tube contains a thixotropic gel composed of a mixture of polymers for plasma separation (elimination of red blood-cells) and sodium citrate solution, as an anticoagulant, located above the separator gel. Therefore, after centrifugation, the blood is fractionated, with the red blood cells trapped under the gel and cellular elements settling on the surface of the gel. The content is resuspended by means of a series of gentle inversions of the tube. The total PRP yield of the is then loaded into 1-ml syringes, ready for injection. The activation process includes the addition of calcium gluconate in a 1:9 ratio (0.1 ml calcium gluconate per 0.9 ml of PRP) [17].

29.7 Application of PRP

Before applying the PRP, the scalp is cleansed using a 0.1% octenidine-hydrochloride spray. Local anaesthesia may be applied, if the patient feels pain that he/she is unable to handle. The PRP (0.05–0.1 ml/cm^2) is then injected, using a 27-G needle or 30.5-G, into the androgen-related areas (frontal, parietal, occipital) of the scalp in men and into the problematic areas in women, using BD-Luer-LokTM 1-ml syringes. The nappage technique may be performed [17]. On the basis of the experience of the authors, mesotherapy guns may also be used for greater accuracy in depth, less pain, and less waste of product (e.g., U-225®). The protocol includes three treatment sessions at intervals of 21–28 days. Six months the beginning of the treatment, a booster session should also be performed [17].

29.8 Results

After PRP application, hair loss decreases. An increase in average hair count, in mean hair diameter, and in hair density is also noticed. Improvement in hair volume and coverage may also occur as well as enhancement of hair quality, according to the subjective evaluation of patients [5].

Patient with androgenetic alopecia before treatment. The same patient at 3 months.

Many black dots may be noted.

29.9 Adverse Effects

Due to the autologous nature of PRP and its proper, careful preparation no significant adverse effects are noted, apart from mild pain during application and sensitivity of the scalp. There were no cases of infections, nodules, or cysts [5, 17].

29.10 Monotherapy-Combination Treatment

According to the authors, despite the encouraging results of PRP treatment in androgenetic alopecia, monotherapy is proposed during the early stages of alopecia or as a form of prevention. In cases where the disease progesses, the physician should use PRP as an effective treatment coadjuvant to conventional medication, such as minoxidil or finasteride. Its autologous nature, its regenerative potential, and the lack of adverse effects, constitute an excellent option for patients presenting with adverse effects due to other hair-loss therapies or women of the childbearing age.

29.11 Conclusion

Despite a growing interest in regenerative medicine, very few accounts of trials investigating the efficacy of PRP on hair growth have been published. Most of the studies reviewed presented some grave methodological deficiencies. The main flaws included lack of scientific approval of the devices used for the preparation of the PRP, lack of a reference protocol regarding the frequency of applications, as well as indications of the amount of PRP to be injected, heterogeneity in descriptions of modes of application, lack of controls, small-size sample groups, lack of detailed reports regarding the characteristics of patients, and the statistical methods a applied. Furthermore, very few studies referred to the safety measures to apply to PRP. Platelet-rich plasma may turn out, possibly, to be an asset useful to the treatment of androgenetic alopecia. Nevertheless, it is still a highly controversial form of therapy. Larger, randomised blind, controlled trials, with approved devices for the preparation of the PRP, are urgently needed, as well as evidence-based data regarding parameters indicating concentration and doses and their clinical efficacy. The protocol we present here is easy to apply and yields encouraging results as far as patients are concerned.

29.12 ADSC and Hair Growth

Several reports have pointed out that growth factors such as PDGF, HGF, VEGF, and fibronectin, increase hair growth in animal and clinical models [20–24].

To understand whether the paracrine effects of ADSCs may promote hair growth in humans, Won et al. investigated the effects of ADSCs on the proliferation of cultured human dermal papilla cells (hDPCs) [20]. Treatment with ADSCS significantly improved proliferation of hDPCs by up to 130% at 48 h. The animal study on nude mice established these results. In particular, histologically, the skin on the backs of ADSC-CM-treated mice showed augmented numbers of hair follicles. This study suggests that ADSCs promote hair growth (Figs. 29.1 and 29.2).

Recently, it was reported that treatment with ADSCs (ADSC-CM) media is effective for female pattern hair loss (FPHL). A retrospective, observational study of outcomes in 27 patients with FPHL treated with ADSC-CM was performed. The authors used microneedles to allow ASC-CM to penetrate the human skin. To assess the efficacy of the treatment, the patients' medical records and trichographic photographic images were analysed. ASC-CM proved its efficacy in treating FPHL after 12 weeks of therapy [25]. For example,

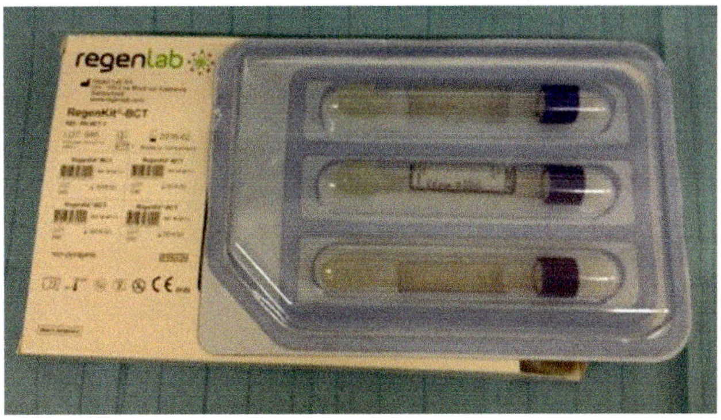

Fig. 29.1 The Regenlab kit. (Published by kind permission of ©Mario Goisis 2018. All Rights Reserved)

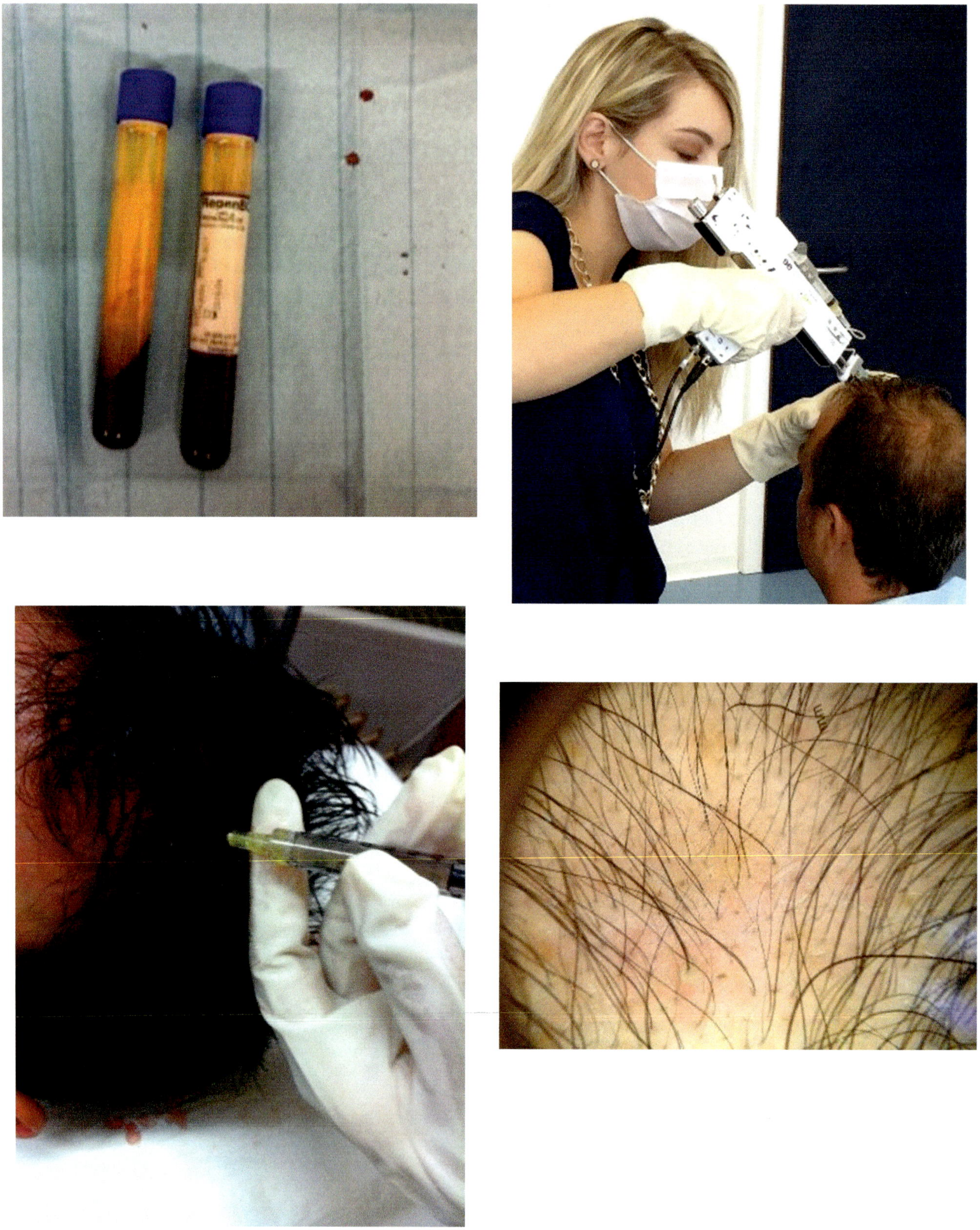

Fig. 29.2 Injection of ADSCs after separation by means of vibration (courtesy of www.microfat.com). (Published by kind permission of ©Mario Goisis 2018. All Rights Reserved)

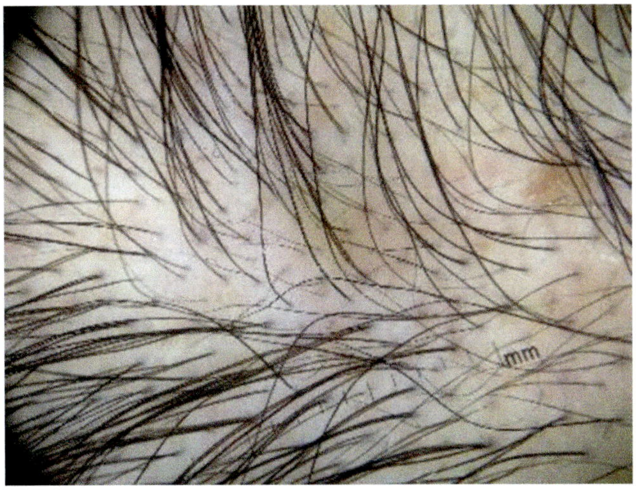

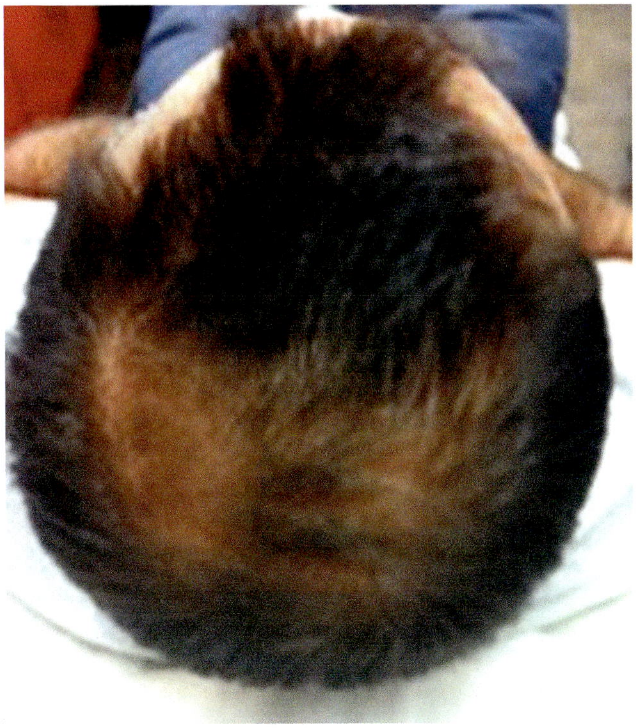

Before Treatment

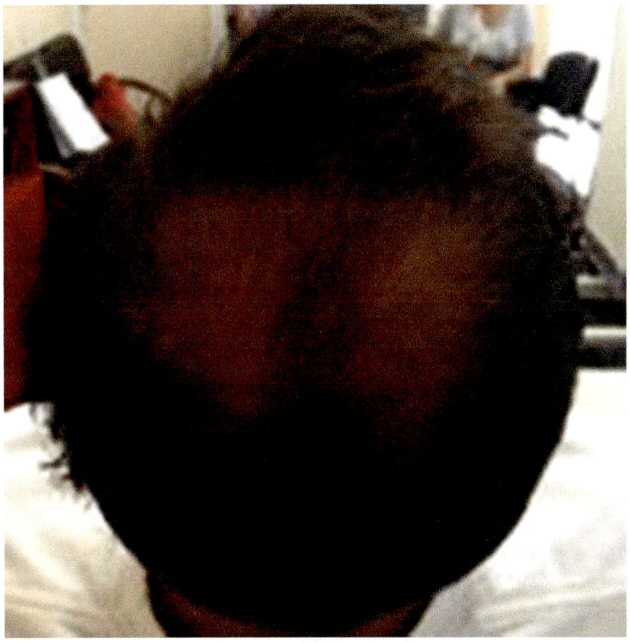

After Treatment

hair thickness and hair density improved significantly, and none of the patients reported adverse reactions.

Fukuoka and Suga also reported the effect of a product containing a protein solution of adipose-derived stem-cell-conditioned medium in hair regeneration. The product was injected intradermally in 22 cases of alopecia [26]. These patients received six treatment sessions every 3–5 weeks, and hair increased significantly in both male and female patients.

29.13 Hair Treatment with Dermal Graft

29.13.1 Indications

Hair loss. Because of dermatologists and trycologists are not allowed to harvest the fat in some countries for specific laws and regulations, a minimally invasive technique of dermal graft (www.dermalgraft.com) is described. Both the donor area, both the recipient area are the dermis. A minimal quantity of local anesthesia is injected: 32mg of lidocaine. In order to do a comparison, it is a similar quantity of lidocaine that the quantity injected with one dose of Ceftriaxone (usually 1gram of ceftriaxone is diluited in 3,5 ml of 1% Lidocaine Solution, which are 35mg of lidocaine).

29.13.2 Operating Time

The procedure usually takes 10 min.

29.13.3 Materials

- An Dermal graft kit (www.dermalgraft.com)
- A 27-G, 3 -cm-long needle
- 40 cc of Klein solution
- 100 cc of saline solution

29.13.4 Procedure

The procedure is illustrated in Figs. 29.3, 29.4, 29.5, 29.6a–c, and 29.7a–d below.

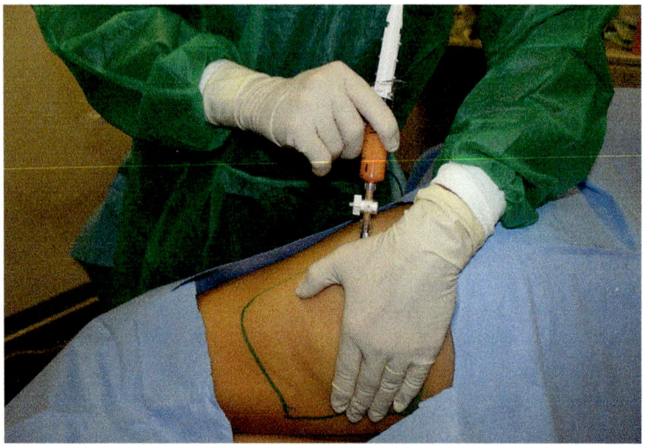

Fig. 29.3 The dermal graft is harvested using an dermal graft kit (www.dermal.bio). (Published by kind permission of ©Mario Goisis 2018. All Rights Reserved)

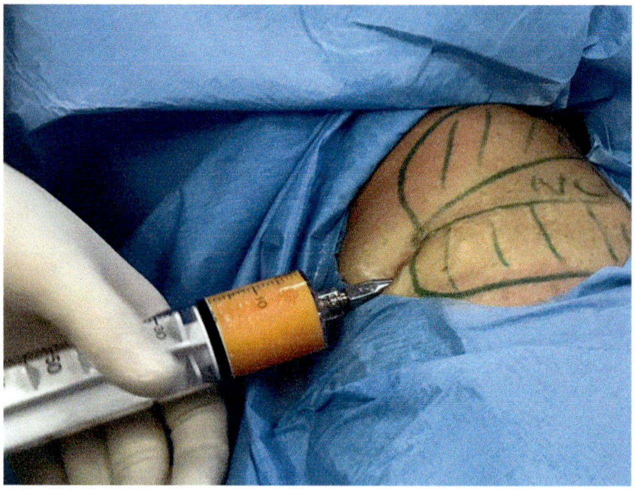

Fig. 29.4 A 60cc syringe is filled by dermal graft mixed with blood

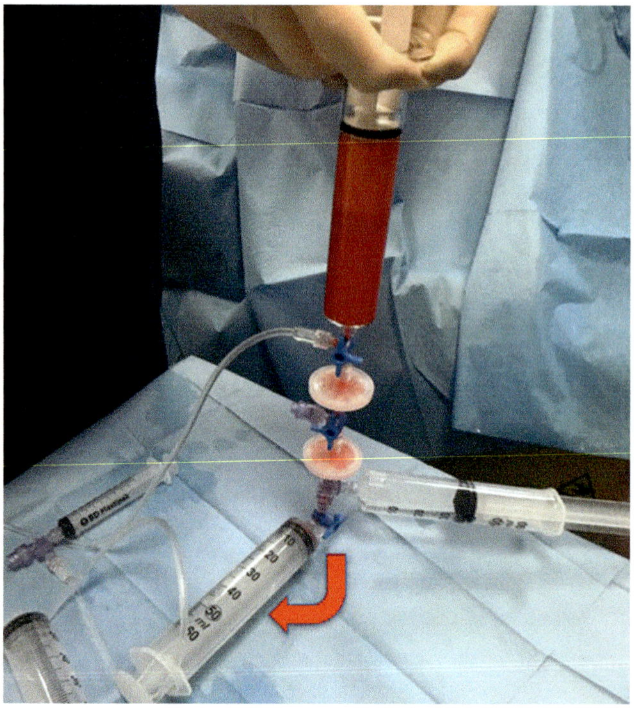

Fig. 29.5 The syringe containing the dermal graft is connected to the dermal system (www.dermal.bio). The system is composed by 2 filters. (Published by kind permission of ©Mario Goisis 2018. All Rights Reserved)

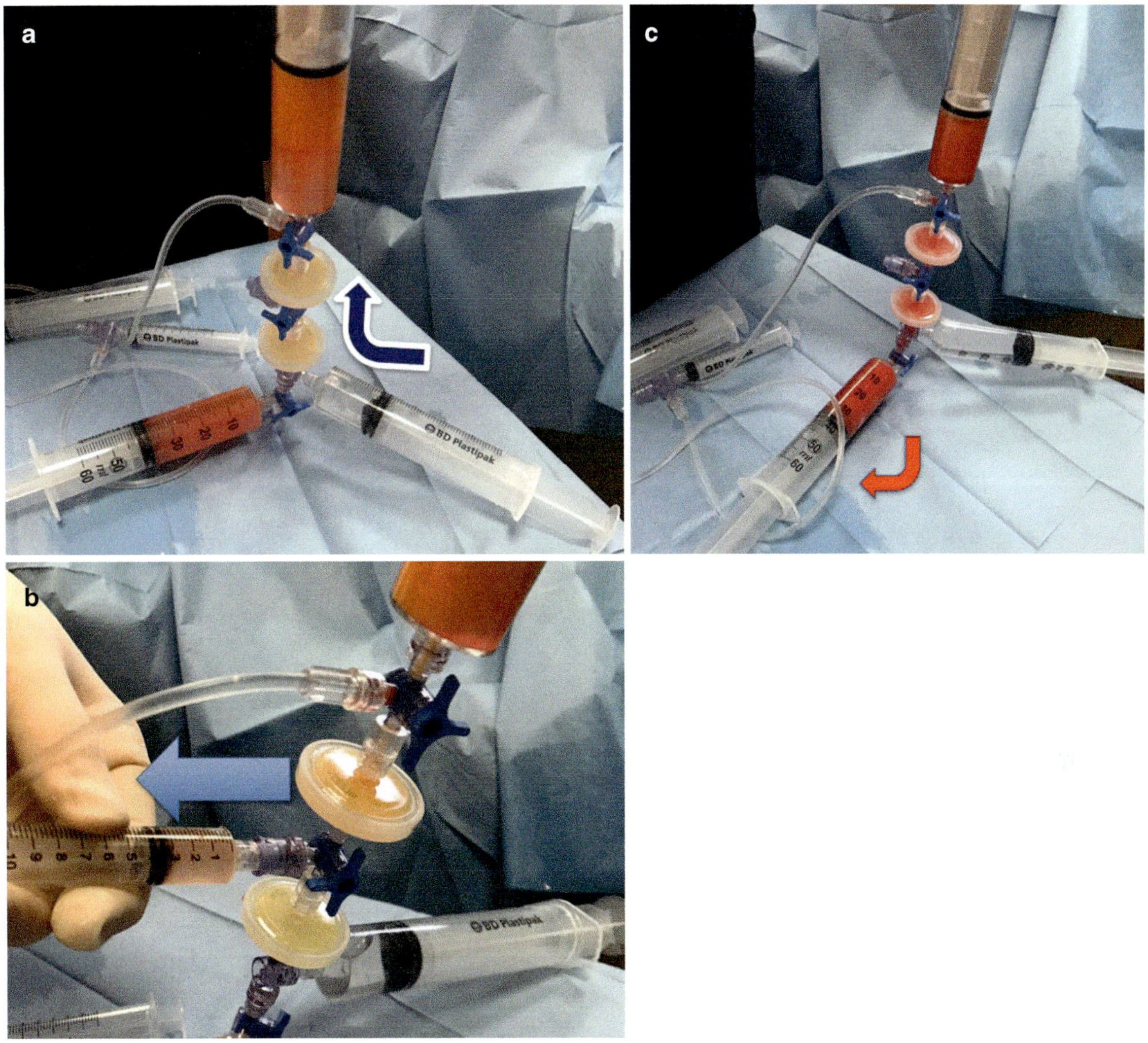

Fig. 29.6 (**a**) The plunger of the syringe is pushed, and the solution together with red cells is automatically filtered and transferred to the second syringe. (**b**) By pushing the plunger of the third syringe filled by saline solution, the content of the first syringe is automatically washed. (**c**) The dermal ultrafiltration is collected. (Published by kind permission of ©Mario Goisis 2018. All Rights Reserved)

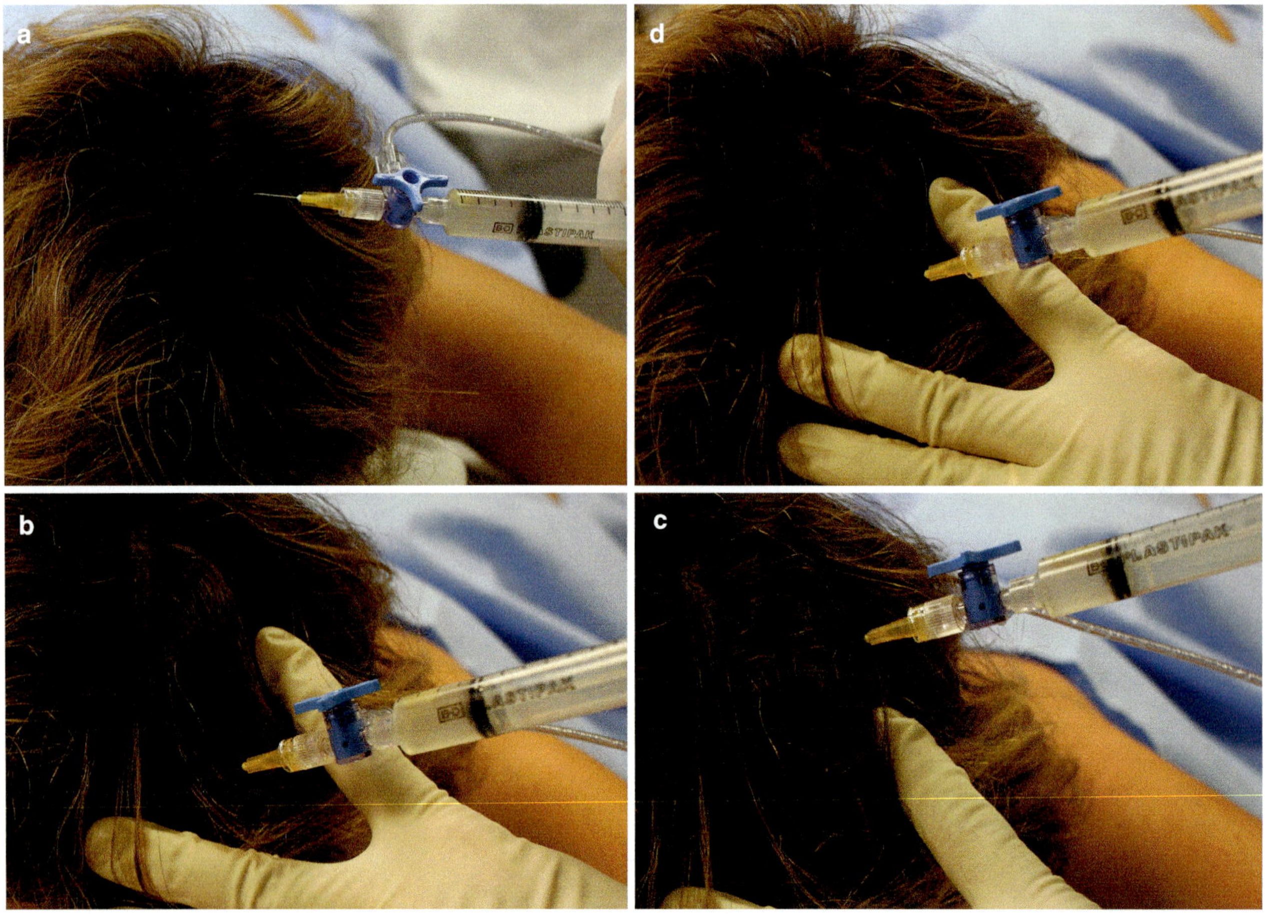

Fig. 29.7 (**a–d**) Ultrafiltration the solution is injected using a 27-G needle. The distance between the different points of injection is 2 cm. The volume injected at the entry-points is 0.2 cc. (Published by kind permission of ©Mario Goisis 2018. All Rights Reserved)

29.14 Hair Treatment with Dermal Nanofat

29.14.1 Materials

- 1–2 cc of nanofat on each side for injection of nanofat: replace with 1-2cc of nanofat for injection on both sides
  - *A 26-gauge needle*
  - *A 27-gauge 3.7 cm blunt cannula*

A standard system for producing nanofat is used, in particular:

- The Nanofat system (www.microfat.com), composed of a connector with a closed system for emulsion of the microfat and filtration
- 2 10-cc syringes

To harvest and process: the dermal graft

A standard system for dermal graft (www.dermal.bio)

- Close dermal graft system (www.dermal.bio)
- 3 syringes 60 cc
- 2 syringes 10 cc
- 1 syringe 1 cc
- 30-gauge needle
- 16-gauge needle
- A 2-mm diameter, 10-cm-long Goisis cannula for fat harvesting

Medications include:

- 100 cc of cold saline solution.
- 40 cc of cold Klein solution.
- One litre of Klein solution is composed of 800 mg of lidocaine, 1 mg of epinephrine, 40 MEq of sodium bicarbonate, and 1000 cc of saline solution.

Location: The dermal graft harvesting can be carried out in a small operating theatre/medical surgery. Oxygen, pulse oximetry, and a crash cart/box should be present.

Assistants: An assistant is useful for the transfer of items to the procedure field in a sterile manner during the first part of the procedure. Despite this, a single doctor may carry out the entire procedure alone.

The procedure is described in photos below (Figs. 29.8, 29.9, 29.10a–c, 29.11, 29.12a, b, 29.13, 29.14, and 29.15).

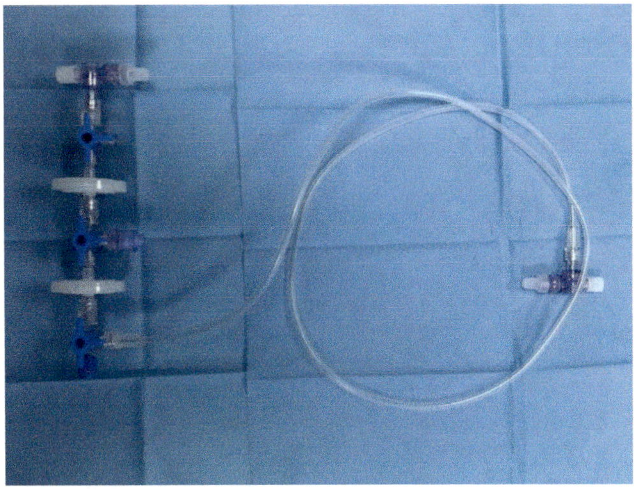

Fig. 29.8 5 cc of microfat are produced using the dermal graft system (www.dermal.bio). (Published by kind permission of ©Mario Goisis 2018. All Rights Reserved)

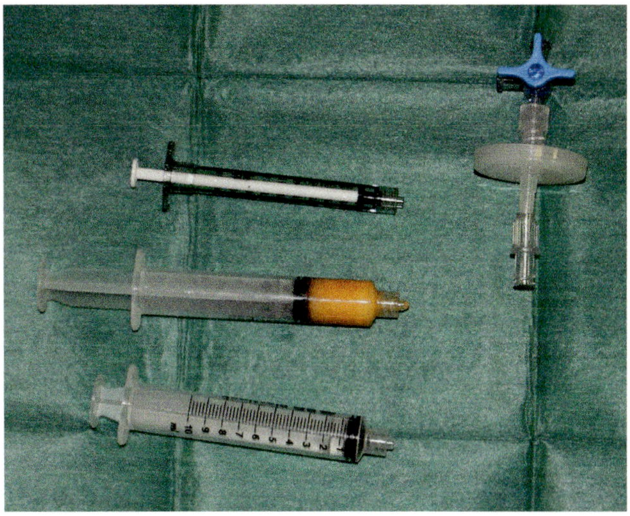

Fig. 29.9 The DE nanofat kit. (Published by kind permission of ©Mario Goisis 2018. All Rights Reserved)

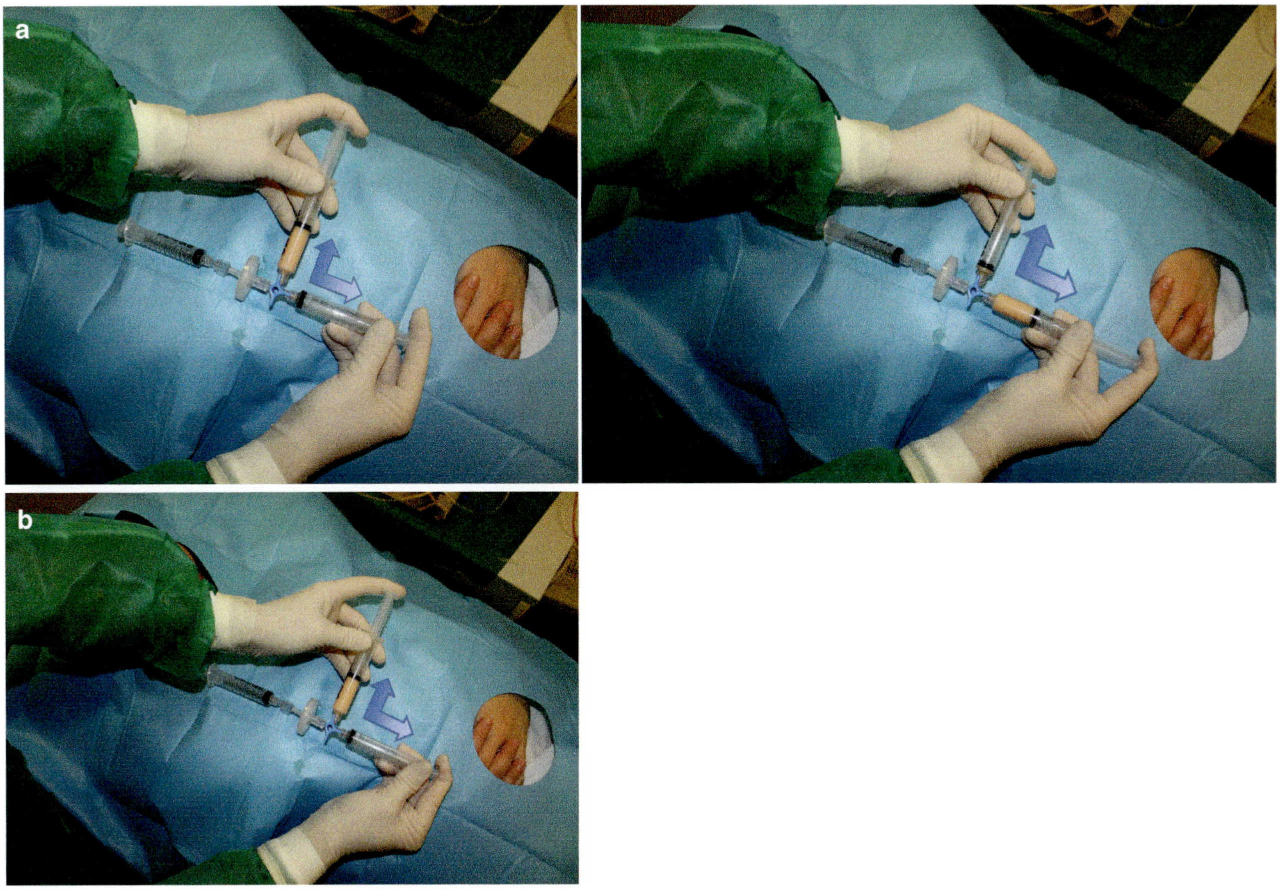

Fig. 29.10 (**a–c**) Three 10-cc syringes are connected to the kit. The fat is moved rapidly between the 2 syringes 30 times. (Published by kind permission of ©Mario Goisis 2018. All Rights Reserved)

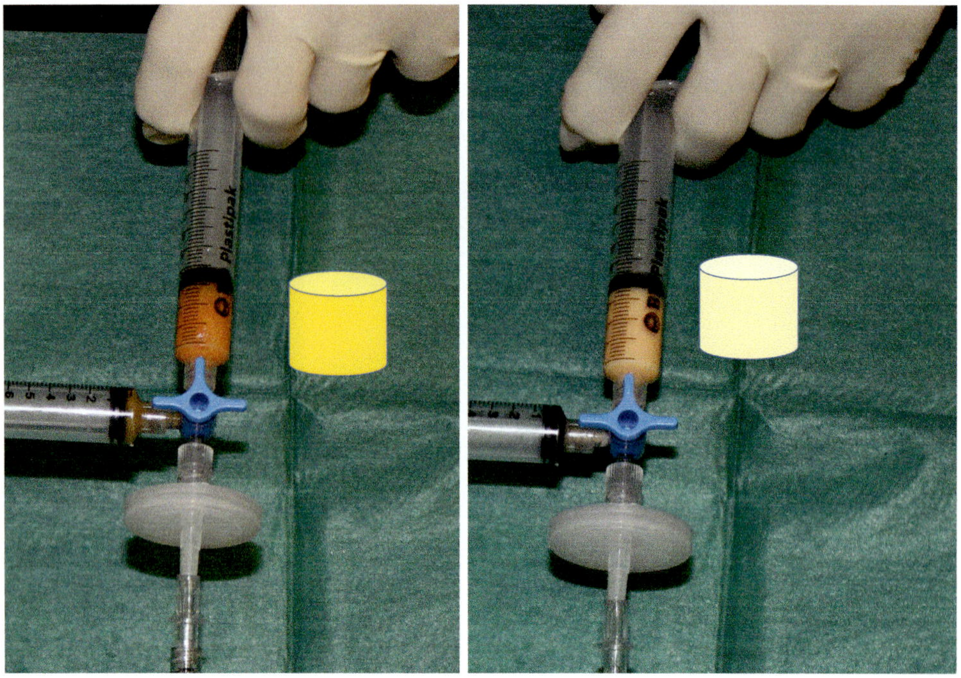

Fig. 29.11 The microfat is yellow in colour. After 30 passages, it is transformed in nanofat, which is whitish. (Published by kind permission of ©Mario Goisis 2018. All Rights Reserved)

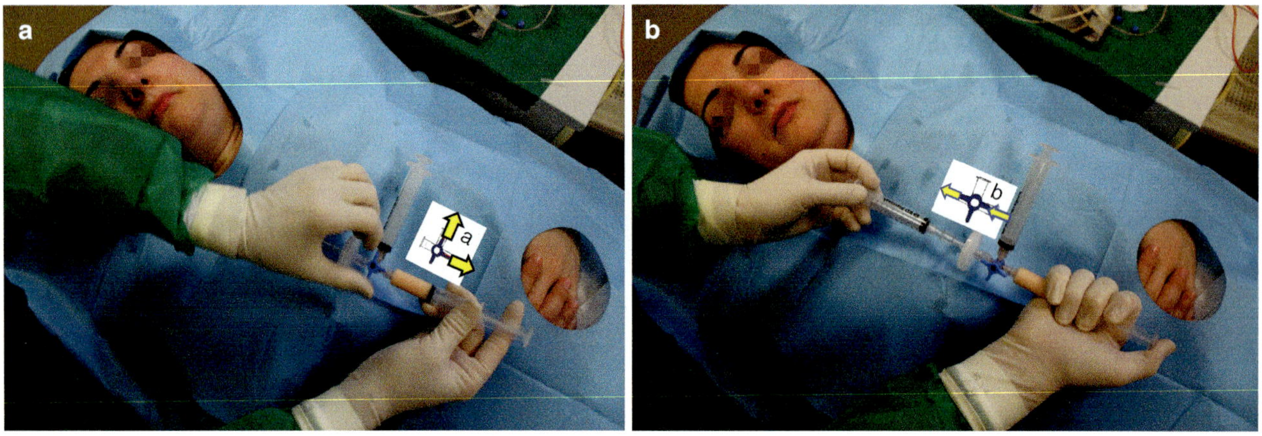

Fig. 29.12 (**a, b**) The stopcock is moved from position "a" to position "b". (Published by kind permission of ©Mario Goisis 2018. All Rights Reserved)

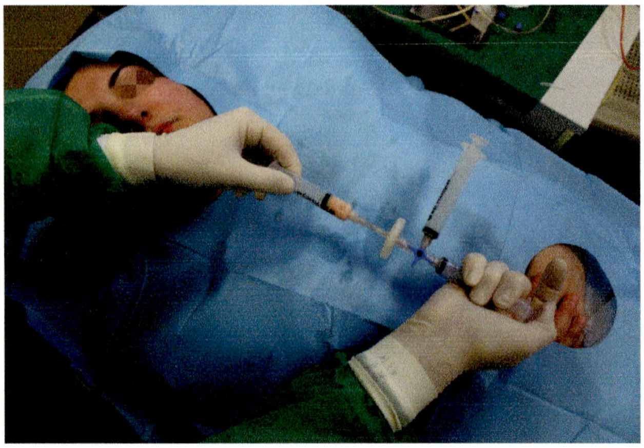

Fig. 29.13 In this way, the fat is filtered and directly transferred in the third syringe. (Published by kind permission of ©Mario Goisis 2018. All Rights Reserved)

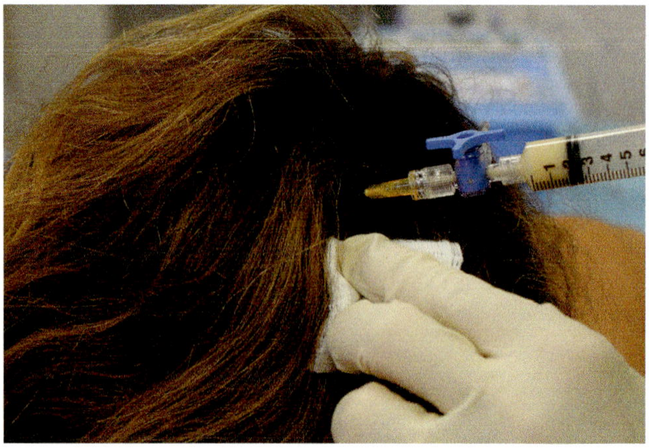

Fig. 29.14 Because of filtration, the fat can be injected directly using a 27-G needle. (Published by kind permission of ©Mario Goisis 2018. All Rights Reserved)

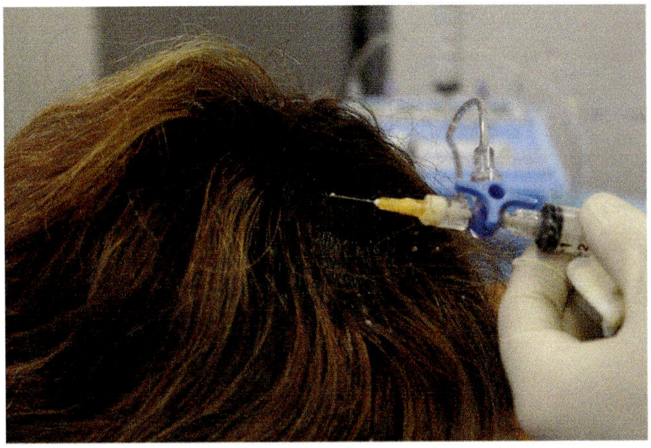

Fig. 29.15 The distance between the different points of injection is 2 cm. The volume injected at the entry-points is 0.2 cc. (Published by kind permission of ©Mario Goisis 2018. All Rights Reserved)

References

1. Arora NS, Ramanayake T, Ren YF, Romanos GE. Platelet-rich plasma: a literature review. Implant Dent. 2009 Aug;18(4):303–10.
2. Marx RE. Platelet-rich plasma: evidence to support its use. J Oral Maxillofac Surg. 2004;62:489–96.
3. Eppley BL, Woodell JE, Higgins J. Platelet quantification and growth factor analysis from platelet-rich plasma: implications for wound healing. Plast Reconstr Surg. 2004;114:1502–8.
4. Weibrich G, Kleis WK, Hafner G, Hitzler WE. Growth factor levels in platelet-rich plasma and correlations with donor age, sex, and platelet count. J Craniomaxillofac Surg. 2002;30:97–102.
5. Gkini MA, Kouskoukis AE, Rigopoulos D, Kouskoukis K. Platelet-rich plasma as a potential treatment for noncicatricial alopecias. Int J Trichology. 2015;7(2):54–63.
6. Uebel CO, da Silva JB, Cantarelli D, Martins P. The role of platelet plasma growth factors in male pattern baldness surgery. Plast Reconstr Surg. 2006;118:1458–66.
7. Marx RE. Platelet-rich plasma (PRP): what is PRP and what is not PRP? Implant Dent. 2001;10:225–8.
8. Rodrigues SV, Acharya AB, Thakur SL. Platelet-rich plasma. A review. N Y State Dent J. 2012;78(1):26–30.
9. Sánchez-González DJ, Méndez-Bolaina E, Trejo-Bahena NI. Platelet-rich plasma peptides: key for regeneration. Int J Pept. 2012;2012:532519.
10. Su HY, Hickford JG, The PH, Hill AM, Frampton CM, Bickerstaffe R. Increased vibrissa growth in transgenic mice expressing insulin-like growth factor 1. J Invest Dermatol. 1999;112:245–8.
11. Tavakkol A, Elder JT, Griffiths CE, Cooper KD, Talwar H, Fisher GJ, Keane KM, Foltin SK, Voorhees JJ. Expression of growth hormone receptor, insulin-like growth factor 1 (IGF-1) and IGF-1 receptor mRNA and proteins in human skin. J Invest Dermatol. 1992;99(3):343–9.
12. Arshdeep, Kumaran MS. Platelet-rich plasma in dermatology: boon or a bane? Indian J Dermatol Venereol Leprol. 2014;80:5–14.
13. Kamp H, Geilen CC, Sommer C, Blume-Peytavi U. Regulation of PDGF and PDGF receptor in cultured dermal papilla cells and follicular keratinocytes of the human hair follicle. Exp Dermatol. 2003;12:662–72.
14. Tomita Y, Akiyama M, Shimizu H. PDGF isoforms induce and maintain anagen phase of murine hair follicles. J Dermatol Sci. 2006;43:105–15.
15. Takakura N, Yoshida H, Kunisada T, Nishikawa S, Nishikawa SI. Involvement of platelet-derived growth factor receptor-alpha in hair canal formation. J Invest Dermatol. 1996;107:770–7.
16. Blumeyer A, Tosti A, Messenger A, Reygagne P, Del Marmol V, Spuls PI, Trakatelli M, Finner A, Kiesewetter F, Trüeb R, Rzany B, Blume-Peytavi U, European Dermatology Forum (EDF). Evidence-based (S3) guideline for the treatment of androgenetic alopecia in women and in men. J Dtsch Dermatol Ges. 2011;9(Suppl 6):S1–57.
17. Gkini MA, Kouskoukis AE, Tripsianis G, Rigopoulos D, Kouskoukis K. Study of platelet-rich plasma injections in the treatment of androgenetic alopecia through an one-year period. J Cutan Aesthet Surg. 2014;7(4):213–9.
18. Mubki T, Rudnicka L, Olszewska M, Shapiro J. Evaluation and diagnosis of the hair loss patient: part I. History and clinical examination. J Am Acad Dermatol. 2014;71(3):415.e1–415.e15.
19. Mubki T, Rudnicka L, Olszewska M, Shapiro J. Evaluation and diagnosis of the hair loss patient: part II. Trichoscopic and laboratory evaluations. J Am Acad Dermatol. 2014;71(3):431.e1–431.e11.
20. Won C. Hair growth promoting effects of adipose tissue-derived stem cells. J Dermatol Sci. 2010;57:132–46.
21. Danilenko DM, Ring BD, Pierce GF. Growth factors and cytokines in hair follicle development and cycling: recent insights from animal models and the potentials for clinical therapy. Mol Med Today. 1996;2:460–7.
22. Limat A, Hunziker T, Waelti ER, Inaebnit SP, Wiesmann U, Braathen LR. Soluble factors from human hair papilla cells and dermal fibroblasts dramatically increase the clonal growth of outer root sheath cells. Arch Dermatol Res. 1993;285:205–10.
23. Kim WS, Park BS, Kim HK, Park JS, Kim KJ, Choi JS, et al. Evidence supporting antioxidant action of adipose-derived stem cells: protection of human dermal fibroblasts from oxidative stress. J Dermatol Sci. 2008;49:133–42.
24. Park BS, Jang KA, Sung JH, Park JS, Kwon YH, Kim KJ, et al. Adipose-derived stem cells and their secretory factors as a promising therapy for skin aging. Dermatol Surg. 2008;34:1323.
25. Shin H, Ryu HH, Kwon O, Park BS, Jo SJ. Clinical use of conditioned media of adipose tissue-derived stem cells in female pattern hair loss: a retrospective case series study. Int J Dermatol. 2015;54(6):730–5.
26. Fukuoka H, Suga H. Hair regeneration treatment using adipose-derived stem cell conditioned medium: follow-up with trichograms. Eplasty. 2015;15:e10.
27. Li ZJ, Choi HI, Choi DK, Sohn KC, Im M, Seo YJ, Lee YH, Lee JH, Lee Y. Autologous platelet-rich plasma: a potential therapeutic tool for promoting hair growth. Dermatol Surg. 2012;38(7 Pt 1):1040–6.

Combined Regenerative and Aesthetic Medicine

30

Mario Goisis and Sara Izzo

The gold standard treatment for correction of many of the aesthetic flaws caused by ageing has been described in this book in terms of the many procedures involved in regenerative treatments. However, as there is a growing interest in a wide range of nonablative interventions that claim being able to rejuvenate skin "safely and successfully" some nonablative treatments such as radio frequency, shock waves, and focused ultrasounds seen as as excellent complements to regenerative medicine, are also dealt with here.

30.1 Radio Frequency for Nonablative Skin Rejuvenation

Facial, neck, or body laxity are some of the major aspects of ageing. Bipolar and monopolar radio frequencies have been used to tighten, by heating, the deep dermis without ablating the skin [1, 2] (Fig. 30.1).

The net result of this is a noninvasive brow lift, face-lift, or neck lift. This modality does not replace current medical regenerative procedures but is an excellent supplement to the and a therapeutic option for patients to consider.

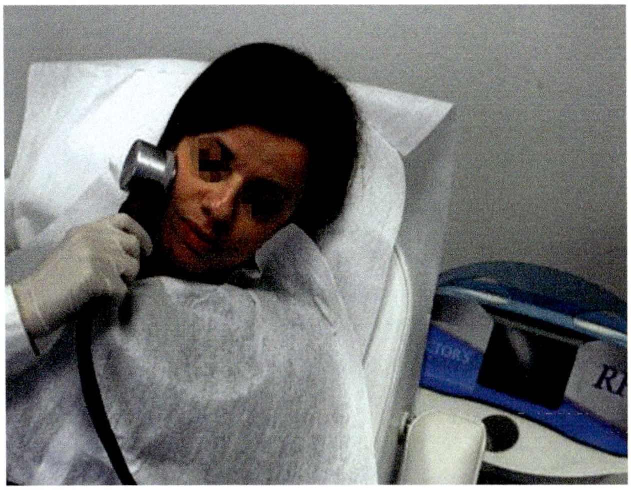

Fig. 30.1 Application of radio frequency to the face (by courtesy of "Injection in aesthetic medicine", Springer). (Published by kind permission of ©Mario Goisis 2018. All Rights Reserved)

30.2 Acoustic Waves

Acoustic waves (AWs) have been used in medicine since 1993 for the treatment of orthopaedic diseases such as disorders of tendons and muscles.

In regenerative medicine as AWs increase blood circulation in the tissue survival of grafts should be significantly enhanced when they are used (Fig. 30.2a, b, and c).

For this reason, AWs represent a noninvasive, easy-to-handle, side-effect-free coadjuvant to filler-injection treatment [3–5].

30.3 Microfocused Ultrasound System (Ulthera)

The Ulthera system uses microfocused ultrasound to cause focal heating of the dermis and stimulate neocollagenesis and elastin remodelling (Figs. 30.3, 30.4, and 30.5).

Goisis and Guareschi have investigated amelioration in terms of tightening and lifting of the malar area and of cheek tissue, and improvement in the definition of the jawline, in patients treated using this system with and without microfat and nanofat injection [6].

A total of 87 adults were enrolled in this prospective nonrandomised clinical trial. Fifty-two of these patients, treatment were treated using the system on the same day/in the

M. Goisis (✉)
Maxillo-Facial and Aesthetic Surgeon, Go Easy Clinic, Milan, Italy

S. Izzo
Department of Plastic Surgery, University of Campania "Luigi Vanvitelli", Naples, Italy

M. Goisis (ed.), *Outpatient Regenerative Medicine*, https://doi.org/10.1007/978-3-319-44894-7_30

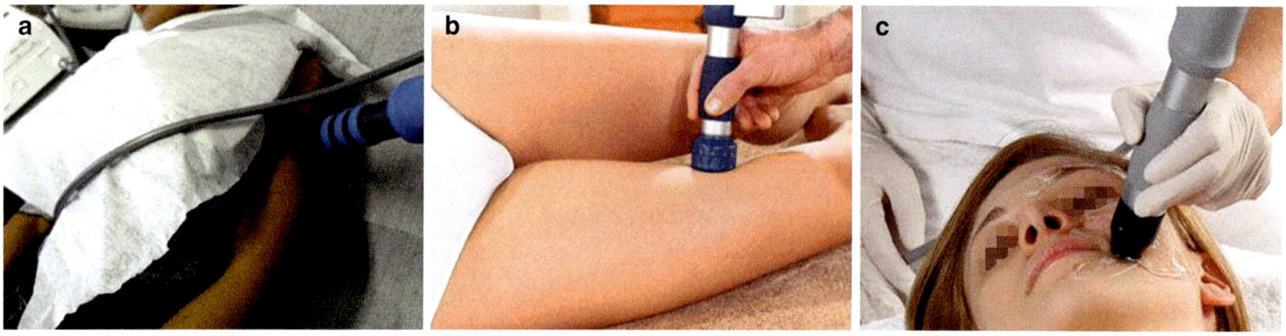

Fig. 30.2 Application of acoustic waves to the arm (**a**), leg (**b**), and face (**c**) (courtesy of Springer, "Injection in aesthetic medicine"). (Published by kind permission of ©Mario Goisis 2018. All Rights Reserved)

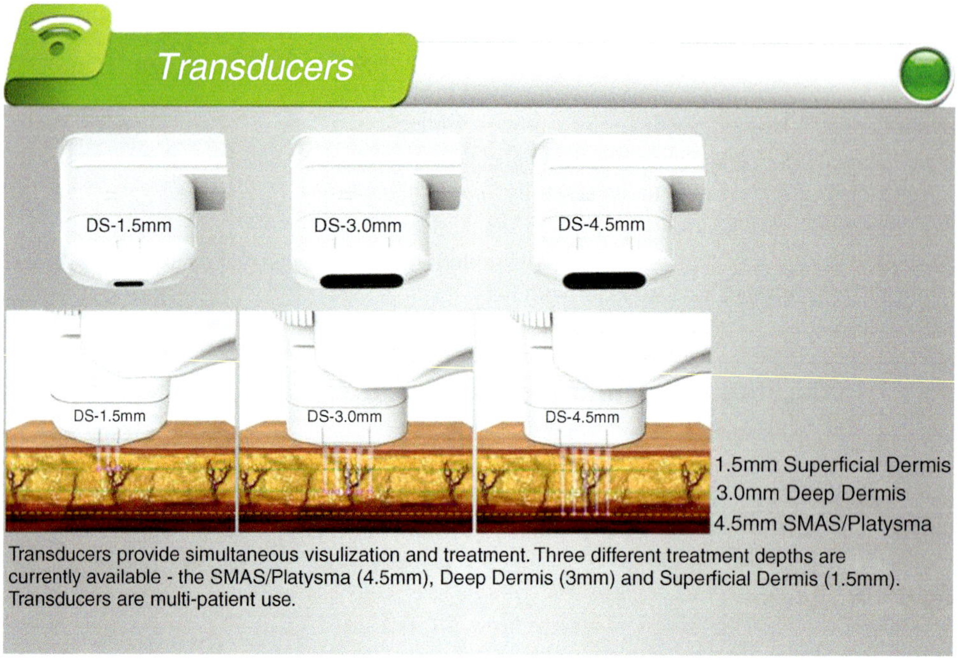

Fig. 30.3 The Ulthera system (courtesy of the Merz Company). (Published by kind permission of ©Mario Goisis 2018. All Rights Reserved)

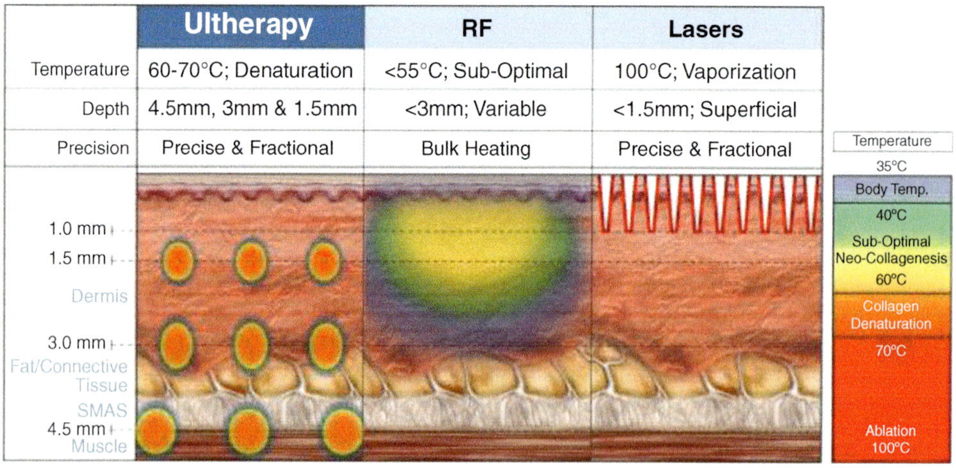

Fig. 30.4 The Ulthera system (courtesy of the Merz Company). (Published by kind permission of ©Mario Goisis 2018. All Rights Reserved)

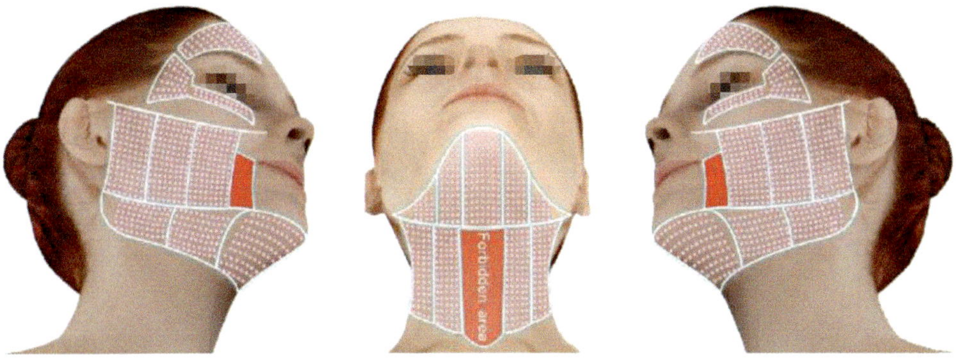

Fig. 30.5 The Ulthera system (courtesy of the Merz Company). (Published by kind permission of ©Mario Goisis 2018. All Rights Reserved)

same month as that of the microfat and nanofat treatment. Thirty-five patients were treated using the system only. Of these patients, 86 Canfield photographs obtained at baseline and at 3 and 12 months after treatment were assessed qualitatively by 3 blinded reviewers. One patient did not turn up for the follow-up. The adverse events of the case were documented.

Eighty-six patients were evaluated. At day 90, blinded reviewers observed improvement in skin laxity in 62% of patients to whom the system only was applied and 91% of the patients who were treated using the system plus microfat and nanofat injection. At 1 year, improvement in skin laxity was observed in 53% of the patients who had used the system only and 94% of the patients who system (one treatment) plus microfat and nanofat treatments (treatment plus touch up).

At days 90 and 120, improvements were reported by the majority of the blinded reviewers. The outcomes were better in the patients who availed themselves of the system plus microfat and nanofat treatment.

References

1. Koch RJ. Radiofrequency nonablative tissue tightening. Facial Plast Surg Clin North Am. 2004;12(3):339–46.
2. Dierickx CCJ. The role of deep heating for noninvasive skin rejuvenation. Lasers Surg Med. 2006;38(9):799–807.
3. Siems W, Grune T, Voss P, Brenke R. Anti-fibrosclerotic effects of shock wave therapy in lipedema and cellulite. Biofactors. 2005;24(1-4):275–82.
4. Adatto MA, Adatto-Neilson R, Novak P, Krotz A, Haller G. Body shaping with acoustic wave therapy AWT(®)/EPAT(®): randomized, controlled study on 14 subjects. J Cosmet Laser Ther. 2011;13(6):291–6.
5. Goisis M, Guareschi M. Combined protocol of acoustic waves plus microfat: preliminary results. IMCAS Congress, Paris, 2016.
6. Goisis M, Guareschi M. Combined treatment of focused ultrasound plus microfat: preliminary results. IMCAS Congress, Paris, 2017.

31 Combination of Regenerative Medicine and Surgery: Fibrin Sealants

Michele Pascali, Davide Quarato, Marco Pagnoni, and Mario Goisis

31.1 Introduction

In blepharoplasty and facelift procedures, different methods may be used to reduce postoperative complications and the need for draining, including the use of complete haemostatic, quilting sutures, heterologous glue, compressive dressing, and tissue sealants. Different types of surgical adhesives have emerged as alternatives capable of fixing and guaranteeing adhesion of tissue. Among these, biological sealants (or fibrin sealants) are produced by recurring to a combination of material from a pool of known donors and bovine thrombin, whereas platelet-rich plasma (PRP) glue is an autologous preparation obtained from the patient's own blood, and which acts as a growth-factor reservoir during treatment.

Platelets are key factors in hard and soft tissue repair-mechanisms. They provide essential growth factors, such as FGF, PDGF, TGF-ß, EGF, and VEGF, which are involved in stem-cell migration, differentiation, and proliferation. They also stimulate fibroblasts and endothelial cells to induce, respectively, new extracellular matrix deposition and neovascularisation. The platelets are concentrates obtained from the patient's own blood plasma. Plasma contains many factors essential for cell survival including nutrients, vitamins, hormones, electrolytes, growth factors such as IGF and HGF, and proteins. The proteins of plasma contain molecules vital for the coagulation process and the generation of the fibrin polymer that serve as a scaffold for cell migration and the generation of new tissue.

Studies investigating the use of PRP in plastic-surgery treatment reveal more rapid restoration of damaged tissues and also a decrease in inflammation and pain. Therefore, the significant enrichment in terms of locally-acting growth factors plays an essential role in cell differentiation and tissue regeneration.

M. Pascali · D. Quarato · M. Pagnoni
Doctor's Equipe, Milan, Italy

M. Goisis (✉)
Maxillo-Facial and Aesthetic Surgeon, Go Easy Clinic, Milan, Italy

Depending on clinical indications, PRP may be either injected in liquid form or applied as a gel (PRP glue). When injected as a gel, PRP needs to be mixed with a gelation inducer immediately before application on the site to be treated. Autologous thrombin serum (ATS) converts soluble fibrinogen into fibrin monomers, which polymerize to form a clot. Addition to the patient's platelet concentrate of autologous thrombin serum (ATS) restarts the coagulation process in a physiological manner. This natural process induces the formation of tri-dimensional fibrin matrix where the platelets become entrapped. This permits a delivery of long-lasting growth factor at the treatment site, and the matrix serves as a scaffold for the construction of new tissue.

Various studies have reported the positive effects of the application of PRP glue in many different clinical fields, especially in orthopaedic, oral and maxillofacial surgery. PRP glue has several potential advantages when it comes to improving the outcome of facelift surgery. The use of PRP glue hinders the formation of hematomas and seromas considerably, permitting faster recovery and return to daily activities, thus leading to higher postoperative patient satisfaction. Haematoma remains the most common complication in rhytidectomy, occurring in 0.3–15% of all cases. It can lead to tissue ischemia and necrosis of the skin, infection, prolonged facial oedema, hyperpigmentation, scar retraction, and the need for further surgery to evacuate and drain the haematoma and/or correct its consequences, the result being decreased patient satisfaction. Furthermore, addition of PRP glue has eliminated the routine use of draining in the majority of cases. Draining is expensive, cumbersome, occlusive and time-consuming when it comes to positioning and removal and may be annoying for patients, so it is reasonable to seek to eliminate them.

Moreover, the cost of the autologous PRP glue obtained with the RegenKit A-PRP Plus is significantly lower than that of industrial glue. Finally, the cost of autologous glue is less than the total cost of the treatment of postoperative complications, including second surgery to drain the haematoma or

M. Goisis (ed.), *Outpatient Regenerative Medicine*, https://doi.org/10.1007/978-3-319-44894-7_31

seroma with additional hospitalisation or multiple consultations aimed at managing similar complications (Fig. 31.1, 31.2, 31.3, 31.4, 31.5, 31.6, 31.7, 31.8, 31.9, 31.10, 31.11, 31.12, 31.13, 31.14, 31.15, 31.16, 31.17, 31.18, 31.19, 31.20, 31.21, 31.22, 31.23, 31.24, 31.25, 31.26, 31.27, 31.28, 31.29, 31.30, 31.31, 31.32, 31.33, 31.34, 31.35, 31.36, 31.37, and 31.38).

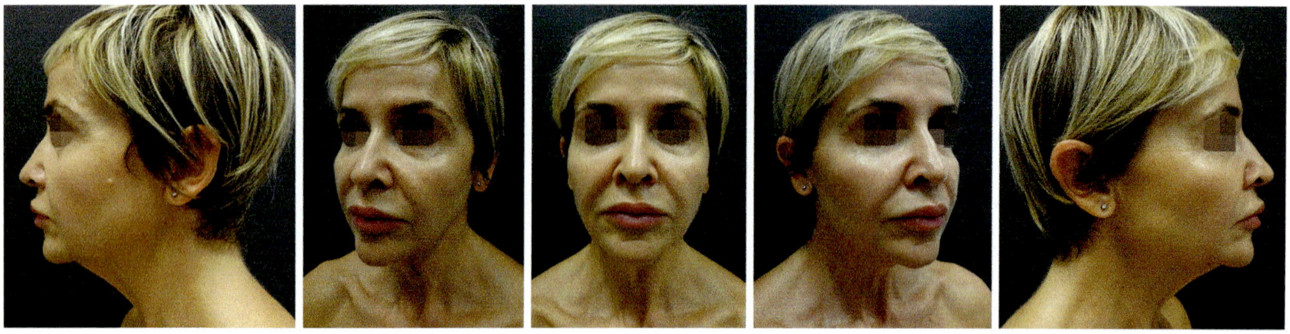

Fig. 31.1 Preoperative pictures. Preoperative frontal, three-quarter, and lateral views of a 43-year-old woman. The pictures show ptosis of the malar tissues; hollowing of the infraorbital area; lengthening of the lower eyelid; deepening of the nasojugal grooves, nasolabial creases and folds, and marionette lines; jowls; neck laxity; and poorly defined and an excessively obtuse cervical-mandibular angle (surgeon: Michele Pascali). (Published by kind permission of ©Michele Pascali 2018. All Rights Reserved)

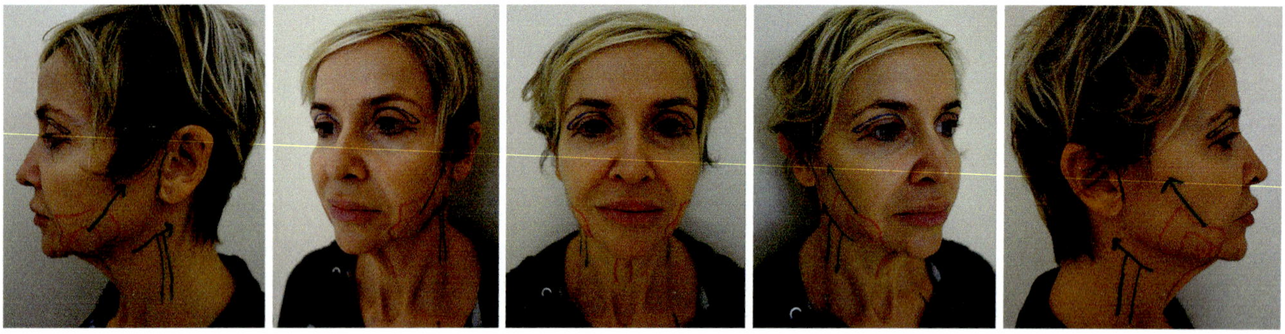

Fig. 31.2 Preoperative marking of the area. Frontal, three-quarter, and lateral view of preoperative markings. The lines where the skin will be incided (temporal, preauricular, retroauricular, occipitomastoid) are marked in blue. The anterior cheek fat pad is marked in red. On the neck, the jugular vein is marked in green and the platysmatic bands in red. Finally, the two traction vectors are marked with two green arrows. (Published by kind permission of ©Michele Pascali 2018. All Rights Reserved)

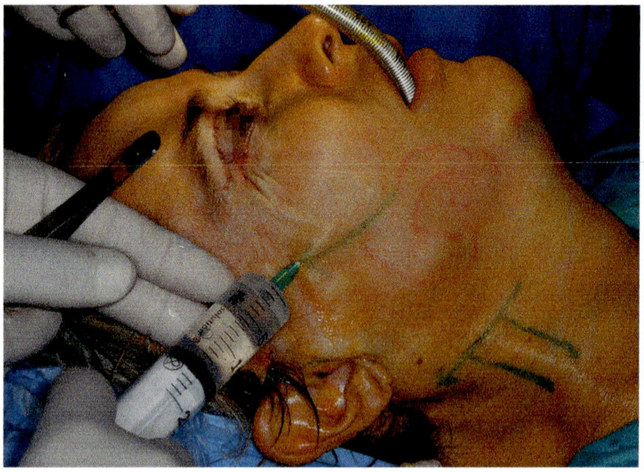

Fig. 31.3 Local anaesthesia. The facelift can be performed under local anaesthesia combined with sedation or general anaesthesia. In this case too, it is necessary to infiltrate the entire area to be treated with anaesthesia: here a saline solution of 0.25% mepivacaine and 1:500.000 epinephrine, in order to obtain adequate hydrodissection and reduce bleeding. (Published by kind permission of ©Michele Pascali 2018. All Rights Reserved)

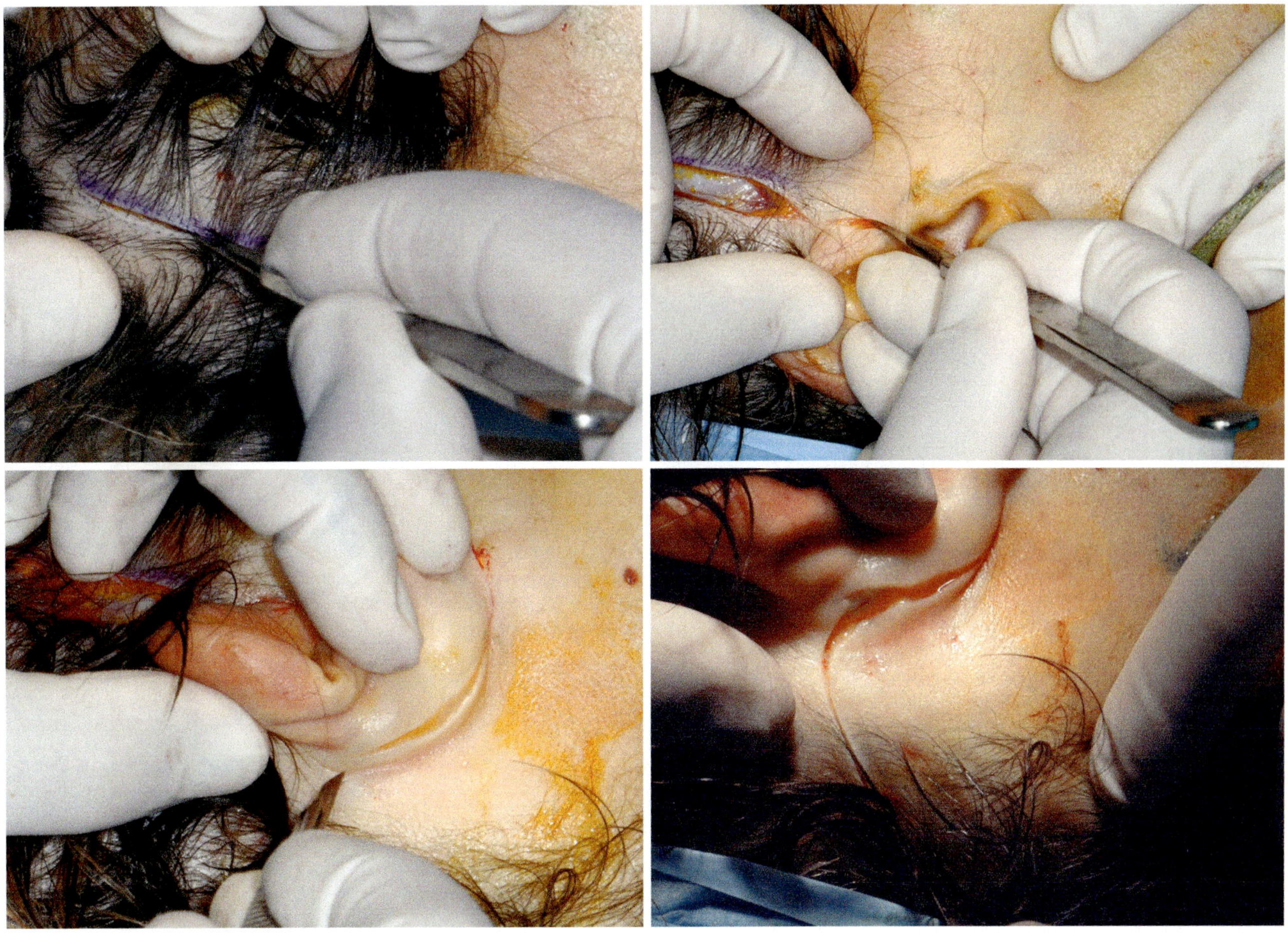

Fig. 31.4 Skin incisions. About 15 min after infiltration, incisions of the skin are performed along the preoperative markings. An incision into the scalp at the temporal region can be made, parallel to the hairline and approximately 3 cm from it. At its cephalad extremity, this incision curves slightly in an inferomedial direction to avoid dog ears. The blade is parallel to the axis of the scalp. The incision is continued down at the preauricular region with the blade perpendicular to the facial plane. In front of the anterior border of the ear, the incision can be pretragal or posttragal, then proceeding inferiorly, around the earlobe, and upward in the retroauricular sulcus, until the hairline is reached, which is then followed for a few centimeters, toward the occipital area, where the blade should go parallel to the axis of the scalp. (Published by kind permission of ©Michele Pascali 2018. All Rights Reserved)

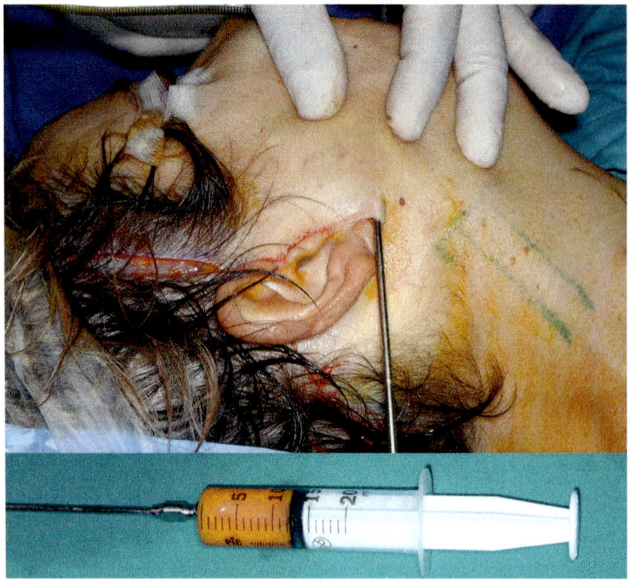

Fig. 31.5 Liposuction. Liposuction of the excess fat of the anterior region of the cheek is performed. This procedure is important to have a few milliliters of autologous fat for an eventual lipofilling and to prepare the subcutaneous undermining. (Published by kind permission of ©Michele Pascali 2018. All Rights Reserved)

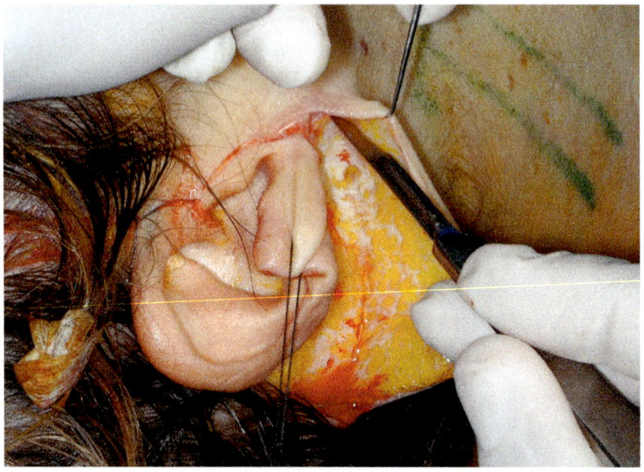

Fig. 31.6 Occipitomastoid dissection. The dissection is initially subcutaneous and usually becomes sub-SMAS only in the cheek and the anterior portion of the neck. It begins from the mastoid area in which the dissection plane can be only subcutaneous, extending caudally until 2 cm below the posterior projection of the gonial angle. After deepening the skin incision until reaching the superficial fascia, tunnels are created in the area to be undermined, trying to stay below the adipose tissue but avoiding to perforate the SMAS and the superficial cervical fascia, in order to prevent any damage to the great auricular nerve. Subsequently, the tunnels are joined to create a uniform dissection plane. (Published by kind permission of ©Michele Pascali 2018. All Rights Reserved)

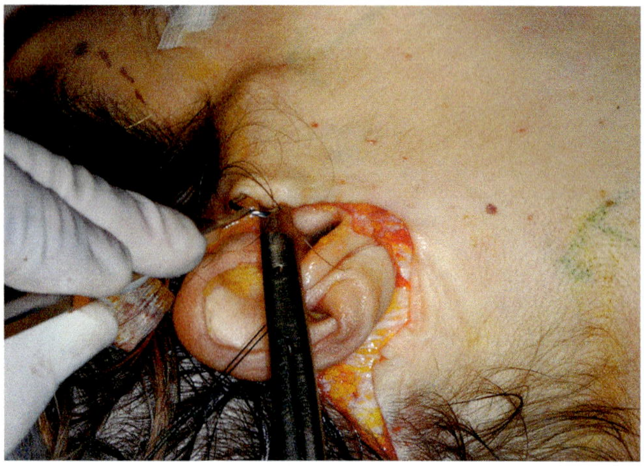

Fig. 31.7 Preauricular dissection. A limited dissection is carried out in the same plane also in the preauricular region. In this area, the dissection is extended 3 cm from the skin incision, except from the area above the zygomatic arch, in which it reaches the orbital rim. In the preauricular area, flap dissection should be conducted in the subcutaneous plane with a scalpel for the first 2 cm and then with blunt scissors or a finger up to the preoperative markings. (Published by kind permission of ©Michele Pascali 2018. All Rights Reserved)

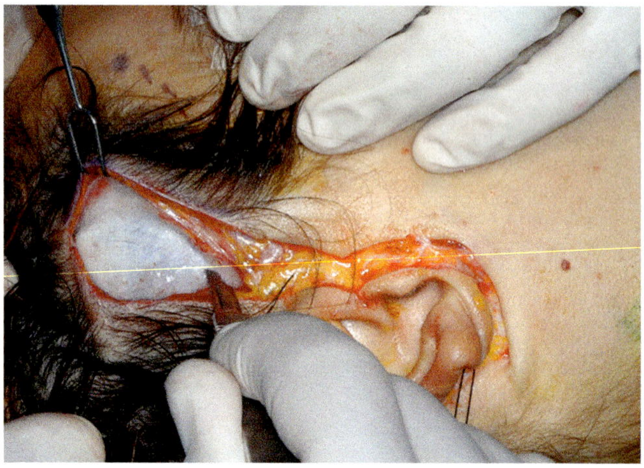

Fig. 31.8 Temporal dissection. The temporal incision is deepened below the galea, which is completely sectioned with scissors. To find the right plane, the incision should start cranial to the temporal muscle, so as to directly reach the periosteum, which, being in direct contact with the bone, provides easy orientation. Once identified the right dissection plane below the galea, dissection is continued initially above the periosteum and then over the aponeurosis of the temporal muscle. At this point, the temporal flap can be easily undermined in an infero-anterior direction by blunt dissection. (Published by kind permission of ©Michele Pascali 2018. All Rights Reserved)

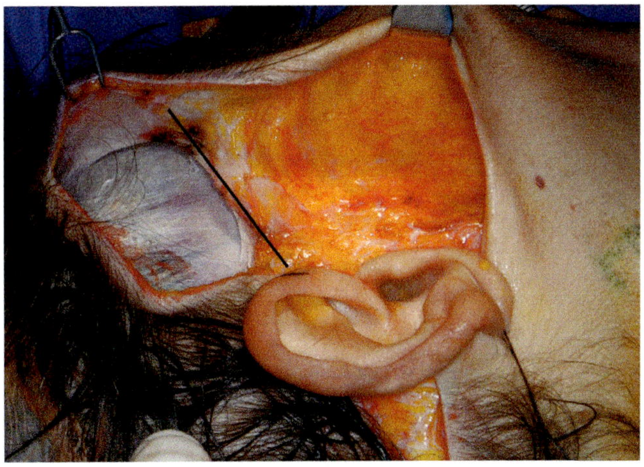

Fig. 31.9 M-M line. The image shows the two different planes of dissection: between galea and periosteum/temporal fascia superiorly; subcutaneous inferiorly. These two areas are separated by the M-M line (represented in the figure by a black line) that is an ideal line running from the root of the helix to a point approximately 4 cm above the outer canthus. The caudal dissection connects the cervical-occipitomastoid area to the preauricular area. The temporoparietal fascia is then incised along the M-M line in order to create a single large flap. (Published by kind permission of ©Michele Pascali 2018. All Rights Reserved)

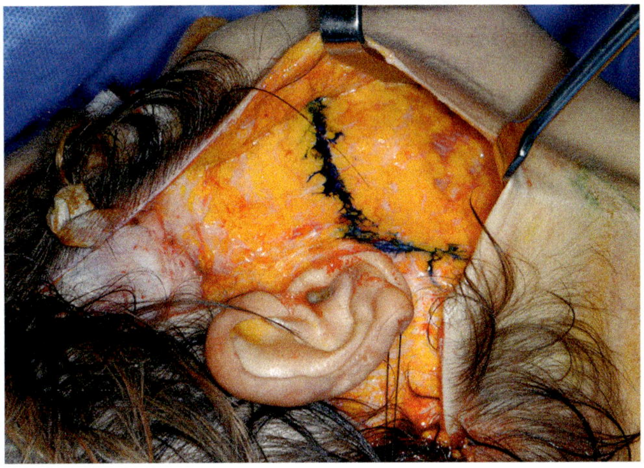

Fig. 31.10 SMAS flap marking. After sectioning the M-M line, unifying the two dissection planes, and before starting sub-SMAS undermining, the SMAS-platysma flap is marked with methylene blue. The horizontal branch lays 1 cm below the zygomatic arch, while the vertical branch descends parallel and 1 cm anterior to the preauricular skin incision and then below the lobe for 6–7 cm along the ear axis. (Published by kind permission of ©Michele Pascali 2018. All Rights Reserved)

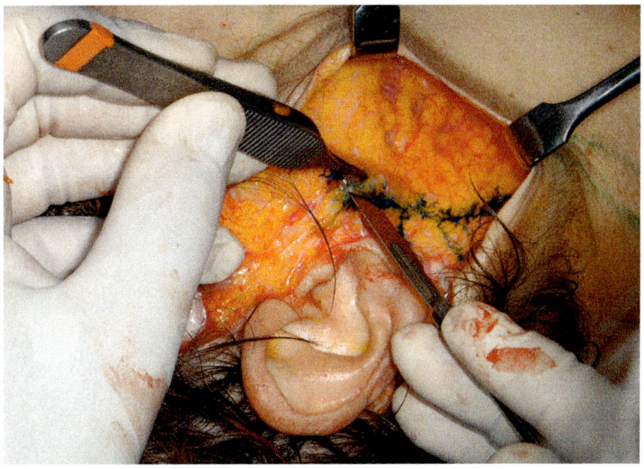

Fig. 31.11 SMAS flap incision. Before starting a sub-SMAS undermining, it is very important to identify the correct level of depth in which to dissect. To accomplish this, it is wise to incise the SMAS over the parotid gland, so the branches of the facial nerve remain totally protected from harm, and the various structures are easily recognizable. It is useful to begin the process elevating the myofascial tissue with tissue forceps 2 cm anteriorly to the earlobe. After verifying the mobility of the flap that is being harvested, a short incision is made posterior to the tips of the forceps. Through this small incision, a tunnel is realized with blunt scissors along the preauricular vertical section of the flap, which is then incised ensuring to not injure vessels or nerves. (Published by kind permission of ©Michele Pascali 2018. All Rights Reserved)

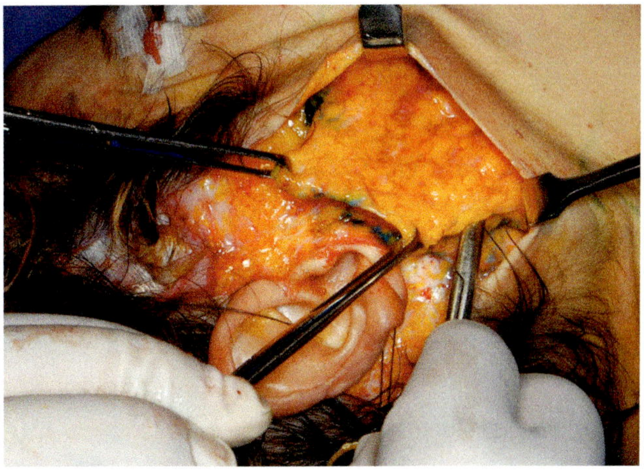

Fig. 31.12 SMAS flap dissection. The SMAS flap is dissected anteriorly for 5–6 cm, spreading the scissors perpendicularly to the facial plane. Particular attention should be taken in order to avoid lesions to the facial nerve branches at the level of the neck and the anterior border of the parotid gland, as well as to the sensitive nerves and vessels. Theoretically, to prevent the chance of meeting the facial nerve, it is possible to limit the SMAS dissection to the parotid area, without passing the anterior border of the gland and avoiding any dissection of the posterior margin of the platysma in the cervical area. (Published by kind permission of ©Michele Pascali 2018. All Rights Reserved)

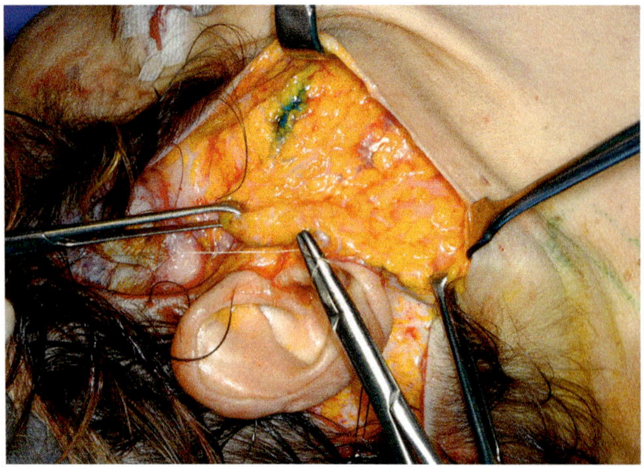

Fig. 31.13 SMAS flap repositioning. The SMAS-platysma flap is mobilized and fixed cranially to the periosteum of the posterior third of the zygomatic arch with two or three 3/0 nylon or PDS sutures. A suture is passed from the SMAS and periosteum of the zygomatic arch through the SMAS flap (posteriorly to anteriorly) and back in a "mattress" fashion, so that the knot remains buried. It is not essential to fix the SMAS flap to the periosteum; superficial fixation to the non-mobilized fascia can also assure sufficient stability. (Published by kind permission of ©Michele Pascali 2018. All Rights Reserved)

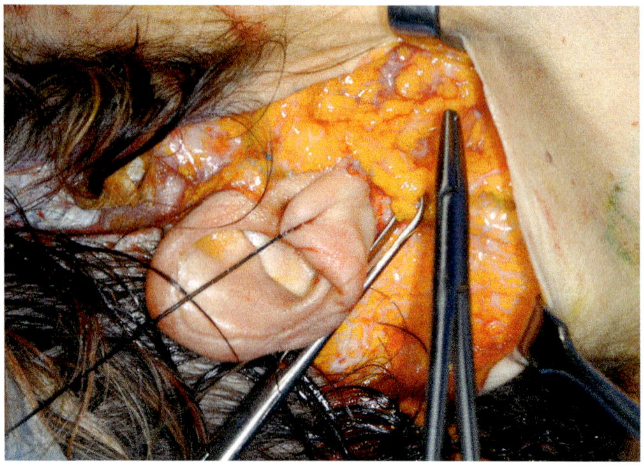

Fig. 31.14 SMAS flap suturing. The SMAS-platysma flap is divided to embrace the ear, and fixation is completed superiorly to the zygomatic arch and infero-posteriorly to the mastoid periosteum. It is wise to place the infra-/retroauricular suspension sutures as far back as possible in order not to engage the great auricular nerve. (Published by kind permission of ©Michele Pascali 2018. All Rights Reserved)

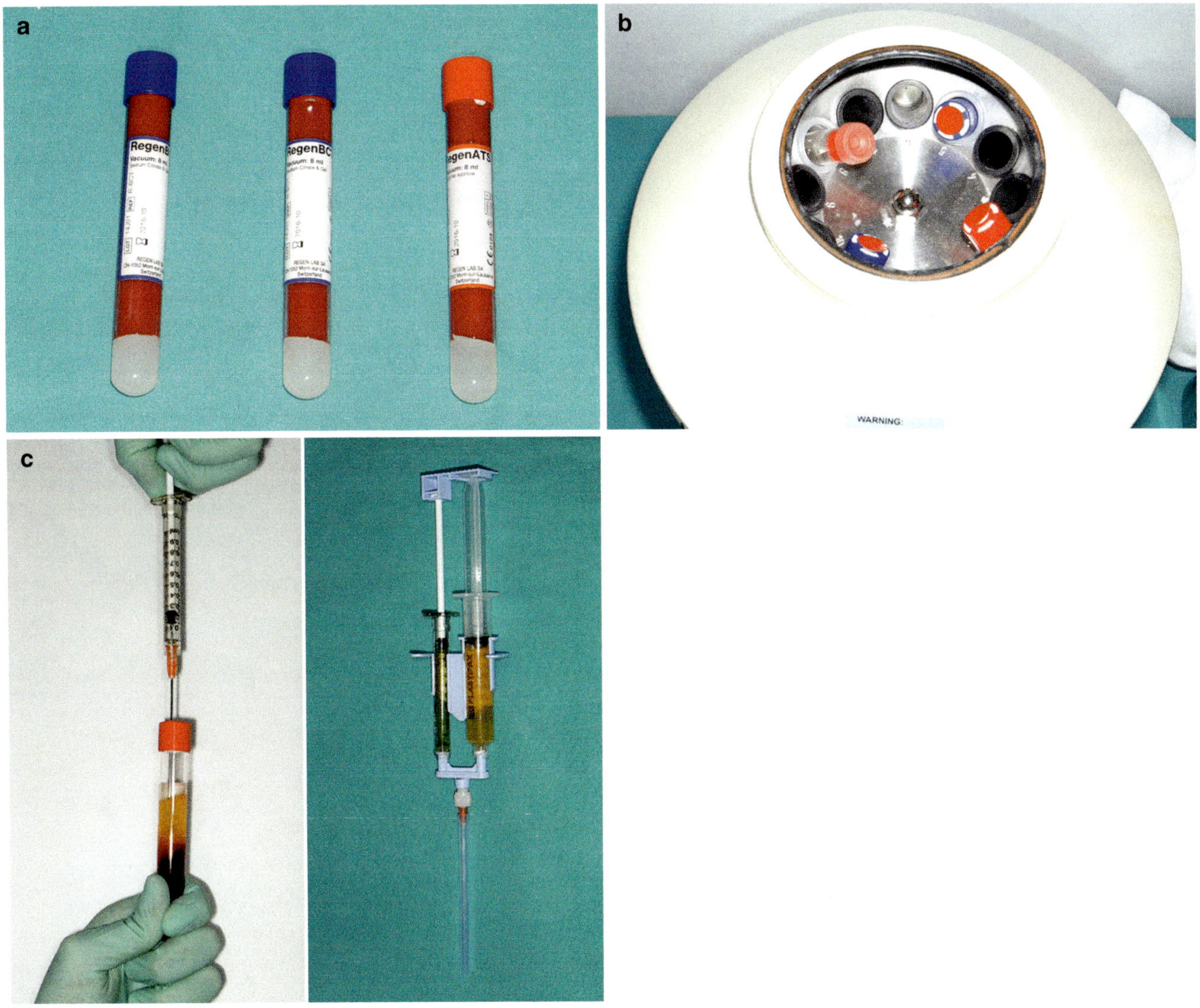

Fig. 31.15 Procedure for preparation of the PRP glue. Only a few steps are required to prepare 4–5 ml of autologous platelet-rich plasma (A-PRP). The RegenLab A-PRP Plus is designed to prepare A-PRP from a small sample of patients' own blood. Each BCT tube (blue tube) draws 8 cc of venous blood and yields 4–5 cc of autologous platelet concentrate, recovering around 80% of the platelets from the whole blood. Regen ATS tube (red tube) draws 8 cc of venous blood and produces a serum of coagulum of PRP with 15 ± 5 IU/ml of activated autologous thrombin. Phase A: collecting whole blood. Perform the venous puncture using butterfly needle connected to the collection holder. Wait for the presence of blood in flexible tube, under the yellow plastic section (the blood is visible over 1–2 mm). Pierce the stopper of the Regen BCT tubes and then do the same with Regen ATS tube to fill them with the whole blood using the internal needle of the collection system. The vacuum within the tubes will enable automatic collection of the necessary volume of blood (about 8 ml). Carefully turn the tubes upside down several times (**a**). Phase B: centrifugation. Insert the previously filled tubes into the centrifuge in a way as to balance the machine (**b**). Adjust the centrifugation values as follows: Time, 5 min; centrifugal force (RCF), 1500 g. Phase C: centrifugation results. The PRP is then mixed and activated with autologous thrombin using the Regen spray applicator with a 9:3 ratio (PRP/thrombin) to form PRP glue (**c**). (Published by kind permission of ©Michele Pascali 2018. All Rights Reserved)

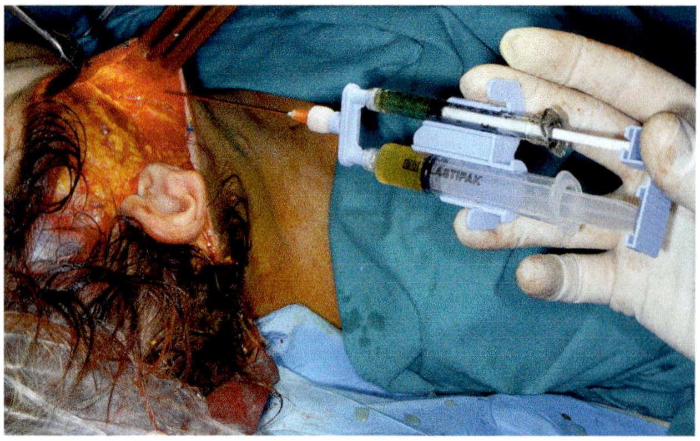

Fig. 31.16 Application of PRP glue. Autologous platelet-rich plasma (A-PRP) and autologous thrombin serum (ATS) together permit the injection of a powerful matrix gel at the targeted area. Platelets then release growth factors over time at the ideal place. This natural process induces the formation of three-dimensional fibrin matrix in which the platelets are entrapped. This allows a long-lasting growth factor delivery at the treatment site, while the matrix serves as scaffold for new tissue reconstruction. The use of PRP glue strongly hinders the formation of hematomas and seromas, allowing for faster recovery and return to daily activities, thus leading to higher postoperative patient satisfaction. (Published by kind permission of ©Michele Pascali 2018. All Rights Reserved)

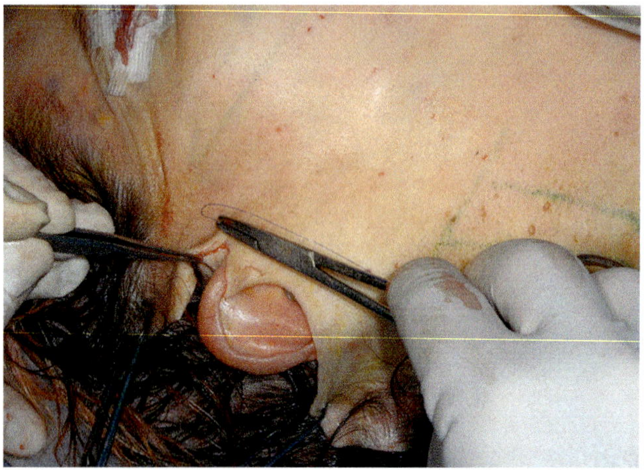

Fig. 31.17 Temporal suspension of the skin flap. Keeping the skin flap stretched supero-posteriorly, a "key point" suture in 3/0 nylon is placed above the ear. If the sideburn migrates too far superiorly, a small triangle of skin can be excised at its base. (Published by kind permission of ©Michele Pascali 2018. All Rights Reserved)

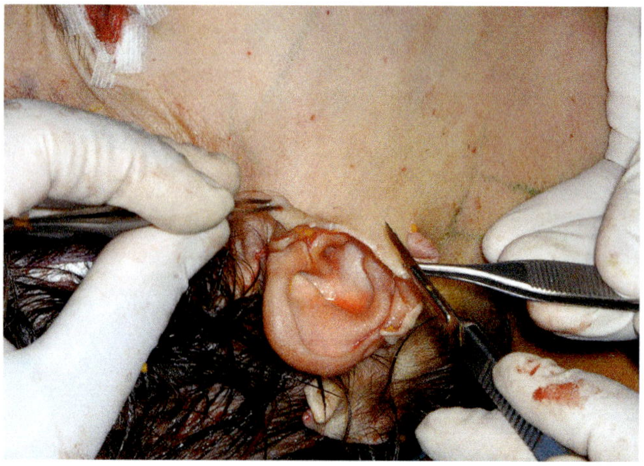

Fig. 31.18 Liberation of the earlobe. The skin flap is carefully incised until the insertion of the earlobe, in order to expose it without distortions. (Published by kind permission of ©Michele Pascali 2018. All Rights Reserved)

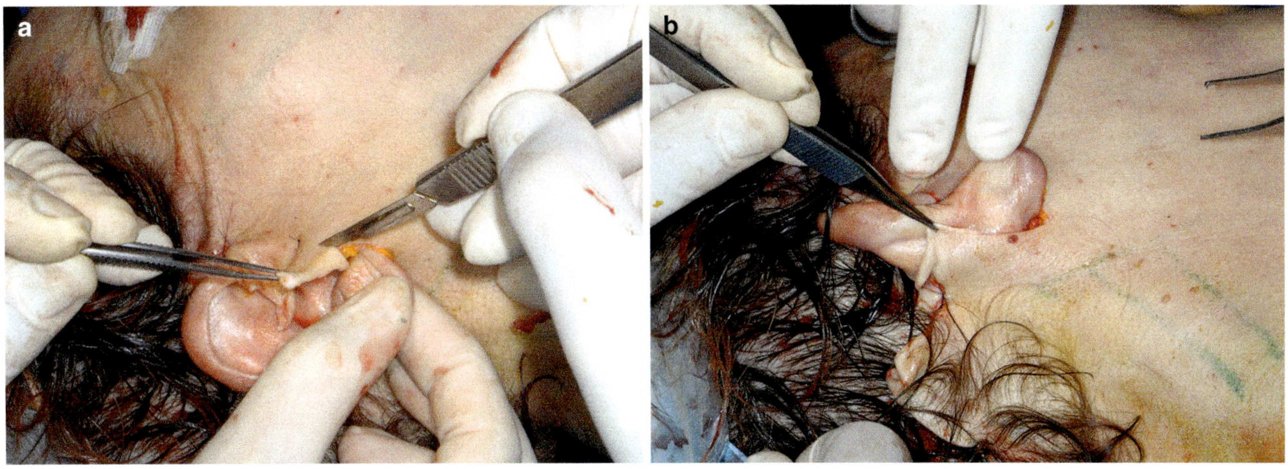

Fig. 31.19 Skin resection. Preauricularly the skin excess is excised directly along the markings left by the Pitanguy (or D'Assumpçao) forceps. Alternatively, for higher safety, small incisions may be performed perpendicularly to the margin of the skin flap until the markings, finally removing the resultant skin triangles (**a**). Postauricularly a "key point" suture in 3/0 nylon is placed, and direct excision of the exceeding skin is performed (**b**). (Published by kind permission of ©Michele Pascali 2018. All Rights Reserved)

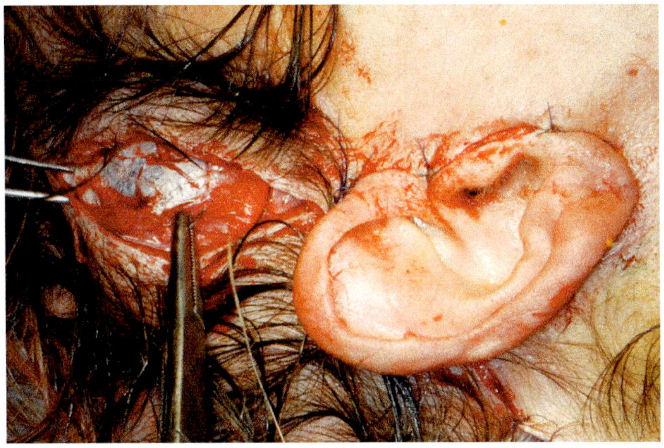

Fig. 31.20 Traction on the temporoparietal fascia. The temporoparietal fascia, previously incised along the M-M line, is pulled upward and fixed to the deep temporal fascia with one or two 3/0 PDS sutures. The cutaneous flap is then pulled with slight traction above the ear, and eventual peripheral irregularities caused by adhesions are released with blunt-tip scissors. (Published by kind permission of ©Michele Pascali 2018. All Rights Reserved)

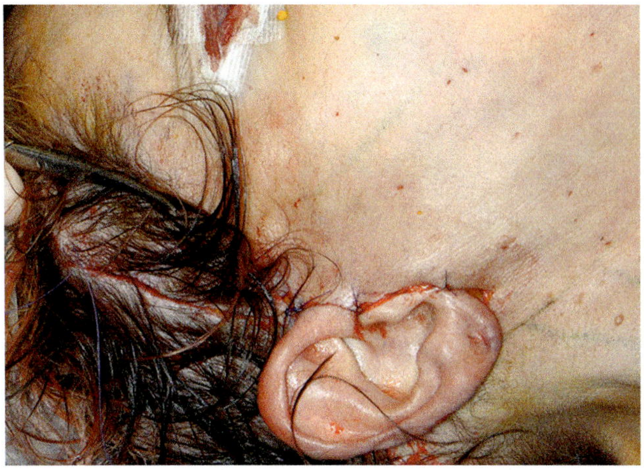

Fig. 31.21 Skin suture. After removing the exceeding skin, the sutures are performed. In the scalp the suture is performed with 3/0 Vicryl or surgical staples. In the preauricular area, a running suture with 6/0 nylon is performed. In the postauricular area, simple interrupted suturing with 4/0 Vicryl is accomplished. (Published by kind permission of ©Michele Pascali 2018. All Rights Reserved)

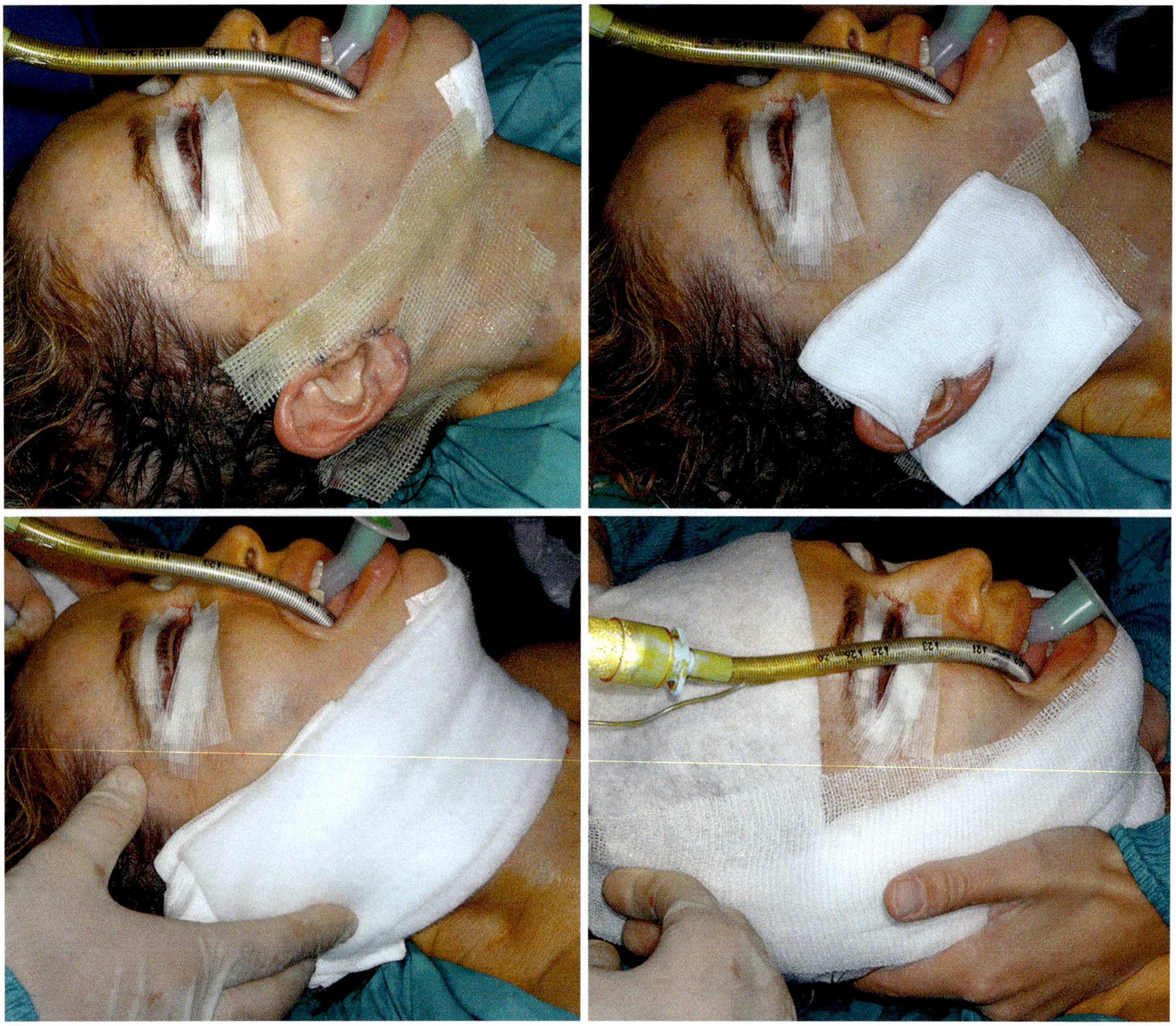

Fig. 31.22 Wound dressing. After the procedure, a dressing is placed around head and neck. It shall not be removed until next day by the physician. It is designed to catch any drainage and provide gentle compression to diminish swelling and allowing the skin to readhere to deeper tissues, thus preventing fluid collection between tissues. A thin elastic compressive dressing (jaw Bra) is sometimes also used to keep tissues compressed increasing healing and comfort. (Published by kind permission of ©Michele Pascali 2018. All Rights Reserved)

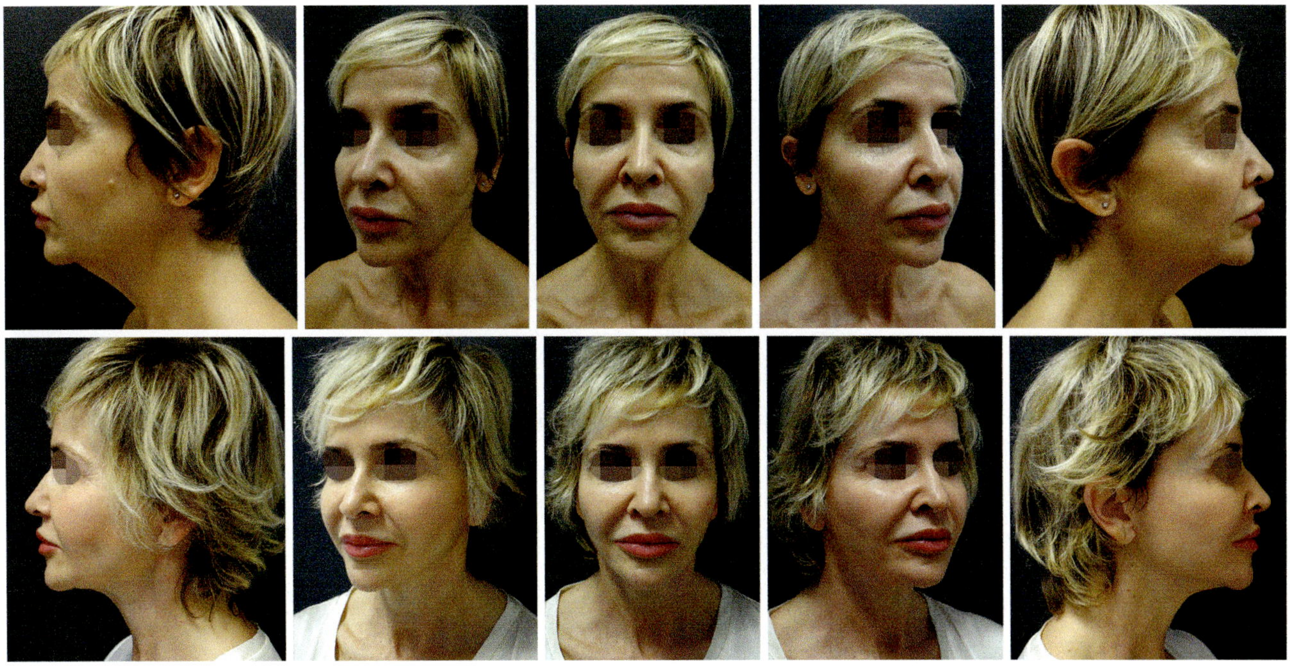

Fig. 31.23 Results. Preoperative and 6 months postoperative frontal, three-quarter, and lateral views of patient. Note the more youthful appearance with firmer and smoother skin tone; the fullness and projection of the malar area; the jowls correction; the improvement of the nasojugal grooves, nasolabial creases, and marionette lines; and the correction of neck laxity with improved definition of the cervical-mandibular angle. (Published by kind permission of ©Michele Pascali 2018. All Rights Reserved)

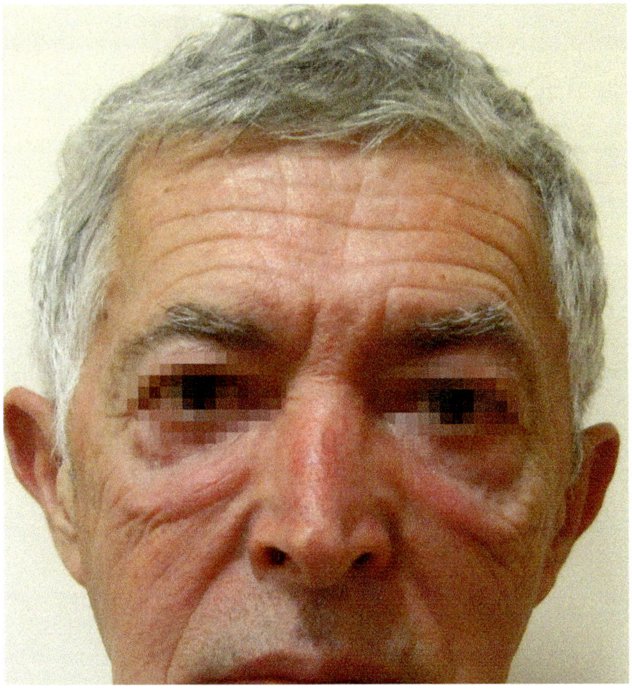

Fig. 31.24 Preoperative photo: upper and lower lid ptosis (surgeon: Mario Goisis, courtesy by Springer, Injection in aesthetic medicine). (Published with kind permission of ©Mario Goisis 2018. All Rights Reserved)

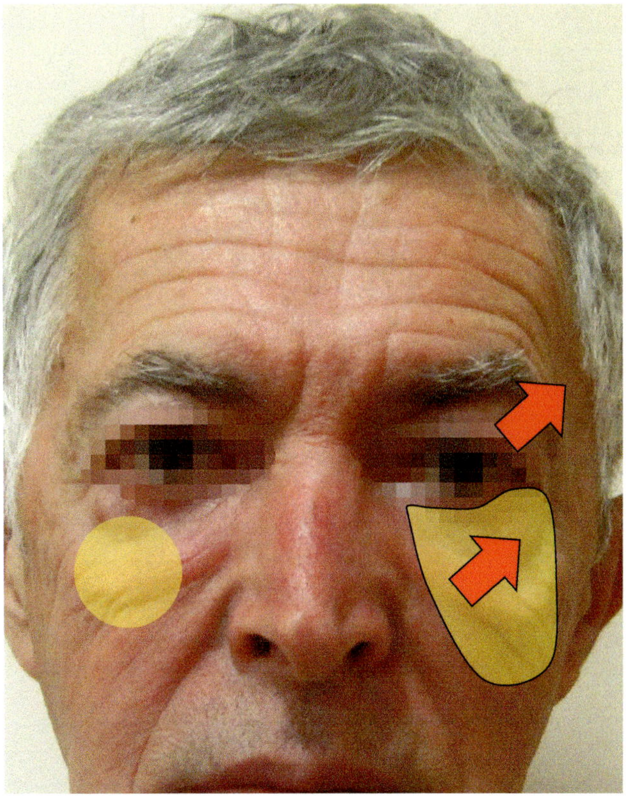

Fig. 31.25 Surgical program: correction of the upper eyelid, midface lift, and malar augmentation with microfat. (Published with kind permission of ©Mario Goisis 2018. All Rights Reserved)

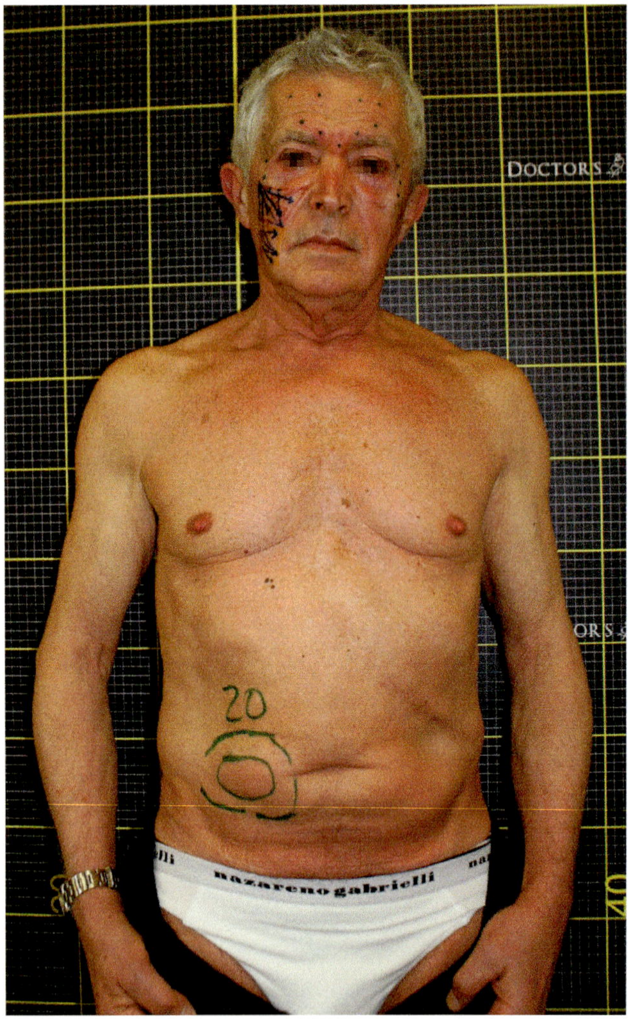

Fig. 31.26 Area of harvesting of microfat. (Published with kind permission of ©Mario Goisis 2018. All Rights Reserved)

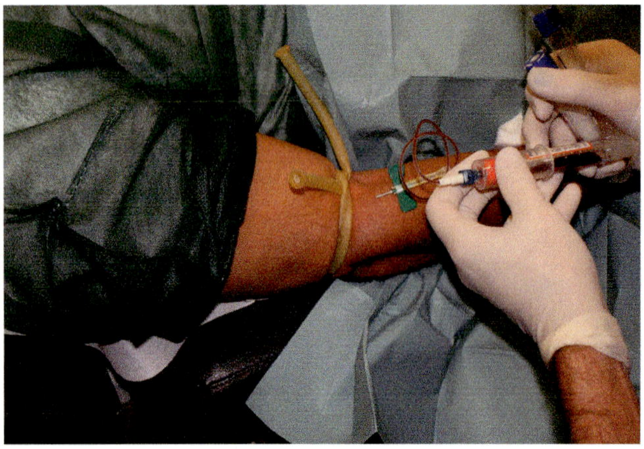

Fig. 31.27 The blood is collected in tube with anticoagulant (blue tube) and without anticoagulant (red tube). (Published with kind permission of ©Mario Goisis 2018. All Rights Reserved)

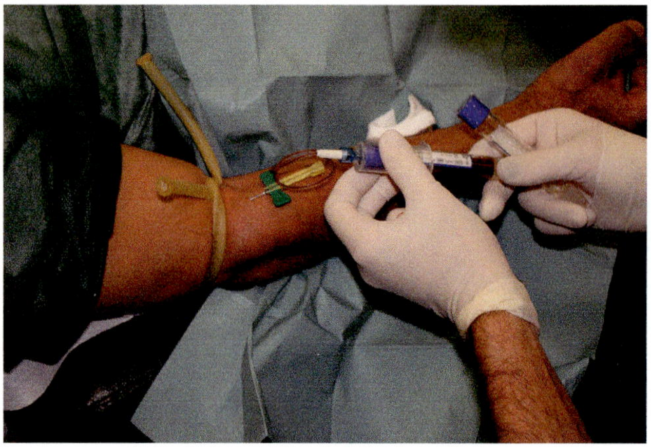

Fig. 31.28 The blood is collected in tube with anticoagulant (blue tube) and without anticoagulant (red tube). (Published with kind permission of ©Mario Goisis 2018. All Rights Reserved)

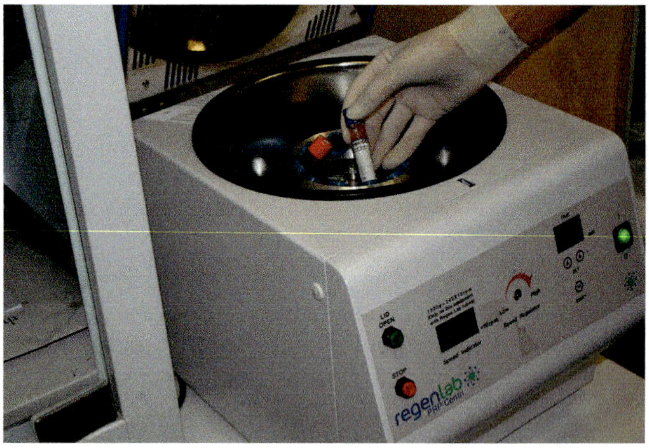

Fig. 31.29 Centrifugation. Insert the previously filled tubes into the centrifuge in a way as to balance the machine (**b**). Adjust the centrifugation values as follows: time, 5 min; centrifugal force (RCF), 1500 g. (Published with kind permission of ©Mario Goisis 2018. All Rights Reserved)

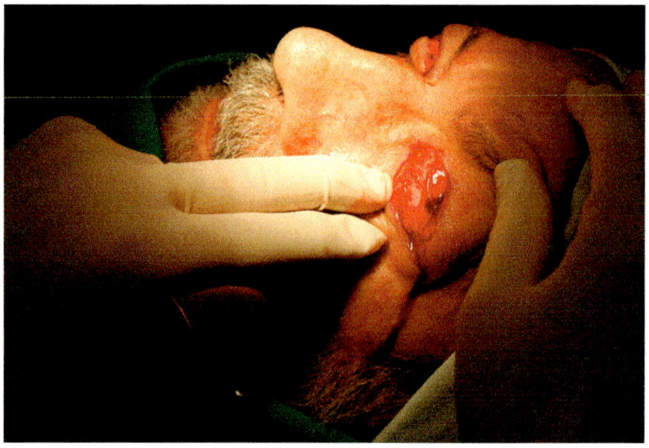

Fig. 31.30 The excess of skin of the upper eyelid is removed. (Published with kind permission of ©Mario Goisis 2018. All Rights Reserved)

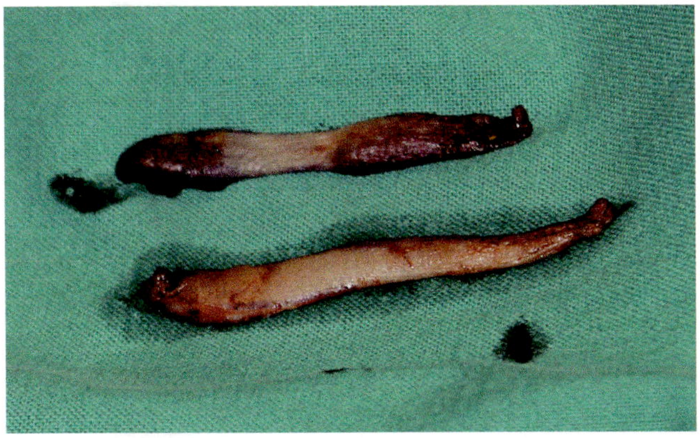

Fig. 31.31 The excess of skin of the upper eyelid is removed. (Published with kind permission of ©Mario Goisis 2018. All Rights Reserved)

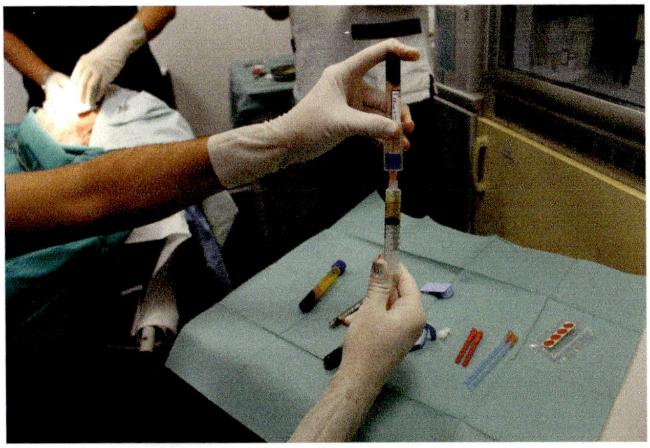

Fig. 31.32 The PRP is mixed and activated with autologous thrombin using the spray applicator with a 9:3 ratio (PRP/thrombin) to form PRP glue. (Published with kind permission of ©Mario Goisis 2018. All Rights Reserved)

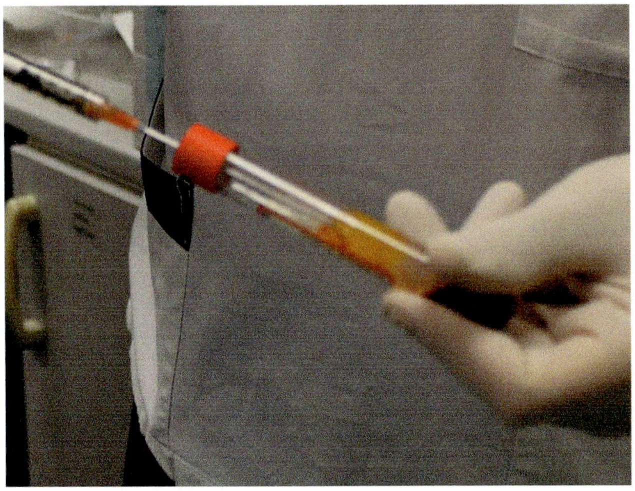

Fig. 31.33 The PRP is mixed and activated with autologous thrombin using the spray applicator with a 9:3 ratio (PRP/thrombin) to form PRP glue. (Published with kind permission of ©Mario Goisis 2018. All Rights Reserved)

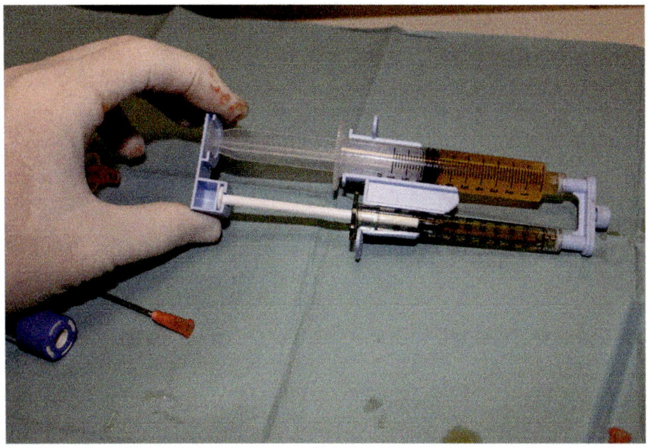

Fig. 31.34 The PRP is mixed and activated with autologous thrombin using the spray applicator with a 9:3 ratio (PRP/thrombin) to form PRP glue. (Published with kind permission of ©Mario Goisis 2018. All Rights Reserved)

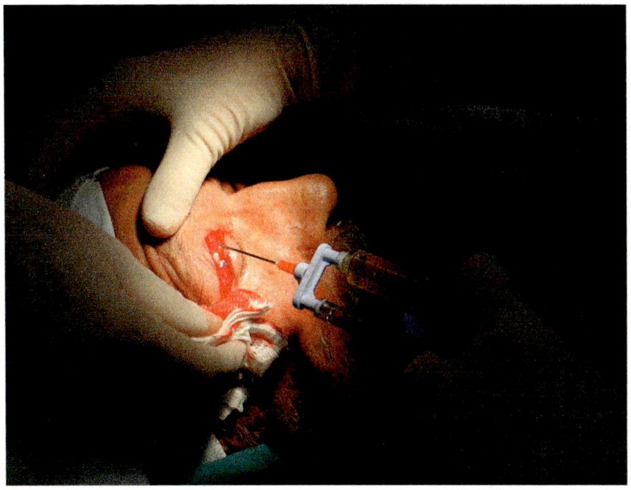

Fig. 31.35 Application of PRP glue. Autologous platelet-rich plasma (A-PRP) and autologous thrombin serum (ATS) together permit the injection of a powerful matrix gel at the targeted area. Platelets then release growth factors over time at the ideal place. This natural process induces the formation of three-dimensional fibrin matrix in which the platelets are entrapped. This allows a long-lasting growth factor delivery at the treatment site, while the matrix serves as scaffold for new tissue reconstruction. The use of PRP glue strongly hinders the formation of hematomas and seromas, allowing for faster recovery and return to daily activities, thus leading to higher postoperative patient satisfaction. (Published with kind permission of ©Mario Goisis 2018. All Rights Reserved)

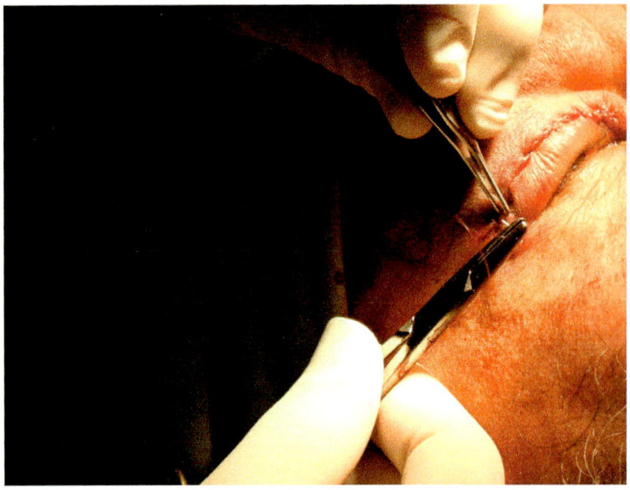

Fig. 31.36 After suture, PRP glue is applied in order to fat the healing process. (Published with kind permission of ©Mario Goisis 2018. All Rights Reserved)

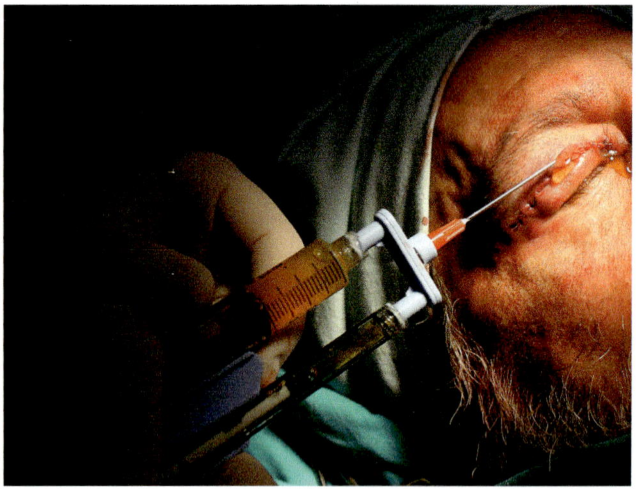

Fig. 31.37 After suture, PRP glue is applied in order to fat the healing process. (Published with kind permission of ©Mario Goisis 2018. All Rights Reserved)

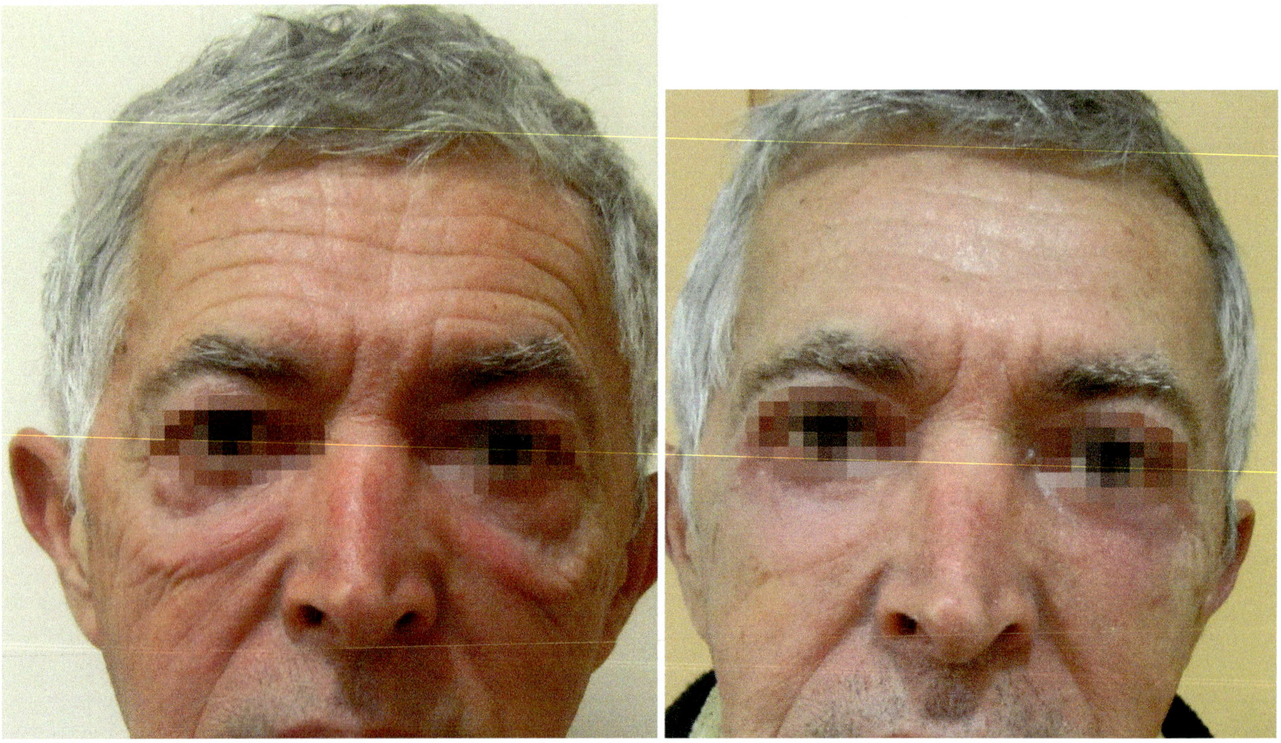

Fig. 31.38 Pre- and 12 months after treatment photo (courtesy by Springer, Injection in aesthetic medicine). (Published with kind permission of ©Mario Goisis 2018. All Rights Reserved)

Regulations and Legal Implications in Outpatient Aesthetic Procedures

32

Mario Goisis and Stefano Fiorentino

32.1 Adipose Tissue and Stem-Cells: The Juridical Aspects

By juridical point of view, when we talk about "adipose tissue" we have to consider three different type of products (Fig. 32.1):

1. *Adipose tissue*: the tissue obtained with a minimal manipulation. In particular, in European Union (EU) the definition is reported in Reg. Eu. 1394/2007 (Reg. Eu. 1394/2007, Annex I: cutting, grinding, shaping, centrifugation, soaking in antibiotic or antimicrobial solutions, sterilization, irradiation, cell separation, concentration or purification, filtering, lyophilization, freezing, cryopreservation, vitrification).
2. *Stromal vascular fraction (SVF)*, a fraction of adipose tissue. It can be obtained with an enzymatic digestion (collagenase). In EU there isn't difference between chemical and mechanical separation, but for EMA/CAT *(the Committee for Advanced Therapies)*, the use of collagenase is considered substantial manipulation: "Enzymatic digestion of tissue to release cells is also considered to be substantial manipulation, when the aim is to dissociate cell-cell contacts" (Committee for Advanced Therapies, Reflection paper on classification of advanced therapy medicinal products, 21 May 2015 EMA/CAT/600280/2010 Rev.1).
3. *Stem-cells*, obtained with cellular manipulation (substantial manipulation) starting from SVF.

At the moment, it's consolidated the autologous use of the adipose tissue for lipofilling in one-step surgery protocols, because by juridical point of view, it's a tissue grafting *not an* advanced therapy medicinal product *(ATMP)*.

In Europe, it's very important to consider the advice of *CAT, the Committee for Advanced Therapies*, because if the biologic product becomes an ATMT, it's considered a drug and is very difficult for the surgeon to use it.

Below you can find the most important and recent advices of CAT on biologic products based on adipose tissue (Fig. 32.2).

1. *Advice 2012, July 24 (EMA/500730/2012): Description*: "The product consists of autologous collagen (AC) derived from human adipose tissue (Cosmetic dermal filling)."

   CAT Position: "The product consists of autologous collagen and does not contain cells. The product does not contain or consist of a recombinant nucleic acid used in or administered to human beings with a view to regulating,

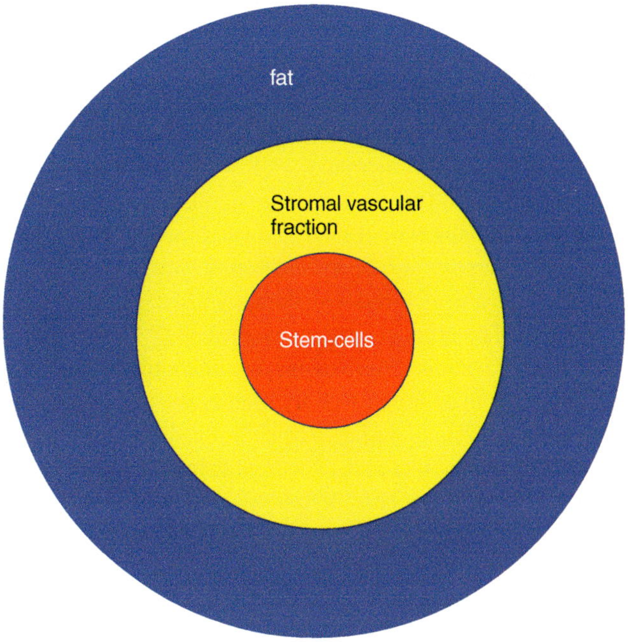

Fig. 32.1 Adipose tissue, SVF, and stem-cells. (Published with kind permission of ©Mario Goisis 2018. All Rights Reserved)

M. Goisis (✉)
Maxillo-Facial and Aesthetic Surgeon, Go Easy Clinic, Milan, Italy

S. Fiorentino
Fiorelaw, Milan, Italy

M. Goisis (ed.), *Outpatient Regenerative Medicine*, https://doi.org/10.1007/978-3-319-44894-7_32

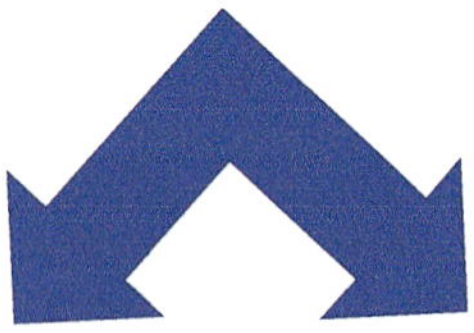

Fig. 32.2 Different classifications of product based on evaluation of the *Committee for Advanced Therapies (CAT)*. (Published with kind permission of ©Mario Goisis 2018. All Rights Reserved)

repairing, adding or deleting a genetic sequence. Based on the above considerations, it is considered that the product does not fall within the definition of an advanced therapy medicinal product as provided in Article 2(1)(a) of Regulation (EC) No 1394/2007."

2. *Advice 2012, July 24 (EMA/500724/2012): Description*: "Autologous, non-manipulated lipoaspirate containing adipocytes and stromal vascular fraction. No medical or therapeutic claims are pursued. The product is intended to act as a natural, autologous lipofiller."

   CAT Position: "The product consists of autologous lipoaspirate, containing adipocytes and stromal vascular fraction. The cells are not subjected to substantial manipulation. The product acts as a natural, autologous filler. Thus the cells cannot be considered 'engineered' by non-homologous use, as the preparation is intended to be used for the same essential function (restoration of subcutaneous fat tissue) in the recipient site as in the donor site. Based on the above considerations, it is considered that the product does not fall within the definition of an advanced therapy medicinal product, as provided in Article 2(1)(a) of Regulation (EC) No 1394/2007."

3. *Advice 2013, February 11 (EMA/90882/2013): Description*: "The isolated autologous human adipose mesenchymal stem-cells, culture-expanded up to passage 4 or 5 when osteogenic differentiation and 3-dimensional structure are induced by demineralised bone matrix (DBM). The product contains viable cells."

   CAT Position: "Autologous mesenchymal stem-cells derived from adipose tissue are used as one of two human-derived starting materials. The cells are subjected to various treatments, including a cell culturing step, during the manufacturing process. It can be concluded that these cells have been subject to substantial manipulation and the cells are considered to be engineered cells. The product is presented as having properties for bone defect treatment when used in human beings with a view to regenerating, repairing or replacing this tissue. The combination of osteogenic cells and DBM promotes angiogenesis and osteogenesis in a bone defect characterized by a lack of spontaneous bone-formation.

   Based on the above considerations, it is considered that the product falls within the definition of Tissue engineered product as provided in Article 2(1)(a) of Regulation (EC) No 1394/2007."

4. *Advice 2013, April 4 (EMA/129099/2013): Description*: "Suspension of viable, adult, autologous, unexpanded, and uncultured regenerative cells of stromal vascular fraction in Autologous Cell-Enriched Matrix of subcutaneous adipose tissue."

   CAT Position: "The product contains viable cells that have not been subjected to a substantial manipulation. The mode of action of the product (contribute to and enhance tissue renewal and turnover of the subcutaneous tissue) is considered to be homologous to the donor fat tissue. Based on the above considerations, it is considered that the product does not fall within the definition of an advanced therapy medicinal product."

5. *Advice 2013, August 2 (EMA/478311/2013): Description*: "Autologous cells of Stromal Vascular Fraction (SVF) of adipose tissue."

   CAT Position: "SVF containing adipose stem-cells (ASCs) is considered to be a substance that is intended to be used in human beings with a view to restoring physiological functions by exerting a pharmacological and/or metabolic action. CAL contains viable cells but these cells have not been subjected to a substantial manipulation.

   The essential function of CAL (formation of adipocytes and vascular cells and maintaining of stem-cells in the administrated fat graft) is considered to be the same as in the donor's fat tissue. Based on the above considerations, it is considered that the product does not fall within the definition of an advanced therapy medicinal product."

6. *Advice 2013, August 2 (EMA/478311/2013): Description*: "Adipose tissue derived mesenchymal stem-cells expanded ex vivo combined with biomaterial betatricalcium phosphate."

   CAT Position: "The product consists of adipose tissue derived mesenchymal stem-cells expanded ex vivo combined with biomaterial β-TCP. The cells are expanded and are therefore considered to be substantially manipulated. The product is presented as a medicinal product having properties for regenerating osteopoiesis and revascularization, i.e. repairing a human tissue. Based on the above considerations, it is considered that the product falls within the definition of an advanced therapy medicinal product, and more specifically a tissue engineered product according to the definition in Article 2(1)(b) of Regulation (EC) No 1394/2007. β-TCP is approved for clinical use according to the requirements set in Directive

93/42/EEC concerning medical devices. β-TCP is an integral part of the ATMP administered to patients. Based on the above consideration, it can be considered that the product falls within the definition of a combined ATMP as defined in article 2(1)(d) of Regulation 1394/2007/EC."

7. *Advice 2014, November 24 (EMA/557278/2015): Description*: "Suspension of non-substantially manipulated autologous differentiated adipocytes in solution for injection (Treatment of primary perianal fistula)."

   CAT Position: "The product consists of autologous differentiated adipocytes in solution for injection.

   There is no device or structural component integrated into the product. The differentiated autologous adipocytes are considered "engineered" as they are not intended to be used for the same essential function or functions in the recipient as in the donor. The product is intended for the treatment of perianal fistula. The claimed mechanism of actions is that upon physiological stimuli the cells from adipose tissue are able to repair, regenerate or replace the injured tissue and promote closure of perianal fistula.

   The EMA/CAT considers that the Product falls within the definition of an advanced therapy medicinal product, a tissue engineered product as provided for in Article 2(1)(b) of Regulation (EC) No. 1394/2007."

8. *Advice 2016, March 21 (EMA/213726/2016): Description*: "Sterile suspension of autologous cells of stromal vascular fraction of adipose tissue in Lactated Ringers (Treatment of Pain associated with joint osteoarthritis)."

   CAT Position: "The committee adopted on 25th November 2015 the following scientific recommendation.

   On the basis that:

   - the product is composed of manipulated cells derived from stromal vascular fraction and;
   - the product is used to treat pain associated with joint osteoarthritis via immunological action.

   the EMA/CAT considers that the Product falls within the definition of a advanced therapy medicinal product (somatic cell therapy medicinal product) for the indication of the treatment of pain associated with joint osteoarthritis, as provided in Article 2(1)a of Regulation (EC) No 1394/2007."

9. *Advice 2016, April 1 (EMA/240965/2016): Description*: "Viable adipose-derived regenerative cells extracted from human abdominal subcutaneous fat (treatment of articular cartilage and bone defects including osteoarthrosis or osteochondral lesions)."

   CAT Position: "The committee adopted on 25th November 2015 the following scientific recommendation.

   On the basis that:

   - the product consists of engineered cells that have been subject to substantial manipulation, so that biological characteristics, physiological functions or structural properties relevant for the intended regeneration, repair or replacement are achieved, and that are not intended to be used for the same essential function or functions in the recipient as in the donor,
   - the product is administered to human beings with a view to regenerating, repairing or replacing a human tissue,
   - the product incorporates, as an integral part of the product a medical devices, hyaluronic acid the EMA/CAT considers that the Product falls within the definition of a combined tissue engineered product."

32.2 Conclusions

(a) *The EU Authorities are oriented to an extension of the legal limits of ATMP.*

(b) *Substantial manipulation, nonhomologous use, and regenerative claims are parameters to qualify the cells as ATMP products.*

(c) *In the next future, many products based on cells will be considered an ATMP (DRUG).*

Printed by Printforce, the Netherlands